CRASH COURSE

Third Edition

Pathology

Series editor

Daniel Horton-Szar
BSc (Hons), MBBS (Hons), MRCGP

Northgate Medical Practice
Canterbury
Kent, UK

Faculty advisor

Professor Rosemary A Walker
MD FRCPath

Department of Cancer Studies &
Molecular Medicine
Leicester Royal Infirmary
Leicester, UK

Atul Anand

BSc (MedSci) Hons

Medical Student, University of Edinburgh, UK

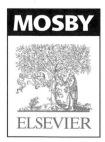

MOSBY

ELSEVIER

Edinburgh • London • New York • Oxford • Philadelphia • St Louis • Sydney • Toronto 2007

MOSBY
ELSEVIER

Commissioning Editor:	**Alison Taylor**
Development Editor:	**Kim Benson**
Project Manager:	**Anne Dickie**
Senior Designer:	**Sarah Russell**
Cover:	**Stewart Larking**
Icon illustrations:	**Geo Parkin**
Illustration Management:	**Bruce Hogarth**

First edition 1999
Second edition 2002
Third edition 2007

ISBN: 978-0-7234-3422-1

British Library Cataloguing in Publication Data
A catalogue record for this book is available from the British Library

Library of Congress Cataloging in Publication Data
A catalog record for this book is available from the Library of Congress

Note

Knowledge and best practice in this field are constantly changing. As new research and experience broaden our knowledge, changes in practice, treatment and drug therapy may become necessary or appropriate. Readers are advised to check the most current information provided (i) on procedures featured or (ii) by the manufacturer of each product to be administered, to verify the recommended dose or formula, the method and duration of administration, and contraindications. It is the responsibility of the practitioner, relying on their own experience and knowledge of the patient, to make diagnoses, to determine dosages and the best treatment for each individual patient, and to take all appropriate safety precautions. To the fullest extent of the law, neither the Publisher nor the Author assumes any liability for any injury and/or damage to persons or property arising out or related to any use of the material contained in this book.

The Publisher

Printed in China

CRASH COURSE
Third Edition

Pathology

WITHDRAWN

WITHDRAWN

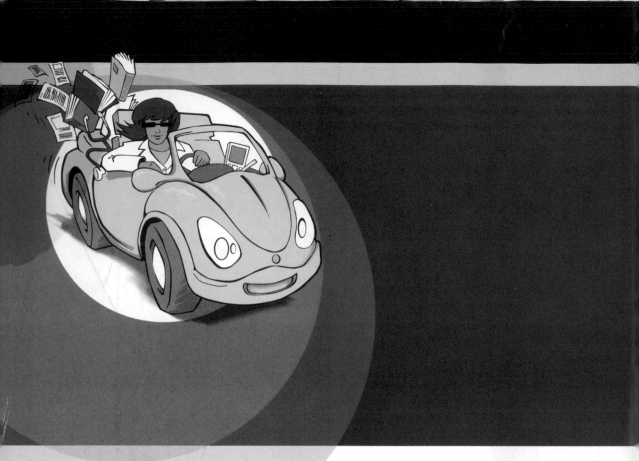

First and second edition authors:

Bethan Goodman Jones

Daniel J O'Connor

Preface

Pathology is the study of disease and is therefore central to all of medicine. Each chapter of this third edition has been updated to reflect the latest advances from a diverse range of research areas. Brand new clinical sketch boxes have been designed to integrate the understanding of pathology with clinical patient management for key diseases. Another new feature is Extended Matching Questions (EMQs) to add to the wide-ranging self-assessment offered by this edition, which should help prepare readers for this increasingly utilised form of examination. I hope this third edition proves a readily accessible but comprehensive tool throughout medical training, from lecture hall to hospital ward. Good luck with your studies!

Atul Anand

There has been an overall revision, with some re-organisation, of both the Principles of Pathology and Systemic Pathology in this third edition of Pathology Crash Course and Atul has ensured that it is up to date and relevant to any medical course. It will provide a very good background to all aspects of pathology and their relevance to clinical medicine. Understanding the pathology of diseases is important for a full appreciation of medicine. This book will certainly help you in all aspects of your medical course.

Professor Rosemary A Walker
Faculty Advisor

More than a decade has now passed since work began on the first editions of the Crash Course series, and over four years since the publication of the second editions. Medicine never stands still, and the work of keeping this series relevant for today's students is an ongoing process. These third editions build upon the success of the preceding books and incorporate a great deal of new and revised material, keeping the series up to date with the latest medical research and developments in pharmacology and current best practice.

As always, we listen to feedback from the thousands of students who use Crash Course and have made further improvements to the layout and structure of the books. Each chapter now starts with a set of learning objectives, and the self-assessment sections have been enhanced and brought up to date with modern exam formats. We have also worked to integrate points of clinical relevance into the basic medical science material, which will not only add to the interest of the text but will reinforce the principles being described.

Despite fully revising the books, we hold fast to the principles on which we first developed the series: Crash Course will always bring you all the information you need to revise in compact, manageable volumes that integrate basic medical science and clinical practice. The books still maintain the balance between clarity and conciseness, and providing sufficient depth for those aiming at distinction. The authors are medical students and junior doctors who have recent experience of the exams you are now facing, and the accuracy of the material is checked by senior faculty members from across the UK.

I wish you all the best for your future careers!

Dr Daniel Horton-Szar
Series Editor

Acknowledgements

I would like to thank everyone who has helped during the writing of this book. I am grateful to the numerous friends who provided moral support and accepted having ideas thrown at them. Particular mentions must go to Alex Adams, David Baker and Chris Kane.

Finally I wish to thank the very helpful people involved in the production of this book, both in Edinburgh and Oxford.

Figure Acknowledgements

Figs 3.3, 3.4, 3.6, 3.7, 5.14, 6.21, 7.17, 11.2 and 13.23 are adapted with permission from General and Systematic Pathology, 3rd and 4th editions, edited by JCE Underwood. Churchill Livingstone, Edinburgh, 2000 and 2004.

Fig. 5.6 is adapted with permission from Pathology, 2nd edition, by A Stevens and J Lowe. Mosby, Edinburgh, 2000.

Figs 5.7 and 5.9 are adapted with permission from Anderson's Pathology, 10th edition, edited by I Damjanov and J Linder. Mosby, St.Louis, 1996.

Fig. 6.16 is adapted with permission from Robbins and Cotran Pathologic Basis of Disease, 7th edition, edited by V Kumar, A Abbas, and N Fausto. Elsevier Saunders, Philadelphia, 2005.

Fig. 7.3 is adapted with permission from Systematic Pathology, 3rd edition volume 5, edited by B Corrin. Churchill Livingstone, Edinburgh, 1990.

Fig. 8.20 is adapted with permission from Clinical Medicine, 3rd edition, edited by P Kumar and M Clark. Baillière Tindall, London, 1994.

Fig. 8.37 is adapted with permission from Principles and Practice of Surgery, 3rd edition, edited by APM Forrest, DC Carter and IB Macleod. Churchill Livingstone, Edinburgh, 1995.

Fig. 8.40 is adapted with permission from Surgery of the Anus, Rectum and Colon, 5th edition, by JC Goligher, HL Duthie and HH Nixon. Baillière Tindall, London, 1984.

Fig. 10.2 is adapted with permission from Brook CGD, Marshall NJ. Essential Endocrinology, 4th edition. Blackwell Publishing; 2001.

Fig. 11.14 is adapted with permission from Lecture Notes on Urology, 5th edition, by J Blandy. Blackwell Scientific, Oxford, 1998.

Fig. 13.4 is adapted with permission from Introduction to Clinical Immunology, by M Haeny. Butterworths, London, 1985.

Figs 13.14 and 13.20 are adapted with permission from Essential Haematology, 3rd edition, by AV Hoffbrand and JE Pettit. Blackwell Scientific, Oxford, 1993.

Figs 13.30 and 13.31 are adapted with permission from Pathology Illustrated, 4th edition, by A Govan, P Macfarlane and R Callander. Churchill Livingstone, Edinburgh, 1995.

Dedication

To Mum, Dad and Pav

Contents

Preface   v
Acknowledgements   vii
Dedication   viii
Glossary   xi

Part I: Principles of Pathology 1

1. **Introduction to pathology** 3
   Disease 3
   Pathology 3
   How pathology is covered in this book 4

2. **Inflammation, repair and cell death** 5
   Inflammation 5
   Acute inflammation 5
   Chemical mediators of inflammation 8
   Chronic inflammation 10
   Cell death 14

3. **Cancer** 17
   Definitions and nomenclature 17
   Molecular basis of cancer 19
   Tumour growth and spread 22
   Carcinogenic agents 24
   Host defences against cancer 27
   Clinical cancer pathology 27

4. **Infectious disease** 29
   General principles of infection 29
   Categories of infectious agent 30
   Mechanisms of pathogenicity 35
   Inflammatory responses to infection 38

Part II: Systematic Pathology . . . 41

5. **Pathology of the nervous system** 43
   Disorders of the central nervous system . . 43
   Disorders of the peripheral nervous
   system 58
   Disorders of the autonomic nervous
   system 61

6. **Pathology of the cardiovascular system** . . . 63
   Congenital abnormalities of the heart . . . 63
   Atherosclerosis, hypertension and
   thrombosis 69

Ischaemic heart disease and
heart failure 78
Disorders of the heart valves 82
Diseases of the myocardium 87
Diseases of the pericardium 88
Aneurysms 91
Inflammatory and neoplastic vascular
disease 93
Diseases of the veins and lymphatics 96

7. **Pathology of the respiratory system** 99
   Disorders of the upper respiratory tract . . 99
   Disorders of the lungs 102
   Infections of the lungs 111
   Neoplastic diseases of the lungs 118
   Diseases of vascular origin 122
   Diseases of iatrogenic origin 126
   Disorders of the pleura 126

8. **Pathology of the gastrointestinal
   system** 129
   Disorders of the upper
   gastrointestinal tract 129
   Disorders of the stomach 134
   General aspects of hepatic damage 139
   Disorders of the liver and biliary tract . . . 146
   Disorders of the exocrine pancreas 158
   Disorders of the intestine 161
   Disorders of the peritoneum 177

9. **Pathology of the kidney and
   urinary tract** 181
   Abnormalities of kidney structure 181
   Diseases of the glomerulus 184
   Glomerular lesions in systemic disease . . 191
   Diseases of the tubules and interstitium . 193
   Diseases of the renal blood vessels 195
   Neoplastic disease of the kidney 198
   Disorders of the urinary tract 200

10. **Pathology of the endocrine system** 205
    Disorders of the pituitary 205
    Thyroid disorders 210
    Parathyroid disorders 216
    Disorders of the adrenal gland 219

Contents

Disorders of the endocrine pancreas . . .223
Multiple endocrine neoplasia
syndromes 227

11. **Pathology of the reproductive system** **229**
Disorders of the vulva, vagina
and cervix 229
Disorders of the uterus and
endometrium 233
Disorders of the ovary and fallopian
tube 237
Disorders of the placenta and
pregnancy 239
Disorders of the breast 244
Disorders of the penis 247
Disorders of the testis and epididymis . .248
Disorders of the prostate 250

12. **Pathology of the musculoskeletal
system** **253**
Disorders of bone structure 253
Infections and trauma 256
Tumours of the bones 259
Disorders of the neuromuscular
junction 261
Myopathies 263
Arthropathies 265

13. **Pathology of the blood and immune
systems** **275**
Autoimmune disease 275
Diseases of immunodeficiency 278
Amyloidosis 282
Disorders of white blood cells 284
Disorders of the spleen and thymus 295
Disorders of red blood cells 297
Disorders of haemostasis 308

14. **Pathology of the skin** **315**
Terminology of skin pathology 315
Inflammation and skin eruptions 317
Infections and infestations 322
Disorders of specific skin structures 329
Disorders of pigmentation 332
Blistering disorders 334
Tumours of the skin 336

Part III: Self-Assessment 343

Multiple-choice questions (MCQs) 345
Short-answer questions (SAQs) 353
Extended-matching questions (EMQs) 355
MCQ answers 359
SAQ answers 369
EMQ answers 373

Index 375

Glossary

Abscess   A localised collection of pus in a tissue, cavity or confined area. Usually associated with infection.

Aetiology   The cause of a disease.

Anaplastic   A lack of cellular differentiation which is characteristic of some cancer cells.

Anhidrosis   The absence of sweating.

Atrophy   Describes the decrease in size (or wasting) of a cell, tissue or organ.

Autocrine   Describes the process whereby a cell secretes a substance whose target for action is the secreting cell itself.

Bursa   A small fluid filled sac that reduces friction on movement between a tendon and bone, or between bone and skin.

Colic   Describes a pain that gradually increases, reaches a peak and then subsides slowly. This pattern may then be repeated.

Contralateral   On the opposite side (to a lesion).

Crypt   A deep pit-like structure found in the wall of the small intestine.

Dysphagia   Difficulty in swallowing.

Dyspnoea   Shortness of breath.

Empyema   The accumulation of pus in a cavity of the body.

Endophytic   Used to describe a tumour that grows inwards and is thus invasive.

Epistaxis   A nosebleed.

Erythrocyte sedimentation rate (ESR)   A non-specific marker of inflammation, based on the rate at which red blood cells settle in a column of liquid.

Exophytic   Used to describe a tumour that grows outwards from an epithelial surface.

Fistula   An abnormal communication between two epithelial lined cavities.

Giant cell   A multinucleated cell formed from the fusion of many cells.

Glossitis   Inflammation of the tongue.

Histiocyte   A resident tissue macrophage which has a long lifespan.

Hyperhidrosis   Excessive sweating.

Hypoxia   A condition where insufficient oxygen reaches the tissues of the body.

Iatrogenic   An inadvertent effect of medical treatment or actions.

Idiopathic   Where the cause is unknown.

Ipsilateral   On the same side (as a lesion).

Paracrine   Describes the process whereby a cell secretes a substance that has an action on nearby cells.

Parenchyma   The functional component of a gland or organ (distinct from support or connective tissue).

Paroxysmal   Describes sudden attacks of a given effect.

Pathogenic   Capable of causing disease.

Petechiae   Small red spots on the skin.

Pruritus   Itchiness.

Ptosis   Drooping of the upper eyelid.

Stroma   Supporting connective tissue of an organ.

Suppurative   Any reaction that produces pus.

Venesection   The removal of blood from a vein.

Xanthoma   A benign yellow-colored lesion common on the eyelid and usually indicating elevated serum cholesterol levels.

PRINCIPLES OF PATHOLOGY

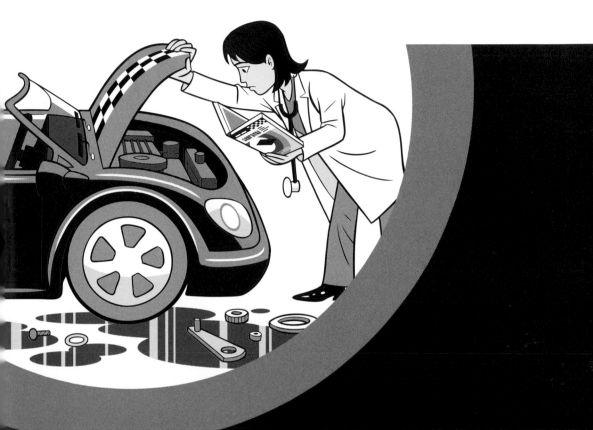

1. Introduction to pathology   3

2. Inflammation, repair and cell
                          death   5

3.   Cancer   17

4.   Infectious disease   29

Introduction to pathology

Objectives

In this chapter, you will learn to:
- Define 'disease'.
- Define 'pathology'.
- Understand the divisions of pathology.
- Understand the characteristics and basic classification of disease.
- Define congenital and acquired disorders.

DISEASE

A disease is an alteration from the normal function/structure of an organ or system, which manifests as a characteristic set of signs and symptoms.

PATHOLOGY

Pathology is the scientific study of disease. It is concerned with the causes and effects of disease, and the functional and structural changes that occur. Changes at the molecular and cellular level correlate with the clinical manifestations of the disease.

Understanding the processes of disease assists in the accurate recognition, diagnosis, and treatment of diseases.

Divisions of pathology

Pathology is traditionally subdivided into five main clinical disciplines:

1. Histopathology—the study of histological abnormalities of diseased cells and tissues.
2. Haematology—the study of primary diseases of the blood and the secondary effects of other diseases on the blood.
3. Chemical pathology—the study of biochemical abnormalities associated with disease.
4. Microbiology—the study of infectious diseases and the organisms that cause them.
5. Immunopathology—the study of diseases through the analysis of immune function.

Classification of disease

The causes of disease are numerous and diverse. For convenience, diseases are often classified as either congenital or acquired disorders. Congenital diseases are present from birth, whereas acquired disorders are incurred as a result of factors originating in the external environment.

Congenital

Congenital causes can be either genetic (e.g. cystic fibrosis) or non-genetic (e.g. thalidomide anomalies).

Acquired

Acquired causes can be any of the following:

- Trauma.
- Infections and infestations.
- Radiation injury.
- Chemical injury.
- Circulatory disturbances.
- Immunological disturbances.
- Degenerative disorders.
- Nutritional deficiency diseases.
- Endocrine disorders.
- Psychosomatic factors.
- Iatrogenic disease.
- Idiopathic disease.

However, many, if not most, diseases are due to a combination of causes, and they are therefore said to have a multifactorial aetiology.

It is important to have a logical and methodical approach to disease description. Fig. 1.1 illustrates the features of disease.

pathological responses. The first part of this book describes the principles of these in relation to our advancing knowledge of the molecular sciences.

HOW PATHOLOGY IS COVERED IN THIS BOOK

Part I: Principles of pathology

A limited number of tissue responses underlie all diseases. These responses are known as basic

Part II: Systematic pathology

As well as an understanding of the basic pathological responses, it is also necessary to understand how they affect individual tissues and organs. The second part of this book describes the common pathology of the specific diseases as they affect individual organs or organ systems. This approach is termed systematic pathology, and it is illustrated by clinical examples of disease.

Fig. 1.1 Features of disease include definition, aetiology, pathogenesis, treatment and prognosis.

Fig. 1.1 Characteristics of disease

Characteristic	Explanation
Definition	A clear, concise and accurate description
Incidence	Number of new cases of disease occurring in a population of a defined size during a defined period
Prevalence	Number of cases of disease to be found in a defined population at a stated time
Aetiology	Cause of disease
Pathogenesis	Mechanism by which a disease is caused
Morphology	Form and structural changes
Complications and sequelae	Secondary consequences of disease
Treatment	Treatment regimens, effectiveness and side effects
Prognosis	Expected outcome of the disease

Inflammation, repair and cell death

Objectives

In this chapter, you will learn to:
- Describe the causes and mechanisms of acute and chronic inflammation.
- Describe the chemical mediators of inflammation.
- Understand the systemic effects of inflammation.
- Define the terms labile, stable and permanent tissue.
- Describe the mechanisms of wound healing.
- Describe necrosis and apoptosis as forms of cell death and understand the differences between them.

INFLAMMATION

Definition

Inflammation is the response of living tissues to cellular injury. It involves both innate and adaptive immune mechanisms.

Purpose

The purpose of inflammation is to localise and eliminate the causative agent, limit tissue injury and restore tissue to normality.

Inflammation can be divided into two types: acute and chronic. The division of inflammation is based according to the time course and cellular components involved. These categories are not mutually exclusive, and some overlap exists (Fig. 2.1).

Causes of acute inflammation

The causes of acute inflammation are:

- Physical agents, e.g. trauma, heat, cold, ultraviolet light, radiation.
- Irritant and corrosive chemical substances, e.g. acids, alkalis.
- Microbial infections, e.g. pyogenic bacteria.
- Immune-mediated hypersensitivity reactions, e.g. immune-mediated vasculitis, seasonal allergic rhinitis (hay fever).
- Tissue necrosis, e.g. ischaemia resulting in a myocardial infarction.

Causes of chronic inflammation

Chronic inflammation usually develops as a primary response to:

- Microorganisms resistant to phagocytosis or intracellular killing mechanisms, e.g. tuberculosis (TB), leprosy.
- Foreign bodies, which can be endogenous (e.g. bone, adipose tissue, uric acid crystals) or exogenous (e.g. silica, suture materials, implanted prostheses).
- Some autoimmune diseases, e.g. Hashimoto's thyroiditis, rheumatoid arthritis, contact hypersensitivity reactions.
- Primary granulomatous diseases—Crohn's disease, sarcoidosis.

Inflammation becomes chronic when it occurs over a prolonged period of time with simultaneous tissue destruction and attempted repair. It may occur secondary to acute inflammation due to the persistence of the causative agent. Fig. 2.2 shows the sequelae of inflammation.

ACUTE INFLAMMATION

Classic signs of acute inflammation

The classic signs of acute inflammation are:

- Redness (rubor).
- Heat (calor).
- Swelling (tumour).

Fig. 2.1 Comparison of acute and chronic inflammation. Note that the acute and chronic categories are not mutually exclusive.

Fig. 2.1 Comparison of acute and chronic inflammation	Acute inflammation	Chronic inflammation
Response	Immediate reaction of tissue to injury	Persisting reactions of tissue to injury
Onset	Rapid	Slow response
Immunity	Innate	Cell mediated
Predominant cell type	Neutrophil	Lymphocytes, plasma cells, macrophages
Duration	Hours to weeks	Weeks/months/years
Vascular response	Prominent	Less important

- Pain (dolour).
- Loss of function (functio laesa).

These classic signs are produced by a rapid vascular response and cellular events characteristic of acute inflammation.

The main function of these events is to bring elements of the immune system to the site of injury and prevent further tissue damage.

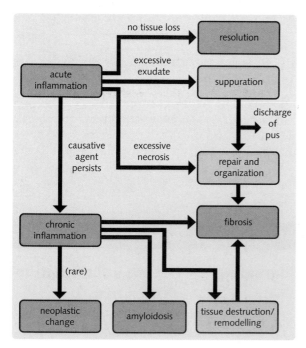

Fig. 2.2 Sequelae of inflammation.

Vascular response

Widespread vasodilatation (hyperaemia)

Blood flow to the capillary bed is normally limited by the precapillary sphincters. In acute inflammation, a phase of vasodilatation occurs when the arterioles and precapillary sphincters relax. This results in increased blood flow to the injured area and increased hydrostatic pressure.

Increased vascular permeability

Endothelial intracellular proteins, such as actin, contract under the influence of chemical inflammatory mediators, such as histamine, bradykinin, nitric oxide and leukotriene B4. Endothelial contraction results in:

- Increased fenestrations (i.e. transient gaps) between endothelial cells.
- Increased permeability of vessels to plasma proteins.

Proteins leak out of the plasma into the interstitial spaces, leading to a decrease in the plasma oncotic pressure. This protein-rich leaking fluid is an exudate. It includes circulating components such as immunoglobulins and coagulation factors.

Inflammatory oedema

The combined increase in hydrostatic pressure (from hyperaemia) and the decreased oncotic pressure (from leakage of proteins into interstitial spaces) causes net fluid movement from plasma into tissues; this is inflammatory oedema. As a result, blood viscosity is increased and blood flow rate is decreased.

Advantages of inflammatory oedema

- Fluid increase in the damaged tissue dilutes and modifies the action of toxins.
- Protein levels increase in the tissue—these include protective antibodies and fibrin.
- Non-specific antibodies act as opsonins for neutrophil-mediated phagocytosis and function to neutralise toxins.
- The formation of a fibrin net acts as a scaffold for inflammatory cells, preventing the spread of microorganisms.
- Circulation of the exudate into the lymphatic system assists in antigen presentation and helps mount a specific immune response.

Cellular events

Neutrophil polymorphs pass between endothelial cell junctions and invade damaged tissue to combat the effects of injury. The movement of leucocytes out of the vessel lumen is termed extravasation, and is achieved in five stages (Fig. 2.3):

1. Margination to the plasmatic zone (Fig. 2.4). This is assisted by the slowing of the blood (leucocytes flow nearer to the vessel wall in the plasmatic zone than the axial stream).
2. 'Rolling' of leucocytes due to the repeated formation and destruction of transient adhesions with the endothelium.

3. Adhesion ('pavementing')—leucocytes eventually firmly adhere to the vascular endothelium, due to the interaction of paired molecules on the leucocyte and endothelial cell surface, e.g. β_2-integrin and ICAM-1.
4. Transmigration (also called diapedesis)—leucocytes pass between the endothelial cell junctions by amoeboid movement through the vessel wall into tissue spaces.
5. Chemotaxis—neutrophils migrate towards, and are possibly activated by, chemical substances (chemotaxins) released at sites of tissue injury. These chemotaxins are thought to be leukotrienes, complement components and bacterial products.

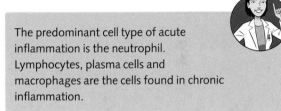

The predominant cell type of acute inflammation is the neutrophil. Lymphocytes, plasma cells and macrophages are the cells found in chronic inflammation.

Phagocytosis and intracellular killing

Neutrophils and monocytes ingest debris and foreign particles at the site of injury (Fig. 2.5). Cellular

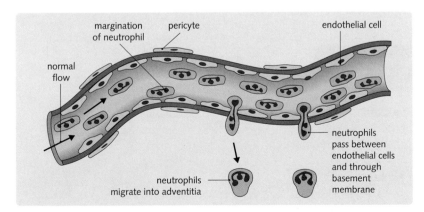

Fig. 2.3 Cellular events in acute inflammation. Neutrophils are the predominant cell type of acute inflammation. They reach the injured tissues by margination, rolling, adhesion and transmigration.

Fig. 2.4 Mechanism of margination of neutrophil polymorphs

Fig. 2.4 Mechanism of margination of neutrophil polymorphs.

Increased plasma viscosity (due to loss of intravascular fluid)	→	Decreased blood flow	→	White blood cells fall out of axial stream into plasmatic zone (margination)

Fig. 2.5 Phagocytosis of foreign particle by leucocyte. (A) Attachment of foreign particle. (B) Pseudopodia engulfing particle. (C) and (D) Incorporation within the cell in a vacuole called a phagosome.

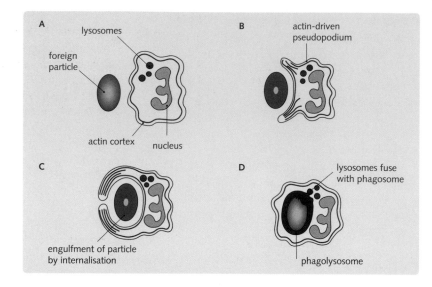

pseudopodia engulf the foreign particle and fuse to produce a phagocytic vacuole or phagosome. Phagocytosis is assisted by opsonisation with immunoglobulins and complement components.

Following phagocytosis, leucocytes attempt to destroy phagocytosed material by:

- Discharge of lysosomal enzymes into the phagosome.
- Oxygen-dependent mechanisms, such as H_2O_2, O_2^-, •OH.
- Oxygen-independent mechanisms, such as lactoferrin, lysozyme and hydrolases.

CHEMICAL MEDIATORS OF INFLAMMATION

Several different inflammatory mediator systems interact to produce inflammation. No chemical mediator alone can be entirely responsible for any single feature of the inflammatory response.

Regulatory mechanisms exist in all mediator systems.

The complement system

This cascading sequence of serum proteins is made up of more than 20 components; the activated product of one protein activates another (Fig. 2.6). The complement proteins have numerous functions in the body's response to infection (Fig. 2.7). The system can

be activated in four ways during the acute inflammatory response:

1. Necrotic cells release enzymes that are capable of activating complement.
2. Antibody–antigen complexes activate complement through the classical pathway.
3. Gram-negative bacterial endotoxins activate complement through the alternative pathway.
4. Products of the kinin and fibrinolytic systems activate complement.

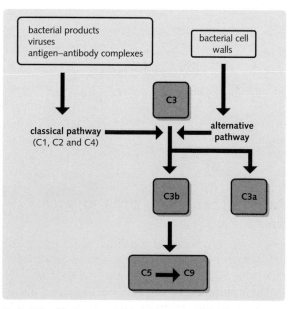

Fig. 2.6 Simplified version of the complement cascade showing how the activated product of one protein activates another.

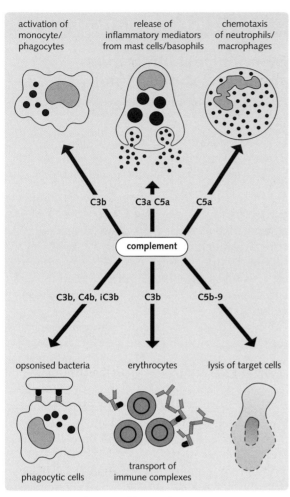

Fig. 2.7 The major functions of the complement system.

Corticosteroids (e.g. prednisolone) are very effective anti-inflammatory drugs but long-term use is associated with numerous side effects, including reduced bone density (osteoporosis), diabetes mellitus, increased blood pressure and cataracts. The prolonged use of corticosteroids is therefore carefully controlled, the lowest possible effective dose is prescribed and prophylaxis is often used against side effects (e.g. supplementary calcium as bone protection).

Platelet activation factors

Platelet activation factors are released from mast cells and neutrophils during degranulation. They have the following effects:

- Induce platelet aggregation and degranulation.
- Increase vascular permeability.
- Induce leucocyte adhesion to the endothelium.
- Stimulate synthesis of arachidonic acid derivatives.

Vasoactive amines

These are preformed inflammatory mediators and so can be rapidly released by inflammatory cells. The

Kinins

Kinins are small, vasoactive peptides (about 10 amino acids). Bradykinin is the most well known. It exerts its effects by increasing vascular permeability and producing pain. Both effects are cardinal features of acute inflammation.

The kinin system is stimulated by activated coagulation factor XII (the Hageman factor).

Arachidonic acid, prostaglandins and leukotrienes

During acute inflammation, the membrane phospholipids of neutrophils and mast cells are metabolised to form prostaglandins and leukotrienes (Fig. 2.8).

The anti-inflammatory action of drugs (e.g. glucocorticoids, aspirin and aspirin-like drugs) is attributable to their ability to inhibit prostaglandin production.

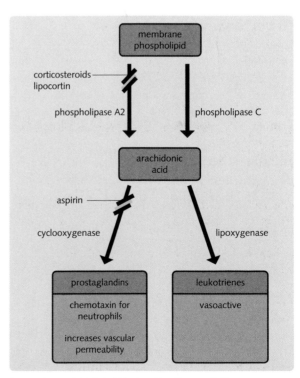

Fig. 2.8 Formation of arachidonic acid and its metabolites.

most notable example is histamine, which is released following the degranulation of mast cells.

Histamine produces the arteriolar vasodilatation and increased vascular permeability seen in early inflammation.

Cytokines

Cytokines are a family of chemical messengers that act over short distances (autocrine and/or paracrine) by binding specific receptors on target cell surfaces. They include:

- Lymphokines—cytokines produced by lymphocytes.
- Monokines—cytokines produced by monocytes/macrophages.
- Interleukins—cytokines that act between leucocytes (more than 15 types).
- Interferons—inhibit replication of viruses within cells and activate macrophages and natural killer (NK) cells.
- Growth factors.
- Tumour necrosis factors—kill tumour cells but also stimulate adipose and muscle catabolism leading to weight loss.

Tumour necrosis factor alpha (TNFα) and interleukin 1 (IL-1) are key cytokines in acute inflammation.

Nitric oxide

Nitric oxide (NO) is a potent vasodilator that is released from endothelial cells and macrophages. It is produced by the action of nitric oxide synthase on L-arginine. NO acts as a regulator of inflammation, actively reducing the effect of other proinflammatory mediators.

Acute-phase proteins

Proteins whose serum level dramatically increases during inflammation are called acute-phase proteins. These proteins are produced by the liver and induced by circulating levels of IL-1, e.g. the C-reactive protein.

C-reactive protein (CRP) can be measured in the serum as a non-specific marker of inflammation. Serial measurements can be used to monitor progress of an inflammatory disease, e.g. Crohn's disease, acute pancreatitis. Note that CRP alone is insufficient for diagnosis of these conditions.

CHRONIC INFLAMMATION

Mononuclear infiltration and granulation tissue

The site of chronic inflammation is dominated by:

- Lymphocytes.
- Plasma cells (for antibody production).
- Macrophages (for phagocytosis)—some macrophages fuse to form multinucleate giant cells.

Macrophages in inflamed tissue are formed from the transformation of blood monocytes (Fig. 2.9). The number of macrophages gradually increases during acute inflammation until they are the dominant cell type in chronic inflammation. These macrophages are activated by numerous stimuli, including interferon gamma (IFNγ), which is produced by activated lymphocytes.

The macrophages gradually remove damaged tissue by phagocytosis and produce biologically active products (e.g. growth factors) to aid repair through fibrosis. This results in the slow replacement of damaged tissue with granulation tissue, which consists of new capillaries and new connective tissue formed from myofibroblasts (i.e. modified fibroblasts capable of contracting) and the collagen that they secrete.

The prolonged presence of activated macrophages in chronic inflammation leads to the overproduction

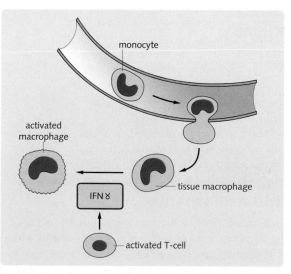

Fig. 2.9 Monocytes and macrophages in chronic inflammation. Note that macrophages may be activated by stimuli other than interferon-gamma, including bacterial endotoxin and fibronectin.

of biologically active products and therefore tissue damage.

Chronic inflammation is a crucial process in many important diseases. Excellent examples are provided later in this book, including atherosclerosis (Chapter 6), tuberculosis (Chapter 7) and rheumatoid arthritis (Chapter 12).

Wound healing

Nature of cells

The regenerative capacity of tissue can be categorised in three main ways: labile, stable and permanent:

- Labile tissue is constantly dividing, usually through stem cell division (unlimited capacity to proliferate). This allows the replacement of ageing tissue, such as the surface epithelia of the skin, gastrointestinal tract and uterus. Blood cells are derived from the labile cells of the bone marrow.
- Stable tissues are in a state of quiescence, meaning that the cells slowly replicate to maintain tissue size. However, such tissue may rapidly regenerate if stimulated. Parenchymal tissue of the liver and kidney are good examples of stable tissues.
- Permanent tissues consist of cells that have left the cell cycle and so are incapable of division. Neurons, cardiac and skeletal muscle cells are good examples.

A good example of stable tissue regeneration is the ability of the liver to regenerate after part of it is surgically removed (partial hepatectomy). In living-donor hepatic transplantations, one lobe of the donor's liver may be removed. Within weeks of the operation, the donor's liver returns to its original size by compensatory growth of the remaining lobes.

The ultimate consequence of tissue injury therefore depends on many factors. Although labile and stable cells may be capable of division, complex tissue architecture might not be replaced. The process of wound healing in the skin depends on the size of the injury; it occurs by two mechanisms:

1. Healing by first intention

Apposed wound margins are joined by fibrin deposition, which is subsequently replaced by collagen and covered by epidermal growth (Fig. 2.10), e.g. surgical incision wound.

2. Healing by second intention

Healing by second intention (Fig. 2.11) involves the following:

- Wound margins are unapposed due to extensive tissue damage.
- Tissue defect fills with granulation tissue.
- Epithelial regeneration to cover surface.
- Granulation tissue eventually contracts resulting in scar formation.

The type of healing process in the skin depends on the extent of tissue damage:
- Minimal tissue loss—involves healing by first intention.
- Extensive tissue loss—involves healing by second intention.

Scar formation

Myofibroblasts within granulation tissue are attached to one another and to adjacent extracellular matrix. Their contraction draws together the surrounding matrix and thus reduces the size of the defect, but in doing so produces a scar.

Patterns of inflammation

Fibrinous inflammation

Fibrinous inflammation is the deposition of increased amounts of fibrin on a tissue surface, e.g. in acute pleurisy secondary to acute lobar pneumonia.

If the fibrin is eventually removed, resolution is said to have occurred. However, if the fibrin persists it may be converted to scar tissue (known as organization).

Suppurative inflammation

Suppurative inflammation is characterised by the production of pus. It is usually caused by infection with pyogenic bacteria such as *Staphylococcus aureus* and *Streptococcus pyogenes*. Pus becomes surrounded by

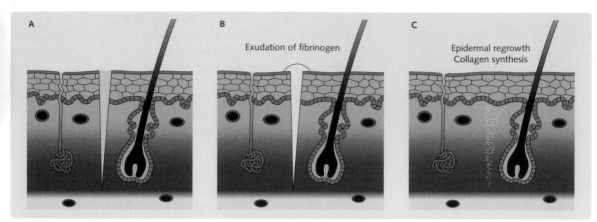

Fig. 2.10 Skin incision healed by first intention. (A) Incision. (B) Weak fibrin join. (C) Strong collagen join.

a 'pyogenic membrane' of sprouting capillaries, neutrophil polymorphs and fibroblasts.

There are two types of suppurative inflammation: superficial (e.g. a boil) and deep-seated (e.g. an abscess within a hollow viscus such as the gall bladder). In the deep-seated type, mucosal layers of outflow tract may become fused with fibrin resulting in empyema. Fistulae (i.e. abnormal passages between mucosal surfaces) might form.

Haemorrhagic inflammation

If damage is severe, blood vessels within the area may rupture, e.g. haemorrhagic pneumonia, meningococcal septicaemia.

Granulomatous inflammation

Granulomatous inflammation is a form of chronic inflammation in which modified macrophages (termed epithelioid histiocytes) aggregate to form small clusters, or granulomas, surrounded by lymphoid cells. It usually occurs in response to indigestible particulate matter within macrophages. Causes of granulomatous inflammation include:

- Microorganisms resistant to intracellular killing mechanisms, e.g. *Mycobacterium tuberculosis* and *Mycobacterium leprae*.
- Foreign bodies—endogenous (e.g. bone, adipose tissue, uric acid crystals) or exogenous (e.g. silica, suture materials, implanted prostheses).
- Idiopathic, e.g. in Crohn's disease, sarcoidosis and Wegener's granulomatosis.
- Drugs, e.g. allopurinol and sulphonamides can cause hepatic granuloma.

Granulomas are aggregates of epithelioid histiocytes but commonly they fuse or divide without cytoplasmic separation to produce multinucleate giant cells. Examples include Langhans' giant cell (typical in tuberculosis), foreign body giant cell (where indigestible foreign body is present) and Touton giant cell (typically seen in xanthomas).

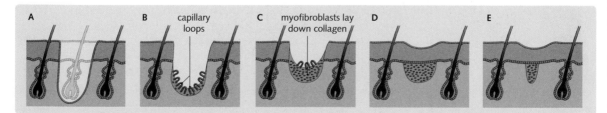

Fig. 2.11 Skin wound repaired by second intention. (A) Loss of tissue. (B) Granulation tissue. (C) Organization. (D) Early fibrous scar. (E) Scar contraction.

Commonly confused terms:
- A *granuloma* is an aggregation of epithelioid histiocytes. It is a feature of some chronic inflammatory diseases.
- *Granulation tissue* is a combination of capillary loops and myofibroblasts. It is a wound-healing phenomenon.

- Pyrexia—polymorphs and macrophages produce pyrogens (e.g. IL-1), which act on the hypothalamus.
- Constitutional symptoms—malaise, nausea and anorexia.
- Reactive hyperplasia of the mononuclear phagocyte system—enlargement of local and systemic lymph nodes.
- Haematological changes—increased erythrocyte sedimentation rate, leucocytosis and acute-phase protein release (e.g. C-reactive protein).
- Weight loss—occurs in severe chronic inflammation such as tuberculosis.

Ulceration

Ulcers are formed when the surface of an organ or tissue is lost because of necrosis and replaced by inflammatory tissue. The most common sites are the alimentary canal and the skin.

Chronic ulceration is a balance between tissue damage, e.g. by gastric acid, and tissue repair by the body's healing response, i.e. the chronic inflammatory response.

Systemic effects of inflammation

Both acute and chronic inflammation can produce a number of systemic effects including:

CELL DEATH

Cells may be damaged either reversibly (sublethal damage) or irreversibly (lethal damage) (Fig. 2.12). The type of damage depends on the:

- Nature and duration of injury.
- Type of cells affected.
- Regenerative ability of tissues.

There are two types of cell death: necrosis and apoptosis. Necrosis tends to occur after severe cellular

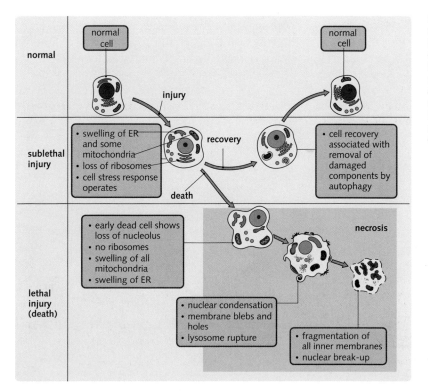

Fig. 2.12 Relationships between sublethal and lethal cell damage. Sublethal damage can be repaired and the cell survives. Lethal cell damage is irreversible and results in cell death, which may occur by necrosis (as shown) or apoptosis. Types of cellular injury include mechanical trauma, loss of membrane integrity, inhibition of metabolic pathways, DNA damage and deficiency of essential metabolites.

injury and is always pathological. Apoptosis can be a physiological process that often follows DNA damage and cell-cycle arrest.

Note that there are no absolute ultrastructural criteria by which reversible and irreversible cellular injury can be distinguished, and that there is a continuum from a reversibly injured cell through to an irreversibly necrotically damaged cell.

Mechanisms of cell death

The initiating mechanisms of cell death depend on the type of injury and are summarised in Fig. 2.13.

Necrosis

Necrosis is the death of cells or tissues that are still part of the living organism. Necrosis is a pathological process following cellular injury, which results in an inflammatory response after the loss of plasma membrane integrity.

Regardless of the cause of cell injury, necrosis occurs with:

- Depletion of intracellular energy systems.
- Disruption of cytoplasmic organelles.
- Liberation of intracellular enzymes.
- Production of oxygen free radicals.
- Disintegration of the nucleus.
- Alterations and failure of the plasma membrane.
- Alteration in ionic transport mechanisms.
- Increased permeability of membrane phospholipids.
- Physical disruption of the plasma membrane.

Histological types of necrosis
Coagulative necrosis

This is the most common form of necrosis, characteristically occurring in the heart, kidney and spleen, although it can occur in most tissues.

Dead tissue is initially swollen and firm, but later becomes soft as a result of digestion by macrophages. Dead cells retain 'ghost' outlines and the necrotic area is highly eosinophilic.

It usually evokes an inflammatory response; damaged tissue is removed by phagocytosis.

Coagulative necrosis is the classic pattern seen in myocardial tissue following a myocardial infarction (MI). It takes several hours to develop. However, the loss of plasma membrane integrity in necrosis allows the leaking of cardiac enzymes into the bloodstream very quickly, making them useful as biochemical markers. The levels of these enzymes (e.g. troponin T) in the blood are routinely used to aid the diagnosis of a MI.

Liquefactive (colliquative) necrosis

This characteristically occurs in the central nervous system (e.g. a hypoxic stroke) due to minimal supporting stroma. Necrotic neural tissue undergoes total liquefaction and a glial reaction occurs around the periphery, with eventual cyst formation.

Fig. 2.13 Mechanisms of cell death. Various cell and tissue types are differentially susceptible to various injurious agents, e.g. the cellular response to ischaemia.

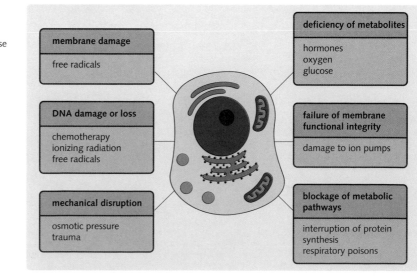

Caseous necrosis (caseation)

This is commonly seen in tuberculosis. Histologically, the complete loss of normal tissue architecture is replaced by amorphous, granular and eosinophilic tissue. There are variable amounts of fat and an appearance reminiscent of cottage cheese, hence the term 'caseation'.

Gangrene

Necrotic tissue is invaded by putrefactive organisms, notably clostridia. The tissue appears green or black because of the breakdown of haemoglobin. There are three main types:

1. Dry gangrene—usually follows gradual arterial occlusion, as seen in the toes of individuals with advanced diabetes ('diabetic foot'). The putrefactive process is very slow and only small numbers of organisms are present.
2. Wet gangrene—occurs when additional bacterial infection produces liquefactive necrosis. An example is the ischaemic necrosis of the bowel (clostridia are common in the bowel).
3. Gas gangrene—is a primary infection of healthy tissue by *Clostridium perfringens*, resulting in putrefactive necrosis.

Fibrinoid necrosis

This occurs in malignant hypertension, where increased arterial pressure results in necrosis of smooth muscle wall. Eosinophilic and fibrinous deposits are seen, although inflammation and actual necrosis are usually inconspicuous.

Fat necrosis

This describes focal adipose tissue destruction, which may be due to:

- Direct trauma—release of triglycerides following trauma elicits a rapid inflammatory response. Fat is phagocytosed by neutrophils and macrophages, which ultimately results in fibrosis.
- Enzymatic lipolysis—in acute pancreatitis, lipases liberated from damaged acini act on fat cells in the peritoneal cavity to release triglycerides.

Apoptosis

Apoptosis is an energy-dependent mechanism of cell death for the deletion of unwanted individual cells; it is a form of 'programmed cell death'. Inhibition of apoptosis results in cell accumulation, e.g. neoplasia (see Chapter 3). The rate of apoptosis must be matched by the rate of cellular division to maintain a stable tissue size. Increased apoptosis results in net cell loss, e.g. tissue atrophy.

Apoptosis can therefore be:

- Physiological—such as in the maintenance of organ size, regulation of the immune system and the shedding of the endometrium at menstruation.
- Pathological—when cellular damage has occurred, often at the nuclear level (i.e. DNA damage). Apoptosis can therefore prevent the perpetuation of a genetically abnormal cell.

A key point: apoptosis is an energy-dependent process that does not result in an inflammatory response. This is in contrast to necrosis, an energy-independent process that can cause inflammation.

Mechanisms of apoptosis

The execution of apoptosis is achieved by the activation of a cascade of proteases known as caspases. Caspase-3 is thought to be a crucial final enzyme in this caspase cascade, which can be initiated by two pathways (Fig. 2.14):

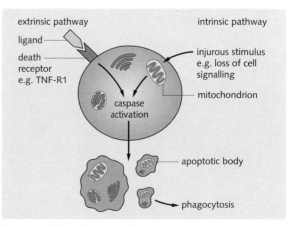

Fig. 2.14 Initiation of apoptosis. The common caspase cascade may be triggered by the extrinsic ('death receptor') pathway or intrinsic (mitochondrial) pathway.

Fig. 2.15 Comparison of cell death by necrosis and apoptosis

Feature	Necrosis	Apoptosis
Induction	Pathological conditions	Pathological or physiological conditions
Number of cells	Groups of cells	Single cells
Plasma membrane	Loss of membrane integrity	Membrane remains intact
Morphology	Cell swelling and lysis	Cell shrinkage and fragmentation, formation of characteristic apoptotic bodies
Inflammation	Inflammatory response	No inflammatory response
Fate of cells	Phagocytosed by neutrophils and macrophages	Phagocytosed by neighbouring cells
Biochemical mechanism	Energy-independent Loss of ion homeostasis	Energy dependent Endonuclease activity

Fig. 2.15 Comparison of cell death by necrosis and apoptosis.

1. The extrinsic pathway—external 'death receptors' (e.g. TNF receptors) are activated by an appropriate ligand.
2. The intrinsic pathway—proapoptotic molecules are released from mitochondria after the breakdown of normal anti-apoptotic signalling (e.g. Bcl-2). Examples of where this occurs include the loss of cellular signalling and exposure to radiation or toxins.

The caspase cascade is the common result of both pathways. Morphologically, an apoptotic cell is characterised by:

- Loss of cell surface markings.
- Cell shrinkage due to cytoskeletal breakdown.
- Nuclear chromatin condensation.
- Formation of apoptotic bodies with intact plasma membrane and organelles. These are eventually phagocytosed by adjacent cells.

A comparison of cell death by apoptosis and necrosis is given in Fig. 2.15.

Cancer

3

Objectives

In this chapter, you will learn to:
- Define tumour, dysplasia, metaplasia, hyperplasia and hypertrophy.
- Understand the differences between benign and malignant tumours.
- Briefly describe the epidemiology of cancer in the UK and worldwide.
- Describe the role of proto-oncogenes and tumour suppressor genes in the development of cancers.
- Understand the multistage model of tumour development.
- Describe the process of tumour growth and angiogenesis, invasion and metastasis.
- Describe the role of chemicals, radiation and viruses as carcinogenic agents.
- Describe the host defences against cancer.
- Understand the importance of tumour markers, grading and staging in clinical cancer pathology.

DEFINITIONS AND NOMENCLATURE

Definitions

Tumour

A tumour can be defined as an abnormal mass of tissue resulting from autonomous disordered growth that persists after the initiating stimulus has been removed. A tumour results from genetic alteration and deregulated growth control mechanisms. There may be an inherited predisposition to tumour development (e.g. breast and ovarian cancer families), although this accounts for only a small proportion of total tumours.

Tumours are:

- Progressive—they are independent of normal growth control and continue to grow regardless of requirements and in the absence of any external stimuli.
- Purposeless—the abnormal mass serves no useful purpose.
- Parasitic—they are endogenous in origin but draw nourishment from the body while contributing nothing to its function.

All tumours have the suffix '—oma', which means a swelling.

Other related definitions are:

- Neoplasm (i.e. new growth)—synonymous with tumour.
- Neoplasia—the process of tumour growth.
- Cancer—a malignant neoplasm.
- Anaplastic neoplasm—a very poorly differentiated neoplasm. Anaplastic specimens highlight the typical changes of a malignant neoplasm: pleomorphism (variation in shape and size) of cells and nuclei, numerous mitoses, abnormal nuclear morphology and cellular disorganization (i.e. loss of cellular polarity).

Dysplasia

Dysplasia is the disordered development of cells resulting in an alteration in their size, shape and organization. It may be reversible but is also known to precede neoplasia. It is, therefore, referred to as a premalignant state in certain circumstances.

Metaplasia

Metaplasia is the change from one type of differentiated tissue to another, usually in response to an irritating stimulus, e.g. a change from mucus-secreting epithelium to stratified squamous epithelium in the bronchial irritation associated with cigarette smoking. Metaplasia is reversible and often represents an adaptive response to environmental stress.

Hyperplasia

This refers to an increase in the number of cells in a tissue or organ, which may result in an increase in the overall size. An example is the hyperplasia of breast tissue during pregnancy.

Hypertrophy

Hypertrophy is an increase in tissue or organ size due to an increase in the size of cells. Crucially, there is no increase in the number of cells in the tissue. Cells that are permanent (e.g. myocardial fibres) cannot divide and so undergo hypertrophy to increase tissue size (e.g. left ventricular hypertrophy as a response to hypertension).

In general, tissues capable of division can undergo both hyperplasia and hypertrophy to increase tissue size.

Benign versus malignant

Tumours are classified as either benign or malignant, according to their appearance and behaviour (Fig. 3.1). Benign tumours are usually well differentiated, localised cancers that do not invade the surrounding tissues or metastasise to other organs. Metastasis is the process whereby malignant cells spread from their site of origin (a primary tumour) to distant sites and grow into secondary tumours.

Malignant tumours are capable of invasion and spread to distant organs. This distinction is crucial in the clinic because metastatic disease is associated with significant morbidity and mortality. Malignant neoplasms can show a range of differentiations.

Nomenclature of tumours

Tumour nomenclature (Fig. 3.2) is based on histological and behaviour patterns. Histology provides information about the type of cell from which the tumour has arisen, whereas behaviour provides information as to whether the cell is benign or malignant.

A few simple rules to follow:
- Carcinomas—malignant tumours of epithelial origin; prefixed by tissue of origin.
- —oma—suffix for tumours, but there are some non-neoplastic '—omas', e.g. granuloma.
- —sarcoma—suffix for malignant tumours of connective tissue origin.

Classification of carcinomas

Carcinomas are malignant tumours of epithelial tissue. Carcinomas of non-glandular epithelium are prefixed by the name of the epithelial cell type. Malignant tumours of glandular epithelium are termed adenocarcinomas. Carcinomas can be further subclassified according to their ability to invade or not, and behavioural information can be gained from histological grading of cellular differentiation.

Intraepithelial neoplasia

This covers the spectrum of changes short of invasive carcinoma:

- Mild dysplasia
- Moderate dysplasia
- Severe dysplasia/carcinoma *in situ*.

Fig. 3.1 Characteristics of benign versus malignant tumours

Benign	Malignant
Localised	Tumour spread
No invasion	Invasion
No metastases	Metastases
Slow growth rate	Rapid growth rate
Good differentiation	Poorly differentiated
Few mitoses	Many mitoses
Normal nuclear chromatin	Increased nuclear chromatin appearance
Uniform size cells	Cells and nuclei vary in size (pleomorphism)
Exophytic	Endophytic
Compression of normal tissue	Invasion and destruction of normal tissue

Fig. 3.1 Characteristics of benign versus malignant tumours. Note that invasion is the only absolute distinguishing feature between benign and malignant neoplasms.

Fig. 3.2 Important tumour nomenclature

Histological type	Benign	Malignant
Epithelial		
Glandular	Adenoma	Adenocarcinoma
Non-glandular	Papilloma	Carcinoma
Connective tissue		
Adipose	Lipoma	Liposarcoma
Cartilage	Chondroma	Chondrosarcoma
Bone	Osteoma	Osteosarcoma
Smooth muscle	Leiomyoma	Leiomyosarcoma
Voluntary muscle	Rhabdomyoma	Rhabdomyosarcoma
Blood vessels	Angioma	Angiosarcoma
Nerve	Neurofibroma	Neurofibrosarcoma
Nerve sheath	Neurilemmoma	Neurilemmosarcoma
Glial cells	Glioma	Malignant glioma
Others		
Haemopoietic	*	Leukaemia
Lymphoreticular	*	Lymphoma
Melanocytes	*	Malignant melanoma
Germinal cell	Benign teratoma	Malignant teratoma

Fig. 3.2 Examples of tumour nomenclature. * represents those tumours that are always malignant and do not have benign counterparts.

Cervical intraepithelial neoplasia (CIN) is a premalignant state that may exist for many years before cervical cancer develops. CIN is categorised according to the level of dysplasia seen in the squamous epithelium of the cervical transformation zone (the area examined on routine 'smear' screening). Three grades are observed:
- CIN I—mildly dysplasic
- CIN II—moderately dysplasic
- CIN III—severely dysplasic (carcinoma *in situ* at high risk of invasion).

Carcinoma *insitu*

This is an epithelial neoplasm with all the cellular features associated with malignancy but which has not yet invaded through the epithelial basement membrane. The in-situ phase may not progress, or it may last for several years before invasion commences.

Invasive carcinoma

This is an epithelial neoplasm that invades through the basement membrane. The tumour gains access to the vascular supply and lymphatics, and will often metastasise to distant tissues.

Epidemiological aspects of cancer

Cancer in the UK

As a cause of mortality in the UK, cancer is the second biggest killer (after cardiovascular disease). Its incidence (Fig. 3.3) is as follows:

- Almost 1 in 3 of the population will develop cancer during their lifetime.
- Almost 1 in 4 of the population will die of cancer.
- Incidence of cancer deaths increases with increasing age.
- Incidence of cancer varies between males and females.

Cancer worldwide

The incidence of different cancers varies from country to country. This variation provides clues to the causes of the cancers. For example, in Japan, gastric carcinoma is 30 times more common than in the UK, whereas pancreatic cancer is much rarer. However, migration of a subset of the Japanese population to different geographical areas (e.g. USA, UK) alters the incidences of these diseases within that population.

These findings suggest that environmental factors (such as diet and occupational, social and geographic effects) rather than genetic causes account for most of the observed differences between countries.

MOLECULAR BASIS OF CANCER

Oncogenes and tumour suppressor genes

Cell proliferation and division is usually tightly regulated by two sets of opposing functioning genes:

1. Growth-promoting genes, called proto-oncogenes.
2. Negative cell-cycle regulators, called tumour suppressor genes (TSGs).

Abnormal activation of proto-oncogenes and loss of function of TSGs leads to the transformation of a normal cell into a cancer cell.

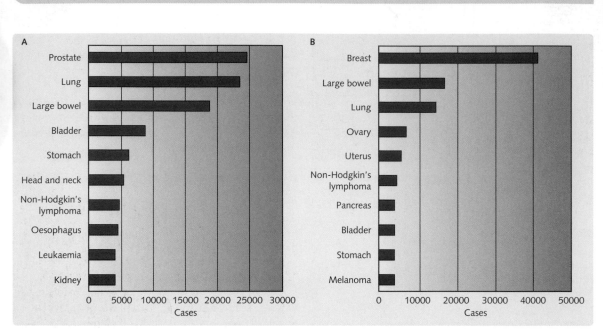

Fig. 3.3 Incidence of the ten most common cancers of (A) men and (B) women in the UK. The data exclude non-melanoma skin cancers (e.g. basal cell carcinoma) because, although common, they are rarely so fatal. Data from Cancer Research UK, 2003. (Adapted from Underwood, 2004.)

Proto-oncogenes

Proto-oncogenes are genes that are expressed in normal cells. They code for oncoproteins, which positively regulate cell growth and differentiation (growth factors, transcription factors and receptor molecules). In healthy cells, the transcription of these genes is tightly controlled. Inappropriate expression of oncoproteins leads to abnormal cell growth and survival. Normally functioning proto-oncogenes can be activated into cancer-causing oncogenes in two ways:

- A mutation can produce an oncoprotein that is functionally altered and abnormally active. For example, intracellular signalling is affected by the hyperactive mutant *ras* protein.
- A normal oncoprotein can be produced in abnormally large quantities because of enhanced gene amplification (e.g. the *myc* oncogene in neuroblastomas) or enhanced transcription (formation of the Philadelphia chromosome from a translocation between chromosomes 9 and 22).

Oncogenes can be classified according to the function of their product. Oncogenes include genes that express:

- Nuclear binding proteins, e.g. *c-myc*.
- Tyrosine kinase proteins, e.g. *src*.

- Growth factors, e.g. platelet-derived growth factor.
- Receptors for growth factors, e.g. c-*erb* B-2/HER-2, which is related to epidermal growth factor receptor.
- GTP binding proteins, e.g. *ras*.

Expression of abnormal oncogene products corresponds to the behaviour and appearance of transformed cells. These include:

- Independence from the requirement of extrinsic growth factors.
- Production of proteases that assist tissue invasion.
- Reduced cell cohesiveness, which assists metastasis.
- Ability to grow at higher cell densities.
- Abnormal cellular orientation.
- Increased plasma membrane and cellular motility.

Tumour suppressor genes

TSGs (e.g. *p53* and *RB1*) encode proteins that prevent or suppress the growth of tumours. Inactivation of TSGs results in increased susceptibility to cancer formation. Genetically increased susceptibility to cancer formation was first proposed by Knudson, who studied the childhood retinal cancer retinoblastoma.

Retinoblastoma is a rare malignant tumour of the retina. In familial cases (bilateral), a germline mutation in the *RB1* gene is present, meaning that only one further somatic mutation is required for tumour formation. Other cases of retinoblastoma are unilateral and sporadic, needing two somatic mutations on an initially fully functioning *RB1* gene. This requirement for separate mutations in both alleles of a TSG has been termed the 'two-hit' hypothesis of oncogenesis.

Examples of dysfunctional TSGs involved in human cancers are:

- *APC*—implicated in colorectal tumours and located on chromosome 5q.
- *NF1*—implicated in neurofibrosarcoma and located on chromosome 17q.
- *RB1*—implicated in retinoblastoma and located on chromosome 13q.
- *BRCA1*—implicated in breast and ovarian cancer and located on chromosome 17q.
- *p53*—implicated in many tumours and located on chromosome 17p.

Loss of function of TSGs or their protein products can result in uncontrolled neoplastic cell growth. TSGs can lose their normal function by a variety of mechanisms:

- Mutations (hereditary or acquired).
- Binding of normal TSG protein to proteins encoded by viral genes, e.g. human papilloma virus proteins E6/E7.
- Complexing of normal TSG protein to mutant TSG protein in heterozygous cells.

TSGs function by maintaining the integrity of the genome through cell-cycle arrest in abnormally dividing cells and repair of DNA damage. They also function to promote cell suicide or apoptosis (see Chapter 2) in cells with sustained DNA damage.

One of the most studied TSGs is the *p53* gene, which is located at 17p; it is called 'the guardian of the genome'. *p53* is mutated or functionally altered in over 50% of all human cancers. In addition, a familial inherited mutation is found in Li-Fraumeni's syndrome, in which there is an increased predisposition to several tumour types.

p53 can recognise damaged DNA and responds either through cell-cycle growth arrest at the G_1 check point or through the initiation of apoptosis. For example, the p53 protein product recognises DNA damage caused by ultraviolet (UV) irradiation and activates apoptotic cell death pathways before the cell can divide and proliferate (Fig. 3.4).

Genes and proteins involved in the process of apoptosis include the death receptor and ligand families, cell-cycle-related genes, the *Bcl-2* family, the caspase family and the caspase substrates.

Cellular proliferation is tightly regulated by two sets of opposing functioning genes. Proto-oncogenes are growth-promoting genes whereas tumour suppressor genes are growth-suppressing genes. Deregulated function of proto-oncogenes and tumour suppressor genes leads to cell transformation and tumourigenesis.

Multistage model of tumour progression

Tumourigenesis is a multistage process that results from accumulated mutation. Tumours arise from single cells, which proliferate to form a clone of cells with identical abnormalities. As tumours develop,

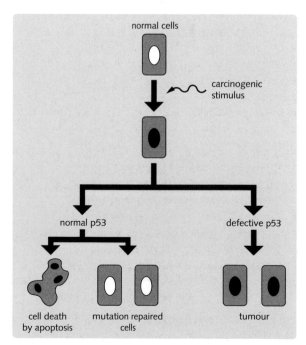

Fig. 3.4 Role of p53 in cells with damaged DNA. Cells either undergo G_1 arrest and DNA repair, or cell death by apoptosis. (Adapted from Underwood, 2000.)

they undergo further somatic mutations, which cause abnormalities in other oncogenes and/or tumour suppressor genes. These additional mutations result in cells that are genetically different from each other but which are part of the same tumour: this is heterogeneity.

Fast-growing, less-differentiated cells take over and eliminate the slower-growing, better-differentiated cells.

Chemotherapy will kill the majority of tumour cells. However, tumour cells that are resistant to chemotherapy will survive and be selected for (because of ablation of competing, non-resistant cells), resulting in the regrowth of a tumour that is resistant to chemotherapy (Fig. 3.5). This highlights the concept of 'minimal residual disease', i.e. the small number of tumour cells that survive an intervention such as chemotherapy.

The progressive nature of tumourigenesis is clearly illustrated in Vogelstein's model of the development of colonic cancer. The accumulation over time of mutations in oncogenes such as *Ki-ras*, and loss of function mutations in tumour suppressor genes such as *APC*, results in the eventual formation of colon carcinoma (Fig. 3.6).

TUMOUR GROWTH AND SPREAD

Kinetics of tumour growth and angiogenesis

Angiogenesis is the formation of new blood vessels and is an important physiological process in normal embryogenesis, the female reproductive cycle and wound healing. However, pathological angiogenesis is a key player in many disorders, including cancer. This is because a solid tumour cannot grow beyond a few millimeters in diameter without a blood supply to maintain nutrient and oxygen provision and remove metabolic waste.

In normal cells, angiogenesis is a highly regulated mechanism. In contrast, tumour cells can release proangiogenic factors, which induce vascular proliferation. This is sometimes called the angiogenic switch. The angiogenic switch results in the production of proangiogenic molecules such as vascular endothelial growth factor.

Eventually, the tumour outgrows its blood supply and areas of necrosis may appear, resulting in slower growth but a more malignant phenotype (Fig. 3.7). This is because only the strongest cells survive the hypoxic conditions.

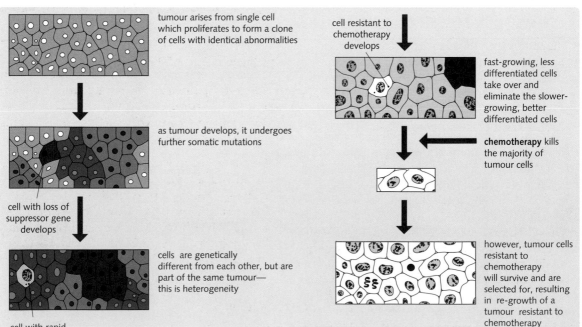

tumour arises from single cell which proliferates to form a clone of cells with identical abnormalities

as tumour develops, it undergoes further somatic mutations

cell with loss of suppressor gene develops

cells are genetically different from each other, but are part of the same tumour—this is heterogeneity

cell with rapid division develops

cell resistant to chemotherapy develops

fast-growing, less differentiated cells take over and eliminate the slower-growing, better differentiated cells

chemotherapy kills the majority of tumour cells

however, tumour cells resistant to chemotherapy will survive and are selected for, resulting in re-growth of a tumour resistant to chemotherapy

Fig. 3.5 Tumour progression and genetic heterogeneity.

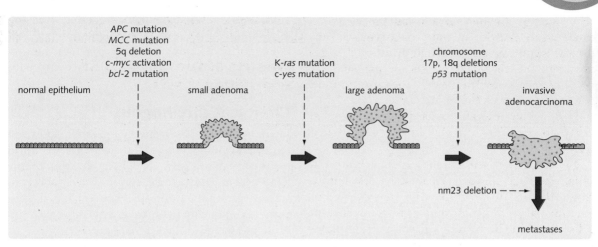

Fig. 3.6 Multistep development of colonic cancer. The accumulation of genetic mutations corresponds to the altered behaviour of the tumour cells. (APC, adenomatous polyposis coli; MCC, mutated in colorectal cancer.) (Adapted from Underwood, 2000.)

Mechanisms and pathways of invasion and metastasis

Invasion

The ability to invade is the only absolute criterion for malignancy. Invading malignant cells have the following properties:

- Abnormal or increased cellular motility—due to loss of contact inhibition.
- Altered cellular adhesion—due to changes in surface adhesion molecules.
- Increased secretion of proteolytic enzymes, e.g. metalloproteinases.

Metalloproteinases, such as collagenases and gelatinases, are the most important enzymes in neoplastic invasion. They digest the surrounding connective tissue, thus aiding invasion.

Metastasis

In metastatic cancer, the total mass of secondary tumours usually exceeds that of the primary lesion. However, only a proportion of neoplastic cells in a malignant tumour are able to metastasise.

It can be impossible to find the primary lesion in some cancer patients who present with extensive secondary metastases.

To metastasise through vessels, neoplastic cells undergo the following sequence of events:

- Detachment of tumour cells from neighbouring cells.
- Invasion of the tissue basement membrane and then surrounding connective tissue.
- Intravasation into blood/lymphatic vessels.
- Evasion of the host's defence mechanisms, often by forming a tumour cell embolus with platelets or host lymphoid cells.
- Adherence to endothelium at a distant site.
- Extravasation of cells from vessel lumen into surrounding tissue.

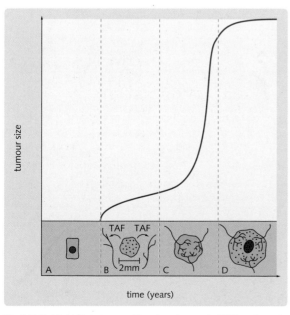

Fig. 3.7 Kinetics of tumour growth and angiogenesis. (A) Transformed cell. (B) Avascular tumour nodule. (C) Vascularised tumour. (D) Vascularised tumour with central necrosis. (TAF, tumour angiogenic factors.) (Adapted from Underwood, 2000.)

Following extravasation, the malignant cells proliferate and secrete more angiogenic growth factors for vascularization. Hence a new tumour is formed.

However, not all cancer cells will grow at all distant sites. This is the seed and soil effect: conditions must be appropriate for cell proliferation.

Main routes of metastasis

There are four main routes of metastasis (Fig. 3.8):

1. Local invasion—most common pattern of spread of malignant tumours is by direct growth into adjacent tissues.
2. Lymphatic spread—forms secondary tumours in lymph nodes.
3. Blood-borne (haematogenous) spread—cells enter the bloodstream and form secondary tumours in organs perfused by blood that has drained from a tumour.
4. Transcoelomic spread—in pleural, pericardial and peritoneal cavities.

It is clinically important to know the major tumours that spread to bone via the blood. These are cancers of the bronchus, breast, thyroid, kidney and prostate. Bone metastases can be evaluated using radionucleotide bone scanning, except in myeloma, where a skeletal survey is needed.

CARCINOGENIC AGENTS

Carcinogens are substances known to cause an increased incidence of cancer.

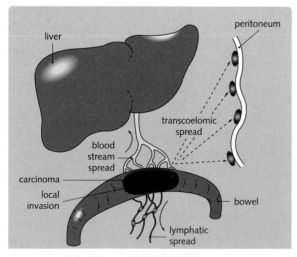

Fig. 3.8 Routes of metastasis exemplified by a carcinoma of the bowel, i.e. via the bloodstream, via the lymphatic spread, through peritoneal cavities and via local invasion.

Carcinogens can exert their effect either by genetic mechanisms (i.e. causing DNA alteration; this is the majority of carcinogens) or epigenetic mechanisms (i.e. acting on the protein product of growth-regulating genes).

Chemical carcinogens

Most chemical carcinogens are procarcinogens and require metabolic conversion into an active form (ultimate carcinogens), usually by the cytochrome P450 system, which shows significant variability in activity (gene polymorphisms) between individuals. Some people are therefore inherently more susceptible to producing ultimate carcinogens.

Some carcinogens act directly to induce cellular damage. Examples of chemical carcinogens are given in Fig. 3.9.

Stages of chemical carcinogenesis

The progressive model of carcinogenesis (Fig. 3.10) is based on observations of the effects of chemical

Fig. 3.9 Examples of chemical carcinogens	
Chemical compound	**Cancer type**
Indirect carcinogens	
Polycyclic hydrocarbons	
• Soot [benzo(a)pyrene; dibenzanthracene]	Skin, colon
• Tobacco smoke	Lung, bladder, oral cavity, larynx, oesophagus
Aromatic amines	
• Benzidine, 2-naphthylamine	• Bladder
Nitrosamines	
• Chemotherapeutic agents	Oesophagus, stomach
• Cyclophosphamide, chlorambucil, thiotepa, busulphan	Leukaemias
Vinyl chloride	Liver (angiosarcoma)
Aflatoxins	Liver
Unknown mechanisms	
Heavy metals	
• Nickel, cadmium, chromium	Lung
• Arsenic	Skin

Fig. 3.9 Examples of chemical carcinogens.

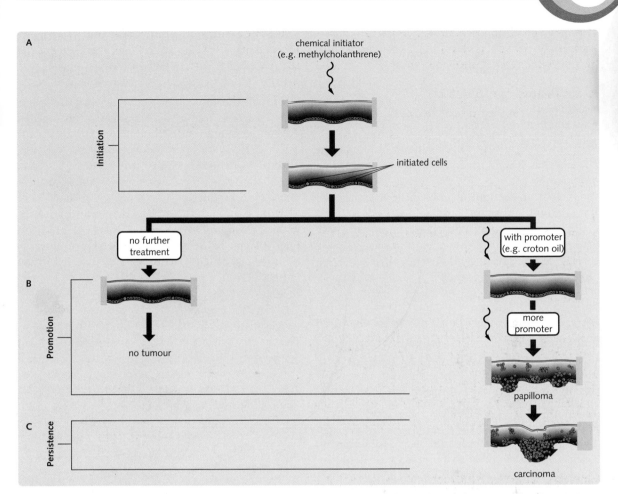

Fig. 3.10 Stages of chemical carcinogenesis. (A) Initiation: induction of genetic changes in cells that result in neoplastic potential. (B) Promotion: induction of cellular proliferation in the initiated cell. (C) Persistence: proliferating tumour cells no longer require the presence of initiators or promoters. Tumour cells exhibit autonomous growth.

carcinogens on laboratory animals. This model proposes three main stages of carcinogenesis:

1. Initiation—induction of a genetic alteration in an oncogene or TSG.
2. Promotion—a stimulus for proliferation of the initiated cell; this may be an external agent or a further random mutational genetic abnormality.
3. Persistence—when proliferation of tumour cells becomes autonomous, i.e. it no longer requires the presence of initiators or promoters.

The stages of chemical carcinogenesis are: initiation, promotion and persistence. The classic examples of initiation and promotion are the effects of methylcholanthrene and croton oil, discovered from experiments in mice. Remember that as humans are likely to be simultaneously exposed to initiators and promoters, chemical carcinogenesis is probably very complex.

Radiation

Radiation can be:

- Ionising—natural radiation, therapeutic radiation and nuclear radiation.
- Non-ionising—UV radiation.

Radiation can result in DNA damage in two ways:

1. Directly—causing strand breaks, base alterations and cross-linking of DNA.
2. Indirectly—ionisation of H_2O with formation of reactive oxygen free radicals, which interact with and damage DNA.

Ultraviolet radiation

UV radiation is associated with many different kinds of skin cancer, particularly:

- Squamous cell carcinoma.
- Basal cell carcinoma.
- Malignant melanoma.

Skin cancer is the most common type of cancer in the UK and USA. It is more common in fair-skinned individuals.

UV light is thought to induce the formation of linkages between pyrimidine bases on the DNA molecule. The risk is greatly increased in patients with xeroderma pigmentosum, a rare, autosomal recessive disease characterised by deficiency of DNA repair enzymes.

Ionising radiation

X-ray radiation

Radiotherapy can cause cancer as well as curing it! It is associated with radiation-induced malignant neoplasms, often sarcomas. These tumours may occur months or years after radiation therapy, in the lungs, CNS, bones, kidneys and liver.

Radioisotopes

Radioactive iodine, which is used to treat thyroid disease, is associated with an increased risk of cancer development as much as 15–25 years after treatment.

Nuclear radiation

Survivors of the Hiroshima and Nagasaki atomic bombs, and of the accident at the Chernobyl nuclear power plant, have shown a greatly increased incidence of cancer, including leukaemia and carcinoma of the breast, lung and thyroid.

DNA repair mechanisms and their failure

DNA is the cellular constituent most sensitive to radiation. Fortunately, cells have DNA repair genes (e.g. *MSH2*) that deal with DNA damage. Repair occurs rapidly in the vast majority of cases but damage is sometimes irreparable and major chromosomal and chromatid alterations occur. If such cells also evade cell-cycle arrest and apoptosis, a tumour may develop.

Repair of single-stranded breaks, particularly in rapidly dividing cells, is error prone and introduces single base mutations.

Double-stranded cleavage leads to chromosome breakage. Attempts to repair multiple breaks result in inappropriate recombination events, e.g. translocation or interstitial deletion.

> An excellent example of failed DNA repair mechanisms is the autosomal dominant condition hereditary non-polyposis colon cancer (HNPCC; discussed in Chapter 8). A DNA repair gene (e.g. *MSH2*, *MLH1*) is inactivated, resulting in failed mismatch repair and predisposition to multiple somatic mutations.

Viruses

Certain DNA viruses and retroviruses (Fig. 3.11) can cause neoplasia, as follows:

- DNA viruses insert DNA directly into the host genome.
- Retroviruses have reverse transcriptase enzyme to produce a DNA copy of viral RNA. The DNA copy is then inserted into the host genome.

Fig. 3.11 Examples of oncogenic human viruses

Type	Virus	Tumour type
Retroviruses	Human T cell leukaemia virus (HTLV)	T cell leukaemia
	Human immunodeficiency virus (HIV)	AIDS-related lymphomas
DNA viruses	Human papillomavirus	Skin papilloma (common wart)
		Cervical carcinoma
	Epstein–Barr virus	Carcinoma of the nasopharynx
		Burkitt's lymphoma
	Hepatitis B virus	Hepatocellular carcinoma

Fig. 3.11 Examples of oncogenic human viruses.

Mechanism of viral carcinogenesis

Inserted viral genes may be viral oncogenes themselves (*v-onc*), expression of which may lead to uncontrolled proliferation, or they may be activators or repressors of important cell-cycle regulating genes.

The mechanism of viral carcinogenesis is understood best in one of the most studied tumour viruses, the human papilloma virus. This double-stranded DNA virus has a tropism for squamous epithelium and subtypes 16 and 18 are implicated in cervical carcinoma. The viral genome incorporates into the host DNA and expresses the E6 oncoprotein, which inactivates the tumour suppressor protein p53. In addition expression of the E7 oncoprotein inactivates the tumour suppressor protein RB1. These oncoproteins, together with other factors, result in cervical intraepithelial neoplasia (CIN).

HOST DEFENCES AGAINST CANCER

Some tumours are known to stimulate both innate (passive) and adaptive (active) immunological reactions in the host.

Innate immunity

Activation of macrophages and natural killer cells can prevent growth of some tumours *in vitro*. Some tumours activate complement via the alternative pathway.

Adaptive immunity

Humoral

Antibodies may have a protective role, through complement activation or opsonisation of tumour cells for cell-mediated destruction. They are more likely to be effective against free cells (e.g. leukaemia or metastasising tumours) than those in solid lumps.

Cell-mediated immunity

Cell-mediated immunity is involved in recognition and monitoring of cells progressing towards malignancy. Therefore, cells that become significantly different to be recognised as 'foreign' may be eliminated by the immune system. This is particularly true of those tumours with a suspected viral aetiology.

The importance of immune surveillance in the prevention of cancer is clearly illustrated in immunocompromised patients. For example, lymphomas associated with Epstein–Barr virus can present 4–7 years post-immunosuppressive therapy following organ transplant.

Cytotoxic T cells are thought to play a role in tumour regression, particularly in virus-associated neoplasms. Infiltration of some tumours by lymphocytes and macrophages is associated with better prognosis.

Although many immune mechanisms are known to be active against tumour cells, most tumours are not distinguishable from normal host cells and so are not easily detected by the immune system. Additionally, tumour cells develop mechanisms to evade the immune system. These are thought to include reducing the expression of the surface major histocompatibility complex (MHC), antigen masking and actually suppressing the host immune system through cytokine release or apoptosis stimulation.

CLINICAL CANCER PATHOLOGY

Tumour markers are increasingly being used for prognostic and management decision processes. These are products derived from the tumour that can be found in the blood and used for diagnosis, assessing response to treatment and detecting recurrence. Examples include the CA125 ovarian tumour marker, the prostate-specific antigen (PSA) marker in prostate carcinoma and the α-fetoprotein in hepatocellular carcinoma and testicular teratoma.

Pathology reports of resected tumours contain macroscopic and microscopic descriptions that give information about the size and type of a cancer, local invasion and lymph node metastasis.

The grade of a tumour is based on morphological study (proliferation, differentiation, pleomorphism) and indicates tumour differentiation. Staging is used to determine how advanced a tumour is. For example, colorectal tumours can be staged by the Dukes classification (A–C/D). The TNM (tumour size, lymph node spread, metastasis formation) system is used to stage many tumours. For an example of the TNM system, see page 121 for the staging of lung cancer.

Infectious disease

Objectives

In this chapter, you will learn to:

- Define infection, colonisation, pathogen, commensals, pathogenicity and virulence.
- Understand the principles of Koch's postulates of disease.
- Outline the categories of infectious agents, their key features and main differences.
- Describe host defences against infection and how microorganisms attempt to evade them.
- Describe the mechanisms of viral and bacterial pathogenicity, and the immune responses of the host.
- Understand how bacterial antibiotic resistance develops and spreads.
- Understand the importance of hospital-acquired infection and the pathogens responsible.
- Describe the inflammatory responses to infection.

GENERAL PRINCIPLES OF INFECTION

Infection and colonisation

Infectious diseases are a common cause of morbidity and mortality. The prevalence of infectious diseases varies considerably between developed and developing nations. The burden of specific diseases depends on the quality of the drinking water, sanitation, healthcare system and the prevailing social and climatic conditions.

Infection is the invasion and proliferation of microorganisms in the tissues of the body. This usually follows the successful breach of host barriers and immune defence mechanisms.

Transmission of infectious agents can be:

- Human to human spread (horizontal and vertical transmission).
- Animal to human (zoonoses).
- Environment to human (airborne, water, fomites).
- Medical institution to patient (nosocomial).

Following invasion, infective organisms can spread to distant tissue sites by:

- Local spread.
- Lymphatic spread.
- Haematogenous spread.
- Dissemination in the tissue fluid.
- Neural spread.

Colonisation is the inhabitation of the external body surfaces—the skin, gastrointestinal (GI) tract, external genitalia and vagina—usually by harmless microorganisms. This generally occurs soon after birth.

Koch's postulates

To establish that a given disease has an infective cause, the postulates stated by the German bacteriologist Robert Koch (1843–1910) must be fulfilled. These are:

- The infectious agent should be found in all cases of the disease and in parts of the body affected by the disease.
- The infectious agent associated with the disease can be isolated from the lesions of an infected person and grown in artificial culture media.
- The cultivated infectious agent can reproduce the disease upon inoculation of a member of the same species.

Be aware that there are certain diseases to which one or more of these criteria cannot be applied but which can still be confidently attributed to a particular organism. For example, *Treponema pallidum*—the cause of syphilis—cannot be grown in culture. Furthermore, Koch's postulates cannot be applied to patients who are immunocompromised.

Pathogens and commensals

Pathogens are microorganisms that are normally absent from the body but which have mechanisms to invade and cause infection. Commensals are those microorganisms that constitute the normal flora of a healthy body. They do not normally cause disease and they are often advantageous to the host by the production of nutrients, such as vitamin B_{12}, and by the exclusion of harmful bacteria. For example, the normal commensal flora of the skin prevents colonisation by pathogenic bacteria.

The distinction between commensals and pathogens is not absolute. Many commensals are potential pathogens, i.e. they are harmless only so long as they are kept at bay by the host's defence mechanisms.

Other characteristics of microorganisms

Pathogenicity

Pathogenicity is the capacity of a particular microorganism to cause disease.

Virulence

Virulence is a measure of the pathogenicity of a microorganism, which can be said to be highly virulent if a small number of microbes can cause severe disease.

Opportunistic infection

Opportunistic infection is an infection by organisms of low pathogenicity, usually due to impaired immune responses. Opportunistic infections are common in immunocompromised patients, such as those with a primary or second immunodeficiency. Examples include:

- Children with severe combined immunodeficiency (SCID), a rare group of inherited syndromes (often X-linked) that require bone marrow

transplantation (or newer gene therapy methods) to prevent death in early infancy.
- Patients infected with human immunodeficiency virus (HIV), which results in the destruction of CD4+ T cells.
- Transplant patients using immunosuppressive drugs, such as ciclosporin A and tacrolimus, which are calcineurin inhibitors that block the proliferation of T cells.

Deficiency of specific immune defences predisposes individuals to characteristic patterns of infection. For example the T-cell-deficient disease, DiGeorge syndrome, results in chronic viral, fungal and intracellular bacterial infections. This syndrome occurs due to the lack of development of the thymus and parathyroid glands.

CATEGORIES OF INFECTIOUS AGENT

There are numerous different categories of infectious agent. The classification of the major pathogens is shown in Fig. 4.1.

Viruses

Viruses carry nucleic acids but lack synthetic machinery. They can therefore replicate only within the host cell, i.e. they are obligate intracellular parasites (Fig. 4.2).

Viruses have the following characteristics:

- They consist of a nucleic acid core and protein coat (capsid), which together constitute the nucleocapsid.
- Some, but not all, viruses are enveloped by a membrane of host-cell origin.
- Morphology is icosahedral, helical or complex.
- Classification is usually based on type of nucleic acid (Fig. 4.3).

Pathogenesis of cell injury

Viruses produce tissue injury by:

- Direct cytopathic effect—viral replication within cells leads to degenerative changes, including cell lysis, e.g. respiratory epithelial cells infected with influenza virus.

Fig. 4.1 Classification of major pathogens

	Viruses	Bacteria	Fungi	Protozoa	Helminths and ectoparasites
Size	20–300 nm	0.1–~5 μm	2–10 μm	2–100 μm	0.5–35 cm
Pro- or eukaryote	Neither	Prokaryote	Eukaryote	Eukaryote	Eukaryote
Nucleic acid	DNA or RNA	DNA + RNA	DNA + RNA	DNA + RNA	DNA + RNA
Replication	Intracellular	Intra- and/or extracellular	Intra- and/or extracellular	Intra- and/or extracellular	Extracellular
External cell wall	No	Yes (usually): peptidoglycan	Yes: rigid chitin	No	No
Reproduction	Assembly	Binary fission	Binary fission and sexually	Binary fission and sexually	Sexually

Fig. 4.1 Classification of major pathogens.

- Induction of an immune response—stimulated by viral proteins on the surface of host cells.
- Incorporation of viral genes into the host genome—often inducing cellular death by apoptosis, e.g. HIV.
- Cellular transformation—some viruses can cause cellular proliferation and transformation to produce cancers, e.g. Epstein–Barr virus, human papillomavirus (see Chapter 3).

Therefore, the harmful effects of viral infections include cell death, acute and chronic tissue damage, triggering of an autoimmune response and transformation of cells to form tumours.

Viral infections can be detected by a variety of methods:

- Direct detection of the virus by electron microscopy.
- Observed specific cellular cytopathic effects.
- Detection of viral proteins by immunofluorescence techniques.
- Detection of host-produced antiviral antibodies by enzyme-linked immunosorbent assay (ELISA).
- Detection of viral nucleic acid by polymerase chain reaction (PCR).

Bacteria

Bacteria are prokaryotes with a single circular DNA chromosome. Bacteria are divided into two broad groups—Gram positive and Gram negative—based on their reaction to the Gram stain (a staining procedure used with light microscopy).

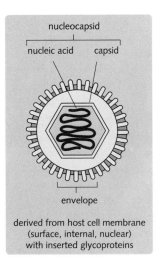

nucleocapsid

nucleic acid   capsid

envelope

derived from host cell membrane (surface, internal, nuclear) with inserted glycoproteins

Fig. 4.2 Structure of an enveloped virus.

Gram staining is a key microbiological test. Crystal violet and iodine are used to stain the bacterial cell wall. Gram-positive bacteria (lots of cell wall peptidoglycan) retain these components on challenge with acetone, and so stain purple. Gram-negative bacteria (little peptidoglycan) lose the iodine and crystal violet colouring with the addition of acetone, instead staining pink from the use of safranin counterstain.

Fig. 4.3 Classification of viruses based on nucleic acid type

Virus type	Mode of replication	Examples
DNA viruses	Utilise host cell polymerases for mRNA synthesis Can remain in infected cell and establish persistent infections (latent, immortalising viruses)	Herpes simplex virus Varicella-zoster virus Adenovirus Papillomavirus
RNA viruses	Encode their own replicative enzymes for formation of more mRNA (Host enzymes cannot replicate RNA)	Measles virus Mumps virus Influenza virus Rabies virus Poliovirus
Retroviruses (RNA)	Contain 'reverse transcriptase' enzyme for production of viral mRNA Viral DNA is inserted into host genome	HIV I and II HTLV I and II

Fig. 4.3 Classification of viruses based on nucleic acid type.

Not all bacteria stain using the Gram method, e.g. *Mycobacterium tuberculosis* requires a special staining technique known as Ziehl–Neelsen.

Further classification is based on practical characteristics, i.e. size, shape, respiration and reproduction. Biochemical and immunological measures can provide further information. For example, Gram-positive cocci can be distinguished by testing for the production of the catalase enzyme; *Staphylococcus* species produce catalase whereas *Streptococcus* species do not.

A generalised structure of a bacterium is shown in Fig. 4.4 and an example of the characteristics used to classify bacteria is shown in Fig. 4.5.

The pathogenic effects of bacteria are the result of the release of endotoxins and exotoxins. These produce acute and chronic inflammation and tissue damage.

Bacterial infections can be diagnosed from a number of different samples obtained from the patient. These include blood, faeces, urine, cerebral spinal fluid and swabs taken from infected wounds. Samples will generally be cultured to determine the species of bacteria and their sensitivity to different antibiotics.

Fungi

Fungi are unicellular, multicellular or multinucleate organisms (Fig. 4.6). They are eukaryotes and contain ergosterol instead of cholesterol in their plasma membranes.

Fungi have a well-defined cell wall composed of polysaccharides and chitin; they can be moulds, yeasts or dimorphic.

Fungal infections are either superficial (e.g. involving the skin, hair, nails and mucous membranes) or systemic (e.g. involving the lungs, brain or heart); the latter are usually found only in the immunocompromised. Such opportunistic fungi include *Aspergillus, Candida* and *Cryptococcus*.

Skin scrapings and tissue swabs are often used in the diagnosis of mycoses.

Some fungi produce toxins termed mycotoxins. For example, *Aspergillus flavus* proliferates on food stored in humid conditions and produces aflatoxins, which are highly carcinogenic mycotoxins. Ingestion of food contaminated with aflatoxins causes an increased risk of hepatocellular carcinoma in humans, particularly where there is underlying hepatitis B infection.

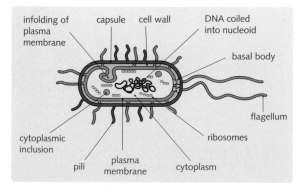

Fig. 4.4 Generalised structure of a bacterium.

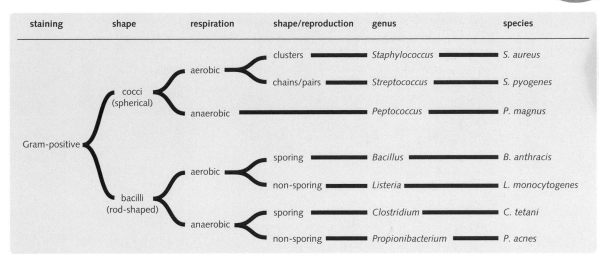

Fig. 4.5 The characteristics used to classify bacteria, using Gram-positive bacteria as an example.

Classification of fungi		
Yeast-like form	**Hyphal form**	**Dimorphic form**
single, rounded cells multiply by budding, e.g. *Candida albicans*, *Cryptococcus neoformans*	branching filaments interlaced to make mycelium or mould produce spores hyphae may be several hundred mm in length, e.g. *Aspergillus fumigatus*, dermatophytes	can assume either yeast or hyphal form depending on environment, e.g. *Histoplasma capsulatum*, *Blastomyces dermatitidis*

Fig. 4.6 Classification of fungi.

Protozoa

Protozoa are unicellular eukaryotes that may develop into cysts in harsh environmental conditions. The main divisions of protozoa are shown in Fig. 4.7. Protozoa species may be capable of replicating intracellularly or extracellularly. The most important protozoal disease worldwide is malaria, which is caused by the *Plasmodium* species.

Identification of protozoa often occurs by microscopy of patient specimens. Specimens include faeces, blood and tissue. Culture methods are not routinely applied for identification purposes.

Helminths and ectoparasites

Helminths are a group of parasitic worms, as shown in Fig. 4.8. Ectoparasites (e.g. bed bugs, crab louse,

Main divisions of protozoa			
Sporozoa	Flagellates	Amoebae	Ciliates
all are intracellular parasites, e.g. Plasmodium in red blood cells	move by beating one or more flagella, e.g. Trypanosoma	move by extending pseudopodia; they have no fixed shape, e.g. Entamoeba	move by beating many cilia, e.g. Balantidium

Fig. 4.7 Main divisions of protozoa.

Main groups of helminths (parasitic worms)		
Nematodes (roundworms)	Cestodes (tapeworms)	Trematodes (flukes)
resistant cuticle; longitudinal muscles; complete digestive system; separate sexed reproductive system, e.g. *Ascaris lumbricoides*, *Strongyloides stercoralis*	cellular epithelium; no digestive system; all hermaphrodites, e.g. *Taenia solium*, *Echinococcus granulosus*	cellular epithelium; circular and longitudinal muscles; incomplete digestive system; mostly hermaphrodites, e.g. *Schistosoma*

Fig. 4.8 Main groups of helminths (parasitic worms).

fleas, etc.) are parasites that live on the outer surfaces of the host.

Microscopy of patient specimens (faeces, blood, tissue) allows the identification of most helminths and ectoparasites.

Chlamydiae, rickettsiae and mycoplasmas

Chlamydiae and *Rickettsiae* are obligate intracellular organisms. *Chlamydia* replicates within vacuoles formed inside epithelial cells. *Chlamydia trachomatis* is an important cause of female infertility (scarring of fallopian tubes) and preventable blindness (corneal scarring and opacification).

Rickettsiae are transmitted by arthropod vectors (e.g. lice, ticks, mites) and replicate in the cytoplasm of epithelial cells to produce injury (usually a haemorrhagic vasculitis).

Mycoplasma lack cell walls and are the smallest free-living organisms known to man (typically 125–300 nm). They can be transmitted between people by aerosol to produce an atypical pneumonia.

Prions

Prions are an abnormal isoform of a normal host protein (the prion protein; PrP). Prions are not microorganisms but are infectious proteins that are highly resistant to decontamination methods, such as standard autoclaving or disinfectants. Humans express normal prion proteins but their function is unknown. However, inoculation of an abnormal prion protein into a normal host induces conformational changes in the normal host prions, resulting in their conversion to abnormal host prions. Disease occurs when the abnormal prion protein is resistant to protease breakdown where the original protein was protease sensitive.

These abnormal host proteins then induce further conformational changes in remaining normal host prions. Thus, the original inoculated prion protein is able to catalyse a chain reaction in which host proteins become conformationally abnormal. Interestingly, there is no evidence of inflammation, immune reaction or cytokine release in the infected host.

The net result is the formation of amyloid plaques of prion protein in the CNS. These plaques result in vacuolar spongiform degeneration of neuronal processes with neuronal loss and glial proliferation.

In humans, two forms of prion protein disease exist—kuru ('laughing death') and Creutzfeldt–Jakob disease, both of which are always fatal, usually within 6 months. The degenerative neurological disease Creutzfeldt–Jakob disease (new variant form) occurs in people under the age of 50. The consumption of offal contaminated with bovine spongiform encephalopathy (BSE) has been implicated in its aetiology.

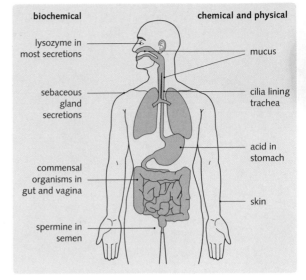

Fig. 4.9 Exterior host defences.

Infective agents include bacteria, viruses, fungi, parasites and prions. Remember, prions are not infective organisms.

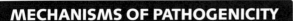

MECHANISMS OF PATHOGENICITY

Host defences and routes of entry

The majority of infectious agents encountered by an individual are prevented from entering the body by a variety of biochemical and physical barriers (Fig. 4.9). For example, anatomical barriers such as the skin, mucous membranes, GI tract and genitourinary tract provide a physical environment of unfavourable growth conditions for bacteria.

Further host defence is provided by the innate and adaptive immune mechanisms. Innate immunity consists of non-specific mechanisms that contribute to resistance and recovery from infection. Innate immunity includes soluble proteins (complement, acute-phase proteins), immune cells [macrophages, neutrophils, natural killer (NK) cells] and receptors (Toll-like receptors). Adaptive immunity is specific and includes cellular immunity (cytotoxic and helper T cells) and humoral immunity (B cells). Adaptive immunity is characterised by antigen specificity and clonal proliferation. In addition, the generation of immunological memory initiates a heightened response to subsequent antigen exposure.

However, despite these defences, pathogenic microorganisms possess efficient mechanisms for attaching to, and often penetrating, the body surfaces where they proliferate and disseminate. If they are to be transmitted to a fresh host, the microorganisms must also exit from the body.

The different routes of entry and exit of microorganisms are outlined in Fig. 4.10.

Virus infections

Viral replication cycles

Fig. 4.11 outlines two types of viral replication cycle.

1. DNA viruses have their own DNA and use the host's cellular machinery to make more DNA,

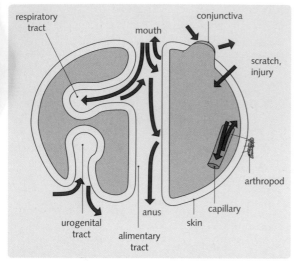

Fig. 4.10 Routes of entry and exit of microorganisms.

protein and glycoprotein. These are then reassembled into new virus particles prior to release from the cell.

2. RNA retroviruses first make viral DNA using the viral reverse transcriptase enzyme. Viral DNA is then inserted into the host genome prior to its transcription to form messenger RNA (mRNA). Viral RNA is in turn translated into viral protein, which is packaged together with the RNA into new virus particles and released.

Release of new virus particles

Cell lysis (cytolysis)

Non-enveloped viruses (e.g. adenoviruses) are released directly into the extracellular environment by lysis of the host cell; their mode of release results in the death of the cell.

Budding

Enveloped viruses (e.g. HIV and herpesvirus) are released by 'budding' from the host cell membrane:

- Nucleocapsid proteins are inserted into the host cell membrane.
- A modified area of host cell membrane extends out from the cell surface and is pinched off (i.e. budded) from the host cell enclosing the new viral particle.

This mechanism does not cause the death of the cell, and so viral replication can continue.

Immune reaction to virally infected cells

Cytotoxic T cells kill virally infected cells as follows:

- Virally infected cells express viral peptides bound to major histocompatibility complex (MHC) class I on their cell surfaces.
- Cytotoxic T cells (T_C) recognize viral antigen via the T-cell receptor.
- T_C cells secrete cytolysins, which results in the lysis of the virally infected cells.

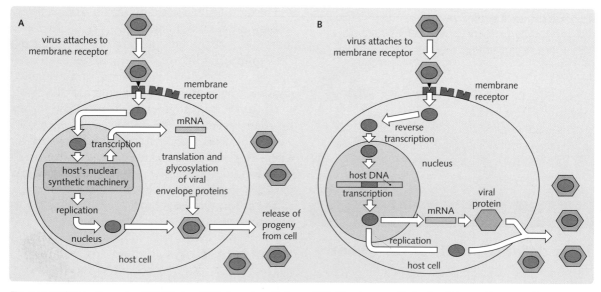

Fig. 4.11 Viral replication cycles. (A) DNA virus: DNA viruses have their own DNA. The viruses use the host's cellular machinery to make more DNA, protein and glycoprotein. These are then reassembled into new virus particles prior to release from the cell. (B) RNA retrovirus: RNA retroviruses first make viral DNA using viral 'reverse transcriptase'. Viral DNA is then inserted into the host genome prior to its transcription to form mRNA. Viral RNA is in turn translated into viral protein, which is packaged together with the RNA into new virus particles and released.

NK cells can do the same, but less effectively. The activity of these cells is enhanced by interferons produced by T_C and helper T cells (T_H). Interferons also prevent adjacent cells from becoming infected by intercellular viral transport.

It is worth noting that as well as spreading infection, immune responses can lead to tissue injury. For example, the liver damage following hepatitis B infection is largely mediated by the strong immune response of T_C cells towards infected hepatocytes.

Bacterial infections

Adherence

Certain bacteria are able to adhere specifically to epithelial cells by means of pili (also called fimbriae), which are slender filamentous processes on the surfaces of some bacteria. Pili are coated with recognition molecules called adhesins. Specific interactions between adhesins of pili and molecules on the surface epithelial cells enable the bacterium to adhere to the host cell membranes. Polymorphisms in host cell-surface glycoproteins may make an individual more susceptible to binding by certain types of bacterial adhesins.

Pili are more common in Gram-negative bacteria, although a few Gram-positive bacteria also possess them. Lipoteichoic acids (Gram-positive bacteria only) can function in a similar manner to pili by binding to fibronectin and epithelial cells.

Exotoxins and endotoxins

Toxins are responsible for many of the local and distant effects of bacterial infection.

Exotoxins

Exotoxins are proteins secreted by bacteria which are highly toxic to the host. The modes of action of some exotoxins are considered below:

- Enzymatic lysis—α-toxin (phospholipase C) of *Clostridium perfringens* breaks down host cell membranes.
- Pore forming—α-toxin of *Staphylococcus aureus* disrupts host cell membrane by pore formation.
- Inhibiting protein synthesis, e.g. diphtheria toxin.
- G protein hyperactivation, e.g. cholera toxin.
- Affecting synaptic transmission at neuromuscular junctions, e.g. tetanus and botulinum toxins.

Treating exotoxin with formaldehyde or high temperatures can denature the toxin to form toxoids, which can be useful for vaccination.

Endotoxins

Endotoxins are integral parts of bacterial cell walls, normally released only when the bacterium dies. They are typically lipopolysaccharides contained within the cell walls of Gram-negative bacteria. (But note that an exception is the 'superantigen' endotoxin TSST1, which is produced by the Gram-positive *Staphylococcus aureus* and causes toxic shock syndrome.)

These endotoxins are not in themselves toxic but can induce toxic effects by their potent activation of:

- The complement cascade, causing inflammatory damage.
- The coagulation cascade, potentially causing disseminated intravascular coagulation.
- Cytokines, notably tumour necrosis factor and interleukin-1 released from leucocytes, causing fever.

In overwhelming infections, the patient is said to suffer from endotoxic shock with fever, hypotension and cardiac and renal failure.

Aggressins

Aggressins are bacterially produced enzymes that act predominantly in the local tissue environment. They include enzymes such as coagulase, streptokinase and collagenases. Aggressins facilitate the growth and proliferation of the bacteria.

Avoiding death by phagocytosis

Successful microorganisms have evolved numerous ingenious antiphagocytic devices:

- Phagocyte killing, e.g. via exotoxin release.
- Prevention of opsonisation—the microbe produces protein that prevents interaction between opsonising antibody and phagocyte.
- Preventing phagocyte contact—some bacteria have an external capsule of polysaccharide, which gives a slimy surface and provides protection against phagocytosis, e.g. *Streptococcus pneumoniae*.
- Protection against intracellular death—this allows the microorganism to survive within the phagocyte by, for example, inhibition of phagosome and lysosome fusion (*Mycobacterium tuberculosis*) or escaping from the phagolysosome into cytoplasm (*Listeria monocytogenes*).

Antibiotic resistance and plasmids

Many bacteria are resistant to antibiotics. Resistance is conferred by genes that encode bacterial enzymes that block the effect of an antibiotic. These genes are not usually contained within the bacterial genome, but rather within extrachromosomal DNA termed 'plasmids'. These plasmids are capable of self-replication and can be transferred from bacterium to bacterium.

Antibiotic-susceptible bacteria (those lacking plasmids conferring antibiotic resistance) can acquire plasmids from resistant bacteria and so gain antibiotic resistance. These newly resistant forms are then differentially selected under antibiotic treatment, with the non-resistant bacteria being deleted from the population.

Mechanisms of antibiotic resistance include:

- Prevention of the drug entering the bacteria.
- Enzyme inactivation.
- Alteration of the antibiotic target site.
- Efflux resistance where the antibiotic is pumped out of the bacteria.

Resistance to antibiotics can be transferred between bacteria by any of the methods of bacterial genetic recombination i.e. conjugation, transduction and transformation.

Hospital-acquired infection

Hospital-acquired infection (nosocomial infection) occurs in up to 10% of uninfected admitted patients. It is thought to be the direct cause of 5000 deaths per year in the UK and it contributes to a further 15 000 deaths. Common pathogens include *Streptococcus pyogenes*, *Staphylococcus aureus*, *Escherichia coli* and *Pseudomonas aeruginosa*. Common sites of nosocomial infections include the:

- urinary tract
- surgical wounds
- lower respiratory tract
- skin
- blood (bacteraemia)—either by direct introduction such as through a venous catheter (primary), or by spread from another site such as a urinary tract infection (secondary).

Such infections can delay recovery, increase complication rates and ultimately result in the death of a patient. Of particular concern is the emergence of multi-drug-resistant infections that do not respond to traditional broad-spectrum antibiotics. Important examples include methicillin-resistant *Staphylococcus aureus* (MRSA) and vancomycin-resistant enterococci (VRE).

Although measures should be put in place to reduce levels of nosocomial infection, it is important to remember that many hospital patients are at inherently high risk of developing an infection in hospital regardless of these measures.

Important measures to reduce levels of hospital acquired infection include hand-washing (staff and visitors), minimising the length of preoperative hospital stays, careful use of prophylactic antibodies before certain procedures, isolating infected patients in side-rooms and using barrier nursing techniques.

INFLAMMATORY RESPONSES TO INFECTION

Suppurative polymorphonuclear inflammation

This is characterised by the production of pus, such as in a boil or abscess, which is usually caused by infection with pyogenic bacteria (e.g. *Staphylococcus aureus*, *Streptococcus pyogenes*).

Chronic inflammation and scarring

This is caused by persisting reactions of tissue to injury and it occurs over weeks, months, or even years. The cell-mediated immune response is characterised by lymphocytes, plasma cells and macrophages.

Examples include hepatitis B viral infection, which may lead to liver cirrhosis.

Granulomatous mononuclear inflammation

This is a form of chronic inflammation in which modified macrophages—epithelioid cells—aggregate to form small clusters or granulomas surrounded by lymphoid cells. It occurs in response to the presence of microorganisms within macrophages that are resistant to intracellular cell killing (e.g. *Mycobacterium tuberculosis*).

Necrotising inflammation

Gangrene

In gangrene, necrotic tissue is invaded by putrefactive organisms, notably clostridia. Tissue appears green or black because of the breakdown of haemoglobin.

SYSTEMIC PATHOLOGY

5.   Pathology of the nervous
     system   43

6.   Pathology of the cardiovascular
     system   63

7.   Pathology of the respiratory
     system   99

8.   Pathology of the gastrointestinal
     system   129

9.   Pathology of the kidney and
     urinary tract 181

10. Pathology of the endocrine system 205

11. Pathology of the reproductive
     system   229

12. Pathology of the musculoskeletal
     system   253

13. Pathology of the blood and
     immune systems 275

14. Pathology of the skin 315

Pathology of the nervous system

Objectives

In this chapter, you will learn to:
- Describe common pathological presentations in the CNS.
- Describe congenital malformations, developmental diseases and perinatal injury of the CNS.
- Recall traumatic injuries to the CNS and describe their effects.
- Understand cerebrovascular disease.
- Describe the infections of the CNS.
- Understand demyelinating and degenerative diseases of the CNS.
- Briefly describe the effect of metabolic disorders and toxins on the CNS.
- Recall the neoplasms that affect the central and peripheral nervous systems, briefly describing them.
- Give examples of peripheral neuropathies of hereditary, traumatic, inflammatory, infectious, metabolic and toxic origin.
- Describe disorders of the sympathetic and parasympathetic nervous system.

DISORDERS OF THE CENTRAL NERVOUS SYSTEM

Common pathological features

Intracranial herniation

Intracranial herniation is the movement of part of the brain from one space to another with resultant damage. It usually occurs following a critical increase in intracranial pressure caused by an expanding lesion, e.g. tumour or haematoma. However, it may be inadvertently precipitated by withdrawing cerebrospinal fluid (CSF) at lumbar puncture.

Figure 5.1 shows a diagrammatical representation of the sites of intracranial herniation.

Cerebral oedema

This is an abnormal accumulation of fluid in the cerebral parenchyma. It may be the result of breakdown of the blood–brain barrier (vasogenic oedema), parenchymal cell membrane injury (cytotoxic oedema) or a combination of the two. Possible causes include:

- Ischaemia, e.g. from infarction.
- Trauma, e.g. from head injury.
- Inflammation, e.g. encephalitis or meningitis.

- Cerebral tumours (primary or secondary).
- Metabolic disturbances, e.g. hyponatraemia or hypoglycaemia.

The condition is associated with raised intracranial pressure and may result in herniation.

Treatment involves minimising the formation of oedema by use of osmotic agents or steroids.

Hydrocephalus

Hydrocephalus is an increase in the volume of CSF within the brain resulting in the expansion of the cerebral ventricles and eventual increase in intracranial pressure. It can occur by one of three mechanisms:

1. Obstruction to flow of CSF (the most common form).
2. Impaired absorption of CSF at arachnoid villi (rare).
3. Overproduction of CSF by choroid plexus neoplasms (very rare).

Obstructive hydrocephalus

This can be congenital or acquired.

Congenital hydrocephalus occurs in 1 per 1000 births, usually due to conditions such as the Arnold–Chiari and Dandy–Walker malformations (see page 45).

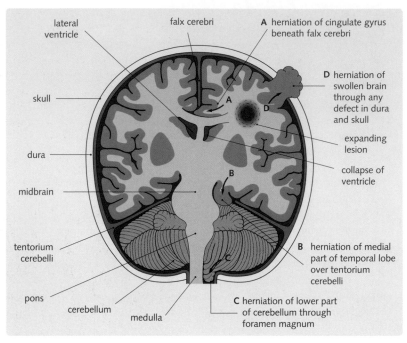

Fig. 5.1 Sites of intracranial herniation. (A) Subfalcine herniation. (B) Transtentorial herniation. (C) Tonsillar herniation. (D) Herniation of swollen brain through any defect in the dura and skull.

Acquired hydrocephalus can result from any lesion that obstructs the CSF pathway such as:

- Tumours—especially of the posterior fossa, as the fourth ventricle aqueducts are easily obstructed.
- Scarring—post-inflammatory fibrosis of the meninges at exit foramina, following meningitis or subarachnoid haemorrhage.
- Haemorrhage—intraventricular or in the posterior fossa.

Further classification of obstructive hydrocephalus is derived from the location of the obstruction:

- Non-communicating hydrocephalus—obstruction within the ventricular system leading to blockage of CSF flow from the ventricles to the subarachnoid space.
- Communicating hydrocephalus—obstruction outside the ventricular system within the subarachnoid space.

Secondary or compensatory hydrocephalus

In this special type of hydrocephalus, an increase in CSF occurs as a compensatory measure following loss of brain tissue, e.g. due to infarction or atrophy. There is no associated increase in CSF pressure.

Congenital hydrocephalus may be diagnosed antenatally via ultrasound (if severe) or present as a considerably enlarged head at birth. In acquired hydrocephalus, enlargement of the head is prevented by the inability of skull expansion (sutures are fused), resulting in increased intracranial pressure. Associated features include dementia, gait disturbances and incontinence. Treatment involves insertion of a ventricular shunt to drain CSF into the peritoneum, attempting to prevent irreversible brain damage.

Normal pressure hydrocephalus (intermittent pressure hydrocephalus)

This is a rare condition of progressive dementia associated with ventricular dilatation. Random sampling shows normal CSF pressure, but continuous monitoring reveals intermittent increases.

Malformations, developmental disease and perinatal injury

Neural tube defects and posterior fossa abnormalities

The aetiology of central nervous system (CNS) malformations includes genetic factors, maternal infections, toxicity, metabolic factors and irradiation *in utero*.

Neural tube defects are the most common congenital abnormalities of the CNS. They are caused by defective closure of the midline structures over the neural tube. The most common forms in the newborn affect the spinal cord (e.g. spina bifida). Screening for neural tube defects can be performed with ultrasound or by measurement of α-fetoprotein in the maternal serum or amniotic fluid. This is raised in 90% of cases.

Posterior fossa abnormalities are the second most common development abnormality of the CNS. Fig. 5.2 illustrates the types of congenital abnormalities.

Syringomyelia and hydromyelia

Syringomyelia is a rare condition in which a cyst (syrinx) develops within the spinal cord, usually posterior to the central canal (Fig. 5.3). The cavity is lined with astrocytes by the process of gliosis. It is most common in the cervical spinal cord, but it may extend into the medulla (syringobulbia).

Hydromyelia is the term used when the ependyma-lined central canal of the spinal cord (containing CSF) is dilatated.

These conditions are usually acquired due to trauma, ischaemia or associated spinal cord tumours. Rarely, they occur because of congenital abnormalities such as the Arnold–Chiari malformation.

Syringomyelia may produce muscle weakness and atrophy in the upper limbs due to compression of the anterior horn cells. There is loss of the sensations of pain and temperature, but preservation of those of position and vibration, due to damage of

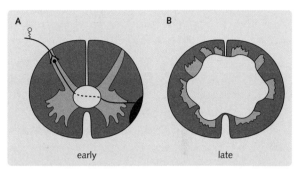

early   late

Fig. 5.3 Syringomyelia. (A) Early effects: damage to the decussating sensory fibres, with loss of temperature and touch in local segments. (B) Late effects: destruction of grey matter and gradual affection of long tracts with loss of local reflexes, severe sensory loss, and spastic paralysis.

Fig. 5.2 Types of congenital abnormality

Condition	Features
Neural tube defects with cranial involvement	
Anencephaly	Absence of the cranial vault and failure in the development of the cerebral hemispheres
Encephalocele	Ossification defects in the bones of the skull result in herniation of the brain and meninges. Most common form is occipital
Neural tube defects with spinal involvement	
Spina bifida occulta	Abnormal development of the vertebral arches but the cord and meninges are normal. Usually asymptomatic
Spina bifida cystica	Abnormal development of the vertebral arches results in cystic outpouching. Presents either with protrusion of CNS tissue through a vertebral column defect (meningomyelocele: 90% of cases) or protrusion of only the meninges (meningocele: 10% of cases)
Posterior fossa abnormalities	
Arnold–Chiari malformation	Prolongation of the cerebellum downwards through the foramen magnum often resulting in obstructive hydrocephalus
Dandy–Walker malformation	Obstruction of the foramina of Luschka and Magendie (exit of the fourth ventricle) results in the formation of a cyst-like structure between the cerebellar hemispheres

Fig. 5.2 Types of congenital abnormality.

nerve fibres crossing the cord in the lateral spinothalamic tracts.

Perinatal injury

This term refers to any brain injury sustained in the period shortly before and after birth. It is an important cause of childhood disability.

Cerebral palsy

Cerebral palsy describes brain malformation or damage affecting motor areas of the brain. It is the leading cause of handicap in children, affecting 2 per 1000 live births. The different presentations of cerebral palsy are outlined in Fig. 5.4.

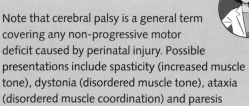

Note that cerebral palsy is a general term covering any non-progressive motor deficit caused by perinatal injury. Possible presentations include spasticity (increased muscle tone), dystonia (disordered muscle tone), ataxia (disordered muscle coordination) and paresis (incomplete paralysis).

Ischaemia and hypoxia

Ischaemia and hypoxia are major causes of severe perinatal brain damage. Perinatal hypoxia is usually due to asphyxiation associated with the trauma of birth, whereas perinatal ischaemia is commonly caused by intracranial haemorrhages.

Premature infants are highly susceptible to developing intracranial haemorrhages because of disturbances in the cerebral circulation, possibly caused by in-utero hypoxia/ischaemia. Mortality is high; one-third of survivors develop cerebral palsy, epilepsy or mental retardation.

In full-term infants, intracranial haemorrhages with the formation of small haematomas may occur during difficult deliveries, although this is less common with modern obstetric care.

Traumatic injuries to the central nervous system

The common types of CNS trauma are summarised in Fig. 5.5 and discussed in more detail below.

Skull fractures

Skull fractures occur in approximately 80% of fatal cases of head injuries. The most common are linear fractures of the vault of the skull; such fractures may extend into the base of the skull causing cranial nerve laceration.

The other types of skull fracture are:

- Penetrating—increased risk of infection due to tearing of the dura.
- Compound—increased risk of infection due to laceration of the scalp and tearing of the dura.
- Depressed—increased incidence of epilepsy.
- Comminuted (fragmented)—increased incidence of massive brain damage.

Parenchymal damage

Concussion

This is an abrupt transient loss of consciousness due to temporal neuronal dysfunction following a relatively slight impact. It is caused by an enormous, but short-lived, increase in pressure within the cranium at time of impact. Full recovery usually ensues, although amnesia for the event often persists.

Contusions and lacerations

A contusion is a bruise with extravasation of blood but with the pia–arachnoid intact. A laceration is

Fig. 5.4 Types of cerebral palsy and their associated characteristics

Type	Characteristics
Spastic cerebral palsy (70%)	Hypertonia, ankle clonus and extensor plantar response
Dystonic (athetoid) cerebral palsy (10%)	Irregular, involuntary muscle movements
Ataxic cerebral palsy (10%)	Hypotonia, weakness, uncoordinated movements and intention tremor
Mixed cerebral palsy (10%)	—

Fig. 5.4 Types of cerebral palsy and their associated characteristics.

Fig. 5.5 Examples of common central nervous system trauma

Level of injury	Pathology
Skull	Fracture
Parenchymal tissue	Concussion Contusions and lacerations Diffuse axonal injury
Vascular system	Extradural (epidural) haemorrhage Subdural haemorrhage Subarachnoid haemorrhage Intracerebral haemorrhage
Spinal cord	Open injuries Closed injuries

Fig. 5.5 Examples of common CNS trauma.

where the pia–arachnoid is torn. Both are focal types of brain damage occurring at the moment of injury, caused by striking the brain against adjacent bone. They are most common at the frontal and occipital poles and mainly affect the crests of gyri. Both lesions are characteristically haemorrhagic.

Types of contusion:

- Fracture contusion—occurs at the site of fracture.
- Coup contusion—occurs at point of impact in absence of fracture.
- Contrecoup contusion—occurs diametrically opposite to the site of impact.
- Herniation contusion—e.g. when the cerebellar tonsils are impacted and bruised by the foramen magnum.
- Gliding contusion—occurs at the superior margins of the cerebral hemispheres; usually caused by interference of the dura with a rotational movement of the brain.

Diffuse axonal injury

This condition is produced as a result of rotational movements of the brain within the skull during angular acceleration or deceleration. It often occurs in the absence of any skull fracture or cerebral contusions.

There are two main features:

1. Small haemorrhagic lesions in the corpus callosum and the dorsolateral quadrant of the brainstem (macroscopic).
2. Widespread tearing of axons, usually at the nodes of Ranvier (microscopic).

Diffuse axonal injuries occur in up to 50% of patients who develop coma shortly after trauma. It is associated with head injuries involving vehicular accidents.

Traumatic vascular injury

Bleeding from craniocerebral trauma is often associated with high mortality. It can occur in one or more of the potential spaces surrounding the brain, e.g. extradural and subdural.

Extradural (epidural) haemorrhage

This type occurs in 2% of all head injuries and in 15% of fatal cases. Haemorrhage occurs into the potential space between the skull and dura, gradually stripping dura from bone to form a large, saucer-shaped haematoma (Fig. 5.6).

This injury is almost always the result of skull fracture, usually of the temporal bone, with laceration of the middle meningeal artery that runs through it (a branch of the maxillary artery).

It is associated with a post-traumatic lucid interval of several hours followed by a rapid increase in intracranial pressure.

Subdural haemorrhage

Haemorrhage occurs into the potential space between the dura and the outer surface of the arachnoid membrane. It is usually caused by a rupture of the small bridging veins or the venous sinuses that exist within the subdural space. The resulting haematoma is often extensive because of the loose attachment of the dura and arachnoid membranes.

Subdural haemorrhage can occur following acute severe head injury or chronically, over days and weeks. Chronic subdural haemorrhage is more common in:

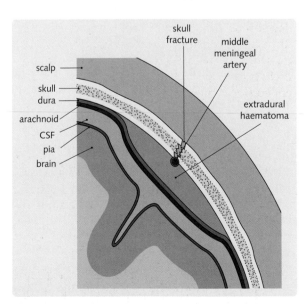

Fig. 5.6 Extradural haemorrhage. (Redrawn with permission from *Pathology* by A Stevens and J Lowe, Mosby.)

- The elderly—even with minimal trauma, due to brain atrophy and the subsequent stretching of bridging veins.
- Infants—because the bridging veins have thin walls.

Subdural haemorrhage may present with focal signs relating to compression of a particular brain area. Personality change, memory loss and confusion are commonly detected.

Subarachnoid haemorrhage

Arterial rupture into the subarachnoid space is usually secondary to superficial contusions or lacerations of the brain. Small amounts of blood can be disposed of by arachnoid granulations. Larger haemorrhages cause arachnoid fibrosis leading to meningeal irritation and raised intracranial pressure. It can also occur as a result of hypertension, aneurysms, embolisms, or infarction.

Intracerebral haemorrhage

This is caused by direct rupture of the intrinsic cerebral vessels at the time of injury.

Resulting haematomas are classified into three types:

1. Solitary—occur in association with cortical contusions; common in temporal and frontal poles.
2. Multiple—associated with severe contrecoup lesions; often fatal.
3. Burst lobe—intracerebral or intracerebellar haematoma in continuity with subdural haematoma; most common in temporal and frontal lobes; rapidly fatal.

Spinal cord injuries

Most spinal injuries occur in males aged under 40 years. Road traffic accidents account for more than 80% of such injuries.

There are two types of spinal cord injury: open and closed.

Open injuries

These are rare. They are a result of direct trauma to the spinal cord and nerve roots and can be either perforating (i.e. with extensive disruption and haemorrhage) or penetrating (i.e. with incomplete cord transection—Brown-Séquard syndrome).

Closed injuries

These are in the majority and are associated with fracture or dislocation of the spinal column causing compression of the cord by distortion of the spinal canal.

The consequences depend mainly on the site and severity of the lesion. Cervical lesions may result in tetraplegia; lower thoracic lesions may result in paraplegia.

Remember that with limited CNS repair mechanisms, the site of trauma is more important than the size of lesion. For example, a small lesion of the frontal lobe may be clinically silent, but would cause tetraplegia if located in the cervical spinal cord, and death if in the brainstem.

Cerebrovascular disease

Cerebrovascular disease is the third leading cause of death in the UK.

Stroke is a common outcome of cerebrovascular disease and it is defined as a sudden event in which neurological deficit develops over minutes or hours and lasts for longer than 24 hours.

If CNS disturbance lasts for less than 24 hours the condition is termed a transient ischaemic attack (TIA).

The incidence of stroke is 1 or 2 per 1000 per year, but is much higher than this in the elderly, affecting males more than females. Causes are:

- Cerebral infarction (80%).
- Intracerebral haemorrhage (10%).
- Subarachnoid haemorrhage (10%).

Pathological effects occur because of extensive hypoxic neuronal damage. The area of brain affected can be readily localised since the blood supply of the brain has a fairly constant anatomic distribution. Fig. 5.7 shows the territories of the major arteries.

Clinical features of stroke depend on localisation and the nature of the lesion. Risk factors are atherosclerosis, ischaemic heart disease, hypertension, and diabetes mellitus.

Hypoxia, ischaemia and infarction

Cerebral infarction is the process whereby a focal area of necrosis is produced in the brain in response to a decreased supply of oxygen (and glucose) in the territory of a cerebral arterial branch.

There are two main causes of infarction:

1. Hypoxia—the reduction of oxygen supply to tissues despite an adequate blood supply, e.g. following respiratory arrest.

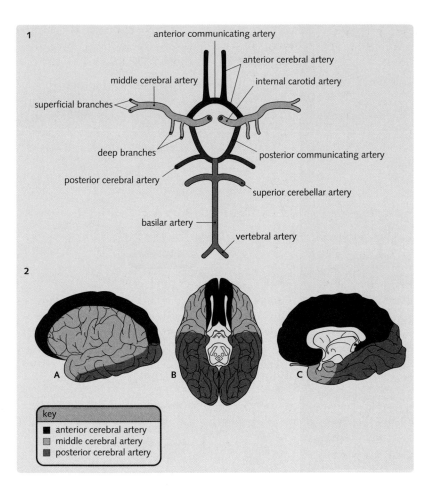

Fig. 5.7 Territories of the major arteries. (1) Main cerebral arteries forming circle of Willis. (2) Their territories: (A) Lateral view. (B) Inferior view. (C) Medial view. (Reproduced with permission from Anderson's Pathology, Damjanou, ed., Mosby.)

2. Ischaemia—blood supply to tissues is absent, or severely reduced, usually as a result of constriction or obstruction of a blood vessel.

Ischaemia accounts for the majority of cases of cerebral infarction.

Mechanisms of ischaemia
Ischaemia may be caused by:

- Vascular disease, e.g. thrombosis, embolic occlusion or vasculitis.
- Cardiac disease, e.g. prolonged hypotension (producing global cerebral ischaemia) or cardiac embolism.
- Trauma—head injury leading to vascular occlusion, dissection or rupture.

Infarcted tissue becomes swollen and soft with the loss of definition between grey and white matter. It undergoes liquefactive (colliquative) necrosis and shows microglial macrophage infiltration. Eventually, the necrotic tissue is completely phagocytosed to leave a fluid-filled cystic cavity with a gliotic wall. Figure 5.8 shows the macroscopic and microscopic pathological features of cerebral infarction.

Atraumatic haemorrhage
Intracerebral haemorrhage
The majority of intracerebral haemorrhages are thought to arise from Charcot–Bouchard microaneurysms associated with hypertension and diabetic vascular disease. These haemorrhages occur most frequently in the basal ganglia.

The resulting haematoma acts as a space-occupying lesion leading to increased intracranial pressure and herniation.

Subarachnoid haemorrhage
This can occur at any age, but it is an important cause of death and disability in the 20- to 40-year age group. The majority of subarachnoid haemorrhages are caused by saccular (berry) aneurysms, which develop at proximal branch points in the major cerebral vessels on the circle of Willis (Fig. 5.9).

Fig. 5.8 Pathological features of cerebral infarction

Time	Macroscopic	Microscopic
Before 24 hours	No naked eye abnormalities	Some neuronal damage
After 24 hours	Softening and swelling (oedema) of affected tissue	Line of demarcation between normal and abnormal myelin in white matter
After a few days	Necrotic tissue	Infiltrating macrophages Proliferating astrocytes and capillaries
After weeks/months	Fluid-filled cystic cavity with gliotic wall	Necrotic tissue removed Thickened capillary walls Only astrocytes remain

Fig. 5.8 Pathological features of cerebral infarction.

These aneurysms occur in 1–2% of the population, but they are more common in the elderly and those with hypertension.

Hypertensive cerebrovascular disease

Systemic hypertension can affect the CNS, resulting in neurological dysfunction:

- Atheroma of the larger cerebral vessels leads to a loss of autoregulation of cerebral blood flow. It may also allow small cavitary (lacunar) infarcts to develop, particularly in the lenticular nucleus and thalamus.

- Aneurysms—both saccular (berry) and microaneurysms—may cause spontaneous intracerebral haemorrhage.
- Encephalopathy—pathogenesis is uncertain but damage to the blood–brain barrier leads to forced cerebral hyperperfusion.

Chronic hypertension may lead to multiple infarct events, often producing a syndrome of dementia and neurological deficit (multi-infarct dementia).

Strokes caused by cerebral infarction clinically present with slowly evolving signs and symptoms depending on the area of the brain affected. Intracerebral haemorrhage commonly gives rise to sudden headache, vomiting, and impairment of consciousness. Mortality is about 80%. Subarachnoid haemorrhage presents with a sudden onset intensely severe headache accompanied by neck pain/stiffness and vomiting. Only 30–40% survive the first few hours and their prognosis remains poor.

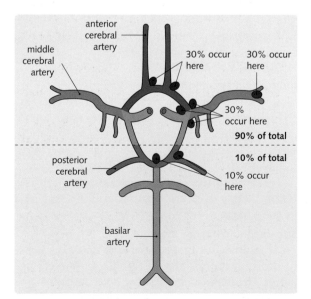

Fig. 5.9 Berry aneurysms: approximate frequency and distribution. The dotted line separates anterior from posterior circulation. (Redrawn with permission from Anderson's Pathology, Damjanou, ed., Mosby.)

Infections of the central nervous system

Meningitis refers to inflammation of the meninges; specifically, the leptomeninges and CSF within the subarachnoid space. Pachymeningitis refers to inflammation centred on the dura, whereas meningoencephalitis is inflammation of the meninges and brain parenchyma.

There are four possible mechanisms of meningeal infection:

1. Direct spread—from penetrating trauma (e.g. compound skull fractures) or adjacent focus of infection (e.g. sinusitis, middle ear or mastoid infection).
2. Blood-borne spread—from septicaemia or septic emboli from other infections such as bacterial endocarditis.
3. Iatrogenic infection—following the introduction of organisms into CSF at lumbar puncture.
4. Congenital abnormalities, e.g. meningomyeloceles.

Aseptic (viral) meningitis

This is the most common cause of meningitis, usually caused by viral infection. The term 'aseptic' is confusing, referring to an absence of recognisable (bacterial) organisms. It is a benign and self-limiting illness, usually less severe than bacterial meningitis.

Common causative organisms

The common causative organisms are enteroviruses (e.g. echoviruses, Coxsackie viruses, polioviruses) and mumps virus. It may occur as a complication of viral infection, e.g. mumps or measles.

Affected individuals present with headache, irritability, and rapid development of meningeal irritation.

The CSF is clear and colourless. It contains excess lymphocytes (lymphocytic pleocytosis) but normal glucose and protein. Complete recovery usually occurs without specific therapy.

Acute pyogenic (bacterial) meningitis

Organisms that typically cause this condition vary between age groups (Fig. 5.10).

The clinical features are headache, photophobia, drowsiness and neck stiffness. These indicators of meningeal irritation usually occur with systemic signs of infection (e.g. fever) and the development of a petechial rash.

In contrast to aseptic meningitis, the CSF is cloudy or frankly purulent due to increased numbers of neutrophils (> 1000 cells/mm^3), with increased protein levels and decreased glucose concentration.

Treatment is with vigorous intravenous antibiotic therapy.

Important complications include:

- Intracerebral abscess (see below).
- Cerebral infarction due to an obliterative endarteritis of local arteries.
- Hydrocephalus due to subarachnoid adhesions blocking CSF flow.
- Epilepsy.
- Disseminated intravascular coagulation (DIC).
- Adrenal haemorrhage (Waterhouse–Friderichsen syndrome).

Mortality varies by bacteria, but may be as high as 60% with *Streptococcus pneumoniae*, particularly affecting the very young and the elderly.

Brain abscess

A brain abscess is a severe focal infection of the brain and is typically 1–2 cm across. It starts as an area of cerebritis—inflammation of the brain parenchyma—and develops into a pus-filled cavity walled off by gliosis and surrounded by cerebral oedema. Multiple abscesses may develop, particularly with haematogenous spread of the causative organism. It often results in raised intracranial pressure.

The aetiology of brain abscesses is as follows:

- Middle ear infection (60%)—temporal lobe and cerebellar abscesses.
- Frontal sinusitis (20%)—frontal lobe abscesses.
- Bacteraemia/septicaemia (10%)—usually frontal lobe abscesses.
- Penetrating skull trauma.

Fig. 5.10 Typical meningitis-causing bacteria by age-group

Neonates	Infants	Young adults	Elderly
Escherichia coli Group B streptococci	*Neisseria meningitidis* *Streptococcus pneumoniae*	*Neisseria meningitidis* *Streptococcus pneumoniae*	*Streptococcus pneumoniae* *Neisseria meningitidis* *Listeria monocytogenes*

Fig. 5.10 Typical meningitis-causing bacteria by age-group.

- Secondary to meningitis.
- Unknown causes.

Common causative organisms are *Streptococcus vividans*, *Staphylococcus aureus* and *Klebsiella* species, but it can also be caused by fungal infection.

Treatment involves antibiotic therapy at an early stage, with surgical aspiration or excision of the capsule. Anticonvulsant medication may be required as epilepsy frequently develops.

Overall mortality is between 10 and 20%, often because of a delay in diagnosis.

Subdural empyema

This is a collection of pus in the subdural space and it is relatively uncommon. In adults, it usually results from frontal sinusitis, whereas in infants it is usually secondary to meningitis.

Clinically, patients with subdural empyema are usually very ill. The pus spreads rapidly on the surface of a hemisphere, producing hemiparesis, raised intracranial pressure, fits, and meningism.

Chronic meningoencephalitis

Tuberculous meningitis

This is meningitis due to infection by *Mycobacterium tuberculosis*. It is rare in the UK but a major problem in developing countries.

The disorder is almost always secondary to tuberculosis elsewhere in the body; infection usually reaches the CNS via the bloodstream.

Pathogenesis—granulomatous inflammation affects the basal meninges, large arteries and cranial nerves, covering the brain in a gelatinous, greenish exudate.

It presents clinically with slow-onset, subacute meningitis. It may be accompanied by isolated cranial nerve palsies.

Hydrocephalus may result from impaired reabsorption of CSF or obstruction of CSF outflow from arachnoid fibrosis.

CSF shows an initial increase in mononuclear cells and polymorphs, with a sharply elevated protein level. Untreated, the disease is usually fatal. Intensive treatment with antituberculous drugs lowers mortality to 15–20%.

Chronic meningitis

This is a rare condition, which usually occurs in the middle-aged and elderly. *Neisseria meningitidis* is the most common cause. The patient can be unwell for weeks or even months with recurrent fever, sweating, joint pains and transient rash.

Neurosyphilis

This is caused by invasion of the CNS by the microorganism *Treponema pallidum*. It can occur weeks, months or years after initial infection (tertiary-stage syphilis). Meningitic illness occurs in only approximately 10% of cases of untreated syphilis. It is usually mild or even asymptomatic, but it may be severe with transient cranial nerve palsies and convulsions.

Lyme disease

This disorder is caused by the tick-borne spirochete *Borrelia burgdorferi*. It is a systemic illness characterised by skin lesions and neurological features.

Viral encephalitis

This is a virally induced diffuse inflammation of the brain, which is usually concomitant with meningoencephalitis. It is a common complication of many viral illnesses. Common causative viruses are:

- Arboviruses.
- Herpes simplex virus I and II.
- Measles.
- Cytomegalovirus.
- Polio and enteroviruses.
- Rabies.
- Human immunodeficiency virus (HIV).

Most cases are mild and self-limiting. However, some cases (e.g. those involving herpes simplex virus type I and rabies) result in extensive tissue destruction and may be fatal.

Mortality for the more severe type is 50%, and the majority of survivors have severe, permanent brain damage.

Fungal infections

These are relatively rare and occur mainly in the immunosuppressed (e.g. associated with chemotherapy, steroid treatment, acquired immune deficiency syndrome; AIDS), but some organisms, e.g. *Cryptococcus neoformans*, can produce disease in the absence of immunosuppression.

The spread can be haematogenous (e.g. from the lungs, which is the most common) or direct (e.g. from the nose and paranasal sinuses, which is rare).

The most common causative organisms are *Cryptococcus neoformans* and *Candida albicans* (causes fungal abscesses).

Protozoal infection

Toxoplasmosis

This is caused by infection with *Toxoplasma gondii*. It may be acquired by eating poorly cooked infected meat or food contaminated with feline faeces. It has two forms: congenital and acquired.

In the congenital form, the organism is transmitted to the fetus through the placenta during maternal infection, potentially leading to:

- Abortion or stillbirth.
- Severe brain damage leading to early death.
- Moderate brain damage and chorioretinitis, compatible with life but with permanent disability.

Acquired toxoplasmosis is the most common opportunistic infection of the CNS in adults with AIDS. It results in:

- Necrotising cerebritis.
- Chronic abscesses.
- Meningoencephalitis.

However, in healthy subjects, it rarely causes cerebral symptoms.

Other protozoan organisms that may cause infection of the CNS are:

- Amoebae.
- *Plasmodium falciparum*.
- Trypanosomes.

Progressive multifocal leucoencephalopathy

Multifocal destruction of oligodendrocytes results in demyelination with minimal inflammation and damage to axons. It is caused by the DNA JC polyomavirus, and it occurs in association with underlying diseases such as AIDS, chronic lymphocytic leucaemia, carcinoma and systemic lupus erythematosus (SLE).

Patients present with progressive dementia. The disease is progressive and death usually occurs within a few months.

Subacute sclerosing panencephalopathy

This subacute encephalitis occurring in children is due to persistent measles infection. It presents with progressive neurological dementia, and death usually occurs within two years of onset. It is now rare due to immunization with the MMR vaccine.

Spongiform encephalitis (Creutzfeldt–Jakob disease)

This presents as rapidly progressive dementia, ataxia and myoclonus; it is rare in the UK (1 per million people per year). Spongiform changes include the formation of intracellular vacuoles in neurons and glia. The infectious agent is a prion protein (PrP; see page 35). The condition has an incubation period of up to 30 years but it is always fatal, usually within 6 months. The disease typically affects people over 70 years old.

Variant Creutzfeldt–Jakob disease (vCJD) is a human disease associated with bovine spongiform encephalopathy that shows the potential for prion transmission between species. Descriptions of the disease are relatively recent but it appears to affect younger individuals than does classic CJD. Neurological decline seems to be slower but fatal progression is—so far—universal. A genetic predisposition may increase susceptibility to vCJD from eating infected beef. Recent estimates have suggested that the disease might be limited to hundreds or thousands of cases.

Demyelinating diseases

This group of diseases has a common factor of primary damage to myelin of nerves while the axons and nerve cells remain relatively intact.

Multiple sclerosis

Multiple sclerosis (MS) is the most common demyelinating disorder of the CNS, affecting 50 per 100 000 in the UK. Peak incidence is between 20 and 40 years, with a slight female predominance.

MS is characterised by relapsing and remitting episodes of immunologically mediated demyelination within the CNS. Recovery from each episode of demyelination is usually incomplete, leading to progressive deterioration. There is an association between the disease and certain human leucocyte antigens (HLA, e.g. A3, B7, DR2 and DQ1). The incidence also increases with distance from the equator, suggesting a possible environmental trigger.

Pathogenesis—activated T lymphocytes cross the blood–brain barrier, reacting to self-antigens against myelin that are presented by microglia. A strong inflammatory reaction follows, enhanced by the release of proinflammatory cytokines. Acute demyelination occurs in the central white matter in discrete areas known as plaques.

Abnormalities are confined to the CNS; the peripheral nervous system (PNS) is usually spared. Common sites are the optic nerve, brainstem, cerebellum, periventricular regions and cervical spinal cord.

Figure 5.11 lists the clinical manifestations of MS and their causes.

> MS diagnosis involves identification of abnormal CNS areas (e.g. by MRI scanning) in the absence of another explanation. The CSF may show increased lymphoid cells and oligoclonal bands of IgG. There is no specific treatment but high-dose intravenous corticosteroids may accelerate remission in relapse. Beta-interferon has also been used to some success. Most follow a relapsing-remitting course with variable disability, but a minority (5%) suffer rapidly progressive (fulminant) disease, which is fatal within 5 years.

Degenerative disorders

These diseases primarily affect the grey matter, with progressive neuronal loss. A common feature of this group is the development of protein aggregates (cellular inclusions) that are resistant to degradation.

Cortical

Alzheimer's disease

This is the most common cause of dementia in Western countries.

Dementia is defined as the progressive loss of cognitive function, independent of the state of attention, and occurs due to degeneration of the cerebral cortex. Alzheimer's disease affects 5% of people over 65 years, and 15% of people over 80 years in the UK; females more than males. Also of significance is the subgroup of early-onset patients (40–60 years).

Genetic studies have shown that there is an increase in incidence of sporadic cases in individuals with ApoEe4 genotype on chromosome 19. The amyloid precursor protein (*APP*) gene on chromosome 21 has been implicated in the familial cases.

The aetiology and pathogenesis are unknown; some cases (5%) are familial but most (95%) are sporadic.

Macroscopically, there is marked cortical atrophy, especially of the frontal lobes; the brain is reduced in weight to 1000 g or less (normal average 1400 g). There is a loss of cortical grey and white matter.

Histological hallmarks are as follows:

- Senile (neuritic) plaques—composed of an extracellular core of amyloid protein (10–150 nm diameter) surrounded by dystrophic neurites; occur most frequently in the hippocampus, cerebral cortex and deep grey matter. The main component of the core is Aβ, a readily aggregating peptide that is thought to be central in the pathogenesis of dementia.
- Neurofibrillary tangles—abnormal tangles of insoluble cytoskeletal-like proteins (paired helical filaments) that form within the cytoplasm of neurons.
- Neuropil threads—distorted, twisted and dilated dendritic processes and axons of cerebral cortex found around amyloid plaques.

Clinically, there is failure of memory and disturbance of emotions. There tends to be progressive physical decline

Fig. 5.11 Clinical manifestations of MS and their causes

Manifestations	Causes
Early clinical symptoms	
Blurring of vision	Optic nerve disease
Incoordination	Cerebellar peduncle disease
Abnormal sensation	Disease of long ascending sensory tracts
Late stages	
Blindness, paraplegia and incontinence	Spinal tract involvement
Ataxia	Spinal and cerebellar involvement
Intellectual dysfunction	Loss of hemispheric white matter

Fig. 5.11 Clinical manifestations of multiple sclerosis (MS) and their causes.

with poor food intake and inability to walk. Death is commonly due to the development of pneumonia.

Basal ganglia

Parkinsonism

This term is used to refer to patients whose clinical presentation typically consists of:

- Akinetic rigidity.
- Stooped posture with slow voluntary movements.
- Diminished facial expression.
- Festinating gait (progressively shortened, accelerated steps).
- Resting ('pill-rolling') tremor.

The causes include:

- Parkinson's disease.
- Postencephalitic parkinsonism (very rare).
- Neuroleptic drugs.
- Cerebral anoxia.

Parkinson's disease

This is characterised by rest tremor, slowness of voluntary movement, and rigidity. It occurs in 1 per 1000 adults but 1 per 200 over the age of 65. The aetiology is unknown.

Pathogenesis:

- The disorder shows degeneration of pigmented dopaminergic neurons of the substantia nigra, the locus caeruleus and several other brainstem nuclei.
- Degeneration of these cells causes disease by reducing the amount of dopamine in the corpus striatum.
- Surviving cells in the substantia nigra contain eosinophilic spherical inclusions (Lewy bodies), which contain cytoskeletal filaments.

The disease can be symptomatically treated with drugs, such as L-dopa, that correct neurotransmitter imbalance. Eventually, there is failure of response to treatment and patients die from wasting and poor nutritional intake. Several genes have been implicated in the development of Parkinson's disease, including those encoding the proteins α-synuclein and parkin.

Motor neurons

Motor neuron disease (amyotrophic lateral sclerosis)

This progressive, neurodegenerative disease is characterised by the selective loss of both upper and lower motor neurons from the spinal cord, brainstem and motor cortex. Its prevalence is 5 per 100 000 of the population, with male incidence greater than female.

The majority of cases are sporadic but 5% of cases are familial—due to mutation of the superoxide dismutase gene.

It eventually progresses to severe paralysis with loss of swallowing and respiration, leading to death in 2–3 years.

Other degenerative disorders are considered in Fig. 5.12.

Metabolic disorders and toxins

Vitamin deficiencies

Vitamin B$_1$ (thiamine) deficiency

This is common in chronic alcoholics, resulting in:

- Wernicke's encephalopathy—memory impairment, ataxia, visual disturbances and peripheral neuropathy.

Fig. 5.12 Additional types of degenerative disease

Degenerative disorder	Features
Pick's disease	Progressive dementia with severe memory and speech loss. Atrophy of cortex in areas of the frontal and temporal lobes. Surviving neurons contain Pick's bodies
Huntington's disease	Autosomal dominant disorder (trinucleotide repeat, chromosome 4) characterised by chorea and progressive dementia. Cerebral atrophy in the caudate nucleus and putamen
Friedreich's ataxia	Autosomal recessive spinocerebellar disease Degeneration of the posterior columns, corticospinal and spinocerebellar tracts

Fig. 5.12 Additional types of degenerative disease.

- Korsakoff's psychosis—confused state, memory loss and confabulation.

If both occur, it is known as Wernicke–Korsakoff syndrome.

Vitamin B$_{12}$ (cyanocobalamin) deficiency

This produces weakness and paraesthesia in the lower limbs resulting from subacute combined degeneration of the spinal cord (Fig. 5.13). Replacement therapy at an early stage reverses the degenerative process, but long-standing cases show irreversible axonal damage with reactive gliosis.

Iodine deficiency

Severe iodine deficiency causes hypothyroidism; it is the most important endocrine disorder to affect the CNS in children. In the fetus, severe iodine deficiency causes cretinism characterised by dwarfism, mental defect, and spastic diplegia. This can be prevented by iodine supplements during pregnancy.

Toxins

Carbon monoxide

Carbon monoxide (CO) binds irreversibly to haemoglobin, rendering erythrocytes incapable of oxygen transport. CO poisoning therefore results in brain damage due to hypoxia. This poisoning may be accidental or associated with attempted suicide.

The amounts of carbon-monoxide-bound haemoglobin (HbCO) with corresponding clinical symptoms are as follows:

- > 20%—dyspnoea and slight headache.
- 30%—severe headache, fatigue and impaired judgement.
- 60–70%—loss of consciousness.
- > 70%—rapidly fatal.

Pathogenesis—hypoxia results in neuronal necrosis with a predilection for globus pallidus. Other selectively vulnerable regions are the hippocampus and the cerebral and cerebellar cortices.

Methanol

Methanol is highly toxic to the CNS, particularly to the retina. It is lipid soluble, so readily diffuses into the CSF and aqueous humour in concentrations higher than in plasma.

Methanol is metabolised into formic acid and formaldehyde. It is the formaldehyde that is thought to be the mediator of toxic effects. There are two types of methanol poisoning:

1. Acute—sudden death with multiple haemorrhagic lesions in the cerebral hemispheres.
2. Chronic—atrophy of retinal ganglion cells with secondary degeneration of the optic nerve.

Ethanol

The consequences of excessive ethanol intake on the CNS are manifold (Fig. 5.14).

Neoplasms of the CNS

Gliomas

Gliomas are tumours that arise from glial supportive tissue of brain. They are the most common primary brain tumours, accounting for 50% of all CNS tumours.

Note that glial cells are the support cells of the CNS. The group includes astrocytes (throughout the CNS), oligodendrocytes (form myelin sheaths), ependymal cells (line the ventricular system) and microglia (act as CNS macrophages).

Astrocytoma

This is a glioma derived from astrocytes. It is more common in children, usually occurring in the cerebellum. It accounts for 10% of all primary tumours in adults, usually in the cerebral hemispheres.

Common types of astrocytomas and their corresponding tumour grading:

- Pilocytic astrocytoma (grade I)—relatively benign, often affecting children.
- Well-differentiated fibrillary astrocytoma (grade II)—small increase in glial cell nuclei.

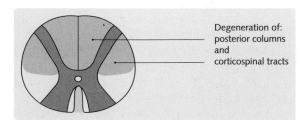

Degeneration of:
posterior columns
and
corticospinal tracts

Fig. 5.13 Subacute combined degeneration of the spinal cord. Degeneration of posterior columns leads to sensory loss (vibration and proprioception) causing ataxia. Degeneration of corticospinal tracts leads to upper motor neuron damage causing spastic paralysis.

Fig. 5.14 Consequences of excess ethanol intake on the central nervous system

Disease	Features	Mechanism
Fetal alcohol syndrome	Cerebral malformations Facial and somatic malformations Growth retardation	Direct toxicity
Acute intoxication	Cerebral oedema Petechial haemorrhages	Direct toxicity
Cerebral and cerebellar atrophy	Neuronal loss	Direct toxicity
Nutritional disorders	Wernicke's encephalopathy Korsakoff's syndrome	Deficiency of vitamin B_1
Hepatocerebral syndromes	Hepatic encephalopathy Chronic hepatocerebral degeneration	Hepatic toxicity with secondary effects on CNS
Demyelinating disorders	Central pontine myelinolysis	Electrolyte disturbances

Fig. 5.14 Consequences of excess ethanol intake on the CNS. (Adapted from Underwood, 2000.)

- Anaplastic astrocytoma (grade III)—densely cellular with nuclear pleomorphism.
- Glioblastoma (grade IV)—relatively poorly differentiated, often occurring with necrosis.

Prognosis depends on the degree of tumour differentiation and the size of the neoplasm. For example:

- Grade I—survival times of 20–30 years are possible.
- Grade IV—20% survive for 1 year.

Oligodendrogliomas

These ill-defined, slow-growing tumours arise from oligodendrocytes in the white matter of the cerebral hemispheres, especially the temporal lobe. They account for 5% of all primary CNS neoplasms in adults, but they are rare in children.

The prognosis is relatively good.

Ependymoma

These tumours arise from the ependymal cells lining the ventricle and central canal of the spinal cord. Ependymoma is the most common tumour of the spinal cord, accounting for 5% of all primary CNS neoplasms. It is common in children and young adults.

Medulloblastoma

This tumour of primitive neuroepithelial cells arises in the cerebellum of children, in whom it is the most common CNS tumour. It is malignant, with a rapid growth rate; obstruction of the fourth ventricle results in hydrocephalus. The tumour is highly radiosensitive, but without treatment it is rapidly fatal.

Other tumours

Primary brain lymphomas

Associated with immunosuppression, especially AIDS, most primary brain lymphomas are high-grade, non-Hodgkin's lymphomas of B-cell type with a poor prognosis.

Germ cell tumours

These rare tumours are seen mainly in children; males more than females. Most arise along the midline, near the pineal gland.

Meningiomas

These account for approximately 15% of adult intracranial tumours; females more than males. Tumours arise from the arachnoid mater. They are usually benign but may invade adjacent bone, resulting in erosion and hyperosteosis. Meningiomas produce symptoms by compression of brain tissue rather than by invasion.

Metastatic tumours

The CNS is a common site for metastasis and tumours are usually multiple. They may arise from hematogenous or direct spread. The cerebellum is the preferred site but they can affect any part of the brain as well as other intracranial structures, especially meninges (hence malignant meningitis). Metastases often occur at the boundary between grey and white matter, surrounded by oedema.

The most common neoplasms to metastasise to the CNS are:

- Breast carcinomas.
- Bronchus carcinomas.

- Kidney carcinomas.
- Colon carcinomas.
- Malignant melanoma.

DISORDERS OF THE PERIPHERAL NERVOUS SYSTEM

Disorders of peripheral nerves are termed neuropathies. They can be predominantly sensory, predominantly motor or mixed, depending on which nerves are affected.

Note that:
- Disorders affecting many peripheral nerves are termed polyneuropathies, and they usually cause symmetrical deficits.
- Disorders affecting only one (mononeuropathy) or a few (multiple mononeuropathies) peripheral nerves typically cause asymmetrical deficits.
- Radiculopathies are disorders of nerve roots.

Hereditary neuropathies

Hereditary motor and sensory neuropathies (HMSN)

Peroneal muscular atrophy (HMSN I+II; Charcot–Marie–Tooth disease)

This disorder is characterised by pronounced atrophy of the calf muscles with associated sensory deficits as a result of slowly progressive symmetric neuropathy. It is the commonest of the hereditary neuropathies,

and it is usually autosomal dominant. It impedes ambulation and causes foot deformities (pes cavus), but it does not shorten the lifespan.

Fig. 5.15 provides a table of the different types of peroneal muscular atrophy and their characteristics.

Hereditary sensory and autonomic neuropathies (HSAN)

This group of autosomal inherited diseases produces mainly sensory and autonomic neuropathies. There are three major types, as described in Fig. 5.16.

Traumatic neuropathies

Laceration

Refers to a jagged tear of the peripheral nerve in which there is partial or complete loss of continuity of the nerve. It occurs most commonly from cutting injuries, misplaced intramuscular injections or fragments of fractured bone.

Avulsion

This is the tearing of nerve fibres from the surface of the spinal cord or from a muscle. It may be partial or complete depending on whether all or only some of the nerve rootlets are involved.

Nerve roots may be avulsed from the spinal cord in two ways:

1. Tensile stresses from cervical plexus transmitted centrally can stretch and finally avulse the nerve roots.
2. A spinal cord injury, such that displacement of the cord acts directly on the nerve roots between their attachment to the cord and their entry into the intravertebral foramen.

Fig. 5.15 Different types of peroneal muscular atrophy and their characteristics

	HMSN I	HMSN II
Type of neuropathy	Demyelinating neuropathy	Axonal neuropathy
Relative occurrence	75%	25%
Type of axonal loss	Large calibre axons	Large and small calibre axons
Nerve conduction velocity	Impaired (< 30 m/s)	Normal (> 45 m/s)
Time of onset	Early (first decade)	Later (second decade)
Effects	Severe distal wasting in legs	Weakness and wasting less marked

HMSN, hereditary motor and sensory neuropathy.

Fig. 5.15 Different types of peroneal muscular atrophy and their characteristics.

Fig. 5.16 Types of hereditary sensory and autonomic neuropathies

	HSAN I	HSAN II	HSAN III
Clinical syndrome	Ulcerative acropathy due to numbness	Congenital sensory neuropathy	Familial dysautonomia
Eponym	Morvan's	Ciacci's	Riley-Day
Inheritance	Autosomal dominant	Autosomal recessive	Autosomal recessive
Affected neurons	Degeneration of large myelinated fibres of both peripheral nerves and posterior columns of spinal cord	Degeneration of large and small myelinated fibres	Degeneration of non-myelinated fibres with preservation of myelinated fibres. Loss of neurons of autonomic ganglia

HSAN, hereditary sensory and autonomic neuropathies

Fig. 5.16 Types of hereditary sensory and autonomic neuropathy.

Both laceration and avulsion injuries cause the severed ends of the damaged nerve to retract and then to undergo Wallerian degeneration to form a traumatic neuroma (a type of benign tumour). Subsequently, the proximal portion of the nerve develops neuritic sprouts which, if sited in proximity to the severed distal nerve, may reinnervate by slow regrowth along the nerve sheath.

If continuity of the nerve is completely interrupted, basal laminae sheaths no longer form continuous tubes to guide regeneration sprouts and so the potential for recovery is limited.

Compression/entrapment neuropathy

Compressed nerves undergo segmental demyelination with decreased nerve conduction velocity. If compression is prolonged or severe, axonal degeneration may occur. Symptoms of nerve compression are paraesthesia, anaesthesia and loss of muscle strength.

Common sites of nerve compression are:
- Nerve roots in the intervertebral foramina by prolapsed intervertebral discs or osteophytes due to osteoarthritis of the spine.
- Median nerve in the carpal tunnel at the wrist.
- Ulnar nerve in flexor carpal tunnel at the medial epicondyle of humerus.
- Common peroneal nerve at the neck of the fibula.

Carpal tunnel syndrome

This is a disorder in which the size of the carpal tunnel is significantly reduced, causing compression of the median nerve. Causes include inflammation of the flexor retinaculum and arthritic changes.

Saturday night palsy

Radial nerve compression (in the middle of the arm), which may result from improper positioning of the upper limb during sleeping, especially in intoxicated persons.

Inflammatory neuropathies

Guillain–Barré syndrome (acute inflammatory demyelinating polyradiculopathy)

This is the most common form of acute neuropathy caused by immune-mediated demyelination of peripheral nerves, usually occurring 2–4 weeks after viral illnesses such as Epstein–Barr infection. The pathogenesis is unclear, but it appears that virus infection triggers a T-cell-mediated autoimmune-like response against peripheral nerves.

Affected patients develop motor neuropathy that rises from the peripheral limbs ('ascending paralysis'), with lesser sensory changes due to widespread demyelination of the peripheral nerves. Recovery (i.e. remyelination) occurs over 3–4 months and is usually complete.

Infectious neuropathies

Leprosy (Hansen's disease)

A chronic granulomatous disease caused by *Mycobacterium leprae*. It is the most common cause of peripheral neuritis worldwide, affecting about 10 million patients in total.

The clinicopathological features of leprosy are dependent on the host's response to infection, with a spectrum of disease ranging from tuberculoid to lepromatous form (Fig. 5.17).

Varicella-zoster virus

An invasion of cutaneous sensory nerves during primary infection with varicella-zoster virus (VZV, the virus that causes chickenpox) leads to infection of the dorsal root ganglia where the virus enters a latent state. Reactivation of VZV may occur years later causing shingles—painful, vesicular skin eruptions in the distribution of sensory dermatomes, usually thoracic or trigeminal. The reason for reactivation is unknown but there is increased incidence in immunocompromised individuals.

Metabolic and toxic neuropathies

Peripheral neuropathy of diabetes mellitus

This occurs in both type I and II diabetes mellitus with a prevalence of 10–60% clinically but up to 100% when evaluated by nerve conduction studies. There is increased prevalence with increased duration of the disease.

Pathogenesis

Vascular occlusion of the blood vessels supplying the nerves results in neuronal atrophy.

There are four types:

1. Symmetrical and predominantly sensory polyneuropathy.
2. Autonomic neuropathy.
3. Proximal painful motor neuropathy.
4. Cranial mononeuritis (mainly CN III, IV and VI).

Metabolic and nutritional causes

Uraemic neuropathy in renal failure

Approximately 60% of patients with chronic renal failure have symptoms of uraemic neuropathy at onset of dialysis. It is typically distal and symmetrical, producing pain and paraesthesia with the lower extremities preferentially involved. Dialysis usually improves symptoms.

Thyroid dysfunction

Mild chronic sensorimotor neuropathy is sometimes seen in both hypothyroidism (more commonly) and hyperthyroidism.

Vitamin deficiencies

Vitamin deficiencies are important causes of peripheral neuropathies. Especially important are deficiencies of vitamins B_1 (thiamine), B_{12}, B_6 (pyridoxine) and E.

Toxic neuropathies

Many toxins cause damage to peripheral nerves. The most common toxins are:

- Drugs—e.g. isoniazides, sulphonamides, vinca alkaloids, dapsone and chloroquine.
- Alcohol—in cases of chronic abuse.

Fig. 5.17 Comparison of peripheral nerve damage by lepromatous and tuberculoid forms of leprosy

	Lepromatous	Tuberculoid
Immune mechanism	Minimal immune response (occurs in patients with low cellular immunity)	Vigorous T-cell mediated (delayed) hypersensitivity
Spread of organisms	Bacteraemia occurs in peripheral sites	Bacteraemia rare
Distribution in nerves	Widely disseminated diffuse nerve involvement	One or a few sites (asymmetrical)
Nerve enlargement and damage	Intense infiltration of nerves by vacuolated macrophages	Hallmark of nerve involvement is discrete, well-formed granulomas
Neurological deficit	Sensory and motor involvement Patchy loss of sensation	Sensory, motor and autonomic involvement Peripheral nerve palsies Anaesthetic areas prone to injury and secondary infection
Prognosis	Progressive and lethal	Progression slow, but immune response produces extensive destruction of tissue resulting in severe disfigurement Eventually heals spontaneously

Fig. 5.17 Comparison of peripheral nerve damage by lepromatous and tuberculoid forms of leprosy.

- Industrial toxins—e.g. acrylamide, hexane, organophosphates, lead, arsenic, mercury.

Most toxins produce a 'dying back' pattern of axonal damage resulting in a distal symmetric pattern of sensorimotor involvement. There is a `stocking glove' distribution at onset but continued exposure to the toxin extends the deficit to the lower calves and forearms.

Neuropathies associated with malignancy (metastatic neuropathy)

Cancer patients frequently have mononeuropathies caused by direct infiltration of individual nerves or plexuses, e.g. brachial plexopathy due to apical lung cancer.

Neoplasms of peripheral nerves

Peripheral nervous system tumours are illustrated in Fig. 5.18.

- Partial ptosis (drooping) of the upper eyelid due to paralysis of smooth muscle fibres contained in the levator muscle of the upper eyelid.
- Enophthalmos (eye sunken into socket).
- Anhidrosis (loss of sweating) on affected side of the face.

Lesions affecting any part of the sympathetic pathway (Fig. 5.19) may produce Horner's syndrome:
- Brainstem—tumours, vascular lesions, or syringobulbia.
- Cervical cord—tumours or syringomyelia.
- Cervical sympathetic chain—pancoast tumours (apical tumours of the lung) frequently invade adjacent sites; invasion of the superior cervical sympathetic ganglion often results in Horner's syndrome.

DISORDERS OF THE AUTONOMIC NERVOUS SYSTEM

Disorders of the sympathetic nervous system

Horner's syndrome

An uncommon condition caused by loss of sympathetic innervation to the eye. It is characterised by:

- Pupillary constriction (miosis) due to unopposed action of the pupillary constrictor.

Trauma/surgical section of the sympathetic trunk

Surgical sympathectomies are sometimes performed for the relief of such conditions as:

- Raynaud's phenomenon—pallor, pain and numbness of the fingers caused by vasospastic constriction of the digital arteries; sympathectomy is occasionally performed to improve limb perfusion.
- Causalgia—severe burning pain that occurs following injury to the major peripheral nerves of

Fig. 5.18 Peripheral nervous system tumours	
Tumour	**Features**
Schwannoma	Benign tumour of schwann cells of the nerve sheaths. Most common site is the vestibular branch of CN VIII
Neurofibroma	A tumour of the neural crest cells derived from the epineurium and endoneurium
Neurofibromatosis type I	An autosomal dominant neurocutaneous syndrome Characterised by multiple neurofibromas
Neurofibromatosis type II	Autosomal dominant disorder affecting CN VIII
Tuberous sclerosis	Autosomal dominant disease causing epilepsy and mental retardation
von Hippel–Lindau disease	Autosomal dominant disease characterised by multiple haemangiomas

Fig. 5.18 Peripheral nervous system tumours.

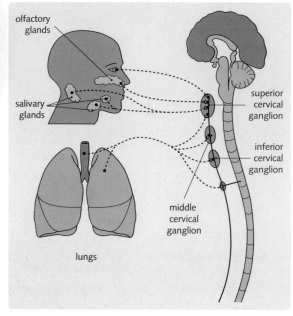

Fig. 5.19 Sympathetic innervation to the eye and face showing the relationship of the sympathetic trunk to the apex of the lungs.

the limbs (e.g. median, ulnar, sciatic) presumed to be due to disturbances of sympathetic reflexes.
- Hyperhidrosis—excessive sweating.

The consequences of either traumatic or surgical section of the sympathetic chain depend on the level of the section, but may cause:

- Loss of blood pressure control → syncope (fainting).
- Impairment of sweating → hyperpyrexia.
- Impairment of bladder and bowel functions.
- Interruption of pathway to erectile tissue → impotence.

Phaeochromocytoma

This is a rare tumour arising from chromaffin cells of the adrenal medulla, occurring in 1 in 1000 cases of hypertension. The majority are sporadic but about 10% are familial. Most are benign but about 5% are malignant.

The effects are those of hypersecretion of catecholamines, i.e. hypertension, hypermetabolism and hyperglycaemia. There is also pallor, headaches, sweating and nervousness.

It may be associated with other endocrine neoplasias, namely:

- Multiple endocrine neoplasia syndrome (especially MEN2 syndromes).
- Von Recklinghausen's disease—associated with neurofibromatosis.
- Von Hippel–Lindau syndrome—associated with renal cell carcinomas and multiple hemangiomas.

It is diagnosed by increased amounts of urinary excretion of catecholamines and their metabolites, such as vanillylmandelic acid (VMA).

Surgical removal of the tumour relieves hypertension and other effects.

Diseases of the parasympathetic nervous system

Effects of ablation of parasympathetic innervation

The most common site of parasympathetic ablation is the vagus nerve (vagotomy) for treatment of duodenal ulcers. This is less common now because of increasing awareness of the bacterial aetiology (*Helicobacter pylori*) of intestinal ulcers.

Beneficial effects

Of benefit is the reduction of acid and pepsin secretion by abolishing direct vagal drive (and to a minor degree by reducing antral gastrin secretion).

Harmful effects

Impairment of antral motility is caused by abolishing receptive relaxation in the gastric corpus, and reducing the power of antral contractions.

The harmful effects of truncal vagotomy can now be largely overcome by performing a selective vagotomy instead, but this is rarely performed due to a lower success rate and higher incidence of ulcer recurrence.

Pathology of the cardiovascular system

Objectives

In this chapter, you will learn to:

- Understand the fetal circulation and how alterations produce congenital abnormalities of the heart.
- Describe the key processes of atherosclerosis, hypertension and thrombosis (arterial and venous).
- Describe the spectrum of ischaemic heart disease and the commonly resulting heart failure.
- Understand the disorders of heart valves, including infective endocarditis.
- Recall the diseases of the myocardium itself.
- Describe the diseases of the pericardium—effusions and pericarditis.
- Understand the development of aneurysms, particularly affecting the aorta.
- Briefly describe the inflammatory and neoplastic diseases of the vasculature.
- Briefly describe other diseases of the veins and lymphatics.

CONGENITAL ABNORMALITIES OF THE HEART

Epidemiology

Congenital heart abnormalities are relatively common, affecting nearly 1% of live births. The incidence is higher in premature babies. Diagnosis of heart abnormalities has been increasing because of improved diagnostic techniques (e.g. Doppler echocardiography).

Causes

Sporadic

These are the majority of cases and no teratogenic factors can be identified.

Maternal factors

There is an increased incidence associated with certain maternal factors including:

- Maternal infection, especially with rubella.
- Maternal alcohol abuse (causes fetal alcohol syndrome).
- Intrauterine radiation.
- Maternal use of teratogenic drugs, e.g. phenytoin, thalidomide.

These factors are of greatest importance between the fourth and ninth week after conception.

Genetic or chromosomal abnormalities

These are associated with an increased incidence of congenital heart malformations. An example of this is Down syndrome.

Clinical features

Most cardiac abnormalities become apparent at or shortly after birth, usually by some manifestation of heart failure such as cyanosis, breathlessness, feeding difficulties, or a failure to thrive. However, it is possible for some conditions to be undetected until adulthood, e.g. atrial septal defects.

Classification

Congenital heart defects may be divided into two main groups depending on whether the lesions cause:

1. Abnormal shunting of blood between the two sides of the heart. A shunt is defined as an abnormal communication between heart chambers or blood vessels. In congenital heart disease there may be either left-to-right (more common) or right-to-left shunts.
2. Obstruction to blood flow by narrowing of chambers, valves or blood vessels. Complete obstruction is termed an atresia.

Fetal circulation

As the fetus does not breathe in the uterus, blood flow is controlled by three unique mechanisms (Fig. 6.1):

- Foramen ovale—this connection from the right atrium to the left atrium allows oxygenated maternal blood from the umbilical vein to bypass the lungs and directly enter the left side of the heart.
- Ductus arteriosus—this connection between the pulmonary artery and aorta allows the small quantity of blood entering the pulmonary circulation to be diverted away from the lungs and to the body. This blood is generally less oxygenated, having entered the heart from the superior vena cava, so avoiding diversion through the foramen ovale. The high resistance of the immature lungs aids flow through this low resistance pathway.
- Aortic isthmus—this constriction in the fetal aorta after the origin of the head and neck arteries ensures that relatively low oxygenated blood

from the ductus arteriosus supplies the immature organ systems of the body, rather than crucial head and neck structures.

After birth, pulmonary vascular resistance drops, allowing the foramen ovale and ductus arteriosus to close. The aortic isthmus also expands shortly after birth.

Left-to-right shunts

These are malformations that result in the shunting of blood from the left side of the heart to the right; they are the most common group of congenital heart abnormalities. Shunting is from left to right because of the higher pressures in the left side of the heart. These defects are not associated with clinical cyanosis as the blood does not bypass the lungs.

Figure 6.2 lists the prevalence of left-to-right shunts.

Ventricular septal defect

This defect of the interventricular septum is the most common cardiac abnormality, accounting for 25–30% of all cases of congenital heart disease (Fig. 6.3). The interventricular septum can be divided into a membranous (fibrous) portion and a muscular portion.

Most congenital defects are perimembranous, i.e. occurring at the junction of the membranous and muscular portions.

There are small and large defects:

- Small defects—often confined to the tiny membranous area, many of which spontaneously close.
- Larger defects—also involve the muscular wall of the septum.

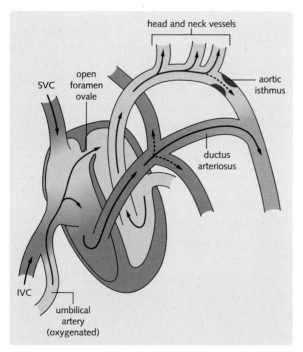

Fig. 6.1 Schematic representation of the fetal circulation. Note the role of the foramen ovale and ductus arteriosus in diverting blood away from the immature lungs. The aortic isthmus ensures that highly oxygenated blood is delivered to the crucial head and neck structures, with less oxygenated blood supplying the immature organ systems. (IVC, inferior vena cava; SVC, superior vena cava.)

Fig. 6.2 Prevalence of left-to-right shunts	
Type	**% of all CHD abnormalities**
Ventricular septal defect	25–30
Atrial septal defect	10–15
Patent ductus arteriosus	10
Atrioventricular septal defect	5

Fig. 6.2 Prevalence of left-to-right shunts. (CHD, congenital heart disease.)

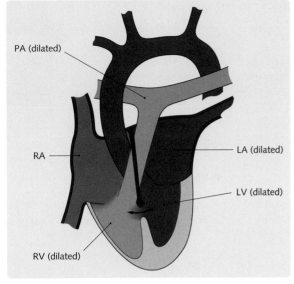

Fig. 6.3 Ventricular septal defect. Larger defects involve the septal muscle but smaller defects may be confined to the maladie de Roger (tiny membranous region). (LA, left atrium; LV, left ventricle; PA, pulmonary artery; RA, right atrium; RV, right ventricle).

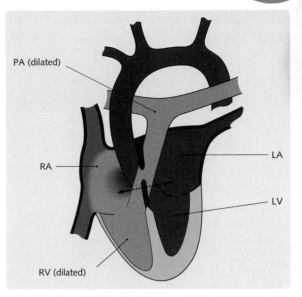

Fig. 6.4 Atrial septal defect. The defect is usually located at the level of the fossa ovalis. (LA, left atrium; LV, left ventricle; PA, pulmonary artery; RA, right atrium; RV, right ventricle).

The size and site of the defect determines the extent of shunting of the blood from left to right. Defects may present as cardiac failure in infants, or as a murmur in older children or adults.

> The clinical presentation of a ventricular septal defect includes:
> - Pansystolic murmur, caused by flow from the high-pressure left ventricle to the low-pressure right ventricle during systole. The smallest defects generally produce the loudest murmurs.
> - Tachypnoea.
> - Indrawing of the lower ribs on inspiration.
> - Right and left ventricular hypertrophy (detectable by ECG changes).
> Small defects need no treatment; larger ones require surgical repair to prevent cardiac failure.

Atrial septal defect

This is a common congenital heart defect, affecting females more than males by 2 : 1. Blood flows from left to right due to the high compliance of the right ventricle. The defect may be of two types (Fig. 6.4):

1. Ostium primum—defect is at the level of the atrioventricular septum and is associated with an abnormal mitral valve (split anterior leaflet).

2. Ostium secundum—the foramen ovale fails to close, remaining patent as the fossa ovalis. This is the most common form of atrial septal defect.

Most children are free of symptoms for many years and the condition is often detected at routine clinical examination or following a chest radiograph. Some children present with dyspnoea, chest infections, cardiac failure or arrhythmia (e.g. atrial fibrillation).

The characteristic physical signs are a systolic flow murmur over the pulmonary valve and wide splitting of the second heart sound.

Atrial septal defects should be closed surgically to prevent shunt reversal (see below). If performed before this develops, the prognosis after surgery is excellent.

Patent (persistent) ductus arteriosus

This persistence of the embryological connection between the aorta and the pulmonary is shown in Fig. 6.5. Patent (open) ductus arteriosus occurs in about 10% of all cases of congenital heart disease, affecting females more than males. There is a recognised association with maternal rubella.

A continuous 'machinery-like' murmur is classically detected, as high volumes of oxygenated blood are shunted from the high-pressure aorta back into the lungs. This can dramatically increase the work of the heart in a large defect, leading to eventual cardiac failure without early surgical correction.

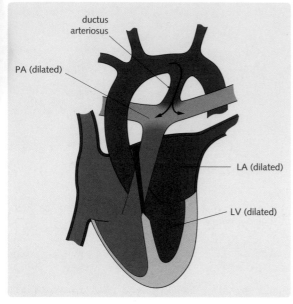

Fig. 6.5 Patent ductus arteriosus. Persistence of the duct is more common in females, and it is associated with maternal rubella.

Understanding the embryonic development of the heart assists in the understanding of congenital abnormalities. For example, the involvement of the embryonic foramen ovale in the development of atrial septal defects, and the congenital abnormality created by a persistent ductus arteriosus.

Atrioventricular septal defect

This is a septal defect with both an atrial and a ventricular component caused by failure of the endocardial cushions to fuse together. An atrioventricular canal persists resulting in a single heart chamber partially separated by abnormal valve leaflets. There is a strong association with Down syndrome.

Eisenmenger's syndrome

All the left-to-right shunts described above have the potential to persistently raise pulmonary flow. Over time, this leads to pulmonary hypertension, partly due to the obliteration of small vessels in the lungs. Eventually, this increase in pulmonary resistance can be so great that reversal to a right-to-left shunt occurs, producing marked cyanosis as deoxygenated blood is pumped around the body (Eisenmenger's syndrome).

Eisenmenger's syndrome is more likely to occur with large left-to-right shunts (e.g. ventricular septal defects or patent ductus arteriosus). The condition is irreversible and usually prevents surgery to correct the original congenital defect.

Right-to-left shunts

These are less common than left-to-right shunts. The result of a right-to-left shunt is that deoxygenated blood bypasses the lungs to enter the systemic circulation. Cyanosis may therefore develop in the early postnatal period with any of these conditions.

Tetralogy of Fallot

This is the most common cause of cyanosis in infancy, occurring in about 1 in 2000 live births. The abnormality consists of four (hence 'tetra—') defects (Fig. 6.6):

1. Ventricular septal defect.
2. Over-riding aorta sitting astride the ventricular septal defect.
3. Pulmonary stenosis, which is usually due to thickening of the subvalvular muscle in the pulmonary outflow tract, but is sometimes associated with valvular stenosis.
4. Right ventricular hypertrophy.

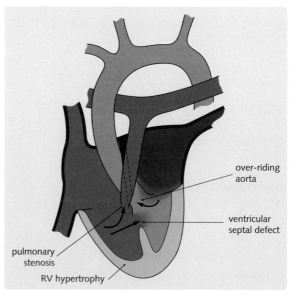

Fig. 6.6 Fallot's tetralogy is an important cause of right-to-left shunting.

Aetiopathogenesis—defects are caused by the abnormal embryological development of the bulbar septum, which normally separates the ascending aorta from the pulmonary artery (and should fuse with the inter-ventricular septum).

Pulmonary stenosis leads to inadequate perfusion of the lungs, and the over-riding aorta receives blood from both the right and left ventricles. The net result is that the systemic circulation contains deoxygenated blood, causing cyanosis in affected individuals.

Clinical features are:

- Cyanosis—especially after feeding or a crying attack. This is termed a 'Fallot's spell', as adrenergic stimulation exacerbates the right ventricular outflow obstruction, so increasing the amount of blood shunted. Squatting after exertion can relieve these symptoms by increasing the afterload of the left heart. In older children, cyanosis causes stunting of growth, digital clubbing and polycythaemia.
- Loud ejection systolic murmur—either from the ventricular septal defect or pulmonary stenosis.

Most cases are now surgically corrected, with a good prognosis if performed in early childhood. Complications include bacterial endocarditis, and consequent cerebral infarction or brain abscess.

Transposition of the great arteries

This is a complex malformation in which connections between the right and left ventricle, aorta, and pulmonary artery are disordered—the aorta emanating from the right ventricle, and the pulmonary artery arising from the left (Fig. 6.7).

Postnatal survival is possible only if one or more of the following shunts exists:

- Atrial septal defect—this is often surgically enlarged in early life to ensure adequate oxygenated blood mixes into the systemic circulation.
- Ventricular septal defect.
- Patent ductus arteriosus.

Surgical correction is possible, at which point all shunts are closed.

Persistent truncus arteriosus

Both the aorta and pulmonary artery develop from a single tube: the truncus arteriosus. Persistence of the truncus results in a single great artery that receives

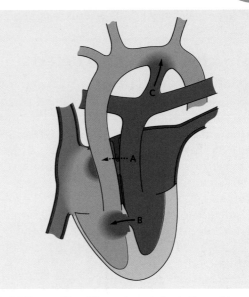

Fig. 6.7 Transposition of the great vessels. Survival is possible only if other shunts are present at either the atrial (A), ventricular (B) or ductus (C) level.

blood from both ventricles. A ventricular septal defect is also present.

Cyanosis occurs due to the mixing of blood from the right and left ventricles.

Tricuspid atresia

This rare disorder is caused by an occluded tricuspid orifice. The defect is always associated with:

- Patent foramen ovale.
- Ventricular septal defect.
- Underdevelopment of the right ventricle.
- Hypertrophy of the left ventricle.

Blood is shunted first from the right atrium to the left, and then a small proportion is shunted from the left ventricle to the right through the ventricular septal defect, so bypassing the obstructed tricuspid valve. Some of the deoxygenated blood enters the systemic circulation resulting in cyanosis.

Surgical correction may be possible, although there is a high neonatal mortality.

Total anomalous pulmonary venous connection

Here, pulmonary veins do not open into the left atrium but into the right atrium, systemic veins or both. There is always an atrial septal defect, resulting in right-to-left shunting with mixing of saturated and desaturated blood in the atria.

The increased pulmonary flow leads to pulmonary vascular disease.

Obstructive congenital defects

Coarctation of the aorta

This is a stenotic narrowing of the aorta, usually located in the region where the ductus arteriosus joins the aorta, i.e. the fetal aortic isthmus (Fig. 6.8). About 50% of affected individuals have an associated bicuspid aortic valve. 'Berry' aneurysms of the cerebral circulation are also more common in these individuals.

This defect accounts for up to 5% of all forms of congenital heart disease, and it affects 1 in 4000 live births, male incidence being greater than female by 2:1.

Clinical features—stricture produces:

- Hypertension proximal to the stenosis, leading to symptoms such as headache and dizziness.
- Hypotension distal to the stenosis, leading to generalised weakness and poor peripheral circulation.

Characteristically, the blood pressure is raised in the upper body but is normal or low in the legs:

- Upper body—abnormally large arterial pulsations may be seen in the neck, and severe hypertension leads to the development of collateral circulations, which may be visible or present on imaging in older children and adults, e.g. pericapsular and intercostal arteries.
- Lower body—femoral pulses are weak and delayed when compared to the radial pulse.

A systolic murmur may sometimes be heard posteriorly over the coarctation.

Pathological complications—in untreated severe cases death may occur in several ways:

- Left ventricular failure, following prolonged hypertension.
- Dissection of the aorta, particularly in patients with associated bicuspid aortic valves.
- Bacterial endocarditis, usually at the site of aortic constriction.
- Cerebral haemorrhage.

A rare variant is the so-called 'infantile preductal coarctation', in which there is stenosis of a long segment of the aorta between the left subclavian artery origin and the ductus arteriosus, which remains patent. Systemic circulation to the lower part of the body often depends on a right-to-left shunt through the patent ductus causing peripheral cyanosis.

Pulmonary artery stenosis or atresia with intact ventricular septum

This presents as a narrowing (stenosis) or fusion (atresia) of the trunk of the pulmonary artery. In atretic cases, the patent foramen ovale forms the only outlet for blood from the right side of the heart. The ductus arteriosus is always patent and represents the only access route to the pulmonary circulation.

Aortic stenosis and atresia

Semilunar aortic valves may be stenosed or atretic. If fusion is complete, the aorta, left ventricle, and left atrium are markedly underdeveloped. This is usually accompanied by an open ductus arteriosus which delivers blood into the aorta. The condition is associated with severe cyanosis.

Figure 6.9 gives a summary of congenital cardiac malformations.

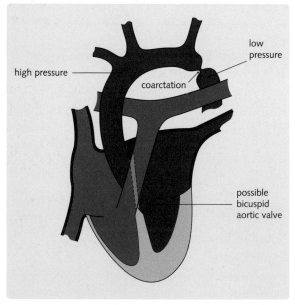

Fig. 6.8 Coarctation of the aorta. Signs and symptoms depend largely on the size of the narrowing.

Fig. 6.9 Summary of congenital cardiac malformations

Left-to-right shunts

- Ventricular septal defect
- Atrial septal defect
- Patent ductus arteriosus
- Atrioventricular septal defects

Right-to-left shunts

- Tetralogy of Fallot
- Transposition of the great arteries
- Persistent truncus arteriosus
- Total anomalous venous connection

Obstructive congenital defects

- Coarctation of the aorta
- Pulmonary artery stenosis/atresia
- Aortic stenosis/atresia

Fig. 6.9 Summary of congenital cardiac malformations.

The terms 'arteriosclerosis' and 'atherosclerosis' are often confused. They are not synonymous and they should not be used interchangeably. Arteriosclerosis is hardening or loss of elasticity of the arteries from any cause, whereas atherosclerosis implies hardening or loss of elasticity due to atheroma.

ATHEROSCLEROSIS, HYPERTENSION AND THROMBOSIS

Definitions and concepts

Arteriosclerosis

This is an imprecise term meaning thickening and loss of elasticity of the arteries caused by any condition. Three patterns of arteriosclerosis exist:

1. Atherosclerosis—the most common form. A degenerative disease involving the intima of large and medium-sized arteries. Atherosclerotic lesions are termed atheromas. This is discussed in greater detail below.
2. Mönckeberg's medial calcific sclerosis—this degenerative disease of older individuals involves the deposition of calcium in the media of medium-sized muscular arteries (forming 'pipe-stem' arteries). These deposits do not reduce the size of the vessel lumen.
3. Arteriolosclerosis—the thickening of small artery and arteriole vessel walls, with subsequent reduction in lumen size. This is associated with systemic hypertension and diabetes mellitus, and particularly affects vessels in the kidney, pancreas, gall bladder, small intestine, adrenals and retina.

Consequences of arteriosclerosis

The consequences particularly of atherosclerosis and arteriolosclerosis are:

- Vessel thickening → narrowing of lumen → poor tissue perfusion.
- Inelasticity of vessels → predisposition to vessel rupture and haemorrhage.
- Alterations in vascular endothelium → increased predisposition to thrombosis.

Arteriosclerosis contributes to the high frequency of cardiac (myocardial infarction, angina pectoris), cerebral (stroke, transient ischaemic attack), colonic (malabsorption, ischaemic colitis) and peripheral (intermittent claudication, rest pain) diseases in the elderly population.

Certain diseases are known to accelerate and aggravate arteriosclerosis, e.g. hypertension and diabetes.

Atherosclerosis

A degenerative, progressive and inflammatory disease of large and medium-sized arteries (but not veins), this is characterised by the focal accumulation of lipid-rich material in the intima of arteries and associated cellular reactions. Although essentially a disease of the vessel intima, atherosclerosis also has an impact on the structure and function of the underlying media.

Atherosclerotic lesions are found to some extent in virtually every adult over the age of 40 as well as in many younger individuals. The consequences of atherosclerosis account for half of all deaths in the Western world.

Commonly affected arteries are:

- Aorta (especially the abdominal aorta).
- Coronary arteries.

- Cerebral arteries.
- Common iliac/femoral arteries.

Atherosclerosis is rare in the arteries of the upper limb and in the pulmonary arteries.

Epidemiological studies have identified risk factors associated with atheroma development. These can be broadly classified into:

- Fixed (constitutional) risk factors, i.e. inherent to an individual.
- Modifiable risk factors, i.e. those that may be controlled (although often to a very limited extent).

Fixed risk factors are:

- Age—atherosclerotic lesions increase in number with increasing age.
- Gender—females have half the incidence of males up to the age of 55, due to the protective effect of oestrogens; over 55 years, the male to female ratio is equal.
- Familial traits—familial increase in predisposition is often associated with familial hyperlipidaemia.
- Race—wide interracial variations exist in the incidence of atheroma, but this may be due to dietary differences. The condition is relatively uncommon in China, Japan and Africa.

Modifiable risk factors lead to an increased severity of atherosclerosis. Such factors are multiplicative rather than additive—this means that combinations of risk factors massively increase the risk of atherosclerosis. Examples are:

- Hypercholesterolaemia [increased serum levels of cholesterol or low-density lipoprotein (LDL)]— usually dependent on diet but may also occur as a result of some forms of familial hypercholesterolaemia. For example, mutation of apoprotein B100 gene on chromosome 2 may result in increased transport of cholesterol into artery walls.
- Hypertension—increased blood pressure, both the systolic and diastolic levels.
- Diabetes mellitus—probably because it results in hypercholesterolaemia.
- Cigarette smoking—there is a strong link between smoking and deaths from coronary artery disease; the mechanism is unclear.
- Sedentary lifestyle—exercise decreases the incidence of sudden death from ischaemic heart

disease but it is not clear whether it directly reduces atherosclerosis formation.

- Obesity—particularly central or truncal obesity, probably a reflection of poor diet and resultant hyperlipidaemia.

Following development of atherosclerosis, factors such as stress, personality traits and coagulation disorders may alter the risk of a related event (e.g. stroke or ischaemic heart disease).

The clinical management of atherosclerosis is based on minimising risk factors:

- Antihypertensive medication, e.g. diuretics, β-blockers.
- HMG CoA reductase inhibitors (statins)—lower cholesterol by inhibiting hepatic synthesis.
- Anticoagulants—75 mg aspirin (low-dose aspirin) daily to minimise thrombotic risk.
- Lifestyle advice, e.g. stopping smoking, healthier diet and increased exercise.

Pathogenesis

The pathogenesis of the characteristic lipid plaques of atherosclerosis is described by the response to injury hypothesis. This states that atherosclerosis is a chronic inflammatory response of the arterial wall to endothelial injury.

Atherosclerosis begins early in life; the first signs of the disorder are termed fatty streaks, which usually occur in areas of altered arterial stress (e.g. bifurcations and sites of endothelial injury). Endothelial dysfunction may also have a role in the early pathogenesis of plaque formation.

Low-grade endothelial injury may be induced by:

- Cigarette smoking.
- Altered haemodynamics—the damaging effect of turbulent blood flow (e.g. at major arterial bifurcations) may be further worsened by hypertension.
- Homocysteine—this amino acid may directly damage the arterial wall. There may be a future role for folate and vitamin B_6 supplementation in reducing levels of circulating homocysteine. Individuals with the rare genetic disorder homocystinuria, which results in raised blood homocysteine levels, develop premature vascular disease.

- Hyperlipidaemia—possibly causing direct endothelial damage and promotion of platelet attachment.
- Others—viruses, other infectious agents and inflammatory cytokines have all been suggested as potential inducers of endothelial injury.

Stages of development in atherosclerosis

The key stages in the development of atherosclerotic plaques (atheromas) are as follows:

1. Chronic endothelial injury results in endothelial dysfunction, causing an increased permeability of the vessel wall, and the expression of receptors for leucocyte adhesion.
2. Plasma proteins (including LDL) diffuse into the arterial intima.
3. Monocytes bind newly expressed receptors and migrate into the intima, differentiating into macrophages. These macrophages take up oxidised LDL to form foam cells. When they die, release of the cellular contents of these cells forms extracellular lipid pools.
4. Adhesion of platelets to the endothelium.
5. Release of cytokines and growth factors (e.g. platelet-derived growth factor) by platelets and activated macrophages results in the migration of smooth muscle cells from the media to the intima (myointimal cells). These muscle cells change from a contractile to repair phenotype, producing collagens in an attempt to stabilise the growing lesion.

The above scheme outlines the formation of a stable atherosclerotic plaque. (see Fig. 6.10, parts A–C). Such a plaque can remain asymptomatic for many years, slowly growing to the point where it may significantly obstruct blood flow.

The maintenance of a stable atherosclerotic plaque depends on the balance between inflammation (macrophage mediated) and repair (smooth muscle mediated). If activated macrophages start producing additional cytokines (e.g. interleukin-1, matrix metalloproteinases), the muscle cells forming the protective fibrous cap may become senescent, resulting in an unstable plaque. Thinning of the cap follows, with potential for erosion, rupture (releasing prothrombotic material) or ulceration (see Fig. 6.10, part D).

Figure 6.11 provides a summary of the events involved in the pathogenesis of atherosclerosis.

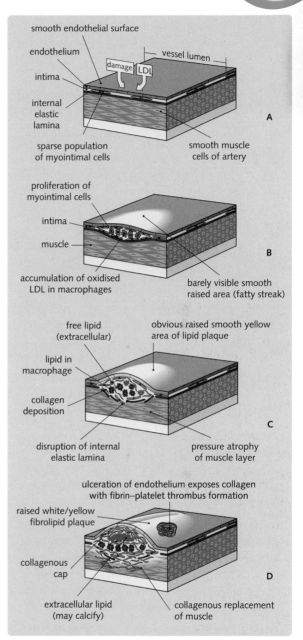

Fig. 6.10 Atheroma formation. (A) Endothelial injury: allows entry of cholesterol-rich, low-density lipoproteins (LDLs) into the intima. (B) 'Fatty streaks': barely visible pale bulges form as a result of phagocytosis and accumulation of lipid by intimal macrophages. (C) Stable plaques: raised, yellow lesions within the intima consisting of free lipid released by macrophages and collagen deposited by myointimal cells (repair phenotype). (D) Unstable plaque with ulceration: allowing platelet aggregation and thrombosis with the potential for embolism to a distant site. Note that pressure atrophy of the underlying media and elastic lamina results in weakening of the arterial wall.

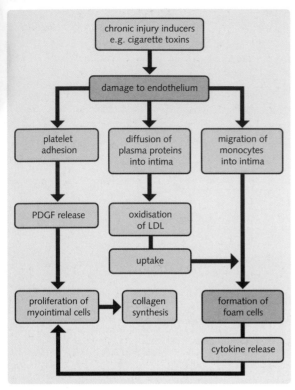

Fig. 6.11 Summary of events involved in pathogenesis of atherosclerosis.

Arterial remodelling

The migration of smooth muscle cells away from the arterial media produces the complex effect of remodelling. Two types have been proposed:

1. Negative remodelling—some arterial segments affected by atherosclerosis constrict, increasing the likelihood of occluding the lumen.
2. Positive remodelling—affected arterial segments dilate, potentially compensating for the plaque and maintaining the size of the lumen.

Thinning of the muscular arterial media predisposes an artery to aneurysm.

Hypertension

Elevated blood pressure is an important and treatable cause of cardiac failure. It is a major risk factor for atherosclerosis and cerebral haemorrhage. Any increase in blood pressure is associated with an increased risk of disease. Consequently, there are no thresholds below which a person has no risk of developing disease in which blood pressure is implicated as a pathogenic factor. Definitions of hypertension are therefore arbitrary.

Functional or operational definition

Hypertension is increasingly being defined by the level at which intervention (e.g. antihypertensive medication) is of proven benefit. Recent research has suggested that a sustained systemic blood pressure above 140 mmHg systolic and/or above 85 mmHg diastolic should be treated to reduce cardiovascular events such as strokes. Target levels for those with diabetes and renal disease are even lower.

Aetiological classification

Hypertension can be classified into two main types according to its aetiology (Fig. 6.12):

1. Primary (essential or idiopathic) hypertension— a complex, multifactorial disease in which blood pressure is elevated with age but with no apparent cause. This accounts for 90% of all cases and probably has a strong genetic determinant. Aetiology may involve increased total peripheral vascular resistance and underlying renal dysfunction.
2. Secondary hypertension—elevated blood pressure due to an identifiable cause. It accounts for 10% of hypertension. Examples include renal hypertension, endocrine causes and coarctation of the aorta.

Pathological classification

Hypertension can also be classified according to the clinical course of disease:

- Benign hypertension—stable elevation of blood pressure over many years.
- Malignant (accelerated) hypertension—a rare condition characterised by a dramatic elevation of blood pressure over a short period of time.

Benign hypertension

Here, vessel changes develop gradually in response to a persistent elevated blood pressure; males are affected more than females. Histologically, it is characterised by:

- Hypertrophy and thickening of muscular media.
- Thickening of elastic lamina.
- Fibroelastic thickening of intima.
- Hyaline deposition in arteriole walls (hyaline arteriolosclerosis).

The effects are:

- Reduced size of vessel lumen leads to tissue ischaemia.

Fig. 6.12 Causes of hypertension	
Primary hypertension: unknown aetiology but probably multifactorial involving . . .	
Genetic predisposition	Strong familial association
Socioeconomic factors	Related to social deprivation
Dietary factors	Obesity, high salt intake, high alcohol, caffeine intake
Hormonal factors	Abnormalities in renin–angiotensin–aldosterone system
Neurological factors	Excessive sympathetic nervous system activity
Secondary hypertension: secondary to . . .	
Renal disease	Parenchymal disease, e.g. chronic pyelonephritis, glomerulonephritis, polycystic kidneys, amyloidosis Vascular disease, e.g. stenosis of renal artery
Adrenal disorders	Pheochromocytoma, Cushing's syndrome, Conn's syndrome (primary hyperaldosteronism), congenital adrenal hyperplasia
Other endocrine disorders	Thyrotoxicosis, hypothyroidism, acromegaly, hyperparathyroidism, diabetes with renal involvement
Cardiovascular disorders	Coarctation of the aorta, arteriovenous fistulae and shunts
Drugs	e.g. Oral contraceptives, anabolic steroids, corticosteroids, epinephrine (adrenaline) and related sympathomimetic drugs
Pregnancy	±Pre-eclampsia

Fig. 6.12 Causes of hypertension are divided into primary and secondary aetiological factors.

- Increased rigidity leads to limited capacity for expansion and constriction.
- Increased fragility of vessels leads to an increased risk of haemorrhage (especially cerebral).

After many years of benign progression, 5% of such patients enter an accelerated malignant phase.

Malignant hypertension
Acute, destructive changes occur in the walls of small arteries when blood pressure rises suddenly and markedly. This results in necrosis of the vessel wall and infiltration of the necrotic media by fibrin (i.e. fibrinoid necrosis of vessels).

The destructive changes result in a cessation of blood flow through small vessels with multiple foci of tissue necrosis, often with intravascular thrombosis. Areas typically affected include the retina (high-grade retinopathy) and the kidneys (glomerular disease).

Figure 6.13 lists the features of malignant and benign hypertension.

Complications and effects of hypertension
Vascular effects
Hypertension accelerates atherosclerosis, which causes thickening of the media of muscular arteries, particularly the smaller arteries and arterioles. Structural changes perpetuate further rises in blood pressure, causing a progressively worsening clinical picture.

The normal flow of protein into the vessel wall is increased resulting in intramural protein deposition termed hyaline in benign hypertension, and fibrinoid in malignant hypertension:

- Hyaline deposition—a common feature of ageing small arteries (< 1 mm diameter); refers to the homogeneous appearance of vessel walls due to infiltration by plasma proteins.
- Fibrinoid deposition—a combination of fibrin infiltration with necrosis of the vessel wall.

Heart
The left ventricle undergoes hypertrophy resulting from the increased workload, causing increased

Fig. 6.13 Features of benign and malignant hypertension

	Benign	Malignant
Incidence	Very common (at least 5% of UK population)	Rare
Age	Begins at < 45 years but prolonged into 6th and 7th decades	Young adults (25–35 years)
Sex	Females > males	Females = males
Aetiology	Majority of cases due to primary hypertension	Majority of cases secondary to renal disease (few cases arise out of benign essential hypertension)
Disease progression	Very slow (many years)	Rapid (months to 1–2 years)
Blood pressure	Very slow rise Diastolic = 90–120 mmHg	Rapid rise Diastolic ≥ 120 mmHg
Arterial changes	Potentiates atheroma → accelerated arteriosclerosis	Intimal fibrous thickening → accelerated arteriosclerosis
Arteriole changes	Hyaline thickening with narrowed lumen	Fibrinoid necrosis of vessel wall Lumen occluded by thrombus Affects mainly kidney and abdominal viscera

Fig. 6.13 Features of benign and malignant hypertension.

susceptibility to spontaneous arrhythmias. Ischaemic heart disease due to accelerated atherosclerosis is a common complication of hypertension.

Brain

Intracerebral haemorrhage is a frequent cause of death in hypertension. Small-vessel damage within the cerebral hemispheres results in the development of micro-infarcts, which form hypertensive lacunae, i.e. small areas of destroyed brain filled with fluid.

Kidneys

Arteriolosclerosis leads to progressive ischaemia of the nephrons and chronic renal failure. This is termed benign hypertensive nephrosclerosis, and it is a common cause of chronic renal failure in the middle-aged and elderly population.

Retina

Hypertension may produce retinal ischaemia and infarction, visible on fundoscopic examination.

Figure 6.14 outlines the complications and effects of hypertension.

Pulmonary hypertension

Definition and causes

This is defined as pulmonary arterial pressure in excess of 30 mmHg. Figure 6.15 lists the causes of pulmonary hypertension.

Effects of pulmonary hypertension

With acute onset, there is a massive transudation of fluid from the pulmonary capillaries into the alveoli (pulmonary oedema), leading to shortness of breath and expectoration of bloodstained, watery fluid.

Chronic onset has three effects:

1. Hyperplastic arteriosclerosis—muscular hypertrophy, intimal fibrosis and dilatation of the pulmonary arteries.
2. Necrotising arteriolitis—increased pressure within the pulmonary arteries causes weakening of the vessel wall with repeated episodes of haemorrhage into the alveolar spaces, which contain haemosiderin-laden macrophages.
3. Cor pulmonale—right ventricular hypertrophy and dysfunction as a result of increased workload.

Fig. 6.14 Complications and effects of hypertension

	Benign	Malignant
Vessels	Hyaline deposition due to infiltration by plasma proteins	Fibrinoid deposition due to combination of fibrin deposition and necrosis of vessel wall
Heart	Hypertrophy of left ventricle → ↑susceptibility to spontaneous arrhythmias Heart failure in 60% of cases Ischaemic heart disease	Hypertrophy of left ventricle → ↑susceptibility to spontaneous arrhythmias Focal myocardial necrosis Acute heart failure Ischaemic heart disease
Brain	Cerebral haemorrhage	Encephalopathy (fits and loss of consciousness) due to cerebral oedema Cerebral haemorrhage
Kidney	Nephrosclerosis, but not usually serious	Severe renal damage; death in uraemia
Retina	Ischaemia and infarction ('cotton wool' exudates) Association with central retinal vein thrombosis	Ischaemia and infarction ('cotton wool' exudates) Association with central retinal vein thrombosis
Other organs	No significant damage	Focal necrosis, e.g. perforation of gut

Fig. 6.14 Complications and effects of hypertension.

Fig. 6.15 Causes of pulmonary hypertension

Mechanism	
Precapillary causes	
Increased pulmonary blood flow	Left-to-right shunts, e.g. atrial septal defects, ventricular septal defects
Capillary causes	
Destruction of lung capillary bed	Emphysema Interstitial fibrosis of lungs
Mechanical arterial occlusion	Recurrent pulmonary emboli
Alveolar hypoxia causing pulmonary vasoconstriction	High altitude Obesity Chronic obstructive airways disease
Postcapillary causes	
Pulmonary venous congestion	Mitral valve disease, e.g. stenosis Chronic left ventricular failure
Idiopathic causes	
Primary pulmonary hypertension	Rare disease of young women due to increased tone in pulmonary vessels → progressive vascular changes and death

Fig. 6.15 Causes of pulmonary hypertension.

Effects of diabetes mellitus on the vessels

Individuals with diabetes suffer from an increased severity of atherosclerosis and capillary microangiopathy, in which thickening of the small-vessel walls is attributed to hyaline arteriolosclerosis and marked expansion of the basement membrane.

Vessel damage is complex and is probably due to the increased plasma levels of cholesterol and triglycerides. Biochemically, there is abnormal glycosylation of protein within the vessel wall. Clinical sequelae of diabetic vessel damage are described in detail in Chapter 10; they include diabetic retinopathy, diabetic nephropathy and peripheral neuropathy.

Thrombosis

Thrombosis is the formation of a solid mass of blood constituents—thrombus—within the vascular system during life. It is not to be confused with a clot, which occurs in non-flowing blood.

Thrombosis can affect both arteries and veins.

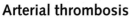

A thrombus is different from a clot! A clot is defined as blood coagulated outside the vascular system or within the vascular system after death.

Arterial thrombosis

This is most commonly superimposed on an atheroma. As the plaque enlarges, it causes turbulent blood flow, which results in the loss of intimal cells. The exposure of vessel collagen predisposes to platelet activation. Turbulence itself will predispose to fibrin deposition and platelet clumping.

The greatest degree of turbulence occurs at the downstream side of the forming thrombus; thrombi therefore grow in the direction of the blood flow (propagation). An arterial thrombosis may result in tissue infarction and ischaemia either directly or through embolisation.

Venous thrombosis

Many venous thrombi begin at damaged valves that produce turbulence. Furthermore, blood stasis during surgery or due to immobilisation may result in the formation of a deep vein thrombosis (risking pulmonary embolism). However, some thrombi form at sites with no known predisposing factors. Often thrombi grow by successive deposition of alternating bands of platelets and red blood cells. These patterns are known as the lines of Zahn.

A thrombosed vein may cause an inflammatory response (thrombophlebitis) or a vein that is inflamed may thrombose (phlebothrombosis). A histological differentiation between the two types is in most cases impossible.

Affected sites
The most commonly affected sites are:

- Deep leg veins (90% of cases), particularly the lower leg.
- Skull and dural sinuses.
- Portal venous tributaries.
- Pelvic veins.

Outcomes
Outcomes of venous thrombosis include:

- Lysis—dissolution of the thrombus by activated fibrinolytic system.
- Propagation—spread of the thrombus proximally in the veins.
- Organization—reparative process with ingrowth of fibroblasts.
- Recanalisation—usually incomplete re-establishment of blood flow.
- Embolism—thrombus migrates to a distant site.

Complications
The most serious acute complication is embolism of the thrombus to the pulmonary arteries, causing a pulmonary embolism (PE). These are divided into massive, major and minor events and are discussed in detail on page 124.

Chronic complications are aching pains due to varicose veins, venous congestion, oedema, venous eczema and ulceration.

Deep vein thrombosis (DVT) is a key clinical topic, as a resulting pulmonary embolus may be life-threatening. High-risk patients should be identified and offered prophylaxis. DVTs typically present as a painful unilaterally swollen calf, which is warm to the touch. Diagnosis is aided by radiographic venograms and non-invasive ultrasound (large veins only). Immediate treatment involves heparin and prolonged warfarin, the latter being used continuously in those with repeated DVTs.

Virchow's triad

Factors that predispose any blood vessel to thrombosis can be classified into three main groups, collectively known as Virchow's triad (Fig. 6.16):

- Changes in the blood constituents—forming a hypercoaguable state.
- Changes in the blood vessel endothelium—usually at the point of injury.
- Changes in the pattern of blood flow—stasis or turbulence.

Hypercoagulability

Primary (hereditary)

Hereditary defects of hypercoagulability lead to a life-long tendency to thrombosis (thrombophilia). They usually affect the venous system:

- Antithrombin III deficiency—autosomal dominant condition characterised by recurrent venous thromboses usually starting in early adult life. Primary defect is a deficiency of antithrombin III, which usually neutralises thrombin and other activated clotting factors.
- Protein C deficiency—autosomal dominant condition resulting in failure of neutralisation of activated factors V and VIII. Protein S is a cofactor for protein C. Therefore, protein S deficiencies produce a similar pathology.

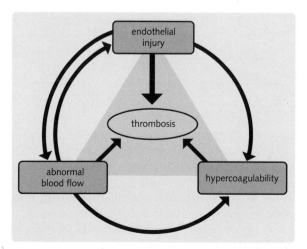

Fig. 6.16 Virchow's triad in thrombosis. Endothelial integrity is the single most important factor: injury can affect local blood flow and/or coagulability. Abnormal blood flow (turbulence or stasis) can, in turn, cause endothelial injury. The elements of the triad may act independently or combine to cause thrombus formation. (Redrawn with permission from Robbins and Cotran Pathologic Basis of Disease, 7th edition, V Kumar, A Abbas, and N Fausto, Elsevier Saunders, 2005).

- Factor V Leiden—point mutation in the factor V gene, which results in factor V protein that is resistant to neutralisation by protein C. This is very common, affecting up to 5% of Caucasians.
- Prothrombin G20210A—this prothrombin gene polymorphism occurs in 2% of the population and is associated with increased levels of prothrombin and venous thromboembolism.

Secondary (acquired)

Defects are as follows:

- Malignancy—patients with carcinoma of the breast, lung, prostate, pancreas or bowel have an increased risk of venous thrombosis.
- Blood disorders, e.g. increased viscosity (especially polycythaemia rubra vera) and thrombocytosis lead to an increased risk of venous thrombosis.
- Oestrogens—associated with raised plasma levels of various clotting factors leading to an increased risk of venous thrombosis.
- Antiphospholipid antibody syndrome—leads to the interaction of antibodies (lupus anticoagulant and anticardiolipin antibodies) with phospholipid-bound proteins involved in coagulation. This causes prolongation of clotting times *in vitro*, with a paradoxical increased risk of venous and arterial thrombosis. Often found in patients with autoimmune disease, especially systemic lupus erythematosus (SLE).
- Cholesterol—partly genetic, partly acquired (diet/lifestyle), leads to an increased risk of arterial thrombosis.
- Smoking—has been implicated as a predisposing risk factor for thrombosis, possibly by causing a hypercoagulable state.

Endothelial injury

Direct injury to the endothelium as seen in trauma (including intravenous cannulation) and inflammation may lead to thrombosis. Damage to the endothelium also occurs in association with atheroma.

Alterations to blood flow

Alterations are:

- Stasis—allows platelets to come in contact with endothelium. Slow flow prevents blood from diluting activated coagulation components, e.g. prolonged immobilisation.
- Turbulence—may cause physical trauma to endothelial cells. Loss of laminar flow may bring platelets into contact with endothelium.

ISCHAEMIC HEART DISEASE AND HEART FAILURE

Ischaemic heart disease (IHD) is a condition caused by a reduction or cessation of the blood supply to the myocardium (myocardial ischaemia). This is usually as a result of atherosclerosis, although in rare cases it may be caused by coronary embolism, arteritis or ostial obstruction. The left ventricle is more prone to ischaemia because of its greater bulk and work requirement, and its higher oxygen demand.

IHD is the most common type of cardiac disease and a leading cause of death in the Western world, accounting for about a third of all male deaths and a quarter of all female deaths. Risk factors for the development of ischaemic heart disease are the same as those for the development of atherosclerosis.

Classification

IHD results in four main syndromes:

1. Stable angina (chronic manifestation).
2. Unstable angina (acute manifestation).
3. Myocardial infarction (acute manifestation).
4. Sudden cardiac death (acute manifestation).

The acute manifestations of cardiac ischaemia form the continuous spectrum of disease termed the acute coronary syndromes (ACS).

Angina pectoris

Angina pectoris is episodic chest pain caused by ischaemia of the myocardium following exercise. Ischaemia is usually the result of stenosis of one or more of the coronary arteries resulting in reduced blood flow to the myocardium.

Stenosis of the coronary arteries is typically the result of atherosclerosis. Atheromatous plaques may lie in two possible positions:

1. Eccentric—fibrolipid plaques affecting only one side of the wall of a coronary artery. Improvement of flow at the site of such plaques may be achieved by the use of vasodilator drugs. These drugs, such as glyceryl trinitrate, produce relaxation of the unaffected part of the vessel wall.
2. Concentric—collagenous plaques affecting the whole of the arterial wall circumference. As the whole wall is abnormal, drug therapy cannot improve flow over a narrowed segment.

Cardiac referred pain

Pain of angina (and myocardial infarction) commonly radiates from the substernal and left pectoral regions to the left shoulder and the medial aspect of the left arm; this is known as cardiac referred pain.

Afferent fibres of the heart, and sensory fibres of affected cutaneous zones, enter the same spinal cord segments (T1 to T4/T5 on the left side) and ascend in the CNS along a common pathway. The brain is unable to discern the origin of the pain, hence the phenomenon of cardiac referred pain.

Less commonly, pain radiates to the right shoulder and arm, with or without concomitant pain on the left side.

Types of angina

Stable angina

This is a predictable angina that occurs at a fixed level of exercise, as a result of an increased demand in myocardial work, usually in the presence of impaired perfusion by blood. It is caused by a fixed obstruction of one or more of the coronary arteries, therefore limiting any increase in coronary blood flow. Pain can usually be relieved by 1 or 2 minutes of rest. A stenosis of at least 75% of the lumen of the arteries is required to produce angina on exercise.

Unstable angina

Unstable anginal pain is unpredictable and not related to exercise. It reflects reversible ischaemia due to variable luminal stenosis of some segments of the coronary arteries: so-called dynamic obstruction.

The condition is usually the result of active fissuring and/or rupture of plaques with intimal surface thrombus deposition, microembolisation and occlusion. Unstable angina is an acute event, often preceding the development of acute myocardial infarction.

Prinzmetal's angina (vasospastic angina)

This is angina at rest caused by an increase in the coronary vasomotor tone. The mechanism for coronary spasm is unknown. The disorder may occur in non-atheromatous arteries (where an increase in tone must be extreme to produce angina) or in atheromatous arteries (where even physiological changes in tone may produce a critical reduction in blood flow).

Prinzmetal's angina is particularly common in the early morning. Attacks are usually self-limiting and, although pain may be severe, they rarely lead on to myocardial infarction.

- Stable angina is predictable (i.e. it occurs at a fixed level of exercise), and it is caused by a fixed arterial obstruction.
- Unstable angina is unpredictable (i.e. it is unrelated to exercise), and it is caused by a variable luminal stenosis of the coronary arteries.
- Prinzmetal's angina is also unpredictable, and this is caused by coronary artery spasm.

Management of angina

Stable angina can be managed as follows:

- Modification of risk factors for atherosclerosis.
- Combination drug therapy with low-dose aspirin and—potentially—nitrates, β-blockers and Ca^{2+} channel blockers.
- Invasive—percutaneous coronary intervention (PCI), using balloon angioplasty to dilate a coronary artery stenosis. If the stenosis is highly progressive or disease is very severe (e.g. involving all three key coronary arteries), coronary artery bypass grafting (CABG) may be indicated.

Patients with unstable angina should be admitted to hospital for ECG analysis and potential thrombolyis or invasive correction of their occlusion. Such active management reduces progression to infarction.

Myocardial infarction

Myocardial infarction (MI) is necrosis of the myocardium as a result of severe ischaemia. MI is extremely common, accounting for 10–15% of all deaths and about 60% of sudden unexpected deaths. It typically affects middle-aged individuals, between 50 and 60 years, but 10% occur in 35- to 50-year-olds. MI affects males more than premenopausal women (by 5 : 1), but there is an increasing incidence in women postmenopausally.

Clinical features are chest pain accompanied by breathlessness, vomiting and collapse or syncope. Pain occurs in the same sites as angina, but it is usually more severe and lasts for longer.

Types

There are two main types of MI:

1. Regional (90% of cases)—infarction occurs in the territory supplied by one major common artery.

2. Diffuse (10% of cases)—relates to problems of overall myocardial perfusion rather than to thrombotic occlusion in any one artery.

Regional myocardial infarction

This involves only one segment of the ventricular wall. The cause of infarction is nearly always thrombus formation on a ruptured or eroded unstable atheromatous plaque.

Patterns of regional MI (Fig. 6.17):

- Full thickness infarct or transmural infarct, due to complete occlusion of an artery (no collateral supply). This is the most common pattern seen in acute MI.
- Subendocardial infarct, due to lysis of thrombus or due to collateral supply. The subendocardium (inner third of the myocardium) is the least well perfused region of the myocardium, and is therefore vulnerable to reduced coronary blood flow.

Diffuse myocardial infarction

An episode of hypotension may produce general hypoperfusion of the main coronary arteries and a critical reduction in blood flow through arteries affected by high-grade atherosclerotic stenoses.

This pattern of diffuse MI differs from that of regional MI in that there is circumferential necrosis of the subendocardial zone resulting from failure of perfusion.

Site of myocardial infarction and vessel involvement

The site of regional MI depends on which vessel is involved, as shown in Fig. 6.18. The majority of

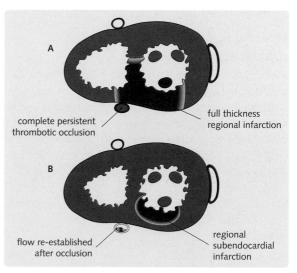

Fig. 6.17 Patterns of regional myocardial infarction (MI). (A) Transmural or full thickness infarct. (B) Regional subendocardial infarct.

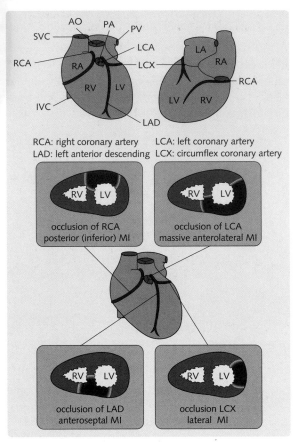

RCA: right coronary artery   LCA: left coronary artery
LAD: left anterior descending   LCX: circumflex coronary artery

occlusion of RCA
posterior (inferior) MI

occlusion of LCA
massive anterolateral MI

occlusion of LAD
anteroseptal MI

occlusion LCX
lateral MI

Fig. 6.18 Site of myocardial infarction (MI) and vessel involvement.

	Morphological changes occurring post MI	
time	macroscopic appearance	microscopic appearance
0-12 hours	not visible	infarcted muscle appears uncoloured on staining with nitroblue tetrazolium due to loss of oxidative enzymes; non-infarcted muscle stains blue
12-24 hours	pale with blotchy discolouration	infarcted muscle is brightly eosinophilic with intercellular oedema
24-72 hours	dead area appears soft and pale with a slight yellow colour	infarcted area excites an acute inflammatory response neutrophils infiltrate between dead cardiac muscle fibres
3-10 days	hyperaemic border develops around the yellow dead muscle	organization of infarcted area replacement with vascular granulation tissue
weeks to months	white scar	progressive collagen deposition infarct is replaced by a collagenous scar

Fig. 6.19 Morphological changes occurring post myocardial infarction (MI).

infarcts affect the left ventricle and septal region; infarction of the right ventricle is relatively rare.

Histological changes following myocardial infarction

MI comprises necrosis and acute inflammation. The necrotic tissue is gradually replaced by a collagenous scar. The entire process from coagulative necrosis to scar formation takes 6–8 weeks, the macroscopic and microscopic appearances of the infarct changing with time (Fig. 6.19). The extensive necrosis of cardiac muscle is associated with the release of cardiac enzymes and proteins that can be used as clinical markers for a MI event. Examples include troponin T, creatinine kinase (CK-MB cardiac isoform) and lactate dehydrogenase.

Sequelae of myocardial infarction

The effects and sequelae of MI are variable, and they can be classified into:

- Immediate effects—sudden cardiac death (described below).
- Short-term complications—occurring in the first 2 weeks post MI.
- Long-term complications.

Short-term complications

There are six short-term complications:

1. Arrhythmias—due to the involvement of conduction tissue, leading to ventricular fibrillation, atrial fibrillation, heart block and sinus bradycardia. Nearly all MI patients have

some form of arrhythmia, usually resolving spontaneously.

2. Left ventricular failure—this is common with large areas of infarction; the necrotic wall softens in organization leading to cardiac dilatation. Ventricular remodelling is the process of thinning and stretching of the infarcted segment, with progressive dilatation and hypertrophy of the remaining ventricle.

3. Rupture, which can be:
   i. external (majority)—blood bursts through the external wall into the pericardial cavity (haemopericardium); the sudden rise in intrapericardial cavity pressure prevents cardiac filling (cardiac tamponade), leading to rapid death
   ii. internal (rarely)—intracardiac rupture through the septum leads to an acquired septal defect, causing a left-to-right shunt and the development of left ventricular failure.

4. Papillary muscle dysfunction—when one or more valve leaflets are unable to close during systole there is mitral valve incompetence.

5. Mural thrombosis—on the inflamed endocardium over the area of infarction; there is a high risk of embolisation producing infarction of various organs, e.g. cerebral, renal, splenic, mesenteric and lower limbs.

6. Acute pericarditis—caused by inflammation over the infarct surface.

Long-term complications

There are four long-term complications:

1. Chronic intractable left-heart failure—the long-term effects of ventricular remodelling result in inadequate left ventricular pumping action; common when the infarct is extensive and full thickness.

2. Ventricular aneurysm (in 10% of long-term survivors)—gradual distension of the weakened fibrotic part of the left ventricular wall with thrombus formation, embolism or severe functional deficit.

3. Recurrent MI—risk of developing a further episode due to underlying coronary artery insufficiency.

4. Dressler's syndrome—a form of autoimmune-mediated pericarditis associated with a high erythrocyte sedimentation ratio (ESR) and persistent fever; develops in a very small number of cases after infarction.

After diagnosis of MI (e.g. ECG changes and cardiac enzymes), management involves:

- Oxygen and analgesia (morphine).
- Aspirin (300 mg), nitrates and β-blockers.
- Early thrombolytic therapy. e.g. streptokinase.
- Percutaneous coronary intervention—primary angioplasty likely to become first-line treatment where resources permit.
- Anticoagulation to prevent reinfarction and reduce thromboembolic risk (e.g. heparin).
- Bed rest for the first 24–48 hours on the coronary care unit.

Long-term therapy—daily low-dose aspirin, β-blockers, angiotensin-converting enzyme (ACE) inhibitors and statins.

Sudden cardiac death

Sudden cardiac death is the most important immediate consequence of myocardial ischaemia. It is usually due to ventricular fibrillation.

This may be the result of:

- Previous ischaemic heart disease, e.g. angina or previous infarction; cardiac arrhythmias can arise from muscle adjacent to an area of old scarring.
- Acute myocardial ischaemia, which, due to a new thrombotic event, may precipitate arrhythmia.

Other causes of sudden death include ruptured or dissecting aneurysms of the aorta and pulmonary emboli.

Heart failure

Heart failure can result from many different types of heart disease. It develops when the heart is no longer able to maintain an adequate cardiac output, or can only do so by increasing the filling pressure. The prognosis of heart failure is worse than many cancers; half of those with severe left ventricular impairment die within 2 years.

Heart failure may develop acutely (e.g. following myocardial infarction) or chronically (e.g. gradually progressing ischaemic heart disease).

Classification

Left-sided heart failure

This occurs due to either reduced output from the left ventricle or increased input pressure from the left atrium. Common causes include:

- Ischaemic heart disease—including the effects of ventricular remodelling after infarction.
- Hypertension—pressure overload produces initial ventricular hypertrophy, but this compensatory change cannot be maintained indefinitely and the ventricle eventually dilates.
- Valve disease—either aortic or mitral.

Eventually, the increased pressure in the left atrium works back through the vasculature resulting in pulmonary hypertension. Pulmonary oedema (also termed pulmonary congestion) and eventual right-sided heart failure may follow.

Right-sided heart failure

The most common cause is progression of left-sided failure, so-called biventricular heart failure. In these cases, the right ventricle has to pump against increased resistance in the pulmonary circulation.

Isolated right heart failure may rarely develop due to:

- Chronic lung disease (cor pulmonale).
- Pulmonary emboli (usually multiple).
- Pulmonary valve stenosis.

Clinical features

Many patients will present with mixed symptoms relating to some failure of both sides of the heart. All heart failure patients are susceptible to the effects of a low cardiac output:

- Fatigue and poor effort tolerance.
- Low blood pressure and cold peripheries.
- Renal failure—due to diversion of blood away from the kidneys.

Left-sided heart failure

In addition to these changes, left-sided failure may present with symptoms of pulmonary congestion:

- Dyspnoea (breathlessness).
- Orthopnoea (breathlessness on lying flat).
- Paroxysmal nocturnal dyspnoea (attacks of extreme breathlessness, usually at night).

Right-sided heart failure

Pure right-sided failure may present with symptoms related to systemic congestion:

- Peripheral oedema.
- Congestive hepatomegaly.
- Congestive splenomegaly.

DISORDERS OF THE HEART VALVES

Concepts of heart valve disease

Types of valve disorder

Valve disorders can be:

- Stenosis—narrowing or abnormal rigidity of a valve.
- Regurgitation (or incompetence)—failure of a valve to close fully.

Both types may coexist in one valve but one type is usually dominant.

Factors that may cause heart valve damage:

- Congenital abnormality.
- Postinflammatory scarring, e.g. after rheumatic heart disease.
- Degeneration with ageing.
- Dilatation of the valve ring, e.g. in dilated cardiomyopathy.
- Degeneration of collagenous support tissue of the valve.
- Acute destruction by necrotising inflammation.

Commonly affected valves

The mitral and aortic valves are the most frequently affected; the tricuspid and pulmonary valves only infrequently.

Figure 6.20 outlines the major causes and basic features of acquired valve disease.

Abnormalities of flow and their effects

Diseased valves often cause regurgitant jets of blood, with concomitant development of endocardial lesions opposite the jet's origin. These lesions (jet lesions) are typically seen on the septum opposite the aortic valve.

Degenerative valve disease

Calcific aortic stenosis

There are two types:

1. Degenerative calcific aortic valve stenosis—calcification of the aortic valve associated with increasing age; typically affects the elderly.
2. Bicuspid calcific aortic valve stenosis—calcification of the congenital bicuspid aortic valve (present in 1% of people); quite common, usually manifesting by 40–50 years of age.

Fig. 6.20 Major causes and basic features of acquired valve disease

Valve lesion	Causes	Effects	Physical findings
Mitral stenosis	Rheumatic	Left-sided cardiac failure with predisposition to atrial thrombosis Left atrial hypertrophy and dilation leads to: • pulmonary vascular congestion • pulmonary hypertension • right ventricular hypertrophy • 'nutmeg liver' and congested kidneys	Loud S_1 Opening snap Diastolic rumble
Mitral regurgitation	Acute: • papillary muscle dysfunction • cusp damage by endocarditis Chronic: • postinflammatory scarring, commonly rheumatic • left ventricular dilation • floppy mitral valve syndrome (prolapse)	Acute: • pulmonary oedema Chronic: • left ventricular hypertrophy and dilation • giant left atrium • progressive left-sided cardiac failure develops with time	Pansystolic murmur Widely split S_2
Aortic stenosis	Calcification of congenital bicuspid aortic valve Rheumatic Senile calcific degeneration	Early: asymptomatic but with slowly progressive left ventricular hypertrophy Late: left ventricular failure low cardiac output → breathlessness coronary artery insufficiency → angina cerebrovascular insufficiency → syncope sudden death	Systolic ejection murmur reaching peak intensity in mid- or late systole Narrow pulse pressure Slow-rising carotid pulse
Aortic regurgitation	Rheumatic Endocarditis Senile calcification Aortic root dilation	Left ventricular hypertrophy Progressive left ventricular failure	Diastolic murmur Wide pulse pressure Collapsing pulse

Fig. 6.20 Major causes and basic features of acquired valve disease.

In both types, the valves become thick and fibrotic with a fusion of the commissures. Large nodular masses of calcium may be found subendothelially within the sinuses of Valsalva, so restricting the opening of the aortic cusps.

Effects

There are two effects:

1. Aortic stenosis—thickening and fusion of valves → decreased valve lumen → reduced systolic flow.
2. Aortic regurgitation—increased rigidity of valves → failure to close properly → backflow into the left ventricle during diastole.

Stenosis and regurgitation result in left ventricular hypertrophy, coronary insufficiency (often angina), and syncope or sudden death due to acute left-sided heart failure.

Mitral annular calcification

This is 'wear and tear' of the mitral valve with calcification of the valve leaflets. Massive calcification can immobilise the valve and predispose to the development of either thrombosis or bacterial endocarditis.

Mitral valve prolapse ('floppy valve syndrome')

The changes here are due to myxomatous degeneration. The leaflets are thickened and redundant, containing large amounts of mucopolysaccharides and abnormal collagen. It most commonly involves the posterior mitral leaflet, which is soft and bulges upwards into the atrium during systole. The net result is mild valvular incompetence and an increased risk of rupture of one of the chordae, which may lead to sudden, severe valvular incompetence.

Mitral valve prolapse can also be a feature of connective tissue disorders such as Marfan's syndrome.

Rheumatic heart disease

Rheumatic fever is an immune disorder that follows 2–3 weeks after a streptococcal infection, usually tonsillitis or pharyngitis.

Epidemiology

This disease occurs mainly in children aged 5–15 years. It was once prevalent in Europe, including the UK, and in the USA. Its incidence has now decreased in the developed world and it is now most frequently seen in parts of central Africa, the Middle East and India. It is associated with poor nutrition and overcrowding.

Pathogenesis

Susceptible individuals develop antibodies to antigens produced by specific strains of group A streptococci; these antibodies then cross-react with host antigens. The disease is a systemic disorder affecting:

- Heart—pericarditis, myocarditis and endocarditis (collectively known as pancarditis).
- Joints—polyarthritis.
- Skin—subcutaneous nodules and erythema marginatum.
- Arteries—arteritis.

The most important target organ is the heart. Repeated attacks of rheumatic fever lead to progressive fibrosis of the endocardium and valves, which is the main cause of chronic scarring of the valves.

Aschoff's nodules

These pathognomonic heart lesions consist of multinucleate giant cells surrounded by activated macrophages and lymphoid cells (predominantly T cells). Lesions stimulate fibroblast proliferation and lead to scarring.

Acute rheumatic heart disease

In the acute phase, rheumatic fever causes a pancarditis, the components of which are:

- Rheumatic pericarditis—acute inflammation of the pericardium.
- Rheumatic myocarditis—mild inflammation with occasional muscle fibre necrosis.
- Rheumatic endocarditis—mitral valves are most prone to the development of severe lesions.

Chronic rheumatic heart disease

The main morbidity of rheumatic fever is the long-term effects of the immune damage causing chronic scarring of valves, particularly the mitral valve. Chronic valvular heart disease develops in about 50% of those affected by rheumatic fever with carditis. Lesions may develop after 10–20 years in Western countries, but much earlier in developing countries.

Pathogenesis

Endocardial valvular damage from the acute phase heals by progressive fibrosis. Valve leaflets and chordae tendineae become thickened, fibrotic and shrunken, often with fusion to their partners; there is frequent secondary deposition of calcium.

Once damage has developed, the altered haemodynamic stresses extend the damage even in the absence of continued autoimmune processes.

Infective endocarditis

This is an acute or subacute disease resulting from infection of a focal area of the endocardium, which usually has pre-existing damage. It can affect almost any age group, but it is increasing in incidence in the elderly population. Predisposing factors in susceptible individuals include genitourinary infection, diabetes, tooth extraction, pressure ulcers and surgical procedures. It is more common in males than females (3 : 1).

Morphological features

The characteristic lesions of endocarditis are termed vegetations. These are formed from deposits of platelets, fibrin and bacteria. The mechanism of formation is outlined in Fig. 6.21. Research suggests that vegetations may form in areas of high-pressure gradients, for example at an incompetent valve.

Almost all vegetation occurs on valve leaflets or chordae tendinae. The size varies from a small nodule to a large mass that may occlude the valve orifice. The mitral and aortic valves are the most commonly affected.

episodes of bacteraemia, organisms become enmeshed in platelet aggregates on the surface of the abnormal endocardium, growing to cause persistent infection.

The main underlying abnormalities in this group are:

- Congenital bicuspid aortic valves.
- Postinflammatory scarring.
- Mitral valve prolapse syndrome.
- Prosthetic valves.

The incidence has increased in Western countries in recent years, mainly as a result of patients surviving with structurally abnormal hearts and heart valves.

Types of infective endocarditis

Acute

The cause is usually a virulent organism, such as *Staphylococcus aureus*. It can affect either normal or abnormal heart valves.

The bacteria proliferate in the valve, causing necrosis and the generation of thrombotic vegetations. Consequently, there is destruction of valve leaflets with perforation and acute disturbance of valve function leading to acute heart failure.

Prognosis—disease is rapidly progressive and often fatal due to the incidence of embolic events, renal failure and heart failure.

Subacute

The typical cause here is poorly virulent organisms, such as *Streptococcus viridans*, infecting structurally abnormal valves.

The bacteria proliferate slowly in the thrombotic vegetation on damaged valve surfaces. Gradual valve destruction occurs, stimulating further thrombus formation with the potential for systemic embolisation.

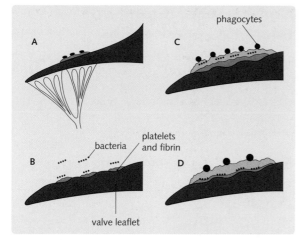

Fig. 6.21 Pathogenesis of vegetation formation in infective endocarditis. (A) Abnormality on endocardium of valve leaflet is coated with small deposits of platelets and fibrin (thrombus). (B) Circulating bacteria or fungi colonise the platelet thrombus. (C, D) Further layers of platelets and fibrin are deposited, and the microorganisms proliferate in the superficial layer of the vegetation. They are separated from blood by a thin layer of fibrinous material, which protects against immune destruction but allows diffusion of nutrients. (Adapted from Underwood, 2000.)

Causative organisms

Bacteria

Pathogens such as *Staphylococcus aureus*, alpha-haemolytic streptococci, pneumococci, meningococci and *Escherichia coli* are commonly responsible.

Fungi

Fungi such as *Candida* and *Aspergillus* can occasionally cause endocarditis, particularly in drug addicts, the immunosuppressed or those with valve prostheses.

The type of causative organism responsible depends on whether the affected valve is structurally normal or abnormal.

Infection of structurally normal valves

Infective organisms are pathogenic and directly invade the valve causing rapid destruction. This is commonly seen in intravenous drug addicts (often affecting the tricuspid valve), after open heart surgery and following septicaemia from other causes. Highly virulent forms of *Staphylococcus aureus* are often responsible for such infections.

Infection of structurally abnormal heart valves

Infective organisms are of low pathogenicity and are derived from normal commensal organisms of the skin, mouth, urinary tract and gut. Following trivial

---

Key clinical features of endocarditis are:
- Systemic symptoms—fever, weight loss and malaise due to cytokines (low-grade infection).
- Skin petechiae and microhaemorrhages in the retina and skin, particularly around the fingernails (splinter haemorrhages), caused by the deposition of immune complexes in small vessels — they also cause glomerulonephritis.
- Finger clubbing (cause unknown), occasionally with characteristic Janeway lesions and/or Osler's nodes.
- Splenomegaly and anaemia due to persistent bacteraemia.

Sequelae

The sequelae are as follows:

- Valvular regurgitation due to gradual destruction of valves leading to cardiac failure.
- Perivalvular abscesses following extension of the infection into the valve ring and myocardium, producing sinuses, fistulae, septal defects and abnormalities of conduction.
- Mycotic aneurysms—infection of the muscular wall of a medium-sized artery caused by emboli to the vasa vasorum.
- Multi-organ infarction—small emboli of infected thrombotic material enter the systemic circulation producing infarction of many organs especially the brain, spleen, and kidneys. Infarcted organs may in turn become infected by organisms within the occluding thrombus.

Complications of infective endocarditis are summarised in Fig. 6.22.

Non-bacterial thrombotic (marantic) endocarditis

Non-bacterial thrombotic endocarditis is inflammation of the valves with the formation of sterile thrombotic vegetations (marantic vegetations) on the closure lines of valve cusps. It occurs in severely debilitated patients with serious systemic disease, particularly malignancy.

Endocarditis of systemic lupus erythematosus (Libman–Sacks disease)

Thrombotic vegetations complicate SLE in 50% or more of fatal cases. The vegetations are small, meaning that valvular changes rarely give rise to any appreciable functional deficiency, but thrombotic material can fragment and cause embolic infarction.

Carcinoid heart disease

Carcinoid syndrome is caused by excess 5-hydroxytryptamine secretion by a carcinoid tumour (usually of the small intestine, which has metastasised to the liver) and can result in endocardial fibrosis of the tricuspid and pulmonary valves, in turn resulting in stenosis or incompetence.

Complications of artificial heart valves

Prosthetic valve diseases

The prosthetic valve diseases are:

- Thrombosis leading to valve obstruction or embolism.
- Valve failure due to breakage of a mechanical prosthesis, or tissue calcification and cusp rupture of bioprosthesis.
- Infective endocarditis from turbulence and prosthetic material; its incidence is 1–2% per year.
- Obstructive gradients—the valve may be too small or there may be tissue ingrowth of the pannus onto the valve ring.
- Haemolysis of red blood cells passing through a mechanical valve, occasionally leading to jaundice.

Precautions necessary to avoid complications of artificial heart valves

The precautions are lifelong anticoagulation (with warfarin) and appropriate prophylactic antibiotic therapy to protect against infective endocarditis, e.g. before dental procedures.

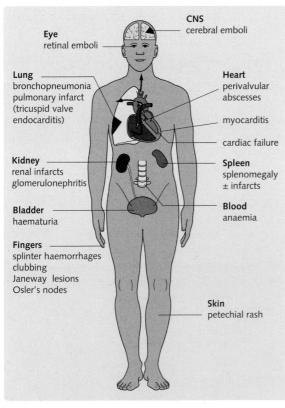

Fig. 6.22 Complications of infective endocarditis.

DISEASES OF THE MYOCARDIUM

Concepts of myocardial disease
Cardiomyopathy
This is a group of disorders in which the structural or functional abnormality primarily affects the myocardium. It should only be considered if all other potential causes of myocardial impairment have been excluded (e.g. hypertension, valvular or coronary artery disease).

Effects of cardiomyopathy
Cardiomyopathies usually cause progressive development of cardiac failure. The time scale varies from weeks to years depending on the specific pathology. In some instances, sudden cardiac death is the first manifestation of disease.

Classification
Cardiomyopathies can be grouped into two types according to aetiology:

1. Primary idiopathic cardiomyopathies—the aetiology is unknown.
2. Secondary cardiomyopathies (also known as specific heart muscle diseases)—diseases of the heart muscle associated with or caused by a systemic disease.

The terms 'cardiomyopathy' and 'myocarditis' are frequently confused: myocarditis refers to inflammation of the myocardium and it is a form of secondary cardiomyopathy, but it is not synonymous with cardiomyopathy.

Primary idiopathic cardiomyopathy
Primary cardiomyopathies follow three main patterns according to the dysfunction of the myocardium—dilated, hypertrophic obstructive or restrictive.

Dilated (congestive) cardiomyopathy
These are abnormalities of the myocardium causing poor systolic contraction. They are characterised by:

- Dilatation of the ventricles—usually left more than right.

- Thin, stretched chamber walls.
- Hypocontractile muscle.

Aetiology is often unidentifiable but the condition may represent end-stage myocardial damage for known causes, including viral myocarditis, alcohol and other forms of secondary cardiomyopathies.

Hypertrophic cardiomyopathy
A familial condition (usually autosomal dominant) resulting in hyperkinetic systolic function with marked reduction in systolic volume and difficulty in diastolic filling. This is characterised by:

- Gross hypertrophy of the heart walls, particularly affecting the interventricular septum.
- Loss of the normal parallel orientation of hypertrophied muscle fibres—disorganized branching.

The genetic mutations identified tend to affect the production of proteins making up the myocardial muscle unit (sarcomere). This condition may present in young adults and juveniles with sudden unexplained death on exertion (hypertrophic obstructive cardiomyopathy, HOCM). Less dramatic presentations include angina and breathlessness on exertion in a young person or repeated fainting attacks.

Restrictive cardiomyopathy
Abnormal stiffness of the myocardium results in impaired ventricular filling during diastole. The stiffness is caused by infiltration of the myocardium, for example:

- Amyloid in amyloidosis.
- Fibrosis in endomyocardial fibrosis (fibrosis of thrombotic material deposited on the endocardial surfaces).
- Haemochromatosis.

The condition causes high atrial pressures resulting in atrial hypertrophy → atrial dilatation → atrial fibrillation.

Secondary cardiomyopathies
Myocarditis
This rare disease is characterised by the presence of inflammatory cells in the myocardium. The clinical picture is highly variable, from an asymptomatic disorder with minor ECG changes, to rapidly progressing heart failure.

Aetiology

The vast majority of cases of myocarditis are either infectious or immune-mediated.

The infectious causes are:

- Viruses—viral infection is the commonest cause of myocarditis in the UK. Coxsackie virus is the most common culprit. Other agents include influenza, echovirus, HIV, CMV, poliomyelitis or mumps virus.
- Bacteria, e.g. *Corynebacterium diphtheriae* (diphtheria), Borrelia (Lyme disease).
- Chlamydiae and rickettsiae.
- Fungi, e.g. Candida.
- Protozoa, e.g. toxoplasmosis, *Trypanosoma cruzi* (Chagas' disease).
- Helminths, e.g. trichinosis.

The immune-mediated causes are:

- Post-streptococcal, e.g. acute rheumatic fever.
- Post-viral.
- SLE.
- Drug hypersensitivity, e.g. sulphonamides, doxorubicin, cyclophosphamide.
- Transplant rejection.

Other less common causes include sarcoidosis (see Chapter 7) and giant cell myocarditis, an acute fulminating form of fatal acute myocarditis.

Other secondary cardiomyopathies

Other causes of secondary cardiomyopathies are listed in Fig. 6.23.

Fig. 6.23 Aetiology of secondary cardiomyopathies

Causes	Example
Infection and inflammation	Myocarditis
Multisystem disease	Diabetes Amyloidosis Thyroid dysfunction Haemochromatosis
Toxic and metabolic disturbances	Alcohol Catecholamines Drugs, e.g. adriamycin
Primary muscle disorders	Muscular dystrophy Mitochondrial cytopathy

Fig. 6.23 Aetiology of secondary cardiomyopathies.

Neoplasms of the heart

Tumours of the heart are extremely rare. Examples include:

- Myxoma—a benign tumour of stellate cells, typically arising from the endocardium (usually of the left atrium).
- Connective tissue tumours, such as lipomas, fibromas and fibroelastomas.
- Malignant tumours, such as rhabdomyosarcomas.
- Metastatic or local-spread tumours.

DISEASES OF THE PERICARDIUM

Accumulation of fluid in the pericardial sac

Pericardial effusion

This is the accumulation of fluid within the pericardial cavity. Effusions may be:

- Serous—transudate has a low protein content (< 2 g/100 mL) and usually contains only very scanty mesothelial cells. Caused by heart failure, hypoalbuminaemia or myxoedema.
- Serosanguinous—exudate with high protein content (> 3 g/100 mL). Occurring with infection, uraemia, neoplasia or connective tissue disorders.
- Chylous—accumulation of lymphatic fluid occurring in the presence of lymphatic obstruction of pericardial drainage, most commonly due to neoplasms and tuberculosis.

The aetiology is of two types: inflammatory (e.g. acute pericarditis) and non-inflammatory. If non-inflammatory, at least one of the following effects must have occurred:

- ↑ Capillary permeability, e.g. severe hypothyroidism.
- ↑ Capillary hydrostatic pressure, e.g. congestive heart failure.
- ↓ Plasma oncotic pressure, e.g. cirrhosis and the nephrotic syndrome.

Clinical effects depend on the increase in pressure within the pericardium which, in turn, depends on:

- Volume of effusion—the greater the volume the greater the increase in internal pressure, and the greater the interference with cardiac function.

- Rate at which the fluid accumulates—sudden increase →marked elevation of pressure → severe cardiac chamber compression. Slow effusion (over weeks to months) → pericardium stretches → no elevation of pressure.
- Compliance characteristics of the pericardium— even small effusions may cause marked elevation of pressure if there is stiffness of the pericardium, e.g. chronic constrictive pericarditis.

The condition is often asymptomatic, but it may present with a dull constant ache in the left side of the chest. Unlike ischaemic cardiac pain, it is accentuated by inspiration, by movement, and by lying flat.

Haemopericardium

This is the accumulation of blood in the pericardial sac. The causes of haemopericardium are outlined in Fig. 6.24. In most cases, death occurs rapidly due to the sudden rise in intrapericardial cavity pressure, which prevents cardiac filling (cardiac tamponade): as little as 200–300 mL usually being sufficient.

Cardiac tamponade

In this condition, fluid (of any kind) accumulates under high pressure, compressing the cardiac chambers to such an extent that filling of the heart is severely limited, resulting in acute heart failure. The condition is often associated with malignant disease.

Diagnosis

The physical signs are:

- Sinus tachycardia.
- Increased jugular venous pulse (often with a further rise on inspiration—Kussmaul's sign).

- Decreased systemic blood pressure (producing shock in severe cases).
- Cyclical decrease in systolic blood pressure during each inspiration—pulsus paradoxus.

Investigations include echocardiography (which shows the presence of pericardial effusion with right ventricular diastolic collapse) and cardiac catheterisation combined with pericardiocentesis.

The management of cardiac tamponade depends on the extent of haemodynamic compromise. Severe cases may be rapidly fatal and require relief by emergency paracentesis; less critical cases require formal surgical drainage.

Pulseless electrical activity (electromechanical dissociation)

Pulseless electrical activity (PEA) is a condition in which electrical activity is normal or near normal on ECG, but there is no effective cardiac output. It is associated with a poor prognosis as it is often due to cardiac rupture, which is rarely amenable to treatment. However, treatable causes of PEA should not be overlooked.

Treatable causes of PEA can conveniently be remembered as the 4Hs and 4Ts:
- 4Hs—hypoxia, hypovolaemia, hypo/ hyperkalaemia and hypothaermia.
- 4Ts—thromboembolism, tamponade, toxins/therapeutics and tension pneumothorax.
Remembering these causes forms an important part of the advanced trauma life support (ATLS) management of critically ill patients.

Fig. 6.24 Aetiology of haemopericardium

Causes	Example
Rupture of heart	Traumatic, e.g. stab wound Spontaneous, e.g. myocardial infarct
Rupture of intrapericardial portion of aorta	Dissecting aneurysm Syphilitic aneurysm Traumatic
Haemorrhagic tendencies	Purpura Scurvy Hypoprothrombinaemia Anticoagulant therapy

Fig. 6.24 Aetiology of haemopericardium.

Pericarditis

Pericarditis, i.e. inflammation of the pericardium, is the main disorder of the pericardium. The condition is often complicated by the development of an effusion.

Acute pericarditis

In acute pericarditis both pericardial surfaces (visceral and parietal layers) are coated with a fibrin-rich acute inflammatory exudate. The loss of smoothness leads to the clinical sign of a friction rub. The causes of acute pericarditis are listed in Fig. 6.25.

Fig. 6.25 Aetiology of acute pericarditis.

Fig. 6.25 Aetiology of acute pericarditis	
Infarction	Myocardial infarction: local pericarditis over infarct is the commonest cause of pericarditis
Infective	Viral infections: second most common cause, usually clinically mild, rarely requiring hospital treatment Pyogenic: e.g.staphylococci, streptococci, haemophilus septicaemia or pneumonia Tuberculosis: spread to pericardium from tuberculous lymph nodes in mediastinum; now rare
Injury	Postoperative: following open heart surgery Pericarditis is diffuse, involving entire pericardial surface Heals by fibrosis → obliteration of pericardial cavity
Invasive	Malignant pericaritis: usually due to infiltration of pericardium by local spread from a primary bronchial tumour; less commonly the cause is blood-borne metastases from a distant site, e.g. malignant melanoma
Immuno-logical	Immune pericarditis: associated with rheumatic fever or may present in patient with systemic autoimmune disease, e.g. SLE, rheumatoid disease

Variants can be:

- Serous, non-bacterial inflammation—the exudate is a clear, straw-coloured and protein-rich fluid.
- Serofibrinous or fibrinous—occurs with MI. The exudate contains plasma protein including fibrinogen. This is the most common form of acute pericarditis.
- Suppurative (or purulent) pericarditis—associated with pyogenic bacterial infection, serosal surfaces are erythematous and coated with thick, creamy pus.
- Haemorrhagic—blood is mixed with inflammatory exudate.
- Caseous—fibrinous exudate with granulation tissue and areas of caseation caused by tuberculosis.

Clinical features

The clinical features of acute pericarditis are:

- Pleuritic chest pain—typically retrosternal pain radiating to the shoulders and neck.
- Fever.
- Pericardial friction rub.
- ECG abnormalities.

Remember the 'Five Is' of possible causes of acute pericarditis: infarctive, infective, injury, invasive and immunological.

Chronic pericarditis

Adhesive pericarditis

Although fibrinous pericarditis may resolve completely, it occasionally results in fibrinous adhesions or even in complete obliteration of the pericardial sac.

Constrictive pericarditis

Progressive fibrosis and calcification of the pericardium cause restriction of ventricular filling and interference with ventricular systole. The heart is effectively encased in a solid shell and filling is impaired. Calcification may extend into the myocardium, producing impaired myocardial contraction.

This condition often follows tuberculous pericarditis, but it can also complicate haemopericardium, viral pericarditis, rheumatoid arthritis and purulent pericarditis.

Clinical features

In chronic pericarditis, the fibrous tissue impairs venous return resulting in symptoms and signs of systemic venous congestion, namely raised jugular venous pressure, enlarged liver, and ascites. Atrial fibrillation is also common.

Rheumatic disease of the pericardium

Rheumatic disease of the pericardium is an acute form of pericarditis occurring with generalised pancarditis following streptococcal infection (see page 84).

ANEURYSMS

Definitions and concepts

Aneurysm

An aneurysm is an abnormal localised, permanent, dilatation of an artery. The term can also be applied to the wall of the heart. Types of aneurysm are shown in Fig. 6.26:

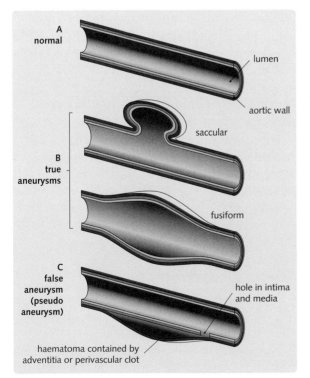

Fig. 6.26 Aortic aneurysms. (A) Normal. (B) True aneurysms. (C) False aneurysm (pseudoaneurysm).

- True aneurysms—the wall is formed by one or more layers of the affected vessel. These can be saccular or fusiform.
- False aneurysms (pseudoaneurysms)—the vascular wall is breached (usually following trauma or infection), allowing communication with an extravascular space that is limited by surrounding tissue (usually an organized haematoma).

True aneurysm morphology

Saccular aneurysms take the form of globular sacs, whereas fusiform aneurysms are spindle-shaped due to long segments of the vessel wall being affected around the whole circumference.

Main causes of aneurysms

Any abnormality that weakens the media may produce an aneurysm:

- Atherosclerosis—the most common cause, typically affecting the abdominal aorta causing thinning and fibrous replacement of media.
- Cystic medial degeneration—focal degeneration of media with the formation of small cyst-like spaces filled with mucopolysaccharide. Aetiology may be idiopathic or associated with connective tissue diseases, e.g. Marfan's syndrome and Ehlers–Danlos syndrome.

The condition is generally confined to the aorta and the origins of its major branches. Extensive disease leads to dissecting aneurysm. These diseases include:

- Infectious aortitis, e.g. syphilitic aortitis (rare, typically affecting the ascending and transverse portions of the aortic arch causing inflammatory destruction of the media with fibrous replacement) and mycotic aneurysms (small saccular dilatations with destruction of the wall caused by bacteria in infected thrombus).
- Vasculitic syndromes (see pages 93–94)—inflammation of the vessels caused by immune complex deposition or cell-mediated immune reactions of the arterial wall leading to a weakening of the vessel wall then aneurysmal dilatations.
- Congenital aneurysms.

Pathogenesis

The majority of aneurysms occur because of a weakening of the arterial wall with loss of elasticity and contractility. Stretching of the weakened wall is gradually progressive due to haemodynamic pressure forces producing an increased thinning of the wall until eventual rupture occurs.

The build-up of layers of thrombus within the lumen of the aneurysmal sac is protective, but not usually sufficient to repair the defect and reconstitute a normal lumen to the artery.

> The most frequent cause of an aneurysm is an atheroma. However, any abnormality that weakens the media may predispose a patient.

Main complications

The main complications of aneurysms are rupture with critical haemorrhage and predisposition to thrombosis. The risk of rupture is usually greater with an increased size of aneurysm; high blood pressure is the most important factor in increasing the rate of growth.

Abdominal aortic aneurysms

Abdominal aortic aneurysms (AAAs) are more common in men, especially over 60 years of age.

Aetiology—Atherosclerosis is the most common cause of abdominal aneurysms. However, they may also arise as a result of inflammation (vasculitis) or infection (mycotic aneurysms). The potential of a genetic predisposition to AAAs is currently being researched as it is thought that many at-risk individuals have poorer quality aortic connective tissue.

Site—80% of AAAs are situated below the origin of the renal arteries and are thus amenable to resection and replacement by graft.

Morphology—Atherosclerotic aneurysms produce a fusiform dilatation of the wall.

Symptoms and signs

The majority of AAAs are asymptomatic, but occasionally patients are aware of a pulsatile mass. It is often first suspected because of aortic dilatation observed on radiographs, especially if the walls of the aneurysm are calcified. It may also come to attention by careful palpation during physical examination.

Symptoms may occur because of compression of neighbouring structures by the expanding aneurysm, e.g. back pain from vertebral compression, or vomiting following duodenal obstruction.

Confirmation of an AAA is achieved by ultrasonography, CT, MRI or arteriography.

Consequences

Rupture is the most devastating consequence and is often fatal. This may occur suddenly without warning or, alternatively, blood may slowly leak into the vessel wall resulting in pain and local tenderness.

Haemorrhage can occur into the retroperitoneal space, abdominal cavity or erode into the intestines resulting in massive gastrointestinal (GI) bleeding.

Thrombus formation on large atheromatous plaques is favoured, increasing the risk of embolic events, e.g. stroke.

Prognostic factors

Fifty per cent of all abdominal aortic aneurysms that are more than 6 cm in transverse diameter rupture within 2 years if not surgically resected. Aneurysms less than 6 cm across may also rupture, albeit less frequently.

Mortalities of emergency and elective surgery

Elective surgical repair has a much lower mortality than emergency surgery for rupture and it is, therefore, recommended for most abdominal aortic aneurysms greater than 5.5 cm in diameter, or those which are rapidly progressing or symptomatic. Mortality for surgical repair of abdominal aneurysms is also lower than that of thoracic aneurysms.

Aortic dissection

An aortic dissection is a tear in the intima of the aorta allowing the entry of blood into media with separation of a 'flap' of intima from the rest of the aortic wall. A false lumen is created, usually between the inner two thirds and outer third of the medial thickness giving the appearance of a double-barrelled aorta.

Types of dissecting aneurysms

There are two types:

1. Type A (67% of dissecting aneurysms)—arise in the ascending aorta with or without extension into the descending aorta.
2. Type B (33% of dissecting aneurysms)—are confined to the descending aorta, distal to the origin of the left subclavian artery.

Epidemiology—there are approximately 600 cases per year in the UK, occurring most commonly in people between 50 and 70 years old and affecting males more than females by 2 : 1.

Predisposing factors are:

- Hypertension.
- Aortic atherosclerosis.
- Aortic aneurysm.
- Connective tissue disorders (e.g. Marfan's syndrome).
- Pregnancy.
- Congenital abnormalities of the aortic valve.

Consequences

The false lumen inevitably ruptures, either:

- Externally—external rupture leads to massive fatal bleed into the thoracic cavity or, less commonly, the pericardial sac, pleural cavity or abdomen.
- Internally—rarely, blood tracks back into the lumen by rupturing through the inner media and intima forming a double-channelled aorta.

Aortic dissection:
- Sudden onset severe chest pain, radiating back between the shoulder blades.
- Usually hypertension.
- Asymmetry of brachial, carotid, or femoral pulses.
- Mediastinal broadening and aortic 'knuckle' distortion on chest radiography.
- Left-sided pleural effusion.

Diagnosis—echocardiography (transthoracic and/or transoesophageal), CT or MRI.

Management:
- Type A—emergency surgical repair.
- Type B—hypertension control with bed rest; surgical intervention may be needed if there is leakage or organ ischaemia.

Prognosis—this condition is fatal without treatment: 25% die within 24 hours, 50% within the week, and almost all by 1 year.

Syphilitic (luetic) aneurysms

Tertiary syphilis is now rare in the Western world. However, cardiovascular complications of untreated syphilis manifest one to three decades after the initial infection. They include:

- Inflammation of the arterial media (aortitis), primarily of the ascending aorta.
- Aneurysm formation (especially thoracic aorta) due to deterioration of elastic fibres and weakening of the media.
- Aortic regurgitation—dilatation of the aortic root weakens aortic valve support.
- Narrowing of the coronary artery ostia by inflammation and aortic intimal proliferation leading to increased myocardial ischaemia.

These complications are now rare due to the early administration of antibiotic therapy.

INFLAMMATORY AND NEOPLASTIC VASCULAR DISEASE

Concepts and classification

Vasculitides

This is a group of disorders characterised by inflammation of the blood vessel walls (vasculitis). Vasculitis can affect capillaries, venules, arterioles, arteries and, occasionally, large veins.

Effects

The effects are:

- Mild cases—transient damage to the vessel wall, which produces leakage of red blood cells.
- Severe cases—irreversible vessel wall destruction resulting in ischaemia and organ damage with associated systemic disturbances, commonly fevers, myalgias, arthralgias and malaise.

Classification

Vasculitis can be classified either according to the size of the vessel affected (Fig. 6.27) or according to the pathogenesis of the inflammation (Fig. 6.28).

Idiopathic vasculitis

The aetiology is unknown but the disorders are as follows:

Fig. 6.27 Classification of vasculitis according to size of affected vessel

Size of vessel	Disorders
Large, medium and small	Syphilitic aortitis Takayasu's disease Giant cell arteritis Kawasaki's disease Rheumatoid disease
Medium and small	Wegener's granulomatosis Polyarteritis nodosa Buerger's disease SLE
Small	Small vessel disease of arterioles, capillaries and venules Henoch–Schönlein purpura

Fig. 6.27 Classification of vasculitis according to the size of the affected vessel.

Fig. 6.28 Classification of vasculitis by pathogenesis

Pathogenesis	Disorders
Idiopathic	Giant cell arteritis Scleroderma (systemic sclerosis) Takayasu's (pulseless) disease Kawasaki's disease Buerger's disease
Immune-mediated	Polyarteritis nodosa Wegener's granulomatosis Rheumatoid vasculitis Systemic lupus erythematosus Henoch–Schönlein purpura
Infectious	Syphilitic aortitis Bacterial aortitis

Fig. 6.28 Classification of vasculitis by pathogenesis.

- Giant cell arteritis (see below).
- Scleroderma (systemic sclerosis)—vascular changes are similar to those of benign or malignant hypertension, but only about 25% of patients are hypertensive. The condition is associated with progressive subcutaneous fibrosis leading to a marked tightening of the skin of the arms and hands; there are no effective treatments.
- Takayasu's (pulseless) disease—a rare chronic inflammatory and granulomatous disorder of the aorta and its proximal branches, typically affecting young or middle-aged females. The condition is characterised by severe necrotising inflammation of all layers of affected vessel walls with fibrous replacement of muscle and a reduction of lumen. It presents clinically with hypertension or ischaemic symptoms of the arms, with loss of arm pulses.
- Kawasaki's disease—a disease of infants, primarily in Japan, affecting the main aortic branch arteries particularly the coronary arteries. It is characterised by medial fibroblastic thickening and, sometimes, aneurysm formation.
- Buerger's disease (thromboangitis obliterans)—a rare disease with a strong association with smoking, usually in young males. The condition mainly affects the small arteries of the arms and lower leg, which show intimal fibrosis, thrombus formation and adventitial tissue changes affecting adjacent veins and nerves. Clinically, peripheral gangrene develops in the fingers and toes; the disease is progressive and amputations are often required.

Immune-mediated vasculitis

Pathogenesis is due to immune complex formation between antigens and antibodies, which become trapped in venule walls and stimulate an acute inflammatory response with neutrophil chemotaxis. Neutrophils release enzymes that destroy the vessel wall.

There are two main types:

1. Hypersensitivity (neutrophilic) vasculitis—most common pattern affecting capillaries and venules; usually manifests as a skin rash, often as a result of an allergy to a drug or occasionally arising as an allergic rash in viraemia or bacteraemia. It also occurs in Henoch–Schönlein purpura, serum sickness and cryoglobulinaemia.
2. Multi-organ autoimmune diseases, e.g. SLE and rheumatoid disease (mainly affects the aorta).

Autoantibodies that react against neutrophils (antineutrophil cytoplasmic antibodies; ANCA) can be detected in 90% of patients with Wegener's granulomatosis and in other types of immune-mediated vasculitis. Identification of these antibodies in serum is used in diagnostic evaluation of patients with possible vasculitis.

Infectious vasculitis

These disorders include:

- Syphilitic aortitis—tertiary manifestation of syphilis typically affecting the ascending and transverse portions of the aortic arch causing inflammatory destruction of media with fibrous replacement.

- Other infections—bacteria in infected thrombi can cause destruction of vessel walls with the development of small saccular dilatations and mycotic aneurysms.

Giant cell (temporal) arteritis

Giant cell arteritis is a systemic disease that mainly involves arteries in the head and neck region, particularly the temporal arteries (hence the alternative name of temporal arteritis).

Epidemiology—the disease is relatively common, affecting 10 per 100 000 per year in the general population in Europe. Incidence increases with age, and it is rare in people under 50 years; it affects females more than males by 2 : 1.

Aetiology—an idiopathic disease with associations with certain types of human leucocyte antigen (HLA) DR (HLA-DR).

The microscopic appearance of vessels is as follows:

- Thickened nodular vessel wall → decreased lumen.
- Necrosis of inner media and gradual replacement with fibrosis.
- Fragmentation of internal elastic lamina.
- Inflammatory cell infiltration—mainly T lymphocytes but also histiocytes and giant cells (hence the name).
- Often complicated by thrombosis.

Clinical features—patients have ill-defined symptoms of:

- Malaise.
- Tiredness.
- Severe headaches.
- Visual disturbance from involvement of the ophthalmic arteries. This is a medical emergency requiring prompt treatment to prevent blindness.
- An association with polymyalgia rheumatica, a musculoskeletal condition causing muscle pain and stiffness classically in the upper body.

Investigations characteristically reveal high ESR and/or C-reactive protein (CRP). Diagnosis is made by biopsy of the temporal artery with histological investigation. Management is with high-dose corticosteroid therapy to control the disease.

Polyarteritis nodosa

This systemic disease is characterised by inflammatory necrosis of the walls of small and medium-sized arteries. Although the disease is systemic, it causes patchy and focal inflammation with only parts of some arteries being involved.

Epidemiology—a rare disease (about 5–10 per million per year in most populations), but it can occur in all age groups; males more than females by 2 : 1.

Aetiology—the cause is unknown but the presence of antineutrophil cytoplasmic antibodies (i.e. ANCA positive) suggests an autoimmune pathogenesis. There is also an association with chronic hepatitis B infection.

Pathogenesis—inflammatory destruction of the vessel wall with necrosis of muscle cells and destruction of the elastic lamina. Healing occurs with fibrous replacement of the muscular media. Extensive damage to the intima predisposes to thrombosis, which is often followed by vessel occlusion and downstream infarction.

Microscopically, the artery wall shows:

- Inflammatory cell infiltration—neutrophils and eosinophils are most numerous.
- Fibrinoid necrosis of segments of artery wall.
- Thrombosis, which is common.

Clinical features include systemic features of inflammation (fever, weight loss, myalgia, and muscle wasting) and the effects of vessel occlusion producing small areas of infarction. Tissues most seriously affected are the kidneys, GI tract and liver.

Diagnosis is by:

- Blood—neutrophilia and raised ESR.
- ANCA, which are present in most cases.
- Tissue biopsy, usually of a kidney or asymptomatic muscle.

Management is by cyclophosphamide with corticosteroids, which has significantly improved the outcome. Antihypertensive drugs reduce morbidity from hypertensive complications.

Prognosis is variable; many patients relapse after treatment.

Neoplastic vascular disease
Benign
Haemangiomas

Haemangiomas are common developmental malformations composed of dilated vascular spaces derived from blood vessels.

There are three types of haemangioma:

1. Capillary haemangiomas (strawberry naevi), which are composed of small, capillary-like vessels.

2. Cavernous haemangiomas, which are composed of cavernous, endothelial-lined spaces (vein-like vessels).

3. Sclerosing haemangiomas, which are fibrous nodules containing iron pigment produced as a result of fibrosis or sclerosis of a capillary haemangioma.

> Haemangiomas are not 'true' tumours, but they are often grouped with neoplasms because they appear as localised tissue masses. They are more accurately described as hamartomas, i.e. non-neoplastic overgrowths of tissue.

Telangiectasias

Dilatations of capillaries are often seen in the elderly and those with irradiated skin or liver failure (spider naevi). Vessels are dilated but histologically normal.

Malignant

Kaposi's sarcoma

Kaposi's sarcoma (KS) is a malignant tumour thought to be derived from lymphatic endothelial cells; it is rapidly becoming more important and common. There are four patterns of disease:

1. Endemic KS (seen in Africa)—is highly malignant in children (through lymphatic spread) with a more indolent course in adults (through blood spread).
2. Classic (chronic) KS—is a rare, low-grade malignant tumour of the skin that develops in the lower limbs of elderly males; there are blood and lymph node metastases.
3. KS in therapeutic immunosuppression, which resembles classic KS. Often develops in transplant recipients.
4. Epidemic KS—is a highly malignant tumour of the skin seen in patients with acquired immune deficiency syndrome (AIDS); spreads to lymph nodes and the visceral organs.

Angiosarcoma

A malignant tumour of blood vessel endothelium. This most commonly occurs as a raised bluish-red patch on the face or scalp of elderly people, which is often confused with a benign haemangioma.

Progressive enlargement of the tumour is accompanied by ulceration and, later, metastasis to regional lymph nodes.

DISEASES OF THE VEINS AND LYMPHATICS

Varicose veins

Varicose veins are persistently distended superficial veins in the lower limbs (long and short saphenous veins). They result from incompetent valves that allow the veins to become engorged with blood under the influence of gravity.

Epidemiology—the condition affects 10–20% of the general population at some age. There is an increasing incidence with age, and it is most common above 50. It affects females more than males by 4 : 1.

Figure 6.29 lists the predisposing factors of varicose veins.

Anatomy of varicose veins—the superficial and deep venous plexuses of the lower limb are connected by perforating veins (Fig. 6.30).

Pathogenesis—the return of blood from the deep veins is aided by normal contraction of the calf and thigh muscles. If the valves in the perforating veins become incompetent, blood is forced from deep venous plexuses to superficial venous plexuses resulting in increased pressure in the superficial

Fig. 6.29 Predisposing factors of varicose veins
Defective support of vessel wall
Familial tendency: in approx. 40% of all cases Sex: significantly increased incidence in females Obesity: adipose tissue = poor venous support; muscle = good venous support Age: degenerative changes in surrounding tissues and decreased activity of muscles → loss of venous support
Increased venous pressure
Standing occupations: increased incidence in occupations involving prolonged standing (venous pressure is greater on standing) Pregnancy Intravascular thrombosis Tumour masses pressing on veins (e.g. uterine fibroids and ovarian tumours) Garters and other constrictions

Fig. 6.29 Predisposing factors of varicose veins.

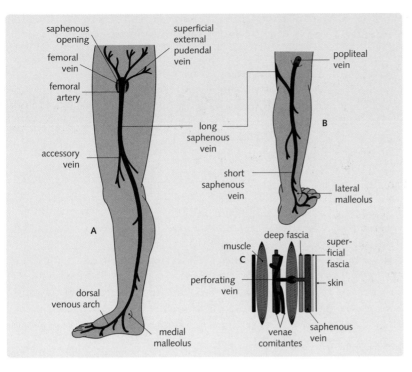

Fig. 6.30 Superficial veins of the right lower limb. (A) Long saphenous vein. (B) Short saphenous vein. (C) 'Venous pump' showing valved perforating veins, which link deep and superficial veins.

veins. Combined with prolonged blood stasis, there is a tendency towards the development of varicosities.

> Varicose leg ulcers are a common clinical condition, and they are associated with chronic venous insufficiency.

Morphological changes

The morphological changes are:

- Increased pressure produces a dilatation of the lumen and an increased tension on vessel walls with compensatory hypertrophy of the muscle and elastic tissues.
- Prolonged increased pressure produces irregular atrophy of muscle and elastic lamina with fibrous replacement leading to stretched, tortuous veins with localised bulging.

Sequelae of varicose veins

The sequelae are:

- Oedema (of lower limbs) due to increased hydrostatic pressure.
- Stasis dermatitis—varicose dermatitis with pigmentation due to haemosiderin deposition.
- Varicose ulcers—dermatitis may proceed to ulceration, which is very slow to heal. Usually on the medial aspect of the ankle or lower leg.
- Thrombosis and embolism are very rare sequelae; these tend to affect deep veins.

Venous thrombosis

This was considered earlier in the chapter (see page 76).

Lymphangitis and lymphoedema

Lymphangitis

Lymphangitis is inflammation of lymphatic channels draining any focus of infection. The channels are dilated and contain inflammatory cells. The condition may result in the spread of the infection in some cases, e.g. in tuberculosis. Rarely, cellulitis or focal abscesses may develop.

Lymphoedema

Lymphoedema is oedema of the tissues caused by obstruction of the lymphatics.

Causes

The causes of obstructive lymphoedema are:

- Metastatic spread of tumours causing mechanical blockage.
- Surgical removal of nodes.
- Post-irradiation fibrosis.
- Filariasis (elephantiasis)—nematode infection of lymph nodes (most common culprit is *Wuchereria bancrofti*); transmitted to man by the bite of an infected mosquito.
- Post-inflammatory thrombosis and scarring, e.g. lymphogranuloma venereum.
- Primary lymphatic disorders (rare).

Effects

The effects of obstructive lymphoedema are:

- Gross swelling.
- Increased predisposition to attacks of lymphangitis and ulceration.
- Severe cases result in thickening of skin and overgrowth of dermal connective tissues leading to elephantiasis.

Pathology of the respiratory system

Objectives

In this chapter, you will learn to:

- Describe common disorders of the upper respiratory tract affecting the nose, nasopharynx and larynx.
- Define the differences between obstructive and restrictive lung diseases.
- Describe the pathological processes in chronic obstructive pulmonary disease, including emphysema and chronic bronchitis.
- Recognise asthma as a common cause of obstructive lung disease and describe the differences between intrinsic and extrinsic forms.
- Describe cystic fibrosis and bronchiectasis.
- Understand the effect of interstitial lung diseases on producing a restrictive pattern of lung function.
- Describe infections of the lung, most notably the pneumonias and tuberculosis.
- Recall the neoplastic diseases of the lung, particularly the four most common pathological patterns.
- Describe lung disorders of vascular and iatrogenic origin.
- Understand disorders of the pleura, notably effusions, pneumothorax and neoplasms.

DISORDERS OF THE UPPER RESPIRATORY TRACT

The nose and nasopharynx

Rhinitis

Rhinitis, inflammation of the nasal mucosa, is the most common nasal disorder seen in family practice. The condition may be either acute or chronic.

Acute rhinitis

Aetiology of acute rhinitis is either:

- Infective.
- Allergic.

Infectious rhinitis is usually of viral origin, e.g. the common cold (rhinoviruses, adenoviruses) and influenza (influenza virus). Virally induced inflammation of surface epithelial cells is followed by exudation of fluid and mucus from the damaged surface ('runny nose'). Later, submucosal oedema produces swelling, which may lead to a partial blockage of the nasal airways.

Allergic rhinitis ('hay fever') is a type I (IgE-mediated) hypersensitivity reaction to inhaled materials such as grass and pollens, producing a mixed serous–mucous exudate and submucosal oedema leading to nasal blockage. Eosinophils are prominent in the inflammatory infiltrate.

Chronic rhinitis

Chronic rhinitis can be caused by repeated attacks of acute rhinitis, which often develop a secondary bacterial infection. It may result in the development of nasal polyps.

Macroscopically, nasal polyps are typically smooth-surfaced, creamy, semi-translucent, ovoid masses.

Microscopically, they have oedematous tissue with scattered infiltrate of chronic inflammatory cells including plasma cells. Eosinophils are often very numerous in allergic polyps.

Sinusitis

This is the acute or chronic inflammation of the sinuses.

Acute sinusitis

The most important type of sinus inflammation is acute maxillary sinusitis (ethmoidal and frontal sinusitis being less common).

Aetiology—usually secondary to acute or chronic rhinitis.

Pathogenesis—rhinitis is usually associated inflammation of the sinus linings; swelling of the mucosa around the drainage foramen of the maxillary sinus in the nasal cavity may cause stasis of maxillary sinus secretions. Stasis predisposes to secondary bacterial infection with alteration of the static maxillary fluid from seromucous to purulent.

In severe cases, the infection may spread into the ethmoid and frontal sinuses with a risk of spread of infection to the meninges. Orbital cellulitis may also complicate acute sinusitis.

Chronic sinusitis

This condition is characterised by chronically thickened and inflamed mucosa of the sinuses and by persistent fluid accumulation.

The condition may arise as a result of:

- Acute sinusitis from failure of drainage of acutely inflamed sinus.
- Chronic inhalation of irritant, e.g. cigarette smoke, industrial exposure.
- Nasal obstruction as a result of a severely deviated nasal septum or from the presence of nasal polyps.

Kartagener's syndrome

This is a syndrome of bronchiectasis, sinusitis and situs inversus (transposition of viscera). Sinusitis is caused by abnormal ciliary function resulting in a failure to clear mucus and bacteria.

Necrotising lesions

Mucormycotic infections

This fulminant opportunistic fungal infection of the nose most commonly affects diabetics or those who are immunosuppressed. It may be rapidly fatal unless treated promptly with systemic antifungals.

Wegener's granulomatosis

An autoimmune granulomatous vasculitis that frequently presents with nasal lesions.

Lethal midline granuloma (lymphoma)

This is a condition presenting with progressive granulomatous inflammation, ulceration and destruction of the structures in the upper respiratory tract, i.e. the nose, nasopharynx, palate and sinuses. It is thought to be a form of lymphoma affecting natural killer cells, and may occur alongside lymphomatous disease elsewhere in the body.

Untreated, death occurs from systemic disease caused by erosion of blood vessels, local infection or the development of pneumonia.

Neoplasms

Nasopharyngeal angiofibroma

This rare benign tumour (also known as juvenile angiofibroma) occurs almost exclusively in males between 10 and 25 years old. The lesions are typically located in the nasopharynx rather than the nose, and may mimic a malignant tumour due to their rapid growth and tendency to erode bone. Ulceration and bleeding are common.

Inverted papilloma

A benign, endophytic (hence 'inverted') tumour of adults, this is associated with human papillomavirus (HPV) infection, probably HPV types 6 and 11. It can be difficult to eradicate and may recur. Malignant transformation occurs in approximately 3%.

Plasmacytomas

This malignant tumour is composed of monoclonal plasma cells. It presents as a soft, haemorrhagic nasal/nasopharyngeal mass, which may rarely progress to disseminated myeloma after many years.

Olfactory neuroblastoma

This is a rare tumour presenting in the upper part of the nasal cavity, often as a haemorrhagic mass with evidence of bone destruction. The tumours usually develop from neuroendocrine cells found in the olfactory mucosa. They are highly malignant and may metastasise widely.

Nasopharyngeal carcinoma

This is a squamous or anaplastic carcinoma of the nasopharynx (part of the pharynx that lies immediately behind the nasal cavities) with characteristic abundant lymphoid tissue in the stroma.

It is strongly associated with Epstein–Barr virus infection, the virus being demonstrable in tumour cells in most cases. The carcinoma is most commonly found in certain parts of Africa and is rare elsewhere in the world.

The tumours often remain small and undetected until metastasis to the lymph nodes in the neck has occurred.

The prognosis is good with radiation therapy: the 5-year survival rate is 80% for localised disease and 50% for advanced disease.

The larynx

Acute laryngitis

This acute inflammation of the larynx may be:

- Infective—the most common form, usually secondary to viral or bacterial upper respiratory tract infection involving the nose, sinuses, etc.

- Allergic—following inhalation or ingestion of an allergen.
- Irritative—following inhalation or ingestion of irritant gases or fluids (e.g. cigarette smoke) or irritation by mechanical factors, e.g. endotracheal intubation.

Sequelae of acute laryngitis

- Resolution—infective causes typically resolve without complications.
- Spread of infection may occur throughout the respiratory tract with the development of tracheobronchitis, bronchopneumonia or lung abscesses; this is more common in the elderly or debilitated due to a poor cough reflex.
- Airway obstruction—laryngeal oedema can result in a life-threatening narrowing of the airway, especially in children (whose airways are narrower) suffering from *Haemophilus influenzae* epiglottitis or in cases of corrosive chemical ingestion.

Croup

Croup is acute inflammation and obstruction of the respiratory tract involving the larynx, trachea and bronchi. It usually affects young children aged 6 months to 3 years.

Aetiology—typically caused by viral infection but secondary bacterial infection can occur.

The condition produces symptoms of laryngitis accompanied by signs of obstruction: harsh difficult breathing (inspiratory stridor), a rising pulse rate, restlessness and cyanosis.

Treatment is by reassurance and humidification of inspired air, which usually reverses the symptoms. In severe cases, the obstruction may require emergency intubation or tracheostomy.

Chronic laryngitis

Chronic inflammation of the larynx is most commonly seen in heavy cigarette smokers. It may lead to a permanent thickening of the laryngeal mucosa and submucosa, particularly where there is associated excess production of keratin ('smoker's keratosis').

Overlying epidermis may also undergo keratotic thickening with dysplastic change in the basal layer; this is a predisposing factor in the development of squamous carcinoma of the larynx.

Reactive nodules

Polyps

This common benign lesion is associated with upper respiratory tract infection or occurs after vocal abuse, e.g. shouting. Presentation is with hoarseness that will not resolve until the polyp is removed.

Singer's nodules

These are smooth, round, minute nodules located at the nodal point (junction between the anterior third and posterior two thirds of the vocal cords). Nodules are especially common in singers and professional voice users, and they can alter the character of the voice even when only a few millimeters in diameter. They consist of oedematous connective tissue with submucosal fibrosis covered by squamous epithelium.

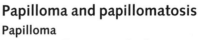

Reactive nodules of the larynx affect men more than women. Remember that polyps are unilateral lesions whereas singer's nodules are bilateral.

Papilloma and papillomatosis

Papilloma

Warty papillomas on the larynx are usually due to infection by the human papillomavirus (HPV 11 and 16). The lesions are usually solitary and confined to the true vocal cords. Papilloma is clinically and histologically difficult to distinguish from early verrucous carcinomas (see below).

Juvenile laryngeal papillomatosis

These multiple, soft, pink papillomas on the vocal cords are largely confined to children. Lesions often extend into other parts of the larynx, sometimes even down the trachea, and they have the histological features of florid viral warts. Spontaneous regression often occurs at puberty, although the lesions are typically difficult to eradicate if this does not happen.

Squamous cell carcinoma of the larynx

This accounts for 1–2% of cancers with an incidence of 1–2 per 100 000 per year worldwide. It typically presents after 40 years of age, affecting males more than females (but the incidence is rising in females). The risk factors are smoking, radiation to the head and neck, carcinoma *in situ* and keratosis (see above).

The affected sites are:

- Supraglottic region (30%), i.e. the lower epiglottis, false cords, ventricles and arytenoids—often presents with dysphagia (difficulty swallowing).

- Glottic region (60%)—true vocal cords and anterior and posterior commissures. The best prognosis follows early detection because this area is alymphatic, which restricts the routes for metastasis. The earliest symptom is hoarseness, which should always be investigated if persisting for more than 4 weeks.
- Subglottic region (10%)—arising below the true vocal cords and above the first tracheal ring; poor prognosis as late presentation is common (rich lymphatic supply to this area).

Macroscopically, they are ulcerated, diffuse, grey, solid or papillary lesions.

Microscopically, the majority are well-differentiated, keratinising squamous carcinomas; a minority are poorly differentiated with spindle cells.

Spread can be:

- Local—to adjacent laryngeal structures but often confined by laryngeal cartilages for a considerable time. The presence of a palpable neck lump usually indicates metastatic disease.
- Lymphatic—to regional lymph nodes.
- Haematogenous—occurs late if at all; lungs are the most common site.

The prognosis depends on location, extent of spread and the presence of lymph node metastasis. The overall 5-year survival is as follows:

- Glottic tumours—80%.
- Supraglottic tumours—65%.
- Subglottic tumours—40%.

Verrucous carcinoma

This is a variant of laryngeal squamous cell carcinoma, often presenting as a large, warty, papillary tumour with all the clinical features of malignancy. It usually affects the true vocal cords, the lesions being composed of benign-looking squamous epithelium with hyperkeratosis. However, the tumour is locally destructive and it requires surgical removal to prevent fatal obstruction or laryngeal destruction. Metastasis is rare.

DISORDERS OF THE LUNGS

Atelectasis

This is a defective expansion and collapse of the lung. It may occur as a result of:

- Obstruction.
- Compression.
- Scarring.
- Surfactant loss.

Obstructive causes

Obstruction of the larger bronchial tubes leads to resorption of air from the lung distal to the obstruction. Causes of obstruction can be within the lung (e.g. mucus plugs in bronchiectasis, inhaled foreign bodies) or outside the lung (enlarged lymph nodes as in tuberculosis or lung cancer).

Patchy atelectasis describes the pattern of atelectasis associated with chronic obstructive airway diseases.

Compressive causes

Compressive atelectasis is the compression of the lung caused by the accumulation of fluid or air in the pleural cavity, e.g. following a pneumothorax.

Scarring

Scarring of the lung may cause contraction of the parenchyma and lung collapse.

Surfactant loss

Surfactant is a surface active agent produced by type 2 pneumocytes (alveolar cells). It reduces surface tension and gives the lung sufficient compliance to expand without collapse. Surfactant loss can be either developmental or acquired and leads to a generalised failure of lung expansion, termed microatelectasis.

Lack of surfactant causes respiratory distress in premature infants; steroids may be administered to the mother to aid fetal lung development (and surfactant production) if premature labour is inevitable.

Consequences of atelectasis

The collapse of a lung has important clinical consequences as respiratory function will be disturbed and there is a predisposition to infection. Expansion can be aided by physiotherapy and bronchoscopy-mediated removal of the obstructive/compressive cause. However, prolonged atelectasis becomes irreversible.

Classification of diffuse lung disease

Obstructive lung diseases

Obstructive lung diseases are those in which there is obstruction to the flow of air within the lungs, although the lungs themselves may be hyperinflated. Disorders include emphysema, chronic bronchitis, bronchiectasis and asthma.

Chronic obstructive pulmonary disease (COPD) is used clinically where emphysema and chronic bronchitis occur together, almost always as the result of long-term cigarette smoking.

Restrictive lung diseases

Restrictive lung diseases are those in which there is obstruction to the expansion of the lungs (e.g. due to fibrosis or oedema) such that they can only take in a limited amount of air. In these diseases, although the lungs are often underinflated, the rate of air flow is unaffected. Causes of this restrictive pattern are covered in more detail later under 'Diffuse interstitial diseases' (see page 109).

Both obstructive and restrictive lung diseases can cause significant respiratory impairment with a characteristic pattern of pulmonary function tests (Fig. 7.1 and Fig. 7.2).

Chronic obstructive pulmonary disease

COPD is a chronic, slowly progressive disease of airflow limitation caused by an abnormal inflammatory response of the lungs to noxious substances (usually from cigarette smoking).

Pathological changes

COPD classically involves three overlapping pathological processes:

1. Chronic bronchitis—this obstructs large airways by increasing mucus production. Smoking also disrupts the 'mucociliary escalator' that lifts mucus out of the airways, so promoting obstruction.

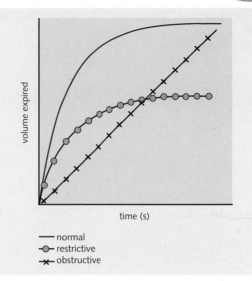

Fig. 7.2 Illustration of a normal, obstructive deficit and restrictive deficit vitalography.

2. Emphysema—this destroys the lung parenchyma.
3. Bronchiolitis—this describes inflammation of the small airways (bronchioles).

Chronic bronchitis and emphysema are considered in more detail in separate sections below.

Diagnosis

Common symptoms of COPD are persistent cough, sputum production and breathlessness. If combined with a strong history of tobacco or pollutant exposure, lung function tests are performed (see Figs. 7.1 and 7.2). These are suggestive of COPD if:

- Forced expired volume in one second (FEV_1) is less than 80% predicted.
- FEV_1/forced vital capacity (FVC) ratio is less than 70% predicted.

Fig. 7.1 Characteristic patterns of lung function tests in obstructive and restrictive lung diseases

	Obstructive lung diseases	Restrictive lung diseases
Vital capacity (VC)	↓ or normal	↓↓
FEV_1	↓↓	↓
FEV_1/VC ratio	↓	Normal or ↑
Peak respiratory flow rate (PEFR)	↓	Normal

Fig. 7.1 Characteristic patterns of lung function tests in obstructive and restrictive lung diseases.

- The limitation is incompletely reversible with bronchodilators (e.g. inhaled salbutamol). This distinguishes the result from asthma, which is fully reversible.

A chest X-ray may show hyperinflation, flat hemidiaphragms, reduced peripheral vascular markings and bullae.

Treating stable COPD involves:
- Bronchodilators—often combinations of inhaled β_2-agonists (e.g. salbutamol), anticholinergics (e.g. tiotropium) and oral theophyllines.
- Help smoking cessation (e.g. nicotine replacement).
- Inhaled corticosteroids if very symptomatic.
- Long-term oxygen if in chronic respiratory failure.
- Nutritional support to maintain weight.
- Influenza and pneumococcal vaccinations.

Remember **SHONA** for the principles of treating an infective exacerbation of COPD:
- **S**teroids (oral)
- **H**eparin (prevent deep vein thrombosis in immobile patients)
- **O**xygen
- **N**ebulised bronchodilators
- **A**ntibiotics

Complications

The frequency of complications increases with progression of the disease:

- Infection—this produces acute exacerbations of symptoms requiring hospital admission (see clinical sketch).
- Pneumothorax—bullae are thin-walled airspaces created by alveolar collapse. Rupture of subpleural bullae may produce a pneumothorax.
- Respiratory failure—with hypoxia and hypercapnia (type 2 failure).
- Cor pulmonale—right-sided heart failure (see Chapter 6).

Note that in COPD, the respiratory centre may become relatively insensitive to CO_2, relying on hypoxic drive to maintain respiratory effort. It is therefore potentially dangerous to give these patients high-concentration oxygen without careful observation, as hypoventilation or apnoea may result.

Emphysema

Emphysema is a permanent dilatation of any part of the air spaces distal to the terminal bronchiole, occurring with tissue destruction but without fibrosis. It is a common condition, which usually forms part of COPD but may occasionally present alone. Emphysema is more common in males than in females.

The aetiology is unclear but risk factors are the same as for COPD, including cigarette smoking, occupational dusts or chemicals and atmospheric pollution. The inherited disorder α_1-antitrypsin deficiency predisposes to early emphysema.

Pathogenesis

In normal individuals, extracellular proteases secreted into the lung by inflammatory cells are inhibited by protease inhibitors (particularly α_1-antitrypsin). In emphysema, these inhibitors are either inactivated (e.g. by cigarette smoke) or absent (inherited disorder), resulting in continued activity of the proteases with destruction of lung parenchyma (Fig. 7.3).

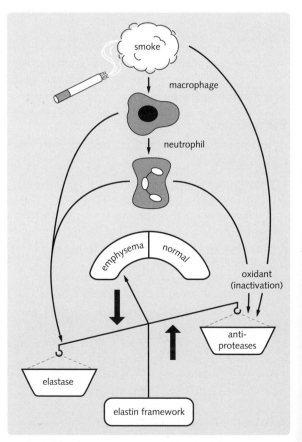

Fig. 7.3 Pathogenesis of emphysema. (Adapted with permission from The Lungs by B Corrin, Churchill Livingstone, 1990.)

Destruction of respiratory tissue leads to a loss of elastic recoil in the lungs and a decreased area available for gaseous exchange. About one-third of lung capacity must be destroyed before clinical symptoms of emphysema appear.

Types of emphysema

There are several forms of emphysema, defined by the location of damage in the respiratory acinus (Fig. 7.4):

- Centrilobular—dilatation of the respiratory bronchioles at the centre of acinus. It is most common in men and is closely associated with cigarette smoking. Lesions are most commonly found in the upper lobes.
- Panlobular—dilatation of the terminal alveoli and alveolar ducts, which later affects the respiratory bronchioles, thereby affecting the whole acinus. Typically affects the lower lobes. This pattern is typically seen in inherited α_1-antitrypsin deficiency.
- Paraseptal—involves air spaces at the periphery of lobules, typically adjacent to the pleura. Usually affects the upper lobes adjacent to areas of scarring or atelectasis.
- Irregular—irregular involvement of the respiratory acinus and almost always associated with scarring. It is thought to be caused by the trapping of air following lung fibrosis and it is, therefore, commonly present around old healed tuberculous scars at the lung apices.

Clinical features

In the early stages of emphysema, a rapid respiratory rate enables individuals to maintain blood oxygenation, such that levels of $Pa\text{CO}_2$ and $Pa\text{O}_2$ are near normal. Patients are breathless but not cyanosed (so-called 'pink puffers'). However, on the slightest exertion patients become increasingly breathless and ultimately hypoxic (type 1 respiratory failure). Complications are the same as described for COPD.

The lungs are hyperinflated, the trachea is often descended (i.e. there is decreased cricosternal distance between the cricoid cartilage and the sternal notch) and the accessory muscles may be hypertrophied. Associated chronic bronchitis may produce cough and sputum. Breath sounds are quiet, especially over bullae, often with crepitations or wheezes.

Chronic bronchitis

Chronic bronchitis is defined as a cough productive of sputum on most days for 3 months of the year for

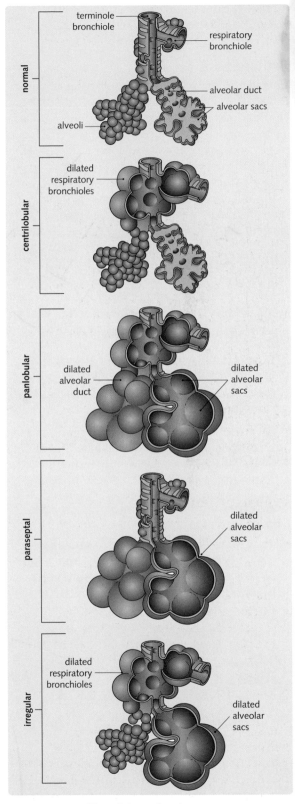

Fig. 7.4 Diagrams of the main types of emphysema.

at least two successive years. It typically affects middle-aged men and normally forms part of COPD; most cases are due to cigarette smoking.

Pathogenesis

Constant irritation by cigarette smoke causes chronic inflammation of the respiratory bronchioles (bronchiolitis) and increased mucus secretion.

Hypersecretion of mucus is associated with hypertrophy and hyperplasia of the bronchial mucus-secreting glands. Proteases stimulate this hypersecretion following their release by neutrophils recruited as part of the inflammatory response. The Reid index gives the ratio of gland to wall thickness in the bronchus, and it is significantly increased in cases of chronic bronchitis.

Clinical features

Bronchiolar obstruction must be extensive and widespread to give clinical symptoms. Eventually, extensive mucus plugging leads to the clinical obstructive features of the disease with typical cough and sputum production.

In later stages of the disease, progressive obstruction may result in patients with hypercapnia, hypoxaemia and cyanosis (so-called 'blue bloaters'). Other complications include:

- Recurrent low-grade bronchial infections caused by bacteria such as *Haemophilus influenzae* and *Streptococcus pneumoniae*, or viruses such as respiratory syncytial virus and adenovirus.
- Squamous metaplasia—loss of ciliated cells as a result of squamous metaplasia can further exacerbate the problem.
- Malignancy—persistent injury by smoking may invoke dysplastic changes in metaplastic squamous epithelium, which may ultimately become malignant (squamous cell carcinoma of the bronchus).

The late complications of COPD discussed previously may also occur.

Asthma

Asthma is an increased irritability of the bronchial tree with paroxysmal narrowing of the airways, which may reverse either spontaneously or after treatment with bronchodilators.

This is a common disorder, affecting around 15% of children and 7% of adults. Its incidence is thought to be rising, possibly due to environmental atmospheric pollution.

There are several known triggers of asthma:

- Allergy—a large number of allergens can precipitate asthma by inducing an IgE-mediated type I hypersensitivity reaction. Examples include pollen, house-dust mites, animal dander, foods and drugs.
- Infection—respiratory tract infection can trigger bronchoconstriction.
- Occupational exposure—some agents act as allergens, others by direct irritation of the airway. Isocyanates, found in substances such as paints, are the most commonly identified factor.
- Drug induced, e.g. β-antagonists and aspirin.
- Irritant gases, e.g. sulphur dioxide, nitric oxide, ozone in smog.
- Psychological stress can exacerbate attacks.
- Cold air.
- Exercise—especially in combination with cold air.

Asthma is associated with other atopic diseases such as eczema, hay fever and some allergies.

Classification

Asthma can be classified into two categories, depending on whether there is an allergic basis to the disease:

1. Extrinsic asthma (atopic)—early-onset asthma triggered by environmental allergens. Individuals often have a family history of allergic disorders. IgE levels are raised and an immediate type 1 hypersensitivity to the allergen is produced on skin challenge. This is the most common type of asthma.
2. Intrinsic asthma (non-atopic)—a late-onset asthma often triggered by infection of the upper respiratory tract. IgE levels are normal, there is no family history of allergic disorders and skin testing is negative.

However, there is often much overlap between the two types and many patients do not fit neatly into any one type.

Pathogenesis

There are three key features in both types of asthma:

1. Airflow limitation—obstruction is caused by a combination of bronchospasm, oedema and mucus plugging. This may be spontaneously reversible, or reversible with bronchodilator treatment.
2. Airway hyper-responsiveness to bronchoconstrictor trigger factors.

3. Airway inflammation—it appears that the allergic inflammation process of extrinsic asthma is driven by type 2 helper T cells (Th2). With time, airway remodelling occurs so that the smooth muscles of the bronchial wall become hypertrophied, increasing airflow limitation.

Remember that both asthma and COPD are obstructive lung diseases, but there are key differences between them:
- Asthma is due to a sensitising agent; COPD is due to a noxious agent.
- Asthmatic airway inflammation is predominated by CD4+ T cells and eosinophils; COPD occurs with predominantly CD8+ T cells, macrophages and neutrophils.
- Asthma airflow limitation is completely reversible with bronchodilator medication; COPD is only partially reversible.

The three phases of extrinsic asthma

- Early (15–20 minutes)—a rapid onset of bronchoconstriction caused by histamine release from mast cells. The allergen binds to IgE antibodies on the surface of mast cells causing cross-linking and degranulation (Fig. 7.5).
- Late (4–6 hours)—following recovery from the early phase, inflammatory mediators released by mast cells cause activation of macrophages and chemotaxis of polymorphs and eosinophils into the bronchial mucosa. These cells release inflammatory mediators causing a secondary wave of bronchoconstriction unrelated to exposure to the original antigen (Fig. 7.6).
- Prolonged hyper-reactivity (over days)—an exaggerated response of the airway on further re-exposure to the allergen or other bronchoconstrictor trigger factors over ensuing days. Persistence of inflammatory cells within the bronchial wall leads to damage and loss of epithelial cells.

Structural changes

The main structural changes that take place in asthmatic airways are listed below and illustrated in Fig. 7.6:

- Immune cell infiltration—the bronchial mucosa is infiltrated by eosinophils, mast cells, lymphoid cells and macrophages.
- Mucosal oedema—extravasation of plasma into submucosal tissues produces a narrowing of the airways.
- Mucus hypersecretion leads to plugging of airways.
- Hypertrophy of bronchial smooth muscle due to recurrent bronchoconstriction.
- Focal necrosis of the airway epithelium, caused by prolonged inflammation.
- Deposition of collagen beneath the bronchial epithelium in long-standing cases.
- Sputum contains Charcot–Leyden crystals (derived from eosinophil granules) and Curschmann's spirals (composed of mucus plugs from small airways).

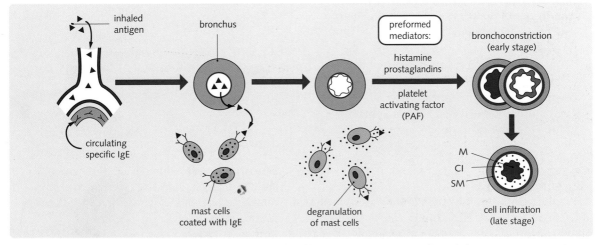

Fig. 7.5 Pathogenesis of the early and late stages of asthma. (CI, cellular infiltration; M, mucus; SM, smooth muscle.)

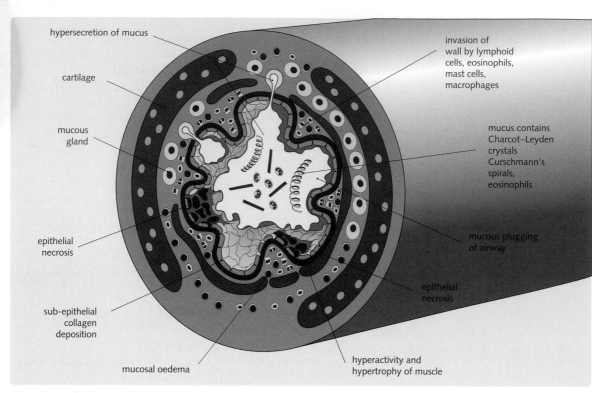

Fig. 7.6 Morphological changes in the airways in asthma.

Clinical features

Clinical features are as follows:

- Mild disease (majority of cases)—acute, intermittent episodes of bronchospasm (wheezing, dyspnoea or coughing) are triggered by well-recognised causes.
- Moderate to severe disease (small percentage)—increasingly severe and irreversible asthma in middle or old age (chronic asthma); patients may present with signs of respiratory distress.
- Acute severe asthma (formerly status asthmaticus)—severe, acute disease usually presenting with tachypnoeic distress, tachycardia and pulsus paradoxus. Air entry may be inadequate to generate any wheeze (the silent chest is an ominous sign) and death may result from acute respiratory insufficiency.

The main complication is cor pulmonale. Pulmonary vasoconstriction caused by chronic alveolar hypoventilation results in pulmonary hypertension leading to right ventricular hypertrophy.

The clinical signs of asthma include widespread, polyphonic, high-pitched wheezes. In severe chronic asthma, a barrel chest may develop.

The disease can usually be controlled by treatment including β_2-agonists, corticosteroids, theophyllines and leukotriene receptor antagonists.

Acute severe asthma can be life-threatening. It requires immediate oxygen, nebulised β_2-agonists and anticholinergics and systemic corticosteroids. Arterial blood gases should be taken to determine severity; if life-threatening, intravenous aminophylline or magnesium sulphate may be of use.

Prognosis

- Remission—approximately 50% of cases of childhood asthma resolve spontaneously but may recur later in life; remission in adult-onset asthma is less likely.
- Mortality—death occurs in approximately 0.2% of asthmatics accounting for about 2000 deaths

per year in the UK. Mortality is usually (but not always) preceded by an acute attack and about 50% are more than 65 years old.

Bronchiectasis

This is an irreversible dilatation of the bronchi or their branches. Its causes are:

- Congenital—cystic fibrosis, primary ciliary dyskinesia and Kartagener's syndrome (bronchiectasis, situs inversus and sinusitis).
- Acquired—infection (especially whooping cough, necrotising pneumonia or measles in childhood) and obstruction (either by an inhaled foreign body or by tumour).

Widened bronchi are more prone to infections, *Haemophilus influenzae* and *Pseudomonas aeruginosa* being the most common pathogens. Patients often cough up purulent sputum, which may contain blood.

Treatment consists of antibiotics (often long-term) for infections and postural drainage physiotherapy to drain sputum.

Cystic fibrosis

Cystic fibrosis (CF) is a hereditary multisystem disease characterised by the production of abnormally thick mucus, and primarily affecting the lung and pancreas. It is the most common autosomal recessive disorder affecting 1 in 2000 newborns. Approximately 1 in 25 Caucasians are heterozygous carriers of the CF gene.

Pathogenesis

The mutated gene is found on chromosome 7 and encodes for a protein termed the cystic fibrosis transmembrane regulator (CFTR). The most common mutation is deletion of the phenylalanine residue at position 508, which is found in 70% of cases. This protein normally enables the transport of chloride ions across cell membranes. In cystic fibrosis, defective CFTR results in impaired chloride transport, which prevents the release of sodium and water to liquefy mucus. The net result is the production of extremely thick and viscous mucus by the exocrine glands.

The epithelial dysfunction of cystic fibrosis affects the following systems:

- Bronchi—abnormally viscid mucus cannot be cleared from the lungs.
- Intestine—causing meconium ileus in newborn babies and distal intestinal obstruction syndrome later in life.

- Pancreas—causing deficiency of the pancreatic enzymes, resulting in malabsorption and failure to thrive.
- Liver—causing biliary cirrhosis.
- Vas deferens—failure to develop leads to male infertility.

In the respiratory tract, the bronchi and bronchioles become obstructed by abnormally viscid mucus, which leads to four main problems:

1. Infections—obstruction and stagnation of secretions leads to repeated bouts of infection, particularly with *Staphylococcus aureus* and *Pseudomonas aeruginosa*. *Burkholderia cepacia* infection is often intrinsically resistant to multiple antibiotics and some forms are transmissible between patients. This has resulted in the segregation of CF patients in hospitals and the community.
2. Bronchiectasis—a frequent complication (see above).
3. Hyperinflation of the lungs due to air trapping behind mucin plugs; increased risk of developing spontaneous pneumothorax.
4. Hypoxia, scarring and destruction of the pulmonary vascular bed, leading to pulmonary hypertension and cor pulmonale.

Prognosis

The median age of survival is just over 30 years, but newly born CF sufferers are now expected to live beyond 40 years. Newer drugs, such as DNAase mucolytics and nebulised tobramycin (an antibiotic), appear to reduce the rate of decline. Future treatment goals include the replacement of the defective gene using gene therapy strategies.

Diffuse interstitial diseases

Interstitial lung diseases are a group of non-infectious, non-malignant disorders in which there is inflammation of the alveolar walls with a thickening of the interstitium between the alveoli, usually with fibrosis. This large group of diseases occurs with a mainly restrictive pattern (see Fig. 7.1).

Disorders can be classified into broad groups, as shown in Fig. 7.7. There are thought to be over 200 distinct diffuse interstitial conditions. The most important of these are discussed below.

Idiopathic pulmonary fibrosis

This disease, of unknown aetiology, is rare but increasing in incidence. It mainly affects the elderly, and

Fig. 7.7 Interstitial (parenchymal) lung diseases

Known cause or association	Connective tissue disease, e.g. rheumatoid disease, scleroderma Drug- or toxin-induced disease, e.g. nitrofurantoin, amiodarone, methotrexate Pneumoconiosis, e.g. coal-worker's pneumoconiosis, silicosis or asbestosis Extrinsic allergic alveolitis, e.g. farmer's lung, bird fancier's lung
Idiopathic interstitial pneumonias	Idiopathic pulmonary fibrosis (IPF) Idiopathic bronchiolitis obliterans organizing pneumonia (BOOP)
Granulomatous disease	Sarcoidosis
Eosinophilic disease	Idiopathic eosinophilic pneumonia Allergic bronchopulmonary aspergillosis
Infections	Miliary tuberculosis Cytomegalovirus *Pneumocystis carinii*
Others	Part of a systemic inflammatory disease, e.g. acute respiratory distress syndrome (ARDS) Acute or chronic radiation pneumonitis Diffuse intrapulmonary haemorrhage, e.g. Goodpasture's syndrome Rare disorders, e.g. alveolar proteinosis, histiocytosis

Fig. 7.7 A classification scheme for diffuse interstitial (parenchymal) lung disease.

males more than females. Fibrosis occurs at the lung bases, resulting in peripheral 'honeycombing'. This describes the appearance of the cut surface of the lung (and can be seen using high-resolution CT scanning).

As with all diseases causing interstitial fibrosis, there is some inflammation involving neutrophil and lymphocyte infiltration. Even the earliest lesions show focal accumulation of fibroblasts; such foci become more collagenous as the disease progresses. Fibrosis results in alveolar wall collapse and the production of cystic spaces.

Macroscopically, the lung is converted into a mass of cystic airspaces separated by areas of dense collagenous scarring.

The clinical feature of the early-stage disease is a slowly increasing respiratory insufficiency due to reduced lung capacity and residual volume, reduced compliance and reduced diffusion capacity.

The characteristic signs are dyspnoea, cough and finger clubbing. There is a restrictive pattern of lung function tests. Median survival is 4 years, although the response to traditional end-stage drug regimes is very variable (usually corticosteroids and azathioprine).

The pneumoconioses

This is a group of interstitial lung diseases resulting from chronic exposure to inorganic dust. The three most common types of pneumoconioses are coal-worker's pneumoconiosis (CWP), silicosis and asbestosis.

In the normal lung, inhaled dust is coughed out, or ingested by macrophages. However, if the dust is toxic to macrophages there is local inflammation, secretion of cytokines and stimulation of fibrosis. The end result is a restrictive pattern of respiratory dysfunction.

Coal-worker's pneumoconiosis

CWP is an interstitial lung disease caused by inhaling coal dust. It has three types of pathology:

1. Simple coal-worker's pneumoconiosis—not usually associated with any clinically significant impairment of respiratory function, despite focal aggregates of dust-laden macrophages. The condition does not progress if the affected individual leaves the mining industry.
2. Progressively massive fibrosis—large nodules and scarring results in severe respiratory impairment. The upper lobes are predominantly affected and there may be cavitation of the nodules. This condition may progress even after leaving the mining industry.
3. Caplan's syndrome—associated with rheumatoid disease, where the nodules appear large, carbon pigmented and rheumatoid.

Silicosis

This is caused by the inhalation of quartz-containing dust (quartz being silicon dioxide), which is abundant in stone and sand.

It is associated with occupations such as slate mining, quarrying and stone masonry.

Pathogenesis—silicates are toxic to macrophages, which stimulate cytokine generation precipitating inflammation with fibrosis and nodule formation.

Tuberculosis is a common complication of silicosis (silicotuberculosis). This is thought to be due to impaired local defences as a consequence of accumulated silica in macrophages.

Asbestosis

This interstitial lung disease is caused by the inhalation of asbestos, a fibrous silicate mineral that was widely used between 1890 and 1970. It is associated with occupations involving asbestos mining/processing, the building industry, insulating and fire-resistant material and shipyard and ship's engine-room work.

There are two main forms of asbestos:

1. Serpentine asbestos (white asbestos)—this is the most common form; fibres persist in the lung for a limited time.
2. Amphibole asbestos (blue and brown asbestos)—fibres persist in the lung for many years and are the main cause of malignant mesothelioma.

Risk of disease depends on the duration and intensity of exposure, and the type of asbestos (short fibres are less pathogenic).

The characteristics of asbestosis are:

- There is usually a latent period of 25 years before clinical symptoms become evident.
- Interstitial fibrosis is maximal at lung bases and asbestos bodies may be seen histologically. Asbestos bodies are fibres coated in acid mucopolysaccharides and haemosiderin.
- The disease progresses with an increasing restrictive defect associated with interstitial fibrosis.
- Pulmonary hypertension and cor pulmonale develop in the late stages.

Sarcoidosis

Sarcoidosis is a multisystem disease of unknown aetiology characterised by the presence of non-caseating granulomas primarily affecting the lymph nodes and lungs.

Maximum incidence is in people between 30 and 40 years of age, affecting slightly more females than males.

Other affected sites are the skin, eyes, liver, spleen, nervous system, phalanges, parotid glands and (rarely) the heart.

The aetiopathogenesis is unknown but thought to involve the type IV hypersensitivity reaction. The disease seems to be less common in smokers and more common with increasing geographical distance from the equator.

Histology shows non-caseating histiocytic granulomas in the lung interstitium. Patients with lung involvement present with slowly progressive dyspnoea and cough and are found to have lung shadowing on chest radiograph with enlargement of the hilar lymph nodes.

Diagnosis—there are no diagnostic blood tests for sarcoidosis, but there is often hypercalcaemia, raised serum angiotensin converting enzyme and a reduced tuberculin skin test. The definitive diagnosis is histological, requiring a tissue sample, e.g. skin lesion biopsy, transbronchial biopsy.

Treatment involves steroid therapy in progressive disease.

Other interstitial lung diseases

Other interstitial lung diseases of note are:

- Goodpasture's syndrome—a diffuse pulmonary haemorrhagic syndrome caused by complement activation following autoantibody binding to the basement membrane.
- Idiopathic pulmonary haemosiderosis—a rare condition with type II pneumocyte hyperplasia.
- Rheumatoid disease—the lung and pleura are affected in 10–15% of patients.
- Extrinsic allergic alveolitis—immune mediated interstitial granulomatous inflammation caused by inhalation of organic agents (type III and type IV hypersensitivity). Examples include farmer's lung and pigeon-fancier's lung.

INFECTIONS OF THE LUNGS

Pneumonia

Pneumonia is defined as the infection of alveolar tissue resulting in the consolidation of lung tissue with an intra-alveolar inflammatory exudate.

Pneumonia is the fifth most common cause of death in the USA. It is most common in the very young and the elderly.

Predisposing factors

Although pneumonia frequently occurs in previously healthy individuals, it is also predisposed by the presence of debility and immobility:

- Suppressed cough reflex, e.g. in coma, anaesthesia and neuromuscular junction disorders.
- Impaired mucociliary clearance, e.g. through cigarette smoke, irritant gases, viral diseases (e.g. influenza) and genetic conditions (e.g. immotile cilia syndrome).
- Pulmonary oedema, e.g. due to right-sided cardiac failure.
- Impaired alveolar macrophages—alcohol, cigarette smoke, oxygen toxicity.
- Retention of secretions due to COPD.
- Immunosuppression, e.g. drugs (cytotoxics and immunosuppressives), AIDS, congenital immunodeficiencies and leukaemias.
- Drugs—previous course of broad-spectrum antibiotics or cytotoxics.
- Instrumentation—endotracheal intubation or mechanical ventilation.
- Prior viral respiratory tract infection.
- Other—prolonged hospitalisation, general debility, immobility.

Remember **INSPIRATION** for the predisposing factors of pneumonia:
- **I**mmunosuppression
- **N**eurological impairment of the cough reflex
- **S**ecretion retention
- **P**ulmonary oedema
- **I**mpaired mucociliary clearance
- **R**espiratory tract infection (viral)
- **A**ntibiotics and cytotoxics
- **T**racheal instrumentation
- **I**mpaired alveolar macrophages
- **O**ther
- **N**eoplasia

Classification

Pneumonia can be classified according to:

- Microbiology—causative organism may be bacterial, viral, fungal or protozoal.
- Pattern of spread of infection—either lobar or bronchopneumonia.
- Clinical classification—according to circumstances surrounding the development of disease, e.g. community acquired, hospital acquired, disease of immunosuppression or aspiration pneumonia.

Causative organisms

Bacterial infection is the most common type of pneumonia, accounting for 80–90% of cases. Knowledge of the circumstances in which a person develops pneumonia is a strong clue as to the likely organism causing the infection (Fig. 7.8).

The clinical features are fever, shortness of breath, cough, pleuritic pain and sputum (occasionally with haemoptysis). There are signs of consolidation with bronchial breathing and/or coarse crackles. Confusion, uraemia, tachypnoea (raised respiratory rate) and hypotension are signs suggestive of severe infection requiring hospital admission.

As a general rule of thumb, community-acquired pneumonia is usually caused by Gram-positive bacteria whereas hospital-acquired pneumonias are mainly due to Gram-negative bacteria.

Bronchopneumonia

Infection is centred on the bronchi but with the extension of the inflammatory exudate into the alveoli, causing a patchy consolidation of the lung (lobular distribution). Bronchopneumonia is illustrated in Fig. 7.9.

The condition primarily affects the very young, very old or debilitated patients.

The infecting organism depends on whether the infection is hospital or community acquired, but it is quite often of the hospital-acquired variety due to underlying disease.

Pathogenesis

Patients develop retention of secretions, which gravitate to dependent parts of the lungs and become infected, hence bronchopneumonia most commonly involves the lower lobes.

Macroscopically, multiple areas of consolidation usually occur distributed bilaterally around bronchi/bronchioles in dependent parts of the lung. Affected areas are firm and airless and have a dark red or grey appearance. Bronchial mucosa is inflamed and pus may be present in the more peripheral bronchi. Patchy collapse is associated with bronchial obstruction. Involvement of the pleura is common with purulent pleuritis.

Fig. 7.8 Common pathogenic bacteria in hospital- and community-acquired pneumonia

Community-acquired infection	Hospital-acquired infection
Streptococcus pneumoniae (> 60%)	*Klebsiella*
Haemophilus influenzae	*Pseudomonas*
Legionella pneumophilus	*Acinetobacter*
Staphylococcus aureus	*Methicillin resistant staphylococcus aureus (MRSA)*
Mycoplasma pneumoniae	*Escherichia coli*
Chlamydia pneumoniae	*Proteus*
Chlamydia psittaci	*Serratia* As well as organisms responsible for community-acquired pneumonia (but much less frequently)

Fig. 7.8 Common pathogens in hospital- and community-acquired pneumonia.

Microscopically, there is acute inflammation of the bronchi and bronchioles with an acute inflammatory neutrophil-rich exudate present in the lumina and extending into the peribronchial alveoli.

Complications and sequelae are as follows:

- Resolution—complete resolution occurs only if treatment is instituted early, before the onset of structural damage.
- Bronchial damage—imperfect repair of the bronchial mucosa results in scarring of the bronchial wall, with increased predisposition to further infection and to bronchiectasis.
- Lung fibrosis—inflammatory exudate is often not completely absorbed but is organized with residual fibrous scarring.
- Lung abscesses—single or multiple areas of suppuration.
- Empyema—pus in the pleural cavity as a result of extension of infection into the pleural cavity.
- Pericarditis—direct extension of infection to the pericardium.
- Death—very common cause of death, particularly as a terminal manifestation of debilitating diseases.

Lobar pneumonia

This is a uniform or homogenous consolidation of part of a lobe or of the whole lobe caused by infection (Fig. 7.10). The condition often affects otherwise healthy adults, primarily between the ages of 20 and 50 years old. Individuals living in poor social conditions, and alcoholics who have reduced access to good medical care, are particularly prone to this pattern of pneumonia, which is often caused by *Pneumococcus* or *Klebsiella* species.

Pathogenesis

Organisms gain entry to distal air spaces without colonisation of bronchi. Infection spreads rapidly

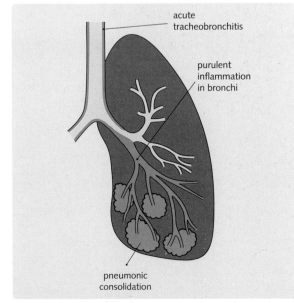

Fig. 7.9 Bronchopneumonia.

113

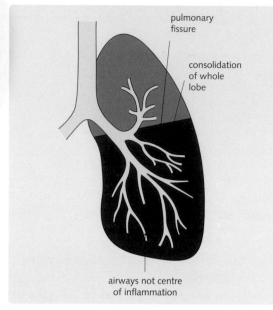

pulmonary fissure

consolidation of whole lobe

airways not centre of inflammation

Fig. 7.10 Lobar pneumonia.

through the alveolar spaces and bronchioles, causing acute inflammatory exudation into air spaces.

Macroscopically, the whole lobe becomes consolidated and airless.

Microscopically, the alveoli are filled with an acute inflammatory exudate, which is limited by the pulmonary fissures.

There are four pathological stages of lobar pneumonia:

1. Congestion—outpouring of protein-rich exudate into the alveolae.
2. Red hepatisation—massive accumulation of red cells and polymorphs in the alveolar spaces, giving a liver-like consistency (hence 'hepatisation')
3. Grey hepatisation—accumulation of fibrin in the lung spaces with red-cell disintegration.
4. Resolution—most patients recover with their lungs returning to normal structure and function.

Complications and sequelae are as follows:

- Lung fibrosis—inflammatory exudate is often not completely absorbed but is organized with residual fibrous scarring and permanent lung dysfunction.
- Bacteraemia—bacterial dissemination of organisms can lead to septicaemia with meningitis, arthritis, endocarditis or pyemic abscesses.
- Lung abscesses—single or multiple areas of suppuration.

- Empyema—pus in the pleural cavity as a result of extension of infection into the pleural cavity.
- Pleural effusion—non-infected effusion is common.
- Death.

Primary atypical pneumonia

This is an inflammation of the alveolar septa by inflammatory cells (acute interstitial pneumonitis) in the absence of any consolidation. Patients develop fever, dry cough and dyspnoea, but there is little sputum and few signs of consolidation, hence the term 'atypical' pneumonia. It may be caused by several factors including infection by viruses, *Mycoplasma*, *Chlamydia* and *Rickettsia* species.

Viral pneumonia

This is a common cause of pneumonia in early childhood but is much less frequent in healthy adults. The majority of viral lung infections cause an atypical pneumonia, which is typically self-limiting (e.g. cytomegalovirus, measles or varicella). However, these infections can prove fatal in an immunocompromised host.

A minority of viruses cause a much more severe pattern of infection. The influenza viruses can cause an acute fulminating pneumonia with pulmonary haemorrhage; the clinical course may be rapidly fatal.

A common complication is secondary infection with pyogenic bacteria, due to the stripping of the respiratory epithelium by the initial viral infection. This can transform a mild viral lung infection into a severe suppurative bronchopneumonia, particularly after influenza infection.

Mycoplasma

Mycoplasma species account for 15–20% of community-acquired pneumonia. It is more common in children between 5 and 15 years old but more serious in adults. The organisms cause a low-grade, chronic, atypical pneumonia that can result in pulmonary fibrosis.

Chlamydia and Rickettsia

A number of chlamydial and rickettsial infections are complicated by the development of pneumonia. Such infections include typhus, psittacosis and Q fever. Fatal cases are rare, except in psittacosis.

Pneumonia in the immunocompromised

The lungs of immunocompromised patients are extremely prone to disease by opportunistic infections, i.e. infections caused by microorganisms that are non-pathogenic to healthy, immunocompetent individuals.

Common opportunistic agents include:

- Viruses—cytomegalovirus, respiratory syncytial virus, varicella-zoster virus, measles (see primary atypical pneumonia, above). Cytomegalovirus pneumonitis is particularly common after bone marrow transplantation.
- Fungi—both *Candida* and *Aspergillus* can cause widespread areas of necrosis with the formation of microabscesses containing characteristic hyphae, e.g. invasive pulmonary aspergillosis. Mortality is high.
- Protozoa—*Pneumocystis carinii* pneumonia (PCP) is common in AIDS patients, affecting 30–50% of cases. Alveoli are filled with a fine, foam-like material in which the minute bodies of the organism can be seen. This disease has a 30% mortality rate in patients with AIDS.

Pulmonary tuberculosis

Pulmonary tuberculosis (TB) is a chronic granulomatous infection of the lung caused by *Mycobacterium tuberculosis*. It is uncommon in the UK and other developed countries (at about 10 per 100 000) but extremely common worldwide (up to 500 per 100 000 in parts of Africa) where it is a leading cause of death.

Rates in the UK are increasing as a result of HIV infection, the increasingly elderly population, overcrowding and social deprivation, immigrant populations and a reduced priority for control. The development of multi-drug-resistant (MDR) tuberculosis has exacerbated this problem.

Spread

Spread is by various means:

- Inhalation of *Mycobacterium tuberculosis* in the form of droplets (by far the most common mode).
- Ingestion of food or milk.
- Inoculation of the skin.
- Transplacental spread, i.e. congenital TB.

Diagnosis

The main form of definitive diagnosis is a positive Ziehl–Nielsen stain of a patient sample (e.g. sputum). Such samples should be cultured and tested to assess drug sensitivity.

Predisposing factors

These are:

- Close contact with infected individuals—increased risk for those living/working in crowded or unhygienic conditions and for healthcare workers.
- Immunosuppression—the very young, very old, immunosuppressive therapy and other diseases of immunodeficiency, particularly AIDS.
- Malnourishment.
- Other diseases—pre-existing chronic lung disease (especially silicosis), diabetes mellitus and alcoholism.

Pathogenesis

The destructive effects of infection are entirely due to the hypersensitivity reaction of the host directed against bacterial cell wall constituents. The following sequence of events occurs:

1. 0–10 days—mycobacteria excite a transient but marked acute inflammatory response. Neutrophils phagocytose the organisms but are unable to destroy them, as the cell walls are resistant to degradation. Instead, engulfed bacteria are drained into local lymph nodes.
2. After 10 days—development of a T-cell-mediated immune response (type IV hypersensitivity reaction) to the bacillary cell wall constituents results in cytokine release and macrophage activation. Gradually a chronic inflammatory pattern develops, which is dominated by aggregates of macrophages called epithelioid cells, which form variable numbers of granulomas (see Chapter 2) with a central core of necrotic caseous tissue containing viable mycobacteria. Tuberculous granulomas are termed tubercles.

Macroscopically, the granulomas appear as pinhead-sized white or greyish foci (tubercles) in the tissues.

Microscopically, granulomas are the histological hallmark of TB infection. A granuloma consists of a central area of amorphous caseous necrosis, surrounded by three cellular layers:

1. An inner layer of activated macrophages (epithelioid cells) with Langhans' giant cells.
2. A middle layer of lymphocytes.
3. An outer layer of fibroblastic tissue, which merges with surrounding structures and increases with the age of the lesion.

The healing of a granuloma occurs slowly, with progressive fibrosis and later calcification. The central necrotic area remains caseous for some time and mycobacteria may remain viable indefinitely within a healed lesion. This is partly due to the ability of the *Mycobacterium tuberculosis* to remain latent within macrophages (inside phagosomes), inhibiting the fusion of lysosomes. Reactivation results in secondary (or post primary) tuberculosis.

TB can be classified into two types, according to the pattern of infection:

1. Primary infection—the first encounter with the organism, resulting in the development of a small parenchymal peripheral focus with a large response in the draining lymph nodes.
2. Secondary infection—reactivation or reinfection of a previously infected individual, resulting in the development of a large, localised, parenchymal reaction but with minimal lymph node involvement.

Primary tuberculosis

The lung is by far the most common site of primary infection, usually occurring in a child or young adult with no specific immunity. Other sites include the pharynx, larynx, skin and intestine.

Inhaled organisms proliferate in the alveoli at the periphery of the lung, often just beneath the pleura. This primary parenchymal tubercle is termed the Ghon focus. It is often associated with enlarged caseous hilar lymph nodes. The combination of lung and lymph node lesions together constitutes the primary complex or Ghon complex.

Primary tuberculosis will either resolve or progress as shown below.

Resolution

This occurs in the majority of cases (85–90%) and the episode is often entirely asymptomatic. The Ghon focus and caseating granulomas in the lymph nodes heal with fibrosis. The disease does not progress due to the confinement of organisms within a fibrotic shell. However, walled-off bacteria may remain viable within the healed primary complex (latent tuberculosis). A tuberculin skin test becomes positive 1–2 months after the onset of infection.

Progression

In patients with poor immunity, the disease is progressive. There is a further spread of mycobacteria with continuing enlargement of the caseating granu-lomas in the lymph nodes (progressive primary TB). Enlarging nodes spread the infection by eroding into adjacent structures in two ways:

1. Bronchus—erosion of an infected lymph node into a bronchus results in tuberculous bronchopneumonia (Fig. 7.11A). The bacilli pass down into the bronchi of one lung where infection can then spread into the opposite lung. There is further spread of infection into the bronchioles and alveoli with the development of extensive, confluent, caseating, granulomatous lesions. This condition is known as 'galloping consumption' and it is usually rapidly fatal.
2. Blood vessel—erosion of an infected lymph node into a blood vessel results in haematogenous spread of mycobacteria to many parts of the body, including the remainder of the lung, causing miliary tuberculosis (Fig. 7.11B).

Direct lymphatic spread (i.e. without erosion) may allow spread to the pleura and pericardium.

Secondary tuberculosis

This occurs as a result of the reactivation of quiescent but viable mycobacteria in hosts with weakened immune responses, or as a result of reinfection by additional organisms. Reactivation occurs in 5–10% of those with latent infection, usually in the lungs.

Caseous granulomas typically develop in the apical segments of the lungs, spreading directly and locally but without lymph node lesions. The initiating apical lesion is often called an Assmann focus, and it is histologically similar to the Ghon focus.

Secondary tuberculosis will either resolve or spread as shown below.

Resolution

Spontaneous healing with fibrosis and calcification occurs, though viable organisms may remain without producing any clinical symptoms.

Spread

In adults with poor immune responses, secondary tuberculosis progresses locally with direct extension and continuing caseation. Further spread of mycobacteria produces various types of progressive tuberculosis:

- Apical cavitation fibrocaseous tuberculosis—a direct extension of the infection. Continuing caseation results in the formation of a large caseous mass surrounded by a thin cellular wall. If caseous material is expectorated, a cavity results. The lesion can heal at this stage but it may

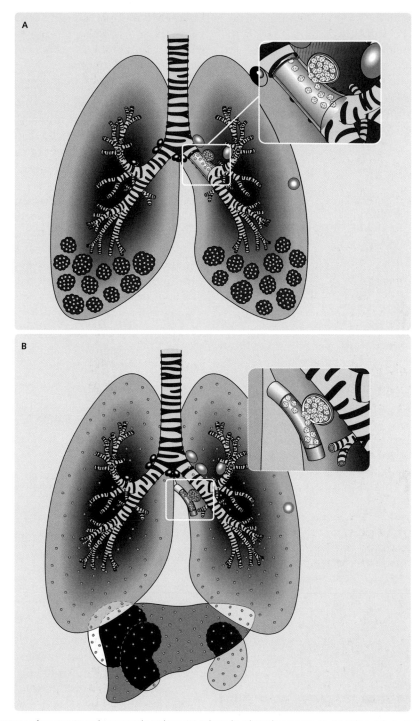

Fig. 7.11 Patterns of progressive pulmonary tuberculosis. (A) Tuberculous bronchopneumonia. (B) Miliary tuberculosis of the lung.

spread further into the bronchi, bloodstream or directly into the pleura.

- Tuberculous pneumonia (see above).
- Miliary tuberculosis—the disease becomes widely disseminated with numerous small granulomas in many organs. Common target tissues are the kidneys, liver, bone marrow and meninges; disease can therefore occur in any of these tissues.

Complications are usually the result of extensive fibrosis involved in the healing process:

- Pulmonary fibrosis—lung lesions typically heal with fibrosis, which may be extensive, producing localised honeycombing. This is common in relapsing and progressive untreated disease.
- Pleural fibrosis with obliteration of the pleural space.
- Bronchiectasis—scarring of the bronchial walls can cause distal pulmonary collapse, secondary infection and bronchiectasis.

Immunization with the BCG vaccine is common practice in the UK, with a protective efficacy of 80%. Treatment of infected individuals involves initial therapy with three drugs (rifampicin, isoniazid and pyrazinamide), followed by continued therapy with rifampicin and isoniazid only. Total treatment lasts 6 months. Ethambutol is added to the regimen where drug resistance is likely (e.g. in HIV-positive patients) and the total treatment time may be extended.

Tuberculosis is a good example of a chronic inflammatory disease. Remember that primary pulmonary tuberculosis has a small granulomatous focus but large lymph node response. By contrast, secondary disease presents with large granulomatous disease (potentially in a number of different tissues) and minimal lymph node involvement.

NEOPLASTIC DISEASES OF THE LUNGS

Bronchogenic carcinoma

Bronchogenic carcinoma is the most common cause of death from neoplasia in the UK, affecting 30 000 people per year. Males are affected more than females,

but there is an increasing incidence in women. The peak incidence is between the ages of 40 and 70 years, reflecting the cumulative exposure to several potential causative carcinogens.

The risk factors include:

- Cigarette smoking—the earlier the age at which smoking starts and the more cigarettes smoked result in an increased risk. Cigarette smoke contains a large number of carcinogens, e.g. polycyclic hydrocarbons. There is a steady decline in risk if smoking stops.
- Occupational factors, such as exposure to radioactive material, asbestos, nickel, chromium, iron oxides and coal gas plants.
- Environmental factors, such as radon (a natural radioactive gas in certain geographic areas).
- Pulmonary fibrosis—somewhat controversial but it appears that there is an increased risk of carcinoma development in areas of lung affected by fibrosis.

There are four main histological types of lung carcinoma:

1. Squamous cell carcinoma—35%.
2. Small cell carcinoma ('oat cell carcinoma')—20%.
3. Adenocarcinoma (including bronchioalveolar carcinoma)—30%.
4. Large cell anaplastic carcinoma—15%.

A small proportion of tumours are mixed adenosquamous carcinoma.

Tumours may be central (all types) or peripheral (mainly adenocarcinomas).

Central or hilar tumours (70%) arise in relation to the main bronchi extending into the bronchial lumen and invading the adjacent lung.

Peripheral tumours (30%) arise in peripheral airways or alveoli, often occurring in relation to scars and frequently extending to the pleural surface.

The routes of spread are as follows:

- Local—central tumours invade locally either through the bronchial wall into the surrounding lung or along the outside of the bronchi (peribronchial spread) to distant parts of the lung. Direct extension into pleura and adjacent mediastinal structures is a feature of advanced disease. Apical lung tumours (Pancoast tumours) may invade local sympathetic ganglia and produce Horner's syndrome.
- Lymphatic spread—carcinomas spread to the ipsilateral and contralateral peribronchial and hilar

lymph nodes. Compression of adjacent tissues by infiltrated nodes may then cause symptoms.

- Transcoelomic spread—tumour cells may seed within the pleural cavity, causing a malignant pleural effusion.
- Haematogenous spread—most commonly to the brain, bone, liver, adrenal glands and skin.

Histological types

Squamous cell carcinoma

This is the most common type of lung cancer. It is thought to be derived from metaplastic squamous epithelium, which develops to line the main bronchi as a result of exposure to agents such as cigarette smoke.

Tumours are typically central and close to the carina, frequently presenting with features related to bronchial obstruction. Compared with other types, they are relatively slow growing and metastasise outside the thorax late; they may be resectable.

Histologically, the tumours show a range of differentiation, from well-differentiated lesions producing lots of keratin through to poorly differentiated lesions with only a few keratin-producing cells.

Small cell (oat cell) carcinoma

These highly malignant tumours arise from the bronchial endocrine or APUD cells. They contain a few dense secretory granules that are also seen in greater numbers in bronchial carcinoid tumours. Therefore, small cell carcinoma is thought to represent a type of neuroendocrine tumour.

Due to their endocrine nature, this form of cancer can be associated with ectopic hormone production.

Macroscopically, these tumours are usually centrally located and they are associated with a rapid rate of growth. Metastases are usually present at the time of diagnosis.

Microscopically, the cells are round to oval and have little cytoplasm. All small cell carcinomas are considered high grade.

Large cell anaplastic carcinoma

This poorly differentiated tumour is thought to be of either squamous or adenocarcinoma origin. Lesions may be central or peripheral and they are composed of large cells with nuclear pleomorphism and frequent giant cell forms. They have a poor prognosis and are frequently widely disseminated at the time of diagnosis.

Adenocarcinoma

This tumour is derived from glandular cells, such as mucous goblet cells, Clara cells, or type II pneumocytes. A proportion of adenocarcinomas are thought to originate in areas of pre-existing lung scarring or fibrosis (scar cancers). Adenocarcinoma has the slowest rate of growth and is the most common form of lung cancer in women. It can be linked to passive cigarette smoking and characteristically develops peripherally.

There are four main histological patterns:

1. Acinar—prominent gland-like spaces lined by columnar epithelium.
2. Papillary—fronds of tumour on thin septa.
3. Solid carcinoma with mucin production—poorly differentiated lesions.
4. Bronchioalveolar carcinoma (see below).

Cigarette smoking is the major risk factor for the development of neoplastic diseases of the lung. It is thought to be responsible for over 90% of all lung carcinomas. Passive smoking has been linked to approximately 5% of all lung cancers.

Clinical features of lung cancer

There are no early symptoms of lung cancer; it is usual for a lesion to have been growing for many years before clinical presentation. The presenting symptoms of lung cancer are outlined in Fig. 7.12 and they can be classified into:

- Pulmonary symptoms—most common types of presenting symptom including cough, dyspnoea, chest pain and haemoptysis.
- Metastatic symptoms—metastatic spread is present in 70% of patients at presentation; 30% present with symptoms caused by metastatic disease.
- Local symptoms—local spread within the thorax can cause several clinical syndromes.
- Non-metastatic extrapulmonary syndromes (paraneoplastic syndromes)—lung cancer frequently causes systemic syndromes that are not associated with metastatic effects and these may rarely be a presenting feature of disease.

Diagnosis is through clinical features (see above), imaging (chest X-ray and CT scans) and histological confirmation techniques:

- Bronchoscopy—tumour biopsy obtained.
- Cytology of pleural effusion.

Fig. 7.12 Clinicopathological features of lung cancer

Cause	Clinical features
Pulmonary involvement	
	Cough (80%): infection distal to airway blocked by tumour Haemoptysis (70%): ulceration of tumour in bronchus Dyspnoea (60%): local extension of tumour Chest pain (40%): involvement of pleura and/or chest wall Wheeze (15%): narrowing of airways Systemic features: weight loss, anorexia and malaise
Local spread	
	Horner's syndrome: local invasion of cervical sympathetic ganglion Hoarseness: spread to the left hilar region may cause recurrent laryngeal nerve palsy Pain in T1 dermatome and wasting of intrinsic hand muscles: caused by brachial neuritis as a result of direct invasion of plexus by apical tumours Pericarditis: due to direct tumour invasion
Metastatic spread	
	Pathological fracture CNS symptoms (brain metastasis) Hepatomegaly or jaundice (liver metastasis)
Non-metastatic extrapulmonary syndromes	
Endocrine disturbances	Inappropriate ADH secretion: by small cell carcinoma and characterised by low sodium and plasma osmolality with high urine osmolality Ectopic ACTH secretion: caused by small cell carcinoma and associated with Cushing's syndrome Hypercalcaemia: caused by secretion of parathyroid hormone-related peptide by a squamous cell carcinoma
Neurological syndromes	Peripheral sensory motor neuropathy Cerebellar degeneration causing ataxia Proximal myopathy Dermatomyositis Lambert–Eaton myasthenic syndrome: associated with small cell tumours
Hypertrophic pulmonary osteoarthropathy (HPOA)	Finger clubbing Swelling of wrists and ankles with periosteal new bone formation (seen in 2–3% of squamous cell carcinomas and adenocarcinomas)

Note: ACTH, adrenocorticotrophic hormone.

Fig. 7.12 Clinicopathological features of lung cancer.

Prognosis and staging

Histological types and the stage of lung cancer determine the outcome and its likely response to treatment. Survival is better for early stage disease, except for small cell carcinoma (very early metastases).

The staging system used for lung cancer is shown in Fig. 7.13.

Treatment

Surgical intervention

Tumours are classified as either operable or inoperable, according to the stage of the disease. For example, distant metastases and advanced local spread are contraindications for surgical resection.

Only 10% of all lung tumours are considered operable at diagnosis. Many patients are unsuitable for

Fig. 7.13 TNM staging of lung cancer

Stage	TNM group	Clinical
Stage I	TI N0 M0 T1 N1 M0	Tumour < 3 cm; distal to origin of lobar bronchus (T1) With (N1) or without (N0) spread to ipsilateral hilar nodes No metastases (M0)
Stage II	T2 N0 M0 T2 N1 M0	Tumour > 3 cm, 2 cm distal to the carina, which invades visceral pleural (T2) With (N1) or without (N0) spread to ipsilateral hilar nodes No metastases (M0)
Stage III	All T3/T4 cases All N3 cases All M1 cases	All tumours involving the carina; involving mediastinal structures (T3/T4) All tumours with spread to contralateral nodes (N3) All cases of metastases (M1)

Fig. 7.13 TNM staging of lung cancer.

surgery due to comorbidities (e.g. poor cardiac status). However, 5-year survival rates are as high as 75% in carefully selected patients with early disease (stage 1).

Radiotherapy and chemotherapy

Tumours are grouped into two categories according to differences in prognosis and response to radiotherapy and chemotherapy:

1. Small cell lung carcinoma—very sensitive to radiotherapy and chemotherapy. However, the disease is usually extensive at diagnosis such that survival is still poor despite local control of tumour growth. Treatment offers good palliation of pain, cough and dyspnoea. Therapy produces a median survival of 11 months (compared with 3 months if untreated) and a 1-year survival of 45%.
2. Non-small cell lung carcinoma (squamous, large-cell and adenocarcinoma); inoperable cases may be treated with radiotherapy depending on clinical circumstances. The role of chemotherapy is limited. Overall prognosis is poor with only a 50% 2-year survival without spread, 10% with spread.

Combination chemotherapy for small cell lung cancer often involves intravenous cyclophosphamide, doxorubicin and vincristine given in cycles lasting 3 weeks each. Although small cell cancer is very sensitive to this therapy, it has almost always metastasised by the time of treatment. Radiotherapy alone is rarely radical (curative) in lung cancer but is of great use in the palliation of symptoms such as superior vena cava obstruction and pain caused by invasion of the chest wall.

Figure 7.14 summarises the main histological types of lung cancer.

Bronchioalveolar carcinoma

This is a special type of adenocarcinoma derived from alveolar or bronchial epithelial cells (Clara cells and type II pneumocytes). There are two types:

1. Multifocal diffuse infiltrative tumours—replace areas of lung in a manner resembling pneumonic consolidation. Cells are tall, columnar, have few mitoses and secrete mucin.
2. Single, grey masses of tumour up to 10 cm in diameter—cells are cuboidal with hyperchromatic nuclei and mitoses. Cells form papillary structures; there is often no mucin secretion. In the absence of metastases, this subtype has a better prognosis than other forms of lung cancer.

Secondary tumours of the lung

Metastatic deposits may spread to the lungs from distant primary sites, most often from carcinomas of the breast, kidney, uterus, ovary, testes and thyroid. Spread is usually via the blood, most commonly resulting in bilateral deposits.

Carcinoid tumours

These are neuroendocrine tumours of the lungs, representing about 5% of all pulmonary neoplasms. The majority are benign, although a minority has the potential for local recurrence or metastasis (atypical pulmonary neuroendocrine tumours).

In contrast to intestinal carcinoid tumours, most pulmonary lesions do not secrete 5-hydroxytryptamine (serotonin).

Fig. 7.14 Summary of histological types of lung cancers

	Small cell	Squamous	Large cell	Adenocarcinoma
Relative incidence	20%	35%	15%	30%
Sex differences	Males > females	Males > females	Males > females	Males = females
Associated with cigarette smoking	Yes	Yes	Yes	No? (passive smoking)
Most common site	Centrally located	Centrally located	Centrally located	Peripherally located; often originating in areas of pre-existing lung scarring
Non-metastatic symptoms	ADH secretion Ectopic ACTH secretion Lambert–Eaton myasthenic syndrome	Hypercalcaemia HPOA	—	HPOA
Rate of growth	Fast; metastases usually present at diagnosis	Slow growing; metastasises late	Fast	Slow growing; metastasises early

Note: ACTH, adrenocorticotrophic hormone; ADH, antidiuretic hormone; HPOA, hypertrophic pulmonary osteoarthropathy

Fig. 7.14 Summary of histological types of lung cancers. (HPOA, hypertrophic pulmonary osteoarthropathy.)

Bronchial hamartomas

These are common but benign lesions of the lung, usually 1–3 cm in diameter and consisting largely of cartilage. They are firm and glistening white in appearance (often termed chondromas). Other elements are bronchial epithelium, fat and muscle. Bronchial hamartomas are asymptomatic and are mainly discovered at post-mortem examination.

Miscellaneous mesenchymal tumours

These tumours can be either benign (e.g. neurofibromas, lipomas) or malignant (sarcomas are extremely rare in the lung).

DISEASES OF VASCULAR ORIGIN

Pulmonary congestion and oedema

Pulmonary oedema is defined as an increase in extravascular fluid in the alveolar walls (pulmonary interstitium), which, if severe, subsequently affects the alveolar spaces.

Pathogenesis

Normally, a balance exists between hydrostatic pressure and colloid osmotic (oncotic) pressure such that only a small amount of fluid passes into the interstitium. This fluid is drained from the lung via lymphatic channels.

In pulmonary oedema, the lymphatic drainage capacity is exceeded, resulting in a net accumulation of fluid within the interstitium. This increases the stiffness of the lungs, giving rise to a subjective sensation of dyspnoea.

Macroscopically, the lungs are heavy and congested. In fatal cases, fluid flows from the cut surfaces and it can often be seen in the large airways.

Microscopically, the interstitium is widened, the capillaries are congested and the alveoli are filled with proteinaceous fluid.

Clinical features and causes

Clinical features of hypoxic respiratory failure may result from a combination of ventilation/perfusion imbalance caused by fluid in the alveoli and airway narrowing from external compression by peri-bronchial fluid.

Pulmonary oedema can result from:

- Altered haemodynamic forces—increased hydrostatic pressure; decreased oncotic pressure.
- Injury to the alveolar capillary wall that increases permeability.
- Blockage of lymphatic drainage.

Altered haemodynamic forces

This is most commonly caused by increased hydrostatic pressure, which may be secondary to:

- Left ventricular heart failure, e.g. after myocardial infarction, or due to aortic valve disease, mitral regurgitation and tachyarrhythmias.
- Pulmonary venous hypertension, e.g. due to mitral stenosis or chronic obstructive lung disease.
- Recurrent pulmonary emboli (see below).
- Fluid overload—excess infusion of crystalloid solutes.

In chronic left heart failure, prolonged increased hydrostatic pressure can lead to rupture of capillaries with leakage of red cells into the interstitium and alveoli. Macrophages of the interstitium and alveoli phagocytose haemoglobin and accumulate iron pigment. These cells are often termed 'heart failure cells'.

Pulmonary oedema due to decreased plasma oncotic pressure is seen in hypoproteinaemia, which may be secondary to:

- Malnutrition.
- Nephrotic syndrome—the triad of hypoalbuminaemia, oedema and proteinuria.
- Hepatic failure—due to a relative decrease in production of plasma proteins.
- Intravenous infusion of hypotonic solutes.

Alveolar capillary injury

Diffuse alveolar damage causes an increased permeability of alveolar capillary membrane leading to pulmonary oedema, haemorrhage, cell necrosis and hyaline membrane formation. These types of damage are seen in acute respiratory distress syndrome (see below).

Blockage of lymphatic drainage

Lymphatic obstruction prevents drainage of fluid to lymphatic channels. Obstruction may be caused by tumour emboli in lymphangitis carcinomatosa.

Acute respiratory distress syndrome

Acute respiratory distress syndrome (ARDS) is a clinical syndrome of diffuse alveolar capillary damage, characterised by pulmonary exudation and oedema with widespread systemic metabolic derangements.

Many conditions predispose to ARDS, most commonly systemic sepsis and severe trauma. The causes are listed in Fig. 7.15.

The exact pathogenesis is unknown in many cases, but events are thought to occur in two phases: an acute exudative phase (with capillary and alveolar endothelium injury) and a late organization phase (cell proliferation and fibrosis).

Fig. 7.15 Causes of ARDS

Cause	Clinical features
Blood borne	Major trauma, especially associated with raised intracranial pressure Septicaemia Major burns Disseminated intravascular coagulation Massive blood transfusion Amniotic fluid embolism Acute pancreatitis Cardiac surgery with bypass Antitumour chemotherapy Paraquat poisoning
Air borne	Pulmonary aspiration of gastric contents Inhalation of toxic fumes or smoke Near drowning Pneumonia from many causes requiring ventilation

Fig. 7.15 Causes of acute respiratory distress syndrome (ARDS).

In severe cases of ARDS, cytokines liberated from the lung vascular bed can enter the systemic circulation and these may cause systemic endothelial activation with massive neutrophil recruitment leading to multiorgan failure.

Figure 7.16 shows the main events and outcomes in ARDS.

Embolism, haemorrhage and infarction

Pulmonary embolism

Pulmonary embolism (PE) is the occlusion of a pulmonary artery, most commonly by thromboemboli

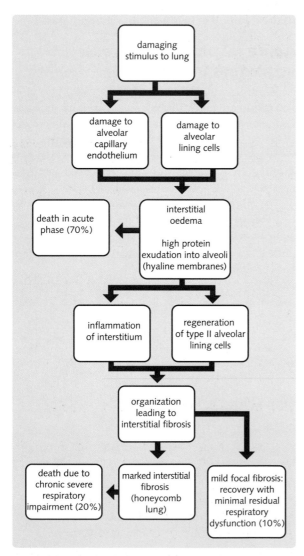

Fig. 7.16 Main events and outcomes in adult respiratory distress syndrome.

originating in the systemic veins (Fig. 7.17). The condition accounts for 1% of all hospital deaths, but this rises to 30% in patients with severe burns or trauma.

The vast majority of cases are caused by emboli arising from thrombosis of the deep leg veins (calf, popliteal, femoral and iliac veins). Venous thrombosis is considered in more detail in Chapter 6.

The consequences of PE are pulmonary hypertension (which puts a strain on the right side of the heart) and infarction of the lung (which occurs in only about 10% of cases of PE, as dual circulation protects against ischaemic necrosis).

Clinical features

The effect of PE depends on the extent of the pulmonary vasculature blockage and the time scale involved:

- Massive PE (5% of cases) is a sudden blockage of more than 60% of the pulmonary vasculature, resulting in electromechanical dissociation of the heart, i.e. the heart continues to beat but there is no output as pulmonary vascular resistance is too high. This results in cardiovascular collapse and rapid death. One example is a saddle embolus at the bifurcation of the left and right pulmonary arteries.
- Major PE (10% of cases) is a blockage of the middle-sized pulmonary arteries. These patients commonly experience breathlessness. Lung infarction develops in about 10% of such cases, which may lead to haemoptysis and pleuritic chest pain, if adjacent to the pleura. If untreated, patients may develop a subsequent massive thromboembolism.
- Minor PE (85% of cases) is a blockage of the small peripheral vessels by small emboli. Patients may be asymptomatic or may experience breathlessness and pleuritic chest pain as a result of small infarcts. As with major pulmonary embolism, patients may develop a subsequent massive thromboembolism if untreated.
- Recurrent minor PE (minority) is a blockage of the many small peripheral arteries over a period of many months by recurrent small emboli. The condition can lead to the obliteration of the vascular bed with the development of pulmonary hypertension and right heart strain.

Prevention and treatment

Pulmonary thromboembolism is the most common preventable cause of death in hospital patients. Prevention involves:

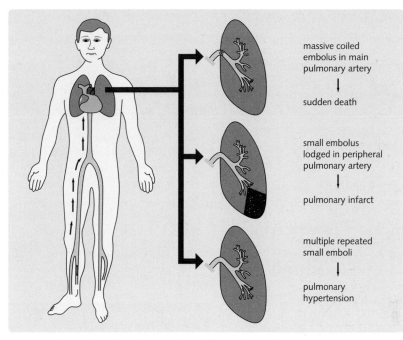

Fig. 7.17 Pulmonary thromboembolism. (Adapted from Underwood, 2000.)

- Mobilising early following surgery.
- Anti-embolic (TED) stockings.
- Heparin prophylaxis.

Treatment is with oxygen, analgesia and anticoagulation therapy (heparin, warfarin).

Non-thrombotic emboli

These are rare, but include:

- Fat, following a bone fracture.
- Amniotic fluid during labour.
- Air (after trauma or surgery).
- Decompression sickness, e.g. in deep sea divers ('the bends' or Caisson disease). Rapid decompression releases nitrogen bubbles, which cause problems in the CNS and bones and can produce functional obstruction of the pulmonary vessels.
- Foreign bodies.
- Tumour embolism—renal or bronchial cell carcinoma.

Pulmonary infarction

Infarction of lung tissue is usually associated with embolism.

The lower lobes are involved in 75% of cases. Macroscopically, pulmonary infarcts are typically haemorrhagic (because of blood entering from the bronchial circulation) and wedge shaped, and there is often an associated pleural reaction, which causes chest pain. With time, the infarct becomes organized to form a fibrous scar.

Microscopically, there is extravasation of blood into the necrotic lung.

Common sequelae include:

- Pulmonary dysfunction due to the loss of lung tissue.
- Pulmonary vascular obstruction leading to right heart failure (cor pulmonale).
- Pleurisy and pleural effusion.
- Healing, with fibrous scarring.
- Septic infarction due to either a primary septic embolism or secondary infection leading to abscess formation.

Pulmonary hypertension and vascular sclerosis

This is increased pressure of the lung vasculature, the main causes of which are listed in Fig. 6.15 (page 75), the most important being:

- Chronic obstructive airways disease.
- Interstitial fibrosis of the lungs.
- Chronic pulmonary venous congestion.

Pulmonary hypertension causes irreversible structural changes to:

- Pulmonary vasculature—medial hypertrophy of the muscular arteries (increased smooth muscle) and pulmonary veins (arterialisation); occlusion of the pulmonary arteries caused by intimal proliferation.
- Lungs; interstitial fibrosis.
- Right side of the heart—increased workload of the right side of the heart causes ultimate development of right heart failure (cor pulmonale).

The clinical effects are breathlessness and the symptoms and signs of right-sided cardiac failure.

Diffuse pulmonary haemorrhagic syndromes

A few interstitial lung disorders may produce diffuse haemorrhage, often with rapid patient deterioration. Important examples include:

- Goodpasture's syndrome—an autoimmune disease resulting in the breakdown of collagen in both lung alveoli and kidney glomeruli.
- Wegener's granulomatosis—an autoimmune granulomatous vasculitis affecting blood vessels of the upper respiratory tract and lung.
- Idiopathic pulmonary haemosiderosis—a rare disorder, probably of immunological origin, that can produce repeated diffuse alveolar haemorrhage, particularly in children.

DISEASES OF IATROGENIC ORIGIN

Drug-induced lung disease

Many drugs have pulmonary side effects, such as some anticancer agents that produce chronic pulmonary fibrosis. The calcium channel blocker and anti-arrhythmic drug amiodarone can have similar effects.

Asthma can by induced by aspirin (the mechanism for this is unknown) and certain β-blockers (by bronchoconstriction caused by an antagonistic effect on β_2-receptors of bronchial smooth muscle).

Complications of radiotherapy

Acute radiation pneumonitis

Excessive exposure to radiation causes diffuse alveolar damage and is an established cause of ARDS.

Chronic radiation pneumonitis

Less severe exposure occurring over a longer period of time results in progressive pulmonary fibrosis with the typical restrictive defect of pulmonary function.

Lung transplants

Heart–lung transplants are usually carried out for cardiac problems associated with pulmonary vascular hypertension.

Single lung transplants may be carried out for cystic fibrosis or pulmonary fibrosis. New surgical techniques have allowed lobar lung transplants from living donors to be used for carefully selected patients. To avoid rejection, all transplant patients require immunosuppression for life.

DISORDERS OF THE PLEURA

Inflammatory pleural effusions

Serofibrinous pleuritis

This acute inflammation of the pleura is accompanied by an accumulation of high-protein fluid (> 30 g protein/L; exudate) containing fibrinogen/fibrin between the pleural surfaces.

The condition is commonly due to infection, infarction or tumour.

Pathogenesis
Effusion is the result of movement of fluid through damaged vessel walls.

In serofibrinous pleuritis, the effusion is typically unilateral, with the pleural surface covered by a fibrinous exudate. The fluid consists of a straw-coloured fibrinous fluid containing mesothelial cells, lymphocytes and polymorphs. In neoplastic diseases, malignant cells can also be identified within the pleural fluid.

Sequelae
Common sequelae include:

- Atelectasis—compression of the lungs causes pulmonary collapse and respiratory impairment.
- Adhesions—formation of fibrous adhesions between the visceral and parietal pleura.
- Fibrosis—obliteration of the pleural space by fibrosis, which is common in long-standing effusions.
- Empyema (see below).

Suppurative pleuritis (empyema)

This is an acute inflammation of the pleura with accumulation of pus in the pleural cavity. Typically caused by pulmonary infection (e.g. pneumonia, tuberculosis, lung abscess), it can also complicate thoracic surgery or penetrating chest wall injury.

Common sequelae include septicaemia (haematogenous spread of infection to other organs) and atelectasis (lung collapse as a result of compression).

Haemorrhagic pleuritis

This acute inflammation of the pleura occurs with the accumulation of a blood-stained exudate and is often caused by tumour or pulmonary infarcts.

Non-inflammatory pleural effusions

Hydrothorax

This collection of low-protein fluid (< 30 g protein/L; transudate) is due to the movement of excess fluid through normal vessel walls. Common causes are:

- Cardiac failure (most common)—increased hydrostatic pressure in pulmonary hypertension.
- Hypoalbuminaemia—decreased oncotic pressure.

Effusions are usually bilateral and the pleural surface appears normal. Fluid is straw coloured and contains occasional lymphocytes and mesothelial cells.

The condition can cause pulmonary collapse (compression of the lungs causing respiratory impairment) or it may resolve completely (resorption of fluid on correction of the cause with no structural alterations).

The difference between 'transudate' and 'exudate' is important. Transudates are characterised by low-protein content (e.g. hydrothorax) in contrast to exudates, which have high-protein content (e.g. serofibrinous pleuritis).

Haemothorax

Bleeding into the chest is called haemothorax. It is most commonly the result of:

- Trauma, especially with rib fractures.
- Surgery.
- Pulmonary infarction.
- Spontaneous rupture of diseased arteries, e.g. atheromatous and dissecting aortic aneurysm.

If blood remains within the pleural cavity, the result is organization and pleural fibrosis.

Chylothorax

The accumulation of chyle (milky white emulsified fat) within the pleural cavity, caused by a leakage from the thoracic duct, is typically the result of malignant infiltration, surgery or trauma.

Pneumothorax

This is the presence of air in the pleural cavity, the causes of which are described in Fig. 7.18.

Spontaneous pneumothorax can be either primary (of unknown cause occurring in otherwise healthy individuals) or secondary (i.e. secondary to lung disease).

Traumatic pneumothorax is a result of chest injury or is iatrogenic.

Complications of pneumothorax include:

- Atelectasis—lung collapse due to compression of the underlying lung.
- Tension pneumothorax—progressive increase in air pressure within the pleural cavity, causing massive collapse of the affected lung, mediastinal shift and compression of the contralateral lung producing life-threatening respiratory insufficiency. The condition occurs as a result of a one way valve-like mechanism at the point at which air enters the pleural cavity. Air that enters the cavity in inspiration is unable to escape during expiration.

Pleural neoplasia

Pleural fibroma

This is a benign tumour of submesothelial connective tissue. The causes are unknown but there is no association with asbestos. The tumour is well circumscribed, localised and attached to the pleural surface by a pedicle. Histologically, it is composed of fibroblast-like cells with abundant collagen fibres.

Metastatic neoplasms

These are the most common pleural tumours, most frequently arising from the lungs, breast or ovary, but they

Fig. 7.18 Causes of pneumothorax

Cause	Type	Clinical features
Spontaneous	Primary	Idiopathic rupture of pulmonary 'bleb'; most common in thin young males
	Secondary	COPD: emphysema, chronic bronchitis and asthma Pneumonia Cystic fibrosis Whooping cough Pleural malignancy
Traumatic	Chest injury	Penetrating chest wounds Rib fractures Oesophageal rupture
	Iatrogenic	Subclavian cannulation Positive pressure artificial ventilation Pleural aspiration Oesophageal perforation during endoscopy Lung biopsy

Note: COPD, *chronic obstructive pulmonary disease.*

Fig. 7.18 Causes of pneumothorax.

can arise from any malignant tumour. They are usually associated with a high-protein exudate (see above).

Malignant mesothelioma

This primary neoplasm of the pleura is rare, but is an important cause of death in people previously exposed to asbestos, such as those from the ship building industry. There is a latent interval between asbestos exposure and disease presentation of between 25 and 45 years. Fibres of crocidolite (blue asbestos) are thought to be most important in the development of mesothelioma. These asbestos fibres become trapped in the lung following inhalation and they are particularly resistant to macrophage and neutrophil destruction.

Macroscopically, the tumours are highly malignant and they spread locally around the pleural cavity and pericardium. However, haematogenous/lymphatic metastasis is rare.

Microscopically, mesotheliomas have spindle cells and glandular patterns.

Clinical features include chest pain and breathlessness and there are commonly recurrent or persistent pleural effusions, which may be blood-stained.

Asbestos exposure also increases risk of lung cancer. Indeed, an individual exposed to asbestos has a far greater risk of dying from lung cancer than mesothelioma, particularly if they also smoke. However, the number of mesothelioma cases has rapidly risen in the UK over the last 20 years and it is estimated that this trend will continue until at least 2010. No curative treatment is possible and death usually occurs within 10 months of diagnosis.

Pathology of the gastrointestinal system

DISORDERS OF THE UPPER GASTROINTESTINAL TRACT

The mouth and oropharynx
Cleft palate and cleft (hare) lip

These are the most common major congenital malformations of the mouth. They frequently occur together as a result of the same process, namely a failure of fusion during the embryonic period.

Aetiology—a few cases are associated with a chromosomal abnormality (e.g. trisomy 13 or 18), but the majority have no identified cause. Retinoic acid (vitamin A) has recently been proposed as having teratogenic activity in the developing palate.

Morphology:

- Cleft lip—may be unilateral or bilateral, involving the lip only or extending upwards and backwards to include the floor of the nose and the alveolar ridge (Fig. 8.1).
- Cleft palate—considerable variation, from a small defect in the soft palate (bifid uvula) that causes little disability, to a complete separation of the hard palate combined with a cleft lip (Fig. 8.2).

The effects are an abnormal facial appearance, defective speech and feeding difficulty with extensive lesions (child is unable to suck).

Management is by artificial feeding, with plastic surgery recommended between 1 and 2 years of age.

Stomatitis

This describes inflammation of the oral cavity, which can be non-infective or infective.

Non-infective stomatitis

Aphthous ulcers are tiny, painful and shallow, occurring on a background of red mucosa typically on the lips, tongue or buccal mucosa. The ulcer crater is covered by a creamy exudate composed of fibrin and inflammatory cells, mainly neutrophils.

Aetiology and pathogenesis are unknown. These ulcers may be associated with Crohn's disease, coeliac disease and Behçet's syndrome; they also occur in 20% of the normal population.

Most aphthous ulcers spontaneously heal within a week, although they often recur. Occasionally, large ulcers may persist for several weeks before healing by fibrosis.

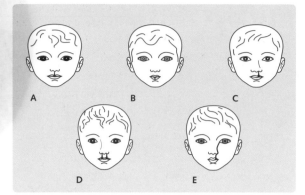

Fig. 8.1 Different types of cleft lip. (A) Median cleft upper lip. (B) Median cleft lower lip. (C) Unilateral cleft lip. (D) Bilateral cleft lip. (E) Oblique facial cleft.

Infective stomatitis

The majority of infections of the lips and buccal cavity are due to either viruses or fungi:

- Herpes simplex virus (herpetic stomatitis)—viral infections of the lips and mouth. Usually manifest as large blisters or crops of small painful vesicles, which eventually erode to form shallow tender ulcers. Severe herpetic stomatitis is important in the immunosuppressed (e.g. HIV-positive patients).
- Oral candidiasis—*Candida albicans* infection of the mouth (also known as 'oral thrush'). Common in infants but less so in adults without diabetes mellitus or immunosuppression. The condition develops as white patches on palatal, buccal and tongue surfaces. Lesions are composed of tangled fungal hyphae mixed with acute inflammatory cells and some desquamated epithelium. Underlying epithelium is acutely inflamed and red.

Glossitis

This inflammation of the tongue arises either as a result of infective stomatitis (see above) or is due to a deficiency of nutritional factors, especially niacin, riboflavin, folic acid and vitamin B_{12}:

- Acute deficiency—tongue is 'beefy-red', raw and painful because of atrophy of papillae.
- Chronic deficiency—tongue appears moist and unduly clean.

Oral manifestation of systemic disease

Many oral pathologies are manifestations of systemic diseases. Examples include aphthous ulcers occurring in Crohn's and coeliac disease, and angular cheilitis/glossitis in iron-deficiency anaemia.

Precancerous and benign neoplastic disease

Leucoplakia (keratosis)

This premalignant epithelial dysplasia may precede the development of carcinoma. The condition is characterised by a white patch or plaque (hyperkeratosis) of the oral cavity that cannot be scraped away. The condition usually affects the tongue. All lesions are considered precancerous unless proven otherwise by histological evaluation.

Erythroplakia (erythroplasia)

Less common than leucoplakia, this is characterised by the presence of red velvety patches of epithelial atrophy and pronounced dysplasia. It is seen mainly in elderly males on the buccal mucosa or the palate.

Malignant transformation is far more common than with leucoplakia. The development of erythroplakia is associated with heavy tobacco use.

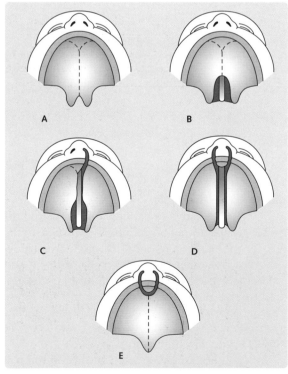

Fig. 8.2 Different types of cleft palate. (A) Cleft uvula. (B) Cleft soft and hard palate. (C) Total unilateral cleft palate and cleft lip. (D) Total bilateral cleft palate and cleft lip. (E) Bilateral cleft lip and jaw.

Malignant neoplastic disease

Squamous cell carcinoma

This is the most common tumour of the mouth, and it is derived from lining epithelium. It may arise from pre-existing dysplasia such as described above. Carcinoma affects 2 per 100 000 in the UK, occurring in men more than women by about 2 : 1. The risk factors are:

- Smoking—direct relationship between number of cigarettes smoked per day and the risk of developing oral cancer.
- Alcohol—moderate intake = decreased risk; excessive intake = increased risk.
- Nutritional deficiencies.
- Viral infections, particularly some forms of human papilloma virus (HPV).

Macroscopically, there are raised nodular lesions and central ulceration with hard raised edges.

Microscopically, the tumour is typically well-differentiated and keratinising.

The sites are:

- Lips (most common)—usually recognised early and amenable to surgery.
- Tongue—typically occurring on the lateral border of the anterior two thirds.
- Cheek or floor of the mouth (less common in the UK)—generally asymptomatic, resulting in extensive local invasion making surgical removal difficult.

Prognosis—may infiltrate locally and metastasise to regional lymph nodes in the neck. Five-year survival is about 50%.

Remember that 95% of all cancers arising in the head and neck are squamous cell carcinomas, most commonly occurring in the oral cavity. These cancers are classically seen in men who are heavy tobacco smokers and alcohol drinkers.

The oesophagus

Congenital abnormalities

Oesophageal atresia

In oesophageal atresia, the upper end of the oesophagus is intact, but it ends in a blind pouch. Oesophageal atresia affects 1 per 4000 live births, and more than 85% of cases are associated with the tracheo-oesophageal fistula—an abnormal communication between the lower oesophagus and trachea (Fig. 8.3).

The effects are:

- Fetus—inability to swallow amniotic fluid results in polyhydramnios, the accumulation of an excessive amount of amniotic fluid.
- Neonate—appears healthy initially but swallowed fluid returns through the nose and mouth and respiratory distress occurs. The condition must be surgically corrected in early life, but is also associated with other congenital abnormalities such as those of the heart.

Oesophageal stenosis

There is a narrowing of the lumen of the oesophagus, usually occurring in the distal third either as a web or as a long segment of oesophagus with a threadlike lumen. The causes are:

- Incomplete recanalisation of the oesophagus during development.
- Failure of blood vessels to develop in affected area → atrophy of a segment.

Webs and rings

These localised constrictions of the oesophagus are caused by mucosal folds or muscular contractions.

In Plummer–Vinson or Paterson–Brown–Kelly syndrome, upper oesophageal webs are associated with dysphagia in patients with iron-deficiency anaemia, cheilosis and glossitis. This is a rare but important condition because of an association with the development of postcricoid oesophageal carcinoma.

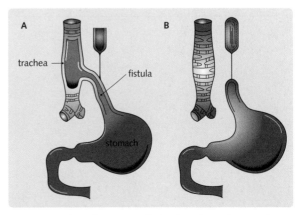

Fig. 8.3 Oesophageal atresia. (A) Blind ending of oesophagus with fistula formed between lower part and trachea. (B) Oesophageal atresia with no fistulous communication: very rare.

Inflammation of the oesophagus (oesophagitis)

Reflux oesophagitis

Inflammation of the oesophagus caused by gastro-oesophageal reflux disease (GORD) is the most common oesophageal abnormality and is caused by reflux of gastric acid through the lower oesophageal sphincter. The condition affects about 5% of adults; it can occur at any age (but with increased incidence over the age of 55 years), and it affects males more than females.

Figure 8.4 lists the predisposing factors of reflux oesophagitis.

Symptoms are a burning pain in the centre of the lower chest commonly known as 'heartburn'.

The complications are:

- Peptic ulceration of lower oesophagus—development of small ulcers which become chronic with fibrosis.
- Lower oesophageal stricture—progressive fibrous thickening of the lower oesophagus wall producing difficulty in swallowing.
- Barrett's oesophagus—metaplasia of lower oesophageal mucosa, with normal squamous epithelium replaced by glandular columnar epithelium composed of tall columnar cells. This increases the risk of oesophageal adenocarcinoma (see below).

Relevant investigations include endoscopy and 24-hour intraluminal pH monitoring.

Management is by:

- Lifestyle alterations—weight loss, stopping smoking, avoiding late meals and decreasing alcohol intake.
- Drug therapy—antacids, alginates, H_2-receptor antagonists and proton pump inhibitors (severe symptoms).

- Surgery—for those not responding to medical therapy, repair of hiatal defects or fundoplication may be appropriate.

Other causes

Other less common causes of oesophagitis are:

- Infective agents—*Candida albicans*, herpes simplex and cytomegalovirus may cause acute oesophagitis in the immunosuppressed.
- Physical agents—irradiation or ingestion of caustic agents (e.g. suicide attempts).
- Desquamative skin diseases, e.g. pemphigoid and epidermolysis bullosa may cause oesophageal ulceration, blistering and eventual erosion.

Lesions associated with motor dysfunction

Achalasia

Achalasia is a condition in which muscular contraction of the oesophagus and relaxation at its lower end are not coordinated, leading to retention of the food bolus. This may occur at any age but it is mainly seen in middle-aged individuals. The cause is unknown but reduced numbers of ganglion cells in the muscle plexus have been noted in long-standing cases.

The consequences are:

- Difficulty in swallowing (dysphagia)—increasing slowly over years.
- Regurgitation of undigested food.
- Occasional severe chest pain caused by oesophageal spasm.
- Mega-oesophagus—oesophageal distension occurs over a period of time.
- Increased predisposition to development of squamous cell carcinoma of the oesophagus.

Chagas' disease

Infection by *Trypanosoma cruzi* is a cause of secondary achalasia due to destruction of the myenteric plexus. It is common in South America.

Fig. 8.4 Predisposing factors of reflux oesophagitis.

Fig. 8.4 Predisposing factors of reflux oesophagitis	
Factors that increase intra-abdominal pressure	Overeating/obesity Pregnancy Poor posture
Factors that render the lower oesophageal sphincter lax or incompetent	Hiatus hernia Smoking Alcohol ingestion

Hiatus hernia

This is a common condition in which the upper part of the stomach herniates through the diaphragmatic oesophageal opening (hiatus) into the thoracic cavity.

The incidence is 5 per 1000 in the UK but it is 50–100 times less common in Asia and Africa. It may rarely be caused by a congenitally short oesophagus but is mainly thought to arise from increased abdominal pressure and loss of diaphragmatic muscular tone.

There are two types (Fig. 8.5):

1. Sliding hiatus hernia (90%)—stomach herniates through oesophageal diaphragmatic hiatus, resulting in the gastro-oesophageal junction moving into the thorax (associated with reflux oesophagitis and peptic ulceration).
2. Rolling (para-oesophageal) hiatus hernia (10%)—the fundus of the stomach protrudes through the hiatus but the gastro-oesophageal junction remains below the diaphragm (less associated with reflux).

Diverticula

Oesophageal diverticula are outpouchings of one or more layers of the oesophageal wall. They can develop by either:

- Pulsion—pressure from within the oesophagus creates a diverticulum. This is common immediately above sphincters.
- Traction—external forces pull on the wall, usually from adherent inflammatory lesions and classically from tuberculous lymph nodes. This is common near the midpoint of the oesophagus.

The site may be:

- Immediately above the upper oesophageal sphincter (Zenker's diverticulum).
- Near the midpoint of the oesophagus (traction diverticulum).
- Immediately above the lower oesophageal sphincter (epiphrenic diverticulum).

The complications are dysphagia (permanently distended diverticula retain food) and an increased risk of oesophageal perforation on endoscopy.

Lacerations

Oesophageal perforation is rare, but it may be caused by:

- Traumatic rupture—usually associated with vomiting.
- Impaction of a sharp foreign body.
- Intubation of strictures.

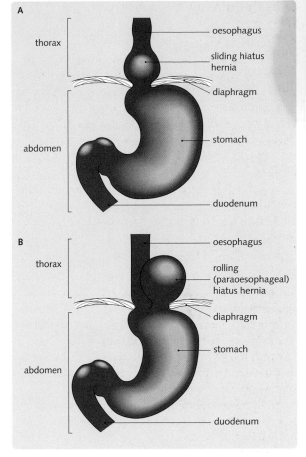

Fig. 8.5 Types of hiatus hernia. (A) Sliding hiatus hernia. (B) Rolling hiatus hernia.

'Mallory–Weiss tear' is a longitudinal oesophageal laceration as a result of severe retching or vomiting. This is most commonly seen in alcoholics, and classically occurs with vomiting of clear fluid (pretearing), followed by vomiting of blood (post-tearing).

Oesophageal varices

Oesophageal varices are varicosed, dilated submucosal veins in the oesophagus.

The condition is caused by portal hypertension (most commonly associated with cirrhosis of the liver).

Pathogenesis

Oesophageal veins normally drain into both systemic and portal venous systems.

Increased pressure in the portal venous system (e.g. as a result of severe diffuse long-standing liver disease) causes dilatation of the oesophageal veins, which often protrude into the lumen.

Rupture of these varices, or ulceration of overlying mucosa, can produce a massive haemorrhage into the oesophagus and stomach, often precipitating vomiting of blood (haematemesis).

Management
There are three stages:

1. Local measures to control bleeding—sclerotherapy, balloon tamponade and transjugular intrahepatic portosystemic stent shunting (TIPSS). TIPSS creates a shunt directly connecting the portal and hepatic veins of the liver, so reducing portal hypertension.
2. Reduction of portal venous pressure—drug therapy with terlipressin and somatostatin.
3. Prevention of recurrent bleeding—sclerotherapy, banding and TIPSS.

Neoplastic disease

Barrett's oesophagus
Definition—metaplastic replacement of normal squamous oesophageal epithelium with glandular columnar epithelium. Three types of mucosa are seen: junctional type, atrophic type and specialised mucosa.

The condition is caused by persistent oesophageal reflux; approximately 10% of these patients will develop Barrett's oesophagus.

Barrett's oesophagus predisposes to the development of adenocarcinoma. Metaplastic glandular epithelium can progress to epithelial dysplasia and then to frank adenocarcinoma.

Barrett's oesophagus is a classic example of metaplasia, and is a good example to quote in an examination.

Benign neoplastic disease
Benign tumours of the oesophagus are rare. The majority are leiomyomas derived from the smooth muscle of muscularis propria; the minority are derived from nerves, i.e. schwannomas and neurofibromas.

Malignant neoplastic disease
The most common malignant tumours of the oesophagus are squamous carcinomas and adenocarcinomas. Incidence is 5–10 per 100 000 per year in the UK. Risk factors are:

- Smoking/alcohol.
- Dietary (tannic acid, food colourings, nitrates and nitrosamines).
- Barrett's oesophagus—10% of these cases will develop adenocarcinoma in their lifetime.
- Corrosives.
- Achalasia.
- Iron-deficiency anaemia.
- HPV infection—this may have a role in the development of some squamous cell carcinomas.

Squamous cell carcinomas are more common than adenocarcinomas. They mostly develop in men who are heavy alcohol drinkers or heavy smokers, and may be preceded by an epithelial dysplastic change. They usually present late, located in the middle and lower oesophagus, and often causing dysphagia.

Adenocarcinomas mainly occur in the lower oesophagus in areas of metaplasia (Barrett's oesophagus). However, some adenocarcinomas are primary carcinomas of the stomach that have infiltrated the lower oesophagus.

Clinical features of oesophageal tumours
- Common—progressively worsening painless dysphagia, anorexia, weight loss, anaemia (acute or chronic).
- Rare—hoarse voice (involvement of larynx or left recurrent laryngeal nerve palsy), supraclavicular lymphadenopathy, tracheo-oesophageal fistula.

Investigations of choice are:

- Upper GI endoscopy—with cytology and biopsy.
- CT of chest and abdomen—stage the tumour and so determine operability.
- Endoscopic ultrasound—especially good for staging disease.

Management is often palliative to relieve pain and dysphagia (intubation, dilatation, bypass, laser treatment). Combinations of surgery, radiotherapy and chemotherapy (often neoadjuvant) may be attempted in early disease. Squamous carcinoma has a slightly better prognosis due to its radiosensitivity, but overall 5-year survival from oesophageal cancer is just 6–9%.

DISORDERS OF THE STOMACH

Congenital abnormalities
Diaphragmatic hernias
These are described in the previous section (page 133).

Pyloric stenosis

Marked narrowing of the pylorus (gastric outflow tract) causes obstruction to the passage of food such that the stomach becomes markedly distended and projectile vomiting occurs. This disorder can be congenital or acquired.

Congenitally, it is a common anomaly, affecting 4 per 1000 live births, males more than females by 5 : 1. Symptoms are caused by hypertrophy of pyloric circular and longitudinal muscle layers; surgical splitting is curative.

Acquired causes are:

- Fibrous stricture from a duodenal ulcer.
- Oedema from a pyloric channel or duodenal ulcer.
- Carcinoma of stomach antrum or compression by pancreatic carcinoma or lymphoma.
- Adult hypertrophic pyloric stenosis.

Symptoms are mainly nausea and vomiting. Signs include wasting, dehydration and a succussion splash, which may be elicited 4 hours or more after the last meal or drink.

Inflammation

Gastritis is the term used to describe inflammation of the gastric mucosa.

Acute gastritis

This superficial acute inflammation is typically caused by ingested chemicals, the most common being alcohol, aspirin and other non-steroidal anti-inflammatory drugs (NSAIDs).

Acute erosive gastritis

Focal loss of the superficial gastric epithelium causes dyspepsia with vomiting and possibly haematemesis, if the erosions are numerous.

Causes are:

- NSAIDs.
- Heavy, acute alcohol ingestion.
- Severe stress or shock (e.g. after major trauma or burns).
- Hypotension—acute hypoxia of surface epithelium.

Chronic gastritis

Chronic inflammation of the gastric mucosa is a common condition. It increases with age and is more common in developed countries. Mucosal atrophy occurs with intestinal metaplasia, increasing the likelihood of gastric carcinoma.

The condition is present in over 90% of patients with duodenal ulceration, in about 70% of those with gastric ulceration, and it is also common in those with gastric cancer.

There are three main aetiological types:

- Infectious—gastritis associated with *Helicobacter pylori*.
- Immune—pernicious anaemia and atrophic gastritis without pernicious anaemia.
- Reactive—after gastrectomy or adjacent to erosions/ulcers.

Helicobacter-associated gastritis

This is the most common form of chronic gastritis, accounting for more than 90% of cases, and it may arise at any age. The pyloric antrum is the most severely affected area, but damage is also seen in the fundus.

Pathogenesis is as follows:

- Colonisation—*Helicobacter pylori* colonises epithelial surface beneath thin layer of mucus. This causes an initial acute neutrophilic gastritis, which gives way to chronic gastritis.
- Urease production—the bacterium produces the enzyme urease, which breaks down urea to give CO_2 and ammonia.
- Immune response—the presence of the organism results in an immune response → epithelial damage.
- Persistence of infection—once established, infection may persist for years.

The morphological features are:

- Mucin depletion leading to damage to the underlying epithelium.
- Atrophy of gastric glands.
- Mixed acute and chronic inflammatory cell reaction in lamina propria and superficial epithelium.
- Intestinal metaplasia—normal gastric epithelium is replaced by a type similar to that of the small intestine.

The tests available for diagnosis of *Helicobacter pylori* infection are listed in Fig. 8.6.

Autoimmune chronic gastritis

This organ-specific autoimmune disease associated with pernicious anaemia is generally seen in elderly patients with the development of severe atrophy of the mucosa (atrophic gastritis). It particularly affects the body of the stomach.

Fig. 8.6 Test for diagnosis of *Helicobacter pylori* infection

Type	Test	Diagnosis
Non-invasive	Urea breath test	Radiolabelled urea is administered; urease produced by *Helicobacter pylori* → radioactive CO_2, which can be detected on the breath
	Serology	Antibodies to *Helicobacter pylori* can be detected in serum
	Stool analysis	Bacteria detected in faecal material
Invasive	Histology	Organisms can be seen in biopsy material
	Culture	Can be cultured from biopsy material
	CLO test	Biopsy added to test kit containing urea. If urease present NH_3 produced causes change in colour of indicator

CLO, *Campylobacter*-like organism.

Fig. 8.6 Diagnosis of *Helicobacter pylori* infection.

Antibodies are of two types:

1. Antibodies against gastric parietal cells (90%)—associated with decreased hydrochloric acid production (hypochlorhydria).
2. Antibodies against intrinsic factor (60%) → failure of absorption of dietary vitamin B_{12} → interference with normal erythropoiesis in bone marrow → megaloblastic, macrocytic anaemia (pernicious anaemia).

The most common form occurs without pernicious anaemia, even though antibodies of both types are often present. This is due to a residual ability to absorb vitamin B_{12}, which may be lost with time producing pernicious anaemia.

The morphological features are:

- Loss of specialised cells.
- Fibrosis.
- Infiltrate of plasma cells and lymphocytes.
- Intestinal metaplasia.

Reactive gastritis (reflux gastritis)
In this pattern of mucosal injury the dominant feature is epithelial change with minimal inflammatory cell infiltrates. The causes are threefold:

1. Idiopathic—majority of cases.
2. Reflux of alkaline bile-containing duodenal fluid into the lower part of the stomach. This may be caused by motility disturbances (e.g. due to gallstones or cholecystectomy) or pyloric incompetence (as a result of previous surgery to the pyloric area).
3. Drugs—NSAIDs may cause direct damage to the mucus layer.

Morphological features are:

- Epithelial desquamation.
- Foveolar hyperplasia.
- Vasodilatation.
- Mucosal oedema.

Complications of chronic gastritis
Regardless of cause, all forms of chronic gastritis can cause:

- Intestinal metaplasia—more likely to result in dysplasia and eventual carcinoma
- Peptic ulcerations—caused by damage to the gastric lining by acidic gastric secretions.

Gastric ulceration
Peptic ulcers
Peptic ulcers are ulcers of the oesophagus, stomach or duodenum caused by damage to the epithelial lining by gastric secretions, particularly acid.

It is estimated that about 10% of the Western population experience peptic ulceration at some time. Ulcers usually develop in adulthood and have a natural history of repeated healing and relapse over many years.

Sites of peptic ulceration, in order of decreasing frequency, are:

- Duodenum—classically the first portion due to hypersecretion of acid by the stomach.
- Stomach—usually at the antrum due to regurgitated bile in pyloric incompetence, or surface epithelial damage by *Helicobacter pylori* infection or NSAIDs.

- Gastro-oesophageal junction—due to gastric reflux onto unprotected mucosa.
- Gastro-enterostomy sites.

Aetiology is probably multifactorial but damaging influences include *Helicobacter pylori* infection, NSAIDs and stress. Less commonly, peptic ulcers may be associated with acid hypersecretion (e.g. gastrinoma), infection, duodenal obstruction/disruption, vascular insufficiency or radiation.

Other factors, such as chronic gastritis, smoking and genetic predisposition, are also believed to play a role in the pathogenesis.

Pathogenesis

Upper GI mucosa is normally protected by either squamous epithelium (oesophagus) or an acid-resisting mucus barrier containing neutralising bicarbonate ions. Peptic ulceration occurs when the aggressive action of acid and pepsin is not opposed by adequate mucosal protective mechanisms.

Macroscopically, peptic ulcers are typically 1–2 cm in diameter (but they can be much larger) with sharply defined borders surrounding the ulcer crater.

Microscopically, the ulcer crater usually penetrates into the muscularis propria of the stomach and it has four histological zones, namely:

- Superficial necrotic debris.
- Non-specific acute inflammation.
- Granulation tissue.
- Fibrosis.

Complete healing of the ulcer leads to fibrous replacement of muscle with regrowth of epithelium over the scar. Clinical features include episodic epigastric pain (alleviated by antacids) which is worsened by eating and may occur with nausea and heartburn (oesophageal ulcers).

Sequelae

Complications and sequelae are as follows:

- Healing—slow process hastened by acid-inhibiting agents or mucosal protectants.
- Haemorrhage—may be small and undetected (causing chronic anaemia) or occur as an acute episode of haematemesis.
- Adherence and erosion—ulcer penetrates full thickness of the stomach or duodenal wall, adhering and eroding into underlying tissue, particularly the pancreas or liver.
- Perforation—may lead to peritonitis.

- Fibrous strictures—caused by the healing of peptic ulcers, which may obstruct the oesophagus or stomach (acquired pyloric stenosis).
- Malignant change (very rare).

Peptic ulcer management:
- General—stopping smoking, avoiding NSAIDs, alcohol in moderation.
- Medical—eradication of *Helicobacter pylori* [triple therapy with a proton pump inhibitor (PPI, e.g. omeprazole), plus two antibiotics, e.g. clarithromycin and metronidazole]. If no infection is present, acid suppression medications include antacids, PPI and H_2-receptor antagonists.
- Surgical—rarely in acute ulcer haemorrhage or where medical control is impossible. A partial gastrectomy is used for gastric ulcers but complications are common.

Acute gastric ulcer

Acute peptic ulcers usually develop in areas of erosive gastritis, and they are predisposed by the same factors that promoted erosion (e.g. NSAIDs). In contrast to chronic ulcers, they are generally multiple and shallow with minimal surrounding inflammation or fibrosis.

Acute ulcers may heal without scarring or they may progress to chronicity.

Hypertrophic gastropathy

Ménétrier's disease

This rare disease of unknown cause is characterised by gross hyperplasia of gastric pits, atrophy of glands and a marked overall increase in mucosal thickness. It is associated with hypoalbuminaemia as a result of gastric protein loss via superficial ulcerations (a form of 'protein-losing gastroenteropathy').

Hypertrophic hypersecretory gastropathy

An extremely rare condition, this is characterised by acid hypersecretion and gastric protein loss.

Zollinger–Ellison syndrome

A gastrin-secreting tumour (gastrinoma) of the pancreatic G cells results in gastric gland hyperplasia and gastric hypersecretion (see Chapter 10). Multiple peptic ulcers and diarrhoea also occur.

Neoplastic disease

Benign polyps

Benign gastric polyps are rare compared with the incidence of malignant tumours of the stomach. The types are:

- Hyperplastic polyps—most common polyp of the stomach, formed by regeneration of mucosa, often at the edge of an ulcer in the stomach antrum.
- Adenomatous polyps—true benign tumours of the surface epithelium ranging up to 5 cm in size. Very rare, but dysplasia indicates that malignant change is possible.
- Fundal polyps—cystic glandular lesions seen mainly in women.
- Hamartomatous polyps—occur in Peutz–Jeghers syndrome (hereditary condition of multiple polyps in the small intestine associated with pigmented areas around the lips, inside mouth, and on palms and soles).

Other benign tumours of the stomach are derived from mesenchymal tissues, the most common being leiomyomas. These appear as mucosal or intramural nodules and are usually asymptomatic.

Gastric adenocarcinoma

The vast majority of malignant tumours of the stomach are adenocarcinomas derived from mucus-secreting epithelial cells. Incidence has been falling worldwide, with 17 per 100 000 males and 7 per 100 000 females affected per year in the UK. Males are affected more than females by 3 : 2.

Gastric adenocarcinoma is common in the Far East and certain parts of South America, but less so in Western Europe and North America.

The sites are:

- Pylorus (60%)—often produce symptoms of obstruction to the gastric outlet.
- Fundus (20–30%)—typically a fungating, ulcerating mass.
- Cardia (5–20%)—may produce dysphagia.

Unlike chronic peptic ulcers of the stomach, they are not confined to the lesser curvature.

Aetiology is unknown but dietary factors are suggested to account for geographical variation, e.g. ingestion of smoked and salted preserved foods. Other risk factors include:

- *Helicobacter pylori* infection—chronic *Helicobacter pylori* infection increases gastric carcinoma risk

5- to 6-fold. This is thought to be the result of chronic gastritis producing intestinal metaplasia, with eventual dysplasia and carcinoma. Chronic inflammation creates reactive oxygen species capable of damaging DNA, along with gland atrophy and hypochlorhydria, which favour further bacterial growth. However, the vast majority of those with *Helicobacter pylori* infection do not develop cancer.

- Chronic gastritis and intestinal metaplasia of other cause, e.g. autoimmune gastritis.
- Gastric adenomatous polyps.
- Postgastrectomy patients with persisting gastric inflammation.
- Gastric cancer families (rare).

The sequence of events in the development of gastric carcinomas is as follows:

> Normal mucosa → chronic gastritis → intestinal metaplasia → dysplasia → intramucosal carcinoma (early gastric cancer) → invasive carcinoma.

Several genetic changes have been reported in gastric cancer, including alterations of *p53* and *E-cadherin* expression, along with overexpression of oncogenes such as *c-myc*. *E-cadherin* changes appear unique to diffuse gastric cancer.

Gastric cancers are classified as either early or advanced according to the extent of their spread through the stomach wall.

Early gastric cancer

This is confined to the mucosa and/or submucosa regardless of whether spread has occurred to regional lymph nodes. It is associated with a good prognosis.

The cancer is further divided into three types according to macroscopic appearance (Fig. 8.7).

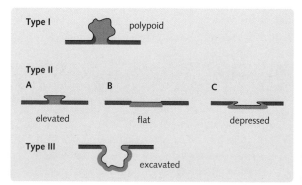

Fig. 8.7 Macroscopic classification of early gastric cancers: type I polypoid; type II is further divided into (A) elevated, (B) flat, and (C) depressed; type III excavated.

Advanced gastric tumours

These extend beyond the submucosa, and are associated with a poor prognosis. They are further divided into three types macroscopically (Fig. 8.8):

1. Polypoid—protrudes into stomach lumen and presents early due to gastric discomfort and bleeding when traumatised. Usually amenable to surgical excision and has the best prognosis.
2. Ulcerating (most common type)—similar to benign peptic ulcers but with a raised edge, necrotic shaggy base and an absence of the radiation folds seen in benign peptic ulcers.
3. Diffuse infiltrative pattern (linitis plastica)—presents late and has the worst prognosis. Tumour spreads extensively within mucosa and submucosa producing a shrunken, inexpansible, rigid stomach. Symptoms are usually non-specific (e.g. vomiting due to small stomach capacity) and metastatic spread is common at the time of diagnosis. Surface ulceration is not a prominent feature and so haematemesis is not common until the later stages.

Other gastric tumours

These are rare but include:

- Lymphomas (see Chapter 13)—a common site for extranodal non-Hodgkin's lymphoma. *Helicobacter pylori* infection is associated with a low-grade lymphoma (so-called 'MALToma').
- Carcinoid tumours (page 121)
- Gastrointestinal stromal tumours (GISTs)—relatively rare tumours that are thought to arise from interstitial cells that control gastrointestinal peristalsis. GISTs may be benign or malignant; it appears that 85% of cases display *c-KIT* mutations.

GENERAL ASPECTS OF HEPATIC DAMAGE

Patterns of hepatic injury

Following hepatic injury, the liver has a limited set of responses:

- Necrosis.
- Inflammation.
- Regeneration.
- Fibrosis.

All pathological processes of the liver result in one or more of the above reactions.

Necrosis

Acute hepatocellular injury can result in variable forms of necrosis. The underlying type of necrosis depends on aetiology.

Coagulative necrosis

This is typically a result of ischaemia (see Chapter 2).

Councilman bodies

During the death of individual liver cells (by apoptosis), single, dead hepatocytes form brightly eosinophilic, shrunken structures known as Councilman bodies.

Hydropic degeneration

This is the ballooning of individual hepatocytes, generally as a result of viral hepatitis. Mild swelling is reversible, but more advanced changes may progress to necrosis.

Focal necrosis

Necrosis of small groups of hepatocytes. Occurs in acute viral- or drug-induced hepatitis.

Zonal necrosis

Necrosis confined to certain zones is seen with particular conditions, e.g. centrilobular area (zone 3) is affected in acetaminophen (paracetamol) toxicity (Fig. 8.9).

Fig. 8.8 Comparison of the types of advanced gastric carcinomas

	Polypoid	Ulcerative	Diffuse infiltrative
Incidence	Common	Very common	Rare
Haemorrhage	Yes	Yes	Not until late stage
Prognosis	Good	Intermediate	Poor
Involvement	Focal	Focal	Diffuse

Fig. 8.8 Comparison of the types of advanced gastric carcinomas.

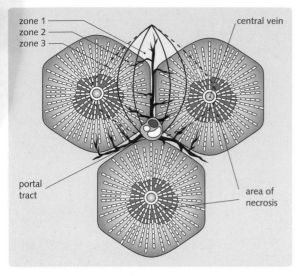

zone 1
zone 2
zone 3
central vein
portal tract
area of necrosis

Fig. 8.9 Centrilobular (zone 3) zonal necrosis. Zone 1 is perivenous (near portal vein) with a good oxygen supply, whereas zone 3 is pericentral (near central vein) with a poorer oxygen supply.

Massive necrosis

Necrosis of the majority of hepatocytes. Occurs with fulminant hepatic damage and is seen in some cases of viral- and toxin-induced damage.

Interface (piecemeal) necrosis

Liver cells at the interface between the periportal parenchyma and inflamed portal tracts are destroyed.

Inflammation

Inflammation of the liver is known as hepatitis, and it is a common response to a wide array of damage, e.g. viral infection, autoimmune disorders, drugs and toxins.

Regeneration

Under normal circumstances there is very little liver cell proliferation. However, following hepatic injury, liver cell regeneration occurs to restore liver function, even if the architectural structure of the liver cannot

be restored. This is a crucial phenomenon for recovery for patients with fulminant or subfulminant liver failure.

Fibrosis

Repeated chronic damage to the liver can result in fibrosis, which is usually considered an irreversible change. Growth factors produced as part of an inflammatory response are thought to stimulate proliferation and differentiation of mesenchymal cells (the normally inconspicuous fat-storing cells of Ito located in the space of Disse) into collagen-secreting fibroblasts.

Development of fibrosis is an important complication of several liver diseases, and it is one of the characteristic features of cirrhosis.

Cirrhosis

Cirrhosis is an irreversible condition in which the liver's normal architecture is diffusely replaced by nodules of proliferating hepatocytes separated by bands of scar tissue. Cirrhosis represents the end-stage of many processes—it is not a specific disease in itself. It involves:

- Long-standing destruction of liver cells.
- Chronic inflammation that stimulates fibrosis.
- Regeneration of hepatocytes to cause nodules.

Macroscopically, the liver is tawny and characteristically knobbly (due to nodules). On a cut surface, parenchyma is replaced by nodules of regenerated hepatocytes separated by fine fibrosis.

Microscopically, the nodules of hepatocytes are separated by bands of collagenous tissue. Bile ducts and portal vessels run in the fibrous septa.

Cirrhosis can be classified either according to the size of regenerative nodules (Fig. 8.10) or according to its aetiology (Fig. 8.11). The aetiological classification is most useful in determining prognosis and treatment. The clinical features of cirrhosis are illustrated in Fig. 8.12.

Fig. 8.10 Classification of cirrhosis according to nodular size.

Fig. 8.10 Classification according to nodular size	
Type	**Nodule size**
Micronodular	≤3 mm
Macronodular	3 mm–2 cm
Mixed micro- and macronodular	Mixture of small and large

Consequences are:

- Liver failure—reduced hepatocyte function (decreased synthesis of proteins, failure of detoxification).
- Portal hypertension and its complications (see below)—a result of impeded blood flow through liver.
- Reduced immune competence → increased susceptibility to infection.
- Increased risk of hepatocellular carcinoma.
- Increased risk of portal vein thrombosis.

Portal hypertension, ascites and splenomegaly

Portal hypertension

This is a continued elevation in portal venous pressure, normal portal venous pressure being less than 2–5 mmHg. Causes of portal hypertension can be classified according to whether the site of obstruction to flow is:

- Prehepatic—blockage of vessels before the hepatic sinusoids.
- Hepatic—blockage in the hepatic sinusoids.
- Posthepatic—blockage in the central veins, hepatic veins or vena cava.

Figure 8.13 lists the causes of portal hypertension.

Complications—portal hypertension causes back-pressure in the portal vascular bed leading to splenomegaly, ascites and varicose venous channels.

The causes and effects of portal hypertension are shown in Fig. 8.14.

Portal hypertension can be controlled with β-blocker drugs (usually propranolol) to reduce the risk of oesophageal variceal haemorrhage.

Portosystemic shunts

Venous communications that link portal and systemic venous systems become enlarged in portal hypertension. The four sites of portal-systemic anastomosis are:

1. Lower third of the oesophagus—left gastric vein (portal tributary) anastomoses with oesophageal veins (systemic tributary).
2. Halfway down the anal canal—superior rectal veins (portal tributary) draining upper half of anal canal anastomose with middle and inferior rectal veins (systemic tributaries).
3. Paraumbilical veins—connect left branch of the portal vein with superficial veins of anterior abdominal wall (systemic tributaries).
4. Veins of ascending colon, descending colon, duodenum, pancreas and liver (portal tributaries) anastomose with renal, lumbar and phrenic veins (systemic tributaries).

Pathogenesis—under normal conditions, portal venous blood traverses the liver and drains into the inferior vena cava of the systemic venous circulation by way of the hepatic veins. In portal hypertension, flow through this direct route is reduced and the portal venous blood is forced through smaller communications that exist between the portal and systemic systems.

Fig. 8.11 Classification according to incidence in the Western world

Common	Alcoholic liver disease Cryptogenic (no cause found) Chronic hepatitis caused by hepatitis B and C viruses
Uncommon	Autoimmune chronic hepatitis Primary biliary cirrhosis Chronic biliary obstruction (biliary cirrhosis) Cystic fibrosis
Treatable but rare	Haemochromatosis Wilson's disease
Rare	α_1-antitrypsin deficiency Galactosaemia Glycogenosis type IV Tyrosinaemia

Fig. 8.11 Classification of cirrhosis according to incidence in the Western world.

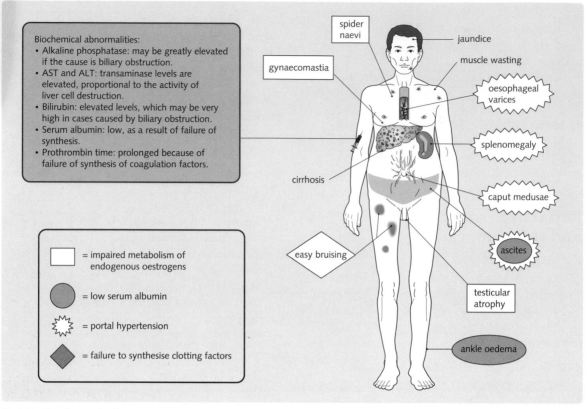

Biochemical abnormalities:
- Alkaline phosphatase: may be greatly elevated if the cause is biliary obstruction.
- AST and ALT: transaminase levels are elevated, proportional to the activity of liver cell destruction.
- Bilirubin: elevated levels, which may be very high in cases caused by biliary obstruction.
- Serum albumin: low, as a result of failure of synthesis.
- Prothrombin time: prolonged because of failure of synthesis of coagulation factors.

□ = impaired metabolism of endogenous oestrogens

● = low serum albumin

✦ = portal hypertension

◆ = failure to synthesise clotting factors

spider naevi

jaundice

gynaecomastia

muscle wasting

oesophageal varices

splenomegaly

cirrhosis

caput medusae

easy bruising

ascites

testicular atrophy

ankle oedema

Fig. 8.12 Clinical signs of cirrhosis.

Anastomotic channels become dilated resulting in the development of varicose venous channels, namely:

- Oesophageal varices (see page 133)—may cause severe bleeding.
- Caput medusae—distension of paraumbilical veins.
- Haemorrhoids—rectal varices develop.

Ascites

Ascites is the accumulation of free fluid in the peritoneal cavity. Common causes are:

- Peritonitis.
- Malignancy in the peritoneal cavity.
- Hypoproteinaemia—e.g. nephrotic syndrome.

Fig. 8.13 Classification of portal hypertension.

Fig. 8.13 Classification of portal hypertension	
Prehepatic	Portal vein thrombosis
Hepatic	Cirrhosis (most common cause of portal hypertension) Idiopathic portal hypertension Hepatic fibrosis: caused by schistosomiasis (important cause in endemic areas) Polycystic disease of the liver
Posthepatic	Disease of hepatic veins and branches, e.g. Budd–Chiari syndrome Severe right-sided heart failure Constrictive pericarditis

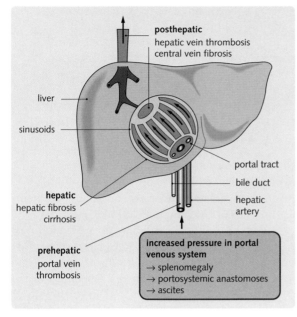

Fig. 8.14 Causes and effects of portal hypertension.

Ascites management:
- Restrict sodium intake.
- Diuretics, e.g. spironolactone.
- Paracentesis—drain 3–5 L over 1–2 hours for immediate relief. Drainage to dryness may be supported by colloid (e.g. albumin).
- LeVeen shunt—a subcutaneous draining tube connecting peritoneum to internal jugular vein via a one-way valve. Complications of infection, thrombosis, and pulmonary oedema limit use.
- TIPSS (see page 134)—relieves portal hypertension.

Prognosis—only 10–20% survive 5 years from onset.

- Portal hypertension—most commonly caused by cirrhosis.
- Heart failure.

Pathogenesis of ascites in cirrhosis—increased transudation of fluid in ascites occurs as a result of:

- ↑ Hydrostatic pressure in portal veins.
- ↓ Plasma oncotic pressure (due to lowered albumin synthesis by damaged liver cells).

Fig. 8.15 describes the types of ascites.

Clinical features are abdominal distension with fullness in the flanks, shifting dullness on percussion and fluid thrill.

Splenomegaly

Increased pressure in the portal vein is transmitted to the splenic vein resulting in splenomegaly. A variety of haematological abnormalities are associated with hypersplenism (see Chapter 13).

Jaundice and cholestasis

Jaundice

This presents as a yellowing of the skin, sclerae or mucous membranes, indicating excess bilirubin in the blood. It is clinically detectable when plasma bilirubin exceeds 50 μmol/L (3 mg/dL), although the biochemical definition refers to any reading above normal levels (approximately 18–24 μmol/L).

The metabolism of bilirubin is illustrated in Fig. 8.16.

Causes of jaundice

The easiest way to classify jaundice is by aetiology (Fig. 8.17):

- Prehepatic—the most common cause is haemolysis associated jaundice, a mild form of which occurs in many neonates due to immature liver function in the first weeks of life.

Fig. 8.15 Types of ascites.

Fig. 8.15 Types of ascites	
Transudate low protein fluid (< 30 g/L)	**Exudate high protein fluid (> 30 g/L)**
Cirrhosis	Malignancy
Constrictive pericarditis	Peritonitis
Cardiac failure	Pancreatitis
Hypoalbuminaemia, e.g. nephrotic syndrome	Budd–Chiari syndrome
	Hypothyroidism
	Lymphatic obstruction (chylous ascites)

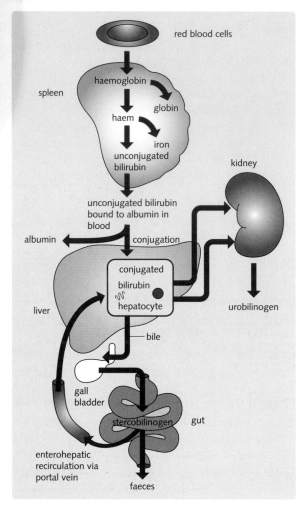

Fig. 8.16 Bilirubin metabolism.

- Intrahepatic—any cause of hepatocellular damage or intrahepatic cholestasis may be responsible. Hereditary enzyme defects may reduce the ability to conjugate bilirubin, so producing jaundice. Gilbert's syndrome is the most common of these conditions; it is not serious and requires no treatment.
- Posthepatic—any obstruction beyond the liver, e.g. gallstones.

Unconjugated versus conjugated hyperbilirubinaemia

An alternative classification system is based on chemical analysis of bilirubin in the blood (Fig. 8.18).

Failure of bile flow caused by the obstruction of either small (intrahepatic) or large (extrahepatic) bile ducts is termed cholestasis. It results in jaundice due to conjugated hyperbilirubinaemia. The high levels of conjugated bilirubin pushed back into the blood result in dark urine (high urobilinogen content), while the lack of bilirubin passing through the liver produces pale faeces. Conjugated bilirubin may be deposited in the skin causing itching (pruritus).

Unconjugated hyperbilirubinaemia is caused by states such as haemolysis, where the excessive release of bilirubin overwhelms the ability of the liver to conjugate it into a water soluble form (bilirubin–glucuronate). Insoluble bilirubin does not enter the urine and so this remains a normal colour, but faeces are darkened by the increased amount of bilirubin excreted through the liver. Pruritus does not usually occur.

Fig. 8.17 Causes of jaundice	
Cause	**Clinical consequence**
Prehepatic causes	Haemolysis (commonest cause)
Intrahepatic causes	Hereditary enzyme defects, e.g. Dubin–Johnson, Rotor's, Gilbert's and Crigler–Najjar syndromes Drugs causing intrahepatic cholestasis Pregnancy-associated cholestatis Hepatocellular damage, e.g. alcohol, virus hepatitis
Posthepatic (obstructive) causes	Large duct obstruction as a result of: • Gallstones • Strictures caused by inflammation or fibrosis • Extrahepatic biliary atresia • Compression by extrinsic masses, e.g. carcinoma of the pancreas, enlarged lymph nodes

Fig. 8.17 Causes of jaundice.

Fig. 8.18 Classification of jaundice according to chemical composition of bilirubin

Cause	Type	Example	Features
Unconjugated hyperbilirubinaemia	Prehepatic	Haemolysis	Urine: normal Faeces: dark
	Intrahepatic	Impaired bilirubin uptake (Gilbert's syndrome) Impaired bilirubin conjugation Crigler–Najjar syndrome Drugs, e.g. rifampicin	Increased risk of pigment gallstones No itching (excess urobilinogen with haemolysis)
Conjugated hyperbilirubinaemia	Intrahepatic non-cholestatic	Impaired bilirubin excretion into bile: • Dubin–Johnson syndrome • Rotor's syndrome	Urine: dark Faeces: pale Itching
	Intrahepatic cholestatic	Small bile duct obstruction: • Acute/chronic hepatitis • Cirrhosis • Intrahepatic tumours • Pregnancy-associated cholestasis • Sclerosing cholestatis • Intrahepatic biliary atresia	Urine: dark Faeces: pale Itching
	Posthepatic	Large bile duct obstruction	Urine: dark Faeces: pale Itching

Fig. 8.18 Classification of jaundice according to chemical composition of bilirubin.

Two important points to note about jaundice:
1. Liver disease is not the only cause of jaundice; there are other causes, e.g. haemolysis.
2. Many patients with significant liver disease are not jaundiced.

Hepatic failure

This is usually the end point of long-standing chronic liver disease, when up to 90% of hepatic function has been lost.

Hepatic encephalopathy

This is a neuropsychiatric syndrome caused by severe liver disease, occurring most often with cirrhosis but occasionally in a more acute form in fulminant hepatic failure.

Pathogenesis is:

• Liver failure—the liver is unable to remove exogenous/endogenous compounds from the circulation. Neurotoxins (e.g. ammonia) accumulate and impair neuronal transmission.
• Shunting—in portal hypertension, there is shunting of portal blood past the liver directly into the systemic circulation.

The overall effect is a biochemical disturbance of brain function. The condition is reversible and rarely shows marked pathological changes in the brain.

Hepatorenal syndrome

Renal failure secondary to liver failure occurs in advanced cirrhosis, and almost always in conjunction with ascites.

The kidneys themselves are normal. Renal failure is thought to result from altered systemic blood flow including diminished renal flow.

Prognosis—recovery depends on improvement of liver function but in chronic liver disease this seldom occurs.

Liver transplantation

Liver transplantation is, necessarily, a treatment for liver failure for which there is no other medical therapy.

Common indications

These are shown below in decreasing order of frequency.

- Chronic liver disease (end-stage), e.g caused by primary biliary cirrhosis, primary sclerosing cholangitis, alcoholic and metabolic liver disease.
- Fulminant hepatic failure—examples of this include rare cases of viral hepatitis and idiosyncratic drug reactions.
- Hepatic tumours—transplantation is only considered in the absence of extrahepatic malignancy.

Signs of end-stage liver disease:

- Sustained or increased jaundice (bilirubin more than 100 μmol/L).
- Ascites not responding readily to medical therapy.
- Malnutrition.
- Hypoalbuminaemia (< 30 g/L).
- Prothrombin time increased.

Risks and prognosis

Risks involved are:

- Rejection—immunosuppressants lower risk.
- Sepsis—prophylactic antibiotic therapy is used.
- Poor biliary drainage due to biliary strictures.

Prognosis is very good and improving. One year survival is 75–85%.

DISORDERS OF THE LIVER AND BILIARY TRACT

Congenital errors of metabolism

Haemochromatosis

This condition is caused by excessive deposition of iron in the tissues, including the liver. There are two types:

1. Primary (hereditary)—an autosomal recessive trait that leads to the production of abnormal HFE protein, which is linked to excessive absorption of iron from the gut. 90% of those affected are male.
2. Secondary—results from excessive iron accumulation caused by other primary diseases (such as sideroblastic anaemia and chronic haemolytic disorders).

Effects of iron accumulation

Iron accumulates as haemosiderin in many tissues including the liver, pancreas, pituitary, heart and skin. Affected tissues appear rusty brown due to haemosiderin within cells, as follows:

- In the liver—hepatocyte necrosis begins in the periportal region and spreads to affect the whole liver. Free radical generation may play a key role in this reaction. Cirrhosis ultimately develops, often with hepatomegaly.
- In the heart—infiltration of cardiac muscle can cause cardiomyopathy with heart failure.
- In the pancreas—damage to pancreatic islets may result in diabetes mellitus.
- In the skin—leaden grey pigmentation of skin due to excess melanin, especially in exposed parts, i.e. the axillae, groin and genitalia.

Diagnosis—there is a high saturation of transferrin in the blood, and high serum iron and ferritin levels. Diagnosis is confirmed by a liver biopsy showing heavy iron deposition and hepatic fibrosis, which may have progressed to cirrhosis.

Management:

- Weekly venesection (bleedings) of 500 mL until serum iron is normal. Followed by venesection as required to maintain normal serum ferritin.
- Therapy for cirrhosis and diabetes mellitus.
- Investigation of first-degree relatives by blood testing and possible genetic screening.

The term 'bronzed diabetes' is often used to describe haemochromatosis due to the combination of diabetes and hyperpigmentation.

Wilson disease

This autosomal recessive disorder of copper metabolism results in chronic destructive liver disease.

Normally, dietary copper is taken up by the liver, complexed to ceruloplasmin (a copper-binding protein) and then the whole complex is secreted into the plasma. Circulating ceruloplasmin is subsequently recycled by the liver, with any remaining excess copper being re-excreted into the bile.

In Wilson disease, a mutation in a copper transport ATPase gene results in failure of the liver to secrete the copper–ceruloplasmin complex into the plasma. The copper complex accumulates within the hepatocytes, saturating the available ceruloplasmin and leaving free copper to overspill into the blood, where it can cause haemolysis or be deposited in various tissues:

- Liver—chronic hepatitis, which progresses to cirrhosis.
- Brain—psychiatric disorders, abnormal eye movements and movement disorders resembling Parkinson disease.
- Eye—development of greenish-brown discolouration around cornea (Kayser–Fleischer rings).

Diagnosis—low levels of serum ceruloplasmin and high free copper in the blood; liver effects confirmed by biopsy.

Management is by copper chelators, e.g. penicillamine.

Alpha$_1$-antitrypsin deficiency

Affected individuals with this inherited condition fail to produce the normal active extracellular protease inhibitor α_1-antitrypsin.

Pathogenesis—α_1-antitrypsin is normally produced and secreted by the liver to inhibit the activity of protease enzymes. Mutations in the genes encoding the inhibitor prevent their secretion such that protease enzymes are not inhibited. The *PiZ* gene is most commonly affected.

In heterozygotes, there is an increased risk of lung damage, especially emphysema in smokers. Homozygotes develop emphysema and liver disease (cholestatic jaundice in the neonate; chronic hepatitis and cirrhosis in adults). This actually occurs due to the accumulation of abnormal α_1-antitrypsin globules in the liver, which cannot be secreted into the bloodstream.

Others

Reye's syndrome

This rare syndrome is characterised by acute encephalopathy with cerebral oedema as a result of sudden severe impairment of hepatic function (associated with microvesicular fatty degeneration). It occurs with high-dose aspirin use in children and adolescents, often following an upper respiratory tract infection.

Neonatal hepatitis

This clinical condition with many causes presents as neonatal jaundice.

Main causes are:

- Idiopathic (50% of cases).
- α_1-antitrypsin deficiency (15% of cases).
- Viral hepatitis.
- Hepatitis due to toxoplasma, rubella, cytomegalovirus or herpes simplex (i.e. TORCH group).
- Metabolic causes, e.g. galactosaemia or cystic fibrosis.
- Extrahepatic biliary atresia.
- Congenital hepatic fibrosis.

Prognosis—children with neonatal hepatitis generally recover. However, cases associated with biliary atresia require a surgical bile drainage operation.

Infectious and inflammatory disease

Viral hepatitis

Viral infection is a common cause of acute hepatitis. The main so-called hepatitis viruses are a group of hepatotrophic viruses. Although all cause a primary hepatitis, they are unrelated and they belong to different viral types.

Clinical features are similar in all forms of acute hepatitis regardless of aetiology.

Symptoms are nausea, anorexia, low-grade pyrexia and general malaise. Signs are hepatomegaly with tenderness, and jaundice 1 week after onset of symptoms, peaking at about 10 days.

Investigations—raised serum levels of conjugated bilirubin and liver aminotransferases (both aspartate and alanine).

Hepatitis A

This RNA enterovirus is prevalent in tropical countries, but uncommon in developed countries.

It is the most common travel related illness in the UK.

Transmission—faecal–oral route, e.g. from:

- Nurseries or institutions where hygiene levels are inadequate (person to person via hand-to-hand contact).
- Recreational activities in waters contaminated by sewage outfalls.
- Ingestion of sewage-contaminated shellfish.
- (Sexual) oral-anal contact.

Time course—illustrated in Fig. 8.19.

Prognosis—the majority of patients recover fully with restoration of normal liver function tests. However, a small minority (1–3 per 1000) develop fulminant hepatic failure with a mortality rate of 85%.

The disease never causes chronic hepatitis and infection confers subsequent immunity. A vaccine is available for long-term immunity.

Hepatitis B

This is a DNA virus of the Hepadna group. It can integrate into host DNA.

Transmission can be:

- Blood-borne—blood transfusions, IV drug abusers, tattooing, acupuncture.
- Sexual—sexual intercourse.
- Vertical—transmission from mother to child; either perinatally (transplacental) or postnatally (breast milk).

There are three clinical patterns of infection (Fig. 8.20):

1. Asymptomatic infection (65%)—transient subclinical infection with complete recovery.
2. Acute self-limiting hepatitis (25%)—symptoms include jaundice, malaise and anorexia, but the majority recover and develop lifelong immunity. There is a 1% mortality associated with fulminant acute hepatitis (massive hepatocyte necrosis).
3. Chronic hepatitis B infection (10%)—the majority enter an asymptomatic carrier state, which carries a future risk of chronic hepatitis.

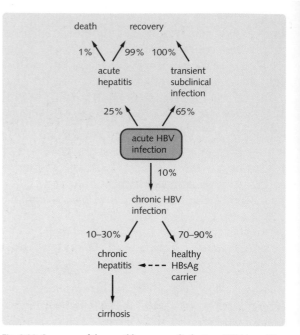

Fig. 8.20 Summary of the possible courses of infection. (HBV, hepatitis B virus; HBsAg, hepatitis B surface antigen.) (Adapted with permission from Clinical Medicine, 3rd edn, by P Kumar and M Clarke, Baillière Tindall, 1994.)

A minority progress to chronic hepatitis after initial infection; chronic hepatitis is a strong risk factor for cirrhosis.

Time course—illustrated in Fig. 8.21.

Complications are cirrhosis (as a result of chronic hepatitis) and hepatocellular carcinoma. Carriers of hepatitis B are 200 times more likely to get liver cancer than non-carriers. However, there is typically a latency period of 20–30 years between infection and cancer.

Treatment—large doses of interferon-α/β for carriers. The role of the antiviral nucleoside drug lamivudine is currently being evaluated. Prophylactic vaccination based on the hepatitis B surface antigen (HBsAg) is available but up to 10% of normal individuals fail to produce protective antibodies.

Hepatitis C

This RNA flavivirus is a major cause of hepatitis worldwide.

Transmission—predominantly blood-borne spread, although sexual and vertical transmissions do occur. Hepatitis C is widespread among intravenous drug abusers and was previously spread by blood transfusions before serological screening of donated samples was introduced.

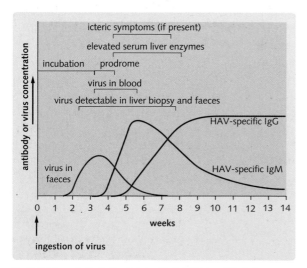

Fig. 8.19 Course of infection in hepatitis A. HAV-hepatitis A virus.

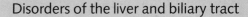

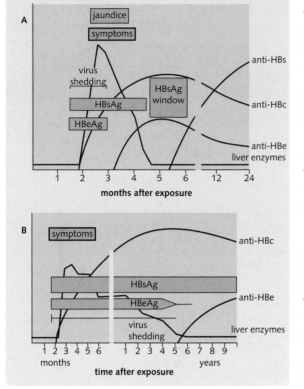

Fig. 8.21 Course of infection in hepatitis B. (A) Acute hepatitis. (B) Chronic hepatitis. (HBsAg, hepatitis B surface antigen; HBeAg, hepatitis Be antigen; anti-HBs, antibody to HBsAg; anti-HBc, antibody to hepatitis B core antigen; anti-HBe, antibody to HBeAg.) HBsAg window is time point where neither HBsAg nor anti-HBs can be detected because of immune complex formation.

Infection is asymptomatic in 10–35% of cases although it may progress to the carrier state. However, the majority of patients develop acute hepatitis (in 65–90% of cases).

Chronic hepatitis develops in 70–80% of those infected, increasing lifelong risk of cirrhosis and hepatocellular carcinoma.

Treatment is with interferon-α and ribavirin, although only half of patients will respond.

Hepatitis D

This RNA virus is incomplete and can only cause infection in the presence of hepatitis B virus; transmission is as for hepatitis B virus. Both viruses may be acquired simultaneously or hepatitis D may be acquired later as a superinfection.

The virus increases the severity of chronic hepatitis, and it may predispose to the development of fulminant hepatitis.

Hepatitis E

This RNA virus has the same transmission pattern as hepatitis A. Infection by hepatitis E is clinically similar to hepatitis A infection.

Other viruses

Non-hepatotrophic viruses may also cause hepatitis. Examples include group B arbovirus (yellow fever), Epstein–Barr virus and cytomegalovirus.

Autoimmune hepatitis

This chronic form of hepatitis is histologically identical to chronic viral hepatitis. It has a prevalence of about 4 per 10 000, and it typically occurs in women (70% of cases) between the ages of 20 and 40 years.

The condition is associated with hyperglobulinaemia and autoantibodies in the serum (antismooth muscle and antinuclear antibodies in type I disease; antiliver–kidney microsomal antibodies in type II). Type I disease (most common) is associated with other autoimmune disorders such as Graves disease and Sjögren's syndrome (dry eyes and mouth).

Clinically, there is insidious onset of anorexia, malaise and fatigue accompanied by abdominal distension and mild jaundice (with dark urine and itching).

Complications are cirrhosis, liver failure and hepatocellular carcinoma.

Investigations:

- Liver function tests—hyperbilirubinaemia, moderately raised aminotransferase levels.
- Hyperglobulinaemia (mainly IgG increases), often with a raised erythrocyte sedimentation ratio (ESR).
- Serology—autoantibodies are useful if titres are high, but low levels may be found in healthy people.

The disease may run a relapsing and remitting course but it progresses inexorably to cirrhosis.

Treatment is with corticosteroids; azathioprine may help to reduce steroid dosage.

Prognosis—patients who do not respond to treatment will almost always progress to cirrhosis. Also, many patients develop cirrhosis despite having a response to treatment. If end-stage liver disease develops, liver transplantation is an effective procedure.

Fulminant hepatitis

This rare syndrome of hepatic encephalopathy results from sudden severe impairment of hepatic function. It is caused by acute, severe liver damage such as:

- Viral infections (most common cause), e.g. hepatitis B.
- Drugs and poisons, e.g. acetaminophen (paracetamol) overdose, carbon tetrachloride.
- Non-viral infections, e.g. *Leptospira, Toxoplasma gondii, Coxiella burnetii*.
- Metabolic—Wilson disease, pregnancy.
- Ischaemic—shock, severe cardiac failure, Budd–Chiari syndrome.

The pathogenesis of hepatic encephalopathy has already been described (see page 145).

Fulminant hepatitis is distinguished from hepatic encephalopathy occurring as a result of deteriorating chronic liver disease by its occurrence within 8 weeks of onset of the precipitating illness, and in the absence of evidence of pre-existing liver disease.

Clinical features are:

- Cerebral disturbance (mental changes progressing from confusion to stupour and coma).
- Weakness, vomiting and nausea.
- Rapidly developing jaundice with fetor hepaticus (distinctive breath odour).
- Asterixis—flapping tremor.
- Ascites and oedema.

The liver may enlarge initially, but later it becomes impalpable; disappearance of hepatic dullness on percussion indicates shrinkage and is a bad prognostic sign.
Complications:

- Oedema—this may be cerebral (causing raised intracranial pressure) or pulmonary (contributing to respiratory failure).
- General vasodilatation—hypotension and hypothermia.
- Infection.
- Coagulation disorders.
- Necrotic cirrhosis.
- Pancreatitis.
- Renal failure—deterioration parallels that of liver failure.
- Metabolic—hypoglycaemia, hypokalaemia, hypocalcaemia, hypomagnesaemia, acid–base disturbance.

There is no specific treatment. Management is by close observation, treating complications as necessary.
Prognosis:

- 66% of patients with minor signs survive.
- Only 10% of patients with coma survive.
- Those who recover from fulminant hepatic failure usually regain normal hepatic structure and function.

Postnecrotic cirrhosis

This rapidly developing cirrhosis follows extensive necrosis, e.g. postfulminant hepatitis.

Liver abscess

This localised collection of pus within the liver is walled off and surrounded by damaged and inflamed liver tissue. Liver abscesses are rare but important as they are inevitably fatal if untreated.

Pyogenic abscesses

The most common causative organisms are *Escherichia coli*, various streptococci and other enterobacteria.
Mode of infection:

- Blood borne—via portal vein (mesenteric infections) or hepatic artery (bacteraemia). Usually solitary abscesses.
- Ascending spread from colonization of biliary tract (most common)—almost always predisposed by biliary obstruction and usually resulting in multiple small abscesses.
- Penetrating trauma.

Symptoms of infection and right upper quadrant pain (may radiate to the right shoulder) are common, along with hepatomegaly and a mild jaundice.

Investigations include ultrasound imaging. Needle aspiration at this time can confirm the diagnosis in addition to providing pus for culture.

Management is by prolonged antibiotics and drainage of the abscess.

Prognosis—the mortality of liver abscesses is 20–40%, usually through failure to make the diagnosis.

Amoebic abscess

The most common causative organism is *Entamoeba histolytica*, which is transmitted from the bowel to the liver via the blood. The disease is rare in the UK but common worldwide, and it must be considered in patients travelling from endemic areas such as Africa, Asia and South America.

Alcohol, drugs and toxins

Alcoholic liver disease

Alcohol abuse is the most common cause of liver disease in Western countries. Women are more prone to alcohol-induced liver damage than men.

Alcohol is metabolised almost exclusively in the liver and liver damage is related to daily alcohol intake. Toxicity of ethanol is probably caused by the generation of its metabolic breakdown product, acetaldehyde, which binds to liver proteins and damages hepatocytes. Alcohol also stimulates collagen synthesis in the liver leading to fibrosis.

Its effects are fatty liver, acute hepatitis and cirrhosis.

Fatty liver (hepatic steatosis)

This is the most common lesion of alcoholic liver disease. The condition is characterised by the accumulation of fat globules within the cytoplasm of hepatocytes. It is reversible on cessation of alcohol ingestion.

It is thought that alcohol stimulates hepatocyte triacylglycerol production, while impairing its excretion from the liver. The condition reflects severe metabolic derangement and it may affect a few or almost all hepatocytes.

Alcoholic hepatitis

This is acute hepatitis with focal necrosis of liver cells. At high concentrations, alcohol causes toxic injury to hepatocytes, evoking a neutrophil-dominant inflammatory reaction, which is reversible on abstinence. Eosinophilic accumulations called Mallory bodies may be seen on liver biopsy. Continued alcohol consumption causes the development of fibrosis around central veins. The result is hepatic fibrosis that may progress to cirrhosis.

The illness resembles acute viral hepatitis (see page 147) and liver function tests show raised levels of aminotransferases and γ-glutamyltransferase (GGT).

Alcoholic cirrhosis

Irreversible architectural disturbance occurs as a result of sustained alcoholic liver injury.

Normal liver architecture is diffusely replaced by nodules of regenerated liver cells separated by bands of collagenous fibrosis. This may develop after episodes of acute alcoholic hepatitis or may be insidious in its onset presenting only as end-stage liver disease.

It affects fewer than 10% of patients suffering from chronic alcoholism.

Fatty change can occur without excessive alcohol intake; it is commonly seen amongst the obese and type 2 diabetic populations. There is predominantly macrovesicular change (large fat globules), although conditions such as pregnancy may be microvesicular (small fat globules). In a minority of individuals, there may be an accompanying inflammatory infiltrate, producing a non-alcoholic steatohepatitis (NASH). This is associated with the same risks of progression to cirrhosis as alcoholic hepatitis.

Drugs and toxins

The liver is the main organ of drug metabolism and, consequently, drugs are a common cause of liver disease. Hepatotoxic drugs may be divided into two main groups: intrinsic hepatotoxins and idiosyncratic hepatotoxins.

Intrinsic hepatotoxins

These have dose-dependent, predictable toxic effects. They are responsible for a high incidence of toxic damage to the liver via either direct toxicity of an unmetabolised drug or normal hepatic conversion to a toxic metabolite.

Idiosyncratic hepatotoxins

These have non-dose-dependent, unpredictable toxic effects. They cause liver disease in a small percentage of exposed individuals as a result of hypersensitivity (drug-mediated autoimmunity) or abnormal drug metabolism.

Circulatory disorders of the liver

Overview

Vascular disorders of the liver (Fig. 8.22) can be classified into one of three categories depending on their pathogenic mechanisms:

1. Obstruction to outflow—hepatic vein obstruction.
2. Lobular compromise.
3. Obstruction to inflow—obstruction of portal vein or hepatic artery occlusion.

Diseases causing obstruction to outflow (hepatic vein obstruction)

- Veno-occlusive disease—widespread occlusion of central hepatic veins.

Fig. 8.22 Vascular disorders of the liver.

Fig. 8.22 Vascular disorders of the liver	
Cause	**Example**
Outflow (hepatic vein) obstruction	Veno-occlusive disease Budd-Chiari syndrome Right-sided cardiac failure
Lobular compromise	Cirrhosis Non-cirrhotic fibrosis: • Infective, e.g. schistosomiasis • Drugs, e.g. alcohol, hypervitaminosis A, vinyl chloride, arsenic • Congenital, e.g. congenital hepatic fibrosis, infantile polycystic disease • Nodular regenerative hyperplasia Systemic circulatory disturbances, e.g. shock
Inflow obstruction	Extrahepatic: • Portal vein obstruction: Portal vein thrombosis Extrinsic compression of portal vein Congenital stenosis • Hepatic artery occlusion: Hepatic artery thrombosis Embolism, e.g. infective endocarditis Intrahepatic: • Occlusion of intrahepatic portal vein branches

- Budd–Chiari syndrome—obstruction occurs in the larger hepatic veins.
- Cardiac disease—right-sided cardiac failure causes congestion of the inferior vena cava.

Clinical manifestations depend on the cause and speed with which obstruction develops, but congestive hepatomegaly and ascites are features in all patients.

Veno-occlusive disease

This condition has clinical features similar to those of Budd–Chiari syndrome (see below).

Causes are hepatic irradiation, cytotoxic drugs and the ingestion of plants containing toxic alkaloids (common in Jamaica and certain areas of Africa in those who drink herbal teas).

Pathogenesis is unclear but involves fibrosis around central veins, which ultimately results in obliteration of the vein lumen.

Budd–Chiari syndrome

This rare condition is caused by occlusion of the main hepatic vein or (more rarely) the intrahepatic vena cava (Fig. 8.23).

Fig. 8.23 Aetiology of Budd–Chiari syndrome.

Fig. 8.23 Aetiology of Budd–Chiari syndrome	
Idiopathic	Underlying cause cannot be found in more than half of cases
Thrombotic causes	Haematological diseases, for example: • Primary proliferative polycythaemia • Paroxysmal nocturnal haemoglobinuria • Deficiencies of antithrombin III, proteins C and S Pregnancy/oral contraceptives
Local compression of hepatic vein (rare)	Obstruction due to tumours, e.g. liver, kidneys or adrenals Congenital venous webs Inferior vena cava stenosis

Obstruction of the hepatic vein causes severe hepatic congestion with atrophy and/or necrosis of liver cells in the affected areas. Fibrous scarring eventually occurs in areas of hepatocyte necrosis. True cirrhosis supervenes in a minority of cases.

Clinical manifestations—patients develop severe acute disease with:

- Painful hepatomegaly.
- Acute portal hypertension.
- Rapid development of ascites.
- Jaundice.

Death results unless a surgical portosystemic vascular shunt is created.

Passive congestion

Congestive cardiac failure causes venous outflow obstruction in the liver due to back pressure transmitted as described below:

Inferior vena cava → hepatic vein → central veins → centrilobular congestion

Centrilobular sinusoids are dilated by blood and the centrilobular hepatocytes undergo atrophy and necrosis (centrilobular necrosis), giving rise to the appearance of what is described as a 'nutmeg liver' (chronic passive venous congestion).

The condition is common in tricuspid valve incompetence when the liver is pulsatile.

Arterial hypotension may increase the congestive effect of right-sided cardiac failure.

Diseases resulting in lobular compromise

- Cirrhosis—distortion and destruction of the hepatic vascular architecture causes sinusoid occlusion.
- Non-cirrhosis fibrosis—where fibrotic damage to the liver does not amount to true cirrhosis, e.g. schistosomiasis infection.
- Systemic circulatory disturbances—shock from any source causes severe hypoperfusion, resulting in zonal necrosis.

Diseases resulting in obstruction to inflow

- Extrahepatic—portal vein obstruction (thrombosis, extrinsic compression) or hepatic artery occlusion (thrombosis, embolism).
- Intrahepatic—occlusion of intrahepatic portal vein branches causes areas of venous infarction.

Portal vein obstruction

Obstruction of the portal vein results in portal hypertension and its associated complications (see page 141). The causes may be thrombotic or non-thrombotic.

Thrombotic conditions (those that predispose to portal vein thrombosis) are:

- Inflammatory—thrombophlebitis and intra-abdominal sepsis (e.g. appendicitis, cholecystitis, pancreatitis).
- Neoplastic—hepatocellular carcinoma, metastatic liver tumours and haematological malignancies (e.g. polycythaemia rubra vera, essential thrombocytosis, myelofibrosis).
- Cirrhosis—leads to portal hypertension and stasis.
- Splenic vein thrombosis (often secondary to pancreatitis) may propagate into the portal vein.

Non-thrombotic conditions are external compression (e.g. by tumour masses) and cirrhosis.

Liver infarction

True infarction of the liver is rare because of its dual blood supply and rich anastomosis of blood flow through the sinusoids. However, hepatic blood flow may be compromised in the following conditions:

- Surgical trauma or accidental ligation of hepatic artery.
- Therapeutic arterial embolisation of the liver or therapeutic hepatic arterial ligation (performed to treat isolated neoplastic masses).
- Bacterial endocarditis—embolism.
- Eclampsia (see below).
- Polyarteritis nodosa—a necrotising vasculitis.

Hepatic disease in pregnancy

Pre-eclampsia

This is high blood pressure (more than 140/90 mmHg) and proteinuria developing during pregnancy in a woman whose blood pressure was previously normal. It occurs in about 10% of pregnancies.

HELLP syndrome

This syndrome of haemolysis, elevated liver enzymes, and low platelets in the blood occurs in approximately 10% of all women with pre-eclampsia. The liver may be destroyed by the development of disseminated intravascular coagulation (see Chapter 13). Irregular areas of necrosis occur as a result of fibrin thrombi deposition in adjacent portal vessels.

Liver function depends on the severity of disease; in severe cases life-threatening haemorrhage into parts of the liver or abdomen may occur.

This disease resolves immediately after delivery and the liver generally heals itself within days to weeks. However, whilst the disease is ongoing, the mother is at risk of complications of liver damage and generalised coagulation disorders, and the fetus is at risk of premature delivery or stillbirth.

Eclampsia

This is the occurrence of one or more convulsions not caused by other conditions such as epilepsy or cerebral haemorrhage in a woman with pre-eclampsia. It is associated with severe epigastric pain, hyper-reflexia, nausea and vomiting, and severe hepatic damage. Fetal and maternal death may occur.

Liver histology shows fibrin deposition and ischaemic necrosis.

Acute fatty liver of pregnancy

This potentially serious but rare condition presents in the third trimester with symptoms ranging from asymptomatic elevation of aminotransferase enzymes, to fulminant hepatitis (jaundice, vomiting, abdominal pain and possibly coma). It affects up to 1 in 4000 pregnancies.

The aetiopathogenesis is unknown, but it is characterised by widespread centrilobular microvesicular fatty change in hepatocytes.

Untreated cases may be associated with a high maternal and fetal mortality. Early recognition of the condition and treatment by caesarean section has greatly improved the outlook.

Intrahepatic cholestasis of pregnancy

Cholestasis occurring as a result of intrahepatic causes appears in the second or third trimester, lasts for the duration of the pregnancy and resolves within 2–4 weeks of delivery.

Aetiology of the syndrome is uncertain but it is probably caused by an inherited susceptibility of a patient's liver cells to oestrogens. The condition is sometimes precipitated by oral contraceptives.

Symptoms are pruritus (almost always starts in third trimester and remits within about 2 weeks of delivery) and jaundice (occurs in about half of the patients).

The fetus remains unharmed but the condition tends to recur in subsequent pregnancies.

Neoplasia of the liver
Benign tumours
Hepatic adenomas

These typically affect premenopausal women, and they are predisposed by oestrogen-containing oral contraceptives.

The macroscopic appearance is of well-circumscribed nodules up to 20 cm in size.

The microscopic appearance closely resembles that of a normal liver, except that no portal structures are seen.

Complications—the majority of lesions are asymptomatic, but subcapsular adenomas are prone to rupture, leading to intra-abdominal bleeding.

Bile-duct adenomas

These are very common lesions composed of abnormal bile ducts in a collagenous stroma that appear as small white nodules, often beneath the liver capsule. They may be mistaken for metastatic tumour deposits at laparotomy.

Haemangioma

These are common hamartomas composed of abnormal vascular channels in a collagenous stroma. They are found at autopsy in 2–5% of the population and are typically seen just beneath the capsule as a dark lesion (usually 2–3 cm in size).

Malignant
Hepatocellular carcinoma (liver cell carcinoma)

Carcinoma of hepatocytes is the commonest primary tumour of the liver. Uncommon in the UK (affects about 1 per 100 000) it is up to 100 times more common in parts of Africa and the Far East, probably because of the higher incidence of hepatitis B and contaminating mycotoxins. Males are affected more than females.

Predisposing factors are:

- Cirrhosis—independent of cause.
- Hepatitis B or C infection—with chronic carrier state.
- Mycotoxins—these contaminate certain foods, e.g. aflatoxins produced by the fungus *Aspergillus flavus*, which frequently contaminates stored nuts and grains in tropical countries.

Tumours may consist of a single mass or multiple nodules. Hepatocellular carcinomas often produce α-fetoprotein, which is secreted into the blood and is useful as a diagnostic marker. Prognosis is very poor with median survival of less than 6 months from diagnosis.

Cholangiocarcinoma

This is an adenocarcinoma anywhere in the biliary tree. Within the liver, it may arise from the intrahepatic bile duct epithelium, accounting for 5–10% of all cases of primary liver tumours.

Many cases are of unknown origin, but predisposing factors include:

- Chronic inflammatory disease of the intrahepatic biliary tree, particularly sclerosing cholangitis.
- Disease caused by Chinese liver flukes (*Clonorchis sinensis*).

Lesions tend to be detected late and are associated with a very poor prognosis; most patients do not survive more than 6 months from diagnosis.

Angiosarcomas

These highly malignant tumours are derived from vascular endothelium, and characterised by multifocal haemorrhagic nodules within the liver. The tumours are rare but can be associated with exposure to substances such as vinyl chloride monomer (used to make PVC) and anabolic steroids.

Secondary tumours

The majority of malignant liver tumours are metastatic. The most common primary carcinomas, which metastasise to the liver, are of the lung, breast, colon and stomach. However, any cancer may spread to the liver, including leukaemias and lymphomas.

Mode of spread is via the bloodstream, through the portal vein (tumours of the GI tract) and the systemic circulation (other tumours). There are usually multiple nodular deposits with a central area of necrosis.

Clinically, the liver is enlarged, hard and craggy on palpation.

Small deposits of tumour have little clinical effect. However, extensive metastases cause compression of the intrahepatic bile ducts leading to obstructive jaundice.

Disorders of the biliary tree

Disorders associated with biliary cirrhosis

Biliary cirrhosis is the result of the long-standing obstruction of bile ducts leading to the development of obstructive jaundice, liver cell necrosis and fibrosis with regenerative nodules. The main causes:

- Primary biliary cirrhosis—intrahepatic bile duct destruction of unknown aetiology.
- Secondary biliary cirrhosis—unrelieved obstruction of the main extrahepatic bile ducts.

- Primary sclerosing cholangitis—inflammation and fibrosis of bile ducts (both intrahepatic and extrahepatic).

Biliary obstruction causes oedema and expansion of intrahepatic portal tracts with portal tract fibrosis. Bile droplets develop in biliary canaliculi, which may rupture and cause death of adjacent hepatocytes (so-called 'bile infarct'). Over a long period of time, liver cell death, regeneration, and fibrosis result in cirrhosis.

Primary biliary cirrhosis

This cirrhosis occurs as a result of a chronic destruction of intrahepatic bile ducts. It affects 5 per 100 000 in the UK, typically among the middle-aged population. Females are affected more than males by 10 : 1.

Aetiology is unknown, but it is thought to involve immune phenomena (antimitochondrial antibodies in more than 90% of cases).

It is often associated with other autoimmune diseases, e.g. rheumatoid arthritis (RA), thyroiditis, systemic lupus erythematosus (SLE), scleroderma and Sjögren's syndrome.

Pathogenesis is progressive, chronic, granulomatous and inflammatory. Inflammatory damage with fibrosis may spread from portal tracts to the liver parenchyma. The condition eventually leads to cirrhosis and its complications over a period of about 10 years.

There are four stages:

1. Florid bile—duct inflammation with non-caseating granulomatous deposits.
2. Ductular proliferation (periportal) upstream from damaged bile ducts.
3. Scarring (bridging fibrosis).
4. Cirrhosis.

Secondary biliary cirrhosis

This occurs as a result of prolonged mechanical obstruction to bile flow in large ducts outside the liver or within the porta hepatis. Causes are:

- Gallstones—impacted in common bile duct (most common cause).
- Tumours, e.g. carcinoma of bile duct, carcinoma of the pancreas.
- Strictures—usually following surgery.
- Congenital diseases—choledochal cyst, extrahepatic biliary atresia.

Histological features—Bile pigment accumulates in hepatocytes, in dilated biliary canaliculi and in Kupffer cells. Prolonged obstruction causes:

Initially, primary biliary cirrhosis causes fatigue, arthralgia, pruritus and mild jaundice. This progresses following cirrhosis to:

- Jaundice.
- Severe pruritus.
- Hepatosplenomegaly.
- Malabsorption.
- Xanthelasma and possible xanthomata.

Investigations involve:

- Liver function tests—features of cholestasis (raised alkaline phosphatase, cholesterol and bile acids).
- Antimitochondrial antibodies.
- Liver biopsy—histological proof.
- Endoscopic retrograde cholangiopancreatography (ERCP)—rules out obstructive causes of cirrhosis.

No specific therapy is available; liver transplantation is often necessary.

- 'Bile infarcts'—extravasation of bile from dilated canaliculi.
- 'Bile lakes'—portal tract lesions from bile extravasation.
- Cirrhosis.

Complications are cholangitis (inflammation of the bile ducts, usually as a result of superimposed infection) and those of cirrhosis (page 140).

Primary sclerosing cholangitis

Chronic inflammation and obliterative fibrosis of bile ducts with stricture formation causes progressive obstructive jaundice. The condition affects 1 per 100 000 with peak incidence between 25 and 40 years, males more so than females. Aetiology is unknown but is probably autoimmune in nature. However, unlike primary biliary cirrhosis, only 10% of patients have detectable autoantibodies.

Ulcerative colitis is also present in 60% of patients with primary sclerosing cholangitis.

The effects are:

- Large intrahepatic and extrahepatic bile ducts—development of fibrous strictures with segmental dilatation causing the 'beaded' appearance on endoscopic retrograde cholangiopancreatography (ERCP).
- Medium-sized ducts and ducts in portal tracts—inflammation with concentric fibrosis around ducts.
- Small bile ducts in portal tracts—replaced by collagenous scarring (vanishing bile ducts).

Clinical features—patients develop cholestatic jaundice (pale stools, dark urine and pruritus) with progression to cirrhosis over a period of about 10 years. There is an increased risk of developing cholangiocarcinomas.

Figure 8.24 summarises disorders associated with biliary cirrhosis.

Diseases of the gall bladder

Gallstones (cholelithiasis)

Gallstones (stones formed in the gall bladder) are the most common cause of disease affecting the biliary tree. They occur in 10% of all adults in the UK, females more often than males by 2.5 : 1. The number of stones per patient has varied from 1 to 26 000.

However, despite the high incidence of gallstones, only about 1% of total patients with gallstones develop complications.

There are two types of gallstone—predominantly cholesterol stones (80% of all stones) and predominantly pigment stones (20% of all stones). Both types also contain calcium salts, e.g. bilirubinate, carbonate, phosphate and palmitate.

Cholesterol stones

The major constituent of the stone is cholesterol, which reaches levels beyond the solubilising capacity of bile (supersaturation). This may occur because of:

- Hypersecretion of cholesterol (most common mechanism).
- Decreased secretion of bile salts, due to either defective bile synthesis or excessive intestinal loss of bile salts.
- Abnormal gall bladder function, usually hypomobility.

Risk factors for cholesterol stones are shown in Fig. 8.25.

Pigment stones

The major constituent of the stones is bile pigment (calcium bilirubinate). These stones are typically found in patients with chronic haemolysis due to increased bilirubin production, hence pigment stones are typically black.

Complications, investigations and management

Gallstones may be asymptomatic (80% of cases), symptomatic (pain and other symptoms) or complicated.

Fig. 8.24 Summary of disorders associated with biliary cirrhosis

	Primary biliary cirrhosis	Secondary biliary cirrhosis	Primary sclerosing cholangitis
Prevalence	5 per 100 000	Unknown	1 per 100 000
Sex association	Females > males by 10 : 1; typically affecting middle-aged population	None	Males > females with peak incidence between 25 and 40 years
Aetiology	Unknown, probably autoimmune	Gallstones Tumours Strictures Congenital diseases Parasitic obstruction (rare)	Unknown
Bile duct changes	Progressive chronic granulomatous inflammatory damage with fibrosis Eventual cirrhosis	Development of bile infarcts and bile lakes Bile duct hyperplasia Eventual cirrhosis	Narrowing and obliteration of intra- and extrahepatic bile ducts Eventual cirrhosis
Laboratory findings			
Liver function tests	Features of cholestasis (increased alkaline phosphatase, cholesterol and bile acids)	Features of cholestasis (increased alkaline phosphatase, cholesterol and bile acids)	Features of cholestasis (increased alkaline phosphatase, cholesterol and bile acids)
Serology	Antimitochondrial antibodies	—	Hypergammaglobulinaemia
ERCP	Patent and non-dilated biliary tree	Dilation of large ducts	Fibrous strictures with segmental dilation → 'beaded' appearance

ERCP, endoscopic retrograde cholangiopancreatography

Fig. 8.24 Summary of disorders associated with biliary cirrhosis.

Fig. 8.25 Risk factors for cholesterol stones

Age	↑ Cholesterol secretion
Female	↑ Cholesterol secretion
Pregnancy	↑ Cholesterol secretion ↓ Bile secretion Impaired gall bladder motility
Obesity	↑ Cholesterol secretion
Rapid weight loss	↑ Cholesterol secretion
Ethnic origin	May ↑ cholesterol secretion
Gallbladder stasis Brief fast Parental therapy Spinal cord injury	Impaired gall bladder motility

Fig. 8.25 Risk factors for cholesterol stones.

Complications include:

- Cholecystitis—inflammation of gall bladder caused by impaction of a stone in the neck of the gall bladder or cystic duct.
- Jaundice—impaction of stone in common bile duct (choledocholithiasis), leading to biliary obstruction and symptoms of biliary colic.
- Cholangitis—inflammation of bile duct usually as a result of biliary obstruction complicated with bacterial infection.
- Pancreatitis—impaction of stone distal to opening of pancreatic duct.
- Predisposition to carcinoma of the gall bladder.

Investigations are:

- Ultrasound (most useful).
- Abdominal X-ray—but stones are calcified in only 10–20% of cases.
- Oral cholecystography and CT scanning.

Management is by:

- Surgery (cholecystectomy).
- Bile acids (e.g. ursodeoxycholic acid)—can dissolve stones in some patients.
- Extracorporeal shock-wave lithotripsy—useful for those patients unsuitable for surgery.

Cholecystitis

This is inflammation of the gall bladder. Aetiology is almost always associated with gallstones. There are two types, acute and chronic.

Acute cholecystitis

This acute inflammation of the gall bladder is precipitated by the chemical effects of concentrated static bile. It is typically due to obstruction of outflow by stones at the gall bladder neck or cystic duct, and it may be exacerbated by secondary infection with enteric organisms such as *Escherichia coli*.

In severe cases, the lumen distends with pus causing increased risk of perforation and peritonitis.

Empyema may occur in an inflamed gall bladder greatly distended with pus.

Chronic cholecystitis

Invariably associated with gallstones. The wall of the gall bladder is thickened and rigid from fibrosis, with variable chronic inflammatory infiltration of the mucosa and submucosa. The thickened wall may contain mucosal outpouches (Rokitansky–Aschoff sinuses).

Hartmann's pouch is a pathological dilatation in the neck of the gall bladder formed by increased intra-luminal pressure or stone.

Mucocele

This is sterile obstruction of the neck by a gallstone. A lack of inflammation permits the gall bladder to distend filled with mucus.

Carcinoma of the gall bladder

This is usually an adenocarcinoma, invariably associated with gallstones and chronic cholecystitis. Most cases are seen in women over the age of 70 years. There is a poor prognosis due to liver invasion.

DISORDERS OF THE EXOCRINE PANCREAS

Acute pancreatitis

This acute inflammation of the pancreas is caused by the destructive effect of enzymes released from pancreatic acini. It is relatively common, affecting 10–20 per 100 000 per year in Western communities. By far the most common causes of acute pancreatitis are gallstones (50% of cases) and alcohol ingestion (20%). These and other causes are classified in Fig. 8.26.

Pathogenesis

Duct obstruction

Impaction of a gallstone distal to the site of union of a common bile duct and pancreatic duct results in:

- Reflux of bile up pancreatic duct → toxic injury to pancreatic acini.
- Increased intraductal pressure → enzymatic leakage from pancreatic ducts.

Pancreatic proenzymes (zymogens) are inappropriately activated at some stage in this process, allowing autodigestion of pancreatic tissue. It is believed that the conversion of trypsinogen to trypsin is central to an activation cascade.

Note—chronic alcohol ingestion may also produce increased intraductal pressure due to production of a

Fig. 8.26 Causes of acute pancreatitis

Cause	Example
Mechanical obstruction of pancreatic ducts	Gallstones Trauma Postoperative
Metabolic/toxic causes	Alcohol Drugs, e.g. corticosteroids, thiazide diuretics, azathioprine Hypercalcaemia Hyperlipidaemia
Vascular/poor perfusion	Shock Atherosclerosis Hypothermia Polyarteritis nodosa
Infections	Mumps

Fig. 8.26 Causes of acute pancreatitis.

protein-rich pancreatic fluid, which can form solid plugs in smaller pancreatic ducts.

Direct acinar injury

Less common causes of pancreatitis (e.g. viruses, drugs and trauma) may produce direct acinar damage.

A useful mnemonic for memorising the causes of pancreatitis is **GET SMASHED**: **G**allstones, **E**thanol, **T**rauma, **S**hock, **M**umps, **A**utoimmune (PAN), **S**corpion bites (rare in the UK!), **H**yperlipidaemia (also hypercalcaemia and hypothermia), **E**RCP and **D**rugs.

Patterns of injury

Irrespective of the cause of pancreatitis, acinar damage leads to the liberation of lytic enzymes (proteases and lipases) causing necrosis of normal tissue. The three patterns of pancreatic necrosis are:

- Periductal—necrosis of acinar cells adjacent to ducts. Typically caused by duct obstruction, particularly associated with gallstones and alcohol.
- Perilobular—necrosis of the periphery of lobules. Caused by poor vascular perfusion usually as a result of shock.
- Panlobular—necrosis affects all portions of the pancreatic lobule. This often develops from initial periductal or perilobular necrosis.

A vicious circle of necrosis occurs in which enzymatic release results in further acinar damage and further enzyme release:

- Lipases → fat necrosis.
- Proteases → destruction of pancreatic parenchyma. Endocrine destruction results in hyperglycaemia.
- Elastase and other enzymes → vascular damage with haemorrhage into pancreas or peritoneum. Extensive haemorrhage is known as acute haemorrhagic pancreatitis.

Clinical features

Clinical features are:

- Symptoms—severe central abdominal pain of sudden onset, often radiating into back. Nausea and vomiting.

- Signs—tachycardia, fever, jaundice, shock, ileus, rigid abdomen, discolouration around the umbilicus (Cullen's sign) or in the flanks (Grey Turner's sign).

Complications, investigations and management

Complications may be:

- Local affecting the pancreas—pancreatic pseudocyst, abscess formation.
- Gastrointestinal—gastric and duodenal erosions, bleeding, intestinal ileus.
- Systemic—shock, renal failure, acute respiratory distress syndrome (ARDS), hyperglycaemia, hypocalcaemia, peritonitis.

Diagnosis of acute pancreatitis is made by an elevated serum amylase (or lipase) alongside evidence of pancreatic swelling (on ultrasound or CT). Liver function tests tend to be deranged ($\uparrow$ bilirubin, $\uparrow$ alkaline phosphatase, $\downarrow$ albumin).

Management is by physiological support and treatment of shock, respiratory failure and pain.

Prognosis

Mortality is about 10–15% (negligible in mild cases, but up to 50% in cases with a severe haemorrhagic pancreatitis).

Death may be from shock, renal failure, sepsis, or respiratory failure with contributory factors being protease-induced activation of complement, kinin and the fibrinolytic and coagulation cascades.

Chronic pancreatitis

This is chronic inflammation and fibrosis of the pancreas with a relapsing and remitting course.

It is a relatively rare disease but with increasing incidence due to a rise in the incidence of alcoholism. Typically, it occurs between the ages of 35 and 45 years; males more so than females.

Aetiology—the main causes of chronic pancreatitis are outlined in Fig. 8.27.

Pathogenesis is thought to be similar to the mechanisms involved in acute pancreatitis. However, there is permanent impairment of function.

Morphological features:

- Chronic inflammation with parenchymal fibrosis.
- Loss of pancreatic parenchymal elements.
- Duct strictures with formation of intrapancreatic calculi (stones).

Fig. 8.27 Main causes of chronic pancreatitis.

Fig. 8.27 Main causes of chronic pancreatitis

	Cause	Pathogenesis
Common	Chronic alcoholism (majority of cases)	Protein plugs form in ducts and become calculi; ducts are obstructed, inflamed and scarred
	Biliary tract disease	Gallstones or anatomical abnormalities of pancreatic ducts
	Idiopathic chronic pancreatitis	Pathogenesis uncertain
Rare	Cystic fibrosis	Protein plugs in ducts
	Familial pancreatitis	Autosomal dominant
	Tropical pancreatitis	Uncertain cause; prevalent in India and Africa

Clinical features:

- Recurrent bouts of severe abdominal pain.
- Malabsorption due to reduced exocrine function (decreased lipase and protease secretion)—steatorrhea (fat in faeces).
- Diabetes mellitus (destruction of pancreatic parenchyma)—this effect on the endocrine pancreas occurs in advanced disease.

Episodes of acute pancreatitis may complicate chronic pancreatitis.

Relevant investigations include imaging and function tests.

Imaging is by plain radiograph (for calcification of the pancreas), ultrasound, CT and ERCP.

Function tests are:

- Secretin/CCK/stimulation test.
- Oral glucose tolerance test.
- Measurement of faecal pancreatic chymotrypsin or elastase.

Management is based on alcohol abstinence, pain relief, dietary fat restriction and surgery for correctable causes.

Pseudocysts

A collection of fluid and necrotic inflammatory debris is localised either within the pancreas itself or more commonly in the adjacent tissue, particularly the lesser sac. They are not 'true' cysts (because they have no epithelial lining) but they are surrounded by a zone of inflammatory granulation tissue and they communicate into the pancreatic duct system. They occur in both acute and chronic forms of pancreatitis.

Although many pseudocysts spontaneously resolve, there is a risk of infection, compression or perforation.

Neoplasms of the pancreas

Cystic tumours

These benign, well-circumscribed masses are composed of multiple cystic cavities lined by either serous or mucin-secreting epithelium.

Carcinoma of the pancreas

This common tumour accounts for 3–5% of cancer deaths in the UK. Most tumours are adenocarcinomas arising from the pancreatic ducts. Incidence rises with age, and the cancer is twice as common in males as in females.

Associations include cigarette smoking, chronic pancreatitis, a diet high in fat and carbohydrate and diabetes in women. Around 10% of cases have a clear genetic association (e.g. hereditary pancreatitis, multiple endocrine neoplasia).

The development of pancreatic cancer follows an adenoma-adenocarcinoma sequence similar to that seen in colonic cancer (see Chapter 3). Precursor lesions with the potential to form adenocarcinomas are termed pancreatic intraepithelial neoplasias.

Macroscopic appearance—gritty, hard, grey nodules invading adjacent gland and local structures.

The tumour arises with different frequencies in different parts of the pancreas: 60% in the head, 15% in the body, 5% in the tail; 20% of pancreatic cancers exhibit a diffuse pattern.

Carcinoma in the head of the pancreas tends to present early with obstructive jaundice. As a result, tumours are on average smaller at diagnosis than in other sites.

Microscopic appearance—lesions are typically moderately differentiated adenocarcinomas composed of glandular spaces in a fibrous stroma.

Routes of spread:

- Local—causes obstructive jaundice, or invasion of the duodenum.
- Lymphatic—spread to adjacent lymph nodes.
- Blood—spread to the liver.

Clinical features:

- Weight loss, anorexia and chronic persistent pain in epigastrium radiating to the back.
- Obstructive jaundice with painless palpable dilatation of gall bladder (Courvoisier's sign).
- Rarely, there may be vomiting (duodenal obstruction), venous thrombosis (migratory thrombophlebitis), acute pancreatitis or diabetes mellitus (destruction of islets of Langerhans with carcinoma).

Management is by:

- Curative resection (Whipple's procedure)—rarely possible due to extensive disease.
- Palliative surgery—often performed to bypass obstruction of the bile duct (relieving jaundice) and obstruction of the duodenum.

Prognosis is extremely poor—5-year survival is just 5%.

DISORDERS OF THE INTESTINE

Congenital abnormalities

Meckel's diverticulum

Diverticulum (outpouching) of the ileum is caused by incomplete regression of part of the yolk stalk (the vitelline duct) during the embryonic period.

Meckel's diverticulum occurs in 2% of the population and in males more than females by about 3 : 1.

Rule of 2s for Meckel's diverticulum:
- Prevalence—2% of the population.
- Site—usually 2 feet (60 cm) from the ileocaecal junction.
- Length—up to 2 inches (5 cm).

Macroscopically, it is up to 5 cm long and located around 60 cm from the ileocaecal junction.

Microscopically, it is true diverticulum, consisting of all three layers of bowel: mucosa, submucosa and muscularis propria. About half of cases also contain heterotopic gastric acid-secreting epithelium or pancreatic tissue.

Complications—the majority of these diverticula are asymptomatic; however, the complications include volvulus, inflammation, peptic ulceration and intussusception (telescoping of one portion of intestine into another).

Congenital aganglionic megacolon (Hirschsprung's disease)

This congenital condition is characterised by dilatation of the colon due to the absence of the normal myenteric plexus distal to the dilatation. It results from the failure of neuroblast cells to migrate from the vagus into the developing gut. It occurs in 1 per 5000 live births.

This condition always involves the rectum, and it may be present in continuity for a variable distance along the bowel.

Macroscopically, there is a narrowing of an abnormally innervated bowel segment, and dilatation and muscular hypertrophy of the bowel segment proximal to this.

Microscopically, there is an absence of normal myenteric and submucosal plexus ganglion cells, and hypertrophy of nerve fibres within submucosa and muscularis mucosae, with extension of abnormal axons up into the lamina propria.

Clinical features—the disease usually presents in early childhood with symptoms of colonic obstruction, i.e. constipation, abdominal distension and vomiting.

Diagnosis—barium enema reveals a small, empty rectum and dilatation above the narrowed segment. A biopsy of the rectal mucosa will confirm the diagnosis.

Treatment is by excision of the abnormal segments of colon and rectum.

Acquired megacolon

Note that megacolon can also be a result of acquired disease. However, acquired megacolon differs macroscopically from Hirschsprung's disease in that there is no narrowed segment, dilatation extends down to the anus, and the rectum is full of faeces.

Causes of acquired megacolon:

- Psychogenic megacolon—disregard for the urge to defaecate (usually in children or the depressed).

- Prolonged stimulant laxative abuse—degeneration of myenteric plexus.
- Smooth muscle disorders—degeneration of colonic smooth muscle, e.g. scleroderma.
- Chagas' disease—infection by *Trypanosoma cruzi* with destruction of myenteric plexus. Common in South America.
- Obstruction—usually by neoplasm or inflammatory stricture.
- Toxic megacolon—complication of ulcerative colitis (see below).

Atresia and stenosis

Atresia refers to complete intestinal obstruction (failure in recanalisation), whereas 'stenosis' (narrowing) implies incomplete obstruction. These defects are most common in the duodenum and small intestine; they are rare in the colon. Thirty per cent of children with Down syndrome have duodenal atresia.

Atresia is more common than stenosis. It is thought that both conditions arise from developmental failures, intussusceptions or an interrupted intrauterine blood supply.

Anorectal anomalies

Numerous anorectal anomalies exist, the most common of which are imperforate anus and anorectal agenesis.

Imperforate anus

This common anomaly affects 1 per 5000 live births, males more so than females. The anus is in the normal position but a thin layer of tissue (the fetal cloacal diaphragm) separates the anal canal from the exterior.

Anorectal agenesis

The rectum ends superior to the puborectalis muscle, accounting for about two-thirds of anorectal defects. There are two types:

1. With fistula (most common)—in males, rectovesical fistula (to bladder) or rectourethral fistula (to urethra), meconium may be observed in the urine; in females, rectovaginal fistula (to vagina) or rectovestibular fistula (to vestibule of vagina). Meconium may be present in the vestibule of the vagina.
2. Without fistula (rectal agenesis)—anal canal and rectum are present but are separated.

Infections and enterocolitis

Diarrhoea and dysentery

Diarrhoea is hard to define. Many consider it to mean frequent bowel evacuation or the passage of abnormal-ly soft or liquid faeces, although it is clinically defined as the passage of more than 200 g of stool per day.

Dysentery is an inflammatory disorder of the intestinal tract causing severe diarrhoea with blood and mucus.

Classification

Diarrhoea can be classified as:

- Secretory—diarrhoea caused by a combined effect of excessive intestinal secretions and decreased absorption. Stool volumes may be very high and diarrhoea persists even when there is total fasting.
- Osmotic—diarrhoea caused by the presence of unabsorbed solute in the colon, which prevents the absorption of fluid. Ceases on fasting long enough to empty the small bowel.
- Exudative—diarrhoea due to inflammatory exudate consisting of extracellular fluid and pus mixed with blood.
- Deranged motility—diarrhoea as a result of either increased or decreased motility of the small intestine.
- Malabsorption—diarrhoea occurring as a result of malabsorption (see below).

The classification and causes of diarrhoea are described in Fig. 8.28.

Infectious enterocolitis

Enterocolitis (inflammation of the colon and small intestine) is common and is often a result of infection.

Viral gastroenteritis

Viruses are the most common cause of gastroenteritis in infants and young children; they account for 10% of all food poisoning outbreaks in the UK. Transmission is typically by a faecal–oral route. Symptoms are cramps, vomiting and fever but no blood in stools.

In children most cases are caused by three viruses:

- Rotavirus—causes 50% of infantile diarrhoea and accounts for some adult cases.
- Adenovirus (especially types 40, 41)—second to rotavirus as cause of acute diarrhoea in young children.
- Astrovirus—most infections occur in childhood and are mild.

In adults, the Norwalk virus accounts for 30% of cases of gastroenteritis. It is responsible for the 'winter vomiting disease'.

Fig. 8.28 Classification and causes of diarrhoea

Type	Causes
Secretory	Infections: bacteria producing enterotoxins, viral diarrhoea, *Giardia* Irritants: laxatives, bile acids, hydroxyl fatty acids Hormonal: VIP, glucagon, medullary carcinoma of the thyroid, Addison's disease Mucosal infiltration: villous adenoma, lymphoma, collagen diseases Congenital: chloridorrhea
Osmotic	Osmotic laxatives, e.g. lactulose, magnesium sulphate Disaccharidase deficiency Malabsorption syndromes Congenital, e.g. chloridorrhea (secretory and osmotic), hexose malabsorption
Exudative	Inflammatory diseases, e.g. ulcerative colitis, Crohn's disease Infections: bacteria causing invasion of the mucosa, i.e. enteroinvasive bacteria such as *Shigella*, *Campylobacter*, enterohaemorrhagic *Escherichia coli*; and *Entamoeba histolytica*
Deranged motility	Decreased motility: • Systemic sclerosis and other collagen disorders • Intestinal pseudo-obstruction • Diabetic autonomic neuropathy Increased motility: • Carcinoid syndrome • Postvagotomy state • Thyrotoxicosis • Unabsorbed bile salts entering colon
Malabsorption	May be a mixture of secretory, osmotic and exudative diarrhoea (see Fig. 8.33)

VIP, vasoactive intestinal polypeptide.

Fig. 8.28 Classification and causes of diarrhoea.

Bacterial enterocolitis

The types of pathogenic mechanisms are as follows:

- Preformed toxin—ingestion of food contaminated with bacterial toxins, e.g. from *Staphylococcus aureus, Bacillus cereus, Clostridium perfringens*. Incubation period is very short (1–7 hours).
- Toxigenic organism—ingestion of bacteria that produce toxins in the gut, e.g. *Vibrio cholerae*, enterotoxigenic *Escherichia coli* (ETEC), and *Clostridium perfringens*. So-called 'traveller's diarrhoea' usually occurs by this mechanism and is extremely common.
- Enteroinvasive organism—ingestion of bacteria that invade the intestinal mucosa and may cause dysentery as a result of severe inflammation, e.g. *Salmonella typhi, Campylobacter jejuni, Shigella*, enterohaemorrhagic *Escherichia coli* (EHEC).
- Antibiotic-associated diarrhoea—occurs as a result of overgrowth of one type of bacteria because of disruption of normal gut flora following antibiotic treatment. Main culprit is *Clostridium difficile*, which causes necrosis of the colonic mucosa and pseudomembranous colitis (a false membrane in the colon). Patients develop fever, abdominal pain and diarrhoea. Clostridial overgrowth is also promoted by surgery, ischaemia, shock and burns. Other pathogens of antibiotic-associated diarrhoea are *Clostridium perfringens* and *Staphylococcus aureus*.
- Necrotising enterocolitis—rare condition arising through a combination of ischaemia and infection. Ischaemia progresses to intestinal infarction and necrosis of the intestines. Infection of infarcted tissue results in gas gangrene (see Chapter 2), sepsis and shock with paralytic ileus. Most cases are seen in neonates. Adult cases are related to *Clostridium perfringens* infection.

Figure 8.29 provides a summary of common bacterial GI infections.

Protozoa

Protozoal infection may result in:

- Chagas' disease—infection by *Trypanosoma cruzi* results in the destruction of the myenteric plexus

Fig. 8.29 Summary of common bacterial GI infections

Mechanism	Bacterium	Incubation period	Duration (days)	V	C	F	B
Preformed toxin	*Staphylococcus aureus*	2–7 hours	1	+	+	±	—
	B. cereus	1–6 hours	1	+	+	—	—
Toxigenic organisms	*Vibrio cholerae*	2–3 days	Up to 7	+	—	—	—
	Escherichia coli (ETEC)	12 hours–3 days	2–4	+	—	—	—
	Clostridium perfringens	8 hours–1 day	0.5–1	—	+	—	—
Enteroinvasive bacteria	Non-typhoidal salmonella	8–48 hours	4–7	+	±	+	±
	Campylobacter jejuni	2–11 days	3–21	—	+	+	+
	Shigella	1–4 days	2–3	—	+	+	+
	Escherichia coli (EHEC)	1–5 days	1–4	+	+	+	+
Antibiotic-associated bacteria	*Clostridium difficile*	—	—	—	+	+	±

B, blood in the stools; C, abdominal cramps; EHEC, enterohaemorrhagic Escherichia coli; ETEC, enterotoxigenic Escherichia coli; F, fever; V, vomiting.

Fig. 8.29 Summary of common bacterial gastrointestinal infections.

over a period of years with resulting dilatation of various parts of the alimentary canal, especially the colon and oesophagus. Common in South America.

- Amoebic dysentery—this infection by *Entamoeba histolytica* is common throughout the tropics where it is spread by faecal–oral transmission of amoebic cysts. The condition follows a chronic course with abdominal pains. Periods of diarrhoea alternating with constipation are common.
- Giardiasis—This disease is caused by the parasitic protozoan *Giardia lamblia* in the small intestine. Infection occurs by eating food or water contaminated with parasitic cysts. Symptoms include diarrhoea, nausea, abdominal pain and flatulence, as well as the passage of pale, fatty stools. The disease occurs worldwide and it is particularly common in children.
- Other protozoal infections include balantidiasis (*Balantidium coli*), cryptosporidiosis (*Cryptosporidium*) and schistosomiasis (*Schistosoma mansoni*).

Inflammatory disorders of the bowel

The most important of these are idiopathic in origin, namely Crohn's disease and ulcerative colitis (together termed 'inflammatory bowel disease'). These conditions are characterised by chronic, relapsing inflammation of the intestinal wall.

Crohn's disease

A granulomatous inflammation of unknown cause that affects the full thickness of the bowel wall anywhere in the GI tract from mouth to anus, this disease is characterised by a relapsing and remitting course. Its incidence is about 5–7 per 100 000 in the UK, but this is increasing.

It usually presents in early adult life, with 90% of patients aged between 10 and 40 years, although a secondary peak occurs in the elderly. Females are affected slightly more than males. There is a higher incidence in northern Europe and the US than elsewhere.

Pathogenesis

Cause and pathogenesis are unknown but several hypotheses have been suggested, most notably that Crohn's patients are genetically susceptible individuals who develop exaggerated and unregulated immune responses to normal commensal flora of the gut. This is likely to involve persistent T-cell activation and inappropriate cytokine production. Infection, dietary deficiencies and smoking have also been proposed.

Macroscopic appearance

Site—most commonly affects the terminal ileum, but it may affect any part of the GI tract from the mouth to the anus in a discontinuous pattern. Two-thirds of cases affect only the terminal ileum, one sixth affect only the colon, and one sixth are in the terminal ileum and colon.

Pattern:

- 'Skip' lesions—normal bowel areas are present between diseased segments, with a sharp demarcation between the two.
- Oedema of submucosa and mucosa.
- Haemorrhagic ulcers—initially small and discrete, these progress to form deep, linear, fissured ulcers ('rose thorn' ulcers).
- Cobblestone pattern of bowel mucosa due to submucosal oedema and interconnecting deep fissured ulcers.
- Thickened bowel wall due to oedema and fibrosis.
- Fibrous strictures may cause partial obstruction.
- Dilatation of normal bowel proximal to diseased segment due to partial obstruction.
- Enlargement of mesenteric lymph nodes.

Microscopic appearance

- Transmural inflammation—all layers of bowel wall are affected. Forms basis of fissures, adhesions, fistulae and sinuses.
- Lymphoid aggregates develop deep in bowel wall.
- Submucosal oedema.
- Ulceration.
- Non-caseating granulomas present in inflamed bowel wall and in mesenteric lymph nodes in about 60% of cases.
- Evidence of persistent and inappropriate T-cell and macrophage activation with increased production of inflammatory cytokines (interleukins: IL-1, IL-2, IL-6, IL-8, interferon-γ and TNFα).

Clinical features

Clinical features are symptoms of abdominal pain, diarrhoea (possibly bloody) and weight loss, with signs of anaemia, clubbing, fever, mouth (aphthous) ulcers and abdominal mass (inflamed bowel loops, abscesses).

Complications

The natural history of Crohn's disease is one of remissions and relapses of inflammation punctuated by complications.

Local complications are:

- Severe inflammation—this may be life threatening, often with dilatation of the colon and passage of bacterial toxins into the bloodstream (toxic megacolon). There is a risk of bowel perforation.

- Fistulae and sinuses—inflammation of serosal layer leads to the formation of adhesions to other bowel loops, to parietal peritoneum of anterior abdominal wall, or to the bladder.
- Strictures and fibrous adhesions lead to intestinal obstruction.
- Perforation of the bowel by deep fissured ulcers leads to intra-abdominal abscesses.
- Carcinoma of bowel—increased incidence after many years.
- Haemorrhage—significant bleeding from areas of ulceration (rare).

Systemic complications, which develop in a minority of patients with Crohn's, are:

- Malabsorption—due to diseased bowel or surgical resections.
- Skin disease—pyoderma gangrenosum, erythema nodosum.
- Eye disease—uveitis.
- Joint disease—polyarthropathy, sacroiliitis, ankylosing spondylitis.
- Chronic liver disease—pericholangitis, gallstones.
- Finger clubbing.
- Systemic amyloidosis (rare).

Ulcerative colitis

This is a diffuse superficial inflammation of the colo-rectum of unknown cause, and characterised by relapses and remissions. It affects about 10 per 100 000 in the UK, with much lower rates in developing countries with warmer climates. Ulcerative colitis has a similar age distribution to Crohn's but the sex incidence is equal.

Aetiopathogenesis

This is unknown, but the same hypotheses as for Crohn's have been proposed with the exception of smoking, which unusually is associated with a decreased risk. Again, inappropriate and persistent T-cell activation may play an important role in the pathogenesis.

Macroscopic appearance

Site—ulcerative colitis usually begins distally as proctitis and then spreads proximally. It may affect the whole of the large bowel (pancolitis), and can therefore reach the terminal ileum ('backwash' ileitis).

The pattern is one of shallow ulceration (which may become confluent), with 'pseudopolyps', hyperaemia and haemorrhage. The diseased bowel is continuous, without gaps of normal tissue.

Microscopic appearance

Inflammation is diffuse and is limited to mucosa, with infiltration of both acute and chronic inflammatory cells. Other features are crypt abscesses with ulceration, crypt atrophy and Paneth cell metaplasia.

Clinical features

Clinical features are symptoms of bloody diarrhoea, mucus, cramping discomfort and weight loss, signs of fever, tachycardia, pallor and abdominal tenderness.

Complications

Acute local complications include perforation, dilatation, haemorrhage and dehydration (blood and fluid loss from extensive ulceration).

Chronic local complications include strictures, dysplasia and carcinoma (higher cancer risk than Crohn's).

Systemic complications are identical to those seen in Crohn's, except for an additional association with primary sclerosing cholangitis.

A comparison of Crohn's and ulcerative colitis

Both Crohn's and ulcerative colitis are examples of inflammatory bowel disease, and they have many features in common. However, in the majority of cases (about 90%), it is possible to distinguish between these two conditions (Figs 8.30–8.32).

Diagnosis

Diagnosis is by colonoscopy, barium and small bowel enema. Colonoscopy is the most sensitive test, and biopsy specimens can be taken for histological examination (see Fig. 8.32 for differences in microscopic

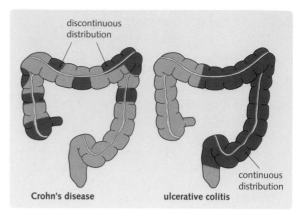

Fig. 8.30 Comparisons of distribution along the bowel.

appearance). This investigation is also important in the surveillance of patients with long-standing colitis as it allows severe dysplasia and early invasive cancer to be detected.

Rectal sparing, discrete patchy ulceration and perianal disease are classically seen on Crohn's colonoscopy. This contrasts with ulcerative colitis, with its confluent ulceration, which is most severe in the distal colon. Long-standing severe disease may show loss of haustral markings with a featureless, shortened hosepipe colon.

Management

Management can be medical or surgical.

Medical:

- Corticosteroids—effective in inducing remission (local, i.e. topical steroid enemas used for

Fig. 8.31 Depth and distribution of lesions in the bowel wall.

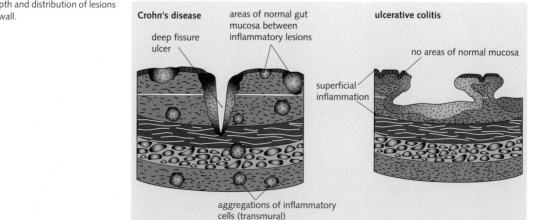

Fig. 8.32 Comparison of the basic features of Crohn's disease and ulcerative colitis

	Crohn's disease	Ulcerative colitis
Incidence in UK	~5–7 per 100 000 in UK	~10 per 100 000
Site	Any part of GI system but typically terminal ileum	Colon and rectum only
Macroscopic		
Disease continuity	Discontinuous	Continuous
Bowel wall	Thickened with strictures and adhesions	Not thickened
Ulcers	Deep fissures form basis of fistulae	Flat based; do not extend to submucosa
Microscopic		
Pattern of inflammation	Transmural Focal Granulomas (in 60% of cases)	Mucosal and submucosal Diffuse No granulomas
Crypt pattern	Little distortion	Distorted in long-standing disease; crypt abscesses
Anal lesions		
	Present in 75%; anal fistulae; ulceration or chronic fissure	Present in <25%
Frequency of fistula		
	10–20% of cases	Uncommon
Risk of developing cancer		
	Slightly increased	Significantly increased

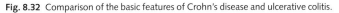

Fig. 8.32 Comparison of the basic features of Crohn's disease and ulcerative colitis.

exacerbations of distal proctocolitis; systemic, i.e. oral prednisolone).

- Mesalazine—can be used to maintain remission once remission has been induced by corticosteroids.
- Azathioprine—helpful to reduce steroid dose and avoid side-effects.
- TNFα blockers (infliximab)—used in active, fistulating Crohn's disease that is unresponsive to other treatments.

Surgical:

- Minimal resections for strictures, fistulae or perforations (more common in Crohn's).
- Colectomy—indicated in cases of extensive disease affecting quality of life, failed medical therapy, fulminant colitis and severe dysplasia or cancer on colonoscopy surveillance. Pouch-forming operations preserve sphincter function and avoid an ileostomy. This is suitable in ulcerative colitis but not in Crohn's, where recurrent disease may affect the pouch.

Miscellaneous intestinal inflammatory disorders

Gastrointestinal manifestations of HIV disease

AIDS is associated with fulminant bowel infection, which often causes severe diarrhoea.

Malabsorptive or colitic syndromes

These are described below.

Diarrhoea in bone marrow transplantation graft-versus-host disease

Bone-marrow transplants contain competent T lymphocytes, which can react against the recipient's human leucocyte antigens (HLA), causing skin rash, liver toxicity and diarrhoea. This may be torrential in severe forms.

Malabsorption syndromes

General aspects of malabsorption syndromes

Malabsorption may be caused by disorders of:

- Intraluminal digestion—assisted by, for example, gastric juices and pancreatic digestive enzymes (these are necessary for breakdown of macromolecules).
- Intraluminal solubilisation—liver secretes bile acids required for solubilisation and absorption of fats.
- Terminal digestion—enzymes located on the brush border of the small intestinal mucosa hydrolyse large molecules for absorption, especially complex sugars (e.g. sucrase for sucrose and lactase for lactose).

- Transepithelial transport—mucosa is specialised for absorption. Transverse mucosal folds and finger-like villi provide a vast surface area.

Systemic effects of the malabsorption syndromes:

- Weight loss and anorexia.
- Abdominal distension and borborygmi (increased bowel sounds).
- Diarrhoea (loose, bulky stools).
- Steatorrhoea—malabsorption of fat, producing pale, foul-smelling stools that characteristically float in water.
- Muscle wasting.

Classification of malabsorption syndromes

This is described in Fig. 8.33.

Fig. 8.33 Causes of malabsorption.

Fig. 8.33 Causes of malabsorption	
Defective intraluminal digestion or solubilisation	Pancreatic insufficiency: • Chronic pancreatitis • Cystic fibrosis • Carcinoma of the pancreas Liver disease: failure of bile secretion into duct
Primary mucosal cell abnormalities	Lactase deficiency
Reduced surface area of small intestine	Conditions that cause villous atrophy: • Coeliac disease • Tropical sprue • Crohn's disease • Malnutrition Iatrogenic: • Extensive small intestine resection • Jejunal ileal bypass procedures • Postradiotherapy
Infection	Parasitic infestation of gut Bacterial overgrowth in blind loops of diverticulae Postinfective malabsorption Giardiasis Whipple's disease
Lymphatic obstruction	Primary lymphangiectasia Lymphoma
Drug-induced	Cytotoxic drugs Drugs that bind bile salts, e.g. cholestyramine and some antibiotics such as neomycin (which causes steatorrhoea)
Miscellaneous	Thyrotoxicosis→increased gastric emptying and motility Zollinger–Ellison syndrome Diabetes mellitus→bacterial overgrowth Hypogammaglobulinaemia→infection

Coeliac disease

This is caused by a chronic inflammatory response to the protein gliadin, a component of gluten (found in wheat, oats, barley and rye). Atrophy of small intestinal villi and crypt hyperplasia are the result. It affects about 1 per 1000 in most Caucasian populations of Western Europe; it is rare in other ethnic origins.

It can present at any age but it is an important cause of failure to thrive in infants and children.

Antigliadin antibodies are present in the majority of cases, although anti-endomyseal antibodies have a greater sensitivity and specificity as a diagnostic aid. Other tests that may be used are small-bowel biopsy and a gluten challenge, in which symptoms improve on a gluten-free diet but relapse once this is stopped.

There is an increased incidence of disease in first-degree relatives of those affected. It sometimes occurs concurrently with dermatitis herpetiformis (itchy, blistering skin disease).

Macroscopically, the luminal surface becomes flattened, developing a mosaic-like pattern of crypt openings (Fig. 8.34).

Microscopically there is:

- Mucosal inflammation with lymphocytic infiltration.
- Loss of villous architecture ranging from blunting (partial villous atrophy) to complete flattening (total villous atrophy) due to a high rate of cell loss.
- Increase in the depth of crypts with epithelial cell hyperplasia to compensate for those lost through damage.

Long-term complications are:

- Chronic ulceration of the small intestine—may lead to strictures.
- Development of primary T-cell lymphoma of the small intestine.
- Development of adenocarcinoma (rare).

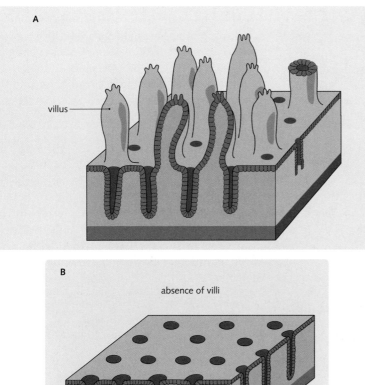

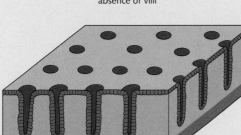

Fig. 8.34 Comparison of normal jejunal mucosa (A) and jejunal mucosa in coeliac disease with total villous atrophy (B).

Management is by the complete withdrawal of gliadin from the diet (i.e. a gluten-free diet), which leads to gradual recovery of the villous structure. This may be partial or complete.

Tropical sprue

This chronic and progressive malabsorption syndrome without a definable cause is seen in patients who live or have lived in the tropics, and in the absence of other intestinal disease or parasites. The disease occurs mainly in the West Indies and Asia.

Aetiology is unclear; however, the condition is thought to be infective, probably toxigenic *Escherichia coli*.

Clinical features and histological appearances resemble those of coeliac disease. However, a gluten-free diet has little beneficial effect.

Whipple disease

Whipple disease is a multisystem disorder involving malabsorption, weight loss, lymphadenopathy and joint pain. The causative agent is the Gram-positive bacillus *Tropheryma whippelii*. This rare condition is characterised by tissue infiltration with foamy macrophages that are periodic acid–Schiff (PAS) reagent positive.

Bacterial overgrowth syndrome

In this syndrome, there is malabsorption secondary to excessive bacteria in the small intestine, usually the jejunum. It is also known as contaminated bowel syndrome, blind loop syndrome, and small intestine stasis syndrome.

Causes of small intestinal bacterial overgrowth are outlined in Fig. 8.35.

Malabsorption is as a result of:

- Deconjugation of bile salts by the bacteria, hence steatorrhoea.
- Damage to the small intestinal mucosa, probably by bacterial products.
- Binding of vitamin B_{12} by bacteria, hence vitamin B_{12} deficiency.

Diarrhoea is both secretory (due to bacterial products affecting mucosa) and osmotic (due to unabsorbed products and deficiency of disaccharidases because of mucosal damage).

Clinical features are weight loss, diarrhoea, and anaemia (due to vitamin B_{12} deficiency).

Management is by antibiotic therapy and surgical resection for a localised abnormality, e.g. stricture, fistula.

Fig. 8.35 Causes of small intestinal bacterial overgrowth

Cause	Example
Excessive entry of bacteria	Achlorydria Infected bile ducts Gastrocolic fistula Gastric surgery Resection of ileocaecal valve
Defective immune mechanisms	Hypogammaglobulinaemia Malnutrition Old age
Stagnant region	Blind loops Enterocolic fistulae Jejunal diverticula Strictures or other obstruction Continent ileostomy
Disturbed motility	Systemic sclerosis Intestinal pseudo-obstruction Diabetic autonomic neuropathy

Fig. 8.35 Causes of small intestinal bacterial overgrowth.

Disaccharidase deficiency

The most important disaccharidase is lactase, which is essential for the digestion of milk sugar (lactose). All babies have lactase in their intestines but the enzyme disappears later in life in about 10% of northern Europeans, 40% of Greeks and Italians, and 80% of Africans and Asians. The presence of undigested lactose in the small intestine (following consumption of raw milk) causes diarrhoea and abdominal pain.

Abetalipoproteinaemia

This rare condition is characterised by the absence of plasma apolipoprotein B.

Dietary fat is taken up by enterocytes but the lack of apolipoprotein B prevents assembly of chylomicrons for further fat transport. This results in fatty infiltration of enterocytes; no low- or very-low-density lipoproteins are present in the plasma. The integrity of lipid membranes throughout the body is affected, causing:

- Abnormally shaped red blood cells with spikes on the surface (acanthocytosis).
- Retinitis pigmentosa leading to blindness.
- Progressive ataxia.
- Diarrhoea and steatorrhoea, with failure to thrive during infancy.

Symptoms are improved by dietary supplementation with medium-chain triglycerides and the fat-soluble vitamins (namely, A, D, E and K).

Obstruction of the bowel

Major causes of bowel obstruction

Obstruction and pseudo-obstruction can be classified as follows:

- Simple mechanical obstruction—the bowel above the obstructing lesion becomes distended with fluid and gas.
- Strangulation obstruction—occlusion of the blood supply by constricting agents.
- Paralytic ileus—may arise as a consequence of peritonitis, pancreatitis or retroperitoneal bleeding.
- Pseudo-obstruction—abnormal gut motility rather than an organic obstructive lesion.

Examples of simple mechanical obstruction, strangulation obstruction, and paralytic ileus types of obstructions are listed in Fig. 8.36.

Hernias

This is the protrusion of the whole or part of a viscus from its normal position through a defect in the cavity wall in which it is contained. About 1 per 100 people has a hernia at some time. Hernias can be congenital or acquired. Acquired hernias are:

- Secondary to increased intra-abdominal pressure—resulting from cough, straining at the stool, cysts, carcinoma, pregnancy.
- Iatrogenic—incisional hernias.

Classification:

- Reducible—contents of sac can be completely returned to abdominal cavity.
- Irreducible/incarcerated—content of sac cannot be completely returned to the abdominal cavity.

Common sites of abdominal hernias are inguinal (70%), femoral (20%) and umbilical (10%). Others are supraumbilical or linea alba, incisional hernias and hiatus hernia (see page 133).

Complications:

- Obstruction—constriction at the neck of the hernial sac causes obstruction of bowel loops within it.
- Strangulation—constriction at the neck of sac prevents venous return leading to venous congestion, arterial occlusion, and gangrene. This may result in perforation leading to peritonitis/groin abscess.

Note that strangulation can occur without obstruction if only one wall of the viscus pouches into the sac (Richter's hernia).

Hernias must be repaired because of potential complications. The principles of surgical repair are identification of the sac and contents, mobilisation of the sac, reduction of the contents, ligation of the sac and repairing the fascial defect.

Inguinal hernia

The most common type of hernia, this is much more prevalent in men than in women. There are two types: indirect inguinal (85%) and direct inguinal (15%).

In indirect cases, the hernial sac enters the inguinal canal through the deep ring (lateral to the inferior epigastric artery) and then traverses through the canal to the superficial ring, where it may eventually reach the scrotum or labium major. It is the result of a congenital abnormality. Strangulation is a common complication due to the narrow neck of the hernial sac.

In direct cases, the hernial sac protrudes through a weakness in the fascia transversalis (medial to inferior epigastric artery) and it does not normally descend into the scrotum or labium major. It originates as a result of weakened abdominal muscles (usually acquired in the elderly). The neck of the sac is wide so strangulation is rare.

Fig. 8.36 Major causes of bowel obstruction

Cause	Example
Simple mechanism obstruction	Intraluminal: • Foreign bodies • Gallstone ileus • Faecoliths • Meconium in cystic fibrosis Bowel wall: • Adhesions • Carcinoma • Strictures • Atresia • Imperforate anus
Strangulation obstruction	Intussusception Infarction Volvulus Internal/external hernias Bands
Adynamic obstruction (paralytic ileus)	Abdominal causes: postoperative, peritonitis, vascular occlusion Systemic causes: electrolyte disorders, uraemia, hypothyroidism Drugs: anticholinergics, opiates

Fig. 8.36 Major causes of bowel obstruction.

Clinically, it is difficult (often impossible) to distinguish between direct and indirect inguinal hernias.

Femoral hernia

The hernial sac protrudes through the femoral canal inferior to the inguinal ligament (Fig. 8.37). There is an increasing incidence with age, and females are affected more than males by 2 : 1 (but inguinal hernia is still more common in both males and females). The most common complication is strangulation.

Adhesions

Adhesions are by far the most common cause of mechanical obstruction in the small bowel, and they are defined as areas of fibrosis between adjacent membranes or organs resulting in their fusion. The causes can be congenital (e.g. bands in small children) or acquired.

Acquired causes are as follows:

- Inflammation, e.g. Crohn's disease, sclerosing peritonitis.
- Infection, e.g. appendicitis, diverticulitis, tuberculosis, peritonitis.
- Trauma, e.g. stab wounds.
- Iatrogenic—postsurgery, irradiation.
- Vascular—infarction/gangrene.
- Malignancies.

Intussusception

This is invagination of one part of the bowel into the adjoining segment (Fig. 8.38). The ileocaecal valve is

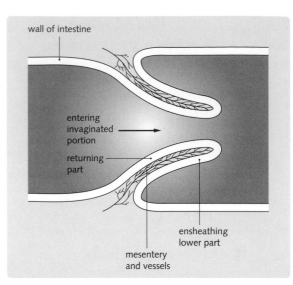

Fig. 8.38 Intussusception.

the most common site, with the ileum invaginating into the caecum. It typically affects children under the age of 4 years.

Adult cases are extremely rare, and they are almost invariably precipitated by an intraluminal mass (e.g. tumour) or structural abnormality (e.g. Meckel's diverticulum).

As the contents of the intestine are pushed onwards by muscular contraction, more and more intestine is dragged into the adjoining bowel. The net effect is venous congestion of the invaginated portion, which may suffer infarction if mesenteric vessels are trapped.

Management is by barium reduction in children or by resection in adults because of the high incidence of organic causes.

Volvulus

This is a twisting of part of the GI tract, usually leading to partial or complete obstruction (Fig. 8.39). It is most commonly seen in redundant loops of the sigmoid colon, but may also occur in the caecum, small intestine and stomach.

The most common complication is strangulation (causing infarction and possibly gangrene).

Management—may untwist spontaneously but surgical manipulation is usually performed.

Colonic diverticulosis

Definitions

A diverticulum is a sac or pouch formed at weak points in the wall of the alimentary tract; diverticulo-

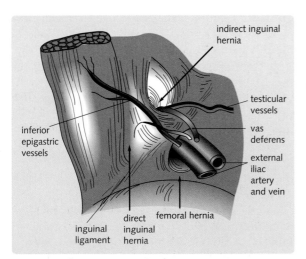

Fig. 8.37 Sites of direct inguinal, indirect inguinal and femoral herniations. (Adapted with permission from Principles and Practice of Surgery, 3rd edn, by APM Forrest, PC Carter and IB Macleod, Churchill Livingstone, 1995.)

Complications are:

- Inflammation (diverticulitis)—may cause severe pain and tenderness in left iliac fossa, alteration of bowel habit, fever, leucocytosis. There may be a palpable mass.
- Perforation—results in peritonitis.
- Obstruction—due to oedema or fibrosis in the inflamed segment of colon or to adherence of small bowel loops.
- Stricture formation—long-standing diverticular disease may cause stricture formation and subacute intestinal obstruction.
- Fistula—most common cause of colovesical fistula.
- Bleeding—common complication.

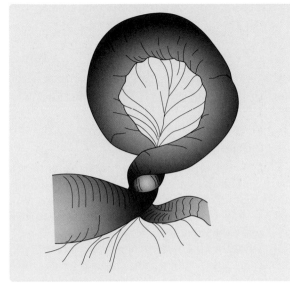

Fig. 8.39 Intestinal volvulus.

The clinical course of colonic diverticular disease may be asymptomatic, but sometimes causes left-sided colicky abdominal pain and alteration of bowel habit (usually constipation) or rectal bleeding.

Diverticula can be visualised and diagnosed by barium enema and/or colonoscopy.

Treatment:
- Conservative—high-fibre diet results in improvement in most patients.
- Surgery—sigmoid colectomy with end-to-end anastomosis if there are persistent symptoms or when carcinoma cannot be excluded by radiology or colonoscopy.

sis means that there is no evidence of inflammation. Diverticulitis is inflammation of a diverticulum, which commonly occurs in one or more colonic diverticula.

Aetiopathogenesis of diverticula

Congenital diverticula are true diverticula containing all three coats of the bowel wall, e.g. Meckel's diverticulum (see page 161).

Acquired diverticula may contain some (false diverticula) or all (true diverticula) coats of the bowel wall. They typically develop during adult life as a result of:

- Pulsion from increased intraluminal pressure (e.g. straining at the stool) causing protrusion at points of focal weakness (e.g. at the sites of penetration of blood vessels).
- Traction due to extrinsic disease.

Colonic diverticulosis is caused by a chronic lack of dietary fibre.

Although rare before 35 years of age, by 65 years of age at least one-third of the population of developed countries is affected. Rare in countries with high-fibre diets.

Diverticula are most common in the sigmoid colon emerging between mesenteric and antimesenteric taeniae.

Vascular disorders of the bowel
Ischaemic bowel disease

Ischaemic bowel disease may affect the small or large bowel, and it is most commonly seen in elderly patients with severe atherosclerosis. The causes are discussed below.

Vessel disease
These are:

- Vascular occlusion—emboli lodge in the superior mesenteric artery, which supplies all the small intestine except for the first part of the duodenum. Emboli are usually derived from cardiac mural thrombus.
- Vascular stenosis (less common)—occurs with thrombosis in a severely atherosclerotic

mesenteric artery. Typically located near its origin from aorta. Resultant small bowel infarction is extensive and usually fatal.

- Vasculitic syndromes (page 93), e.g. polyarteritis nodosa, Henoch–Schönlein purpura, SLE.

Strangulation

Thin-walled veins which drain blood from the small bowel become occluded by extrinsic pressure, e.g. from:

- Loop of bowel in a narrow hernial sac.
- Intussusception.
- Volvulus.
- Adhesions.

Venous occlusion causes congestion and oedema of the bowel wall. Increased pressure prevents entry of oxygenated arterial blood leading to ischaemic necrosis.

Hypoperfusion

In severe hypotension, blood is shunted preferentially away from the superficial mucosa, which is the layer of the wall most susceptible to injury because of its high metabolic requirements.

In infants, poor perfusion of the mucosa followed by infection produces a rapidly fatal condition known as neonatal necrotising enterocolitis. The bowel wall is thickened from congestion, and there is extensive superficial mucosal ulceration. Predisposing factors are prematurity, ARDS, Hirschsprung's disease and cystic fibrosis with meconium ileus.

Classification of severity

Ischaemic infarcts are classified according to the depth of involvement:

- Mucosal infarction—transient or reversible infarction which may be followed by complete regeneration. However, increased permeability to toxic substances can cause gradual progression to a transmural infarct.
- Mural infarction—infarction of mucosa and submucosa up to the muscularis propria. The mucosa is ulcerated, oedematous and haemorrhagic. Healing occurs by granulation tissue formation. Mural infarction may lead to the development of fibrous strictures (occurs in about half of patients with ischaemic bowel disease).
- Transmural infarction—necrosis extends through the muscularis propria. The bowel is flaccid, dilated, and liable to perforation. Surgical resection is an option, but many patients already

have peritonitis, endotoxaemia and severe circulatory problems at the time of diagnosis, so the prognosis is poor.

The splenic flexure is a common and early site of ischaemic damage, as it is a watershed area between the distribution of superior and inferior mesenteric arteries.

Angiodysplasia

In this condition, abnormal venous dilatations develop in the submucosa of the large intestine (typically the right side) often causing occult or massive intestinal bleeding. It occurs in the elderly and is associated with aortic valve disease.

It is thought to be a degenerative process resulting in increasing obstruction of the mucosal veins, which become tortuous and prone to bleeding. Developmental abnormalities of the colon may also be involved in the pathogenesis.

Haemorrhoids (piles)

These are dilated varicose veins forming in the anal canal. The most common of all anal conditions, they affect as much as 40% of the population at some time. Haemorrhoids develop as a result of increased intra-abdominal pressure, e.g. constipation and straining at the stool, pregnancy.

Rarely, raised portal hypertension can cause haemorrhoid formation.

Two anatomical areas are affected, although both are often involved at the same time:

1. Internal haemorrhoids—proximal to superior haemorrhoidal plexus, above the anorectal margin. These most commonly occur at three main points equidistant to the circumference of the anus (Fig. 8.40).
2. External haemorrhoids—below the anorectal margin.

Haemorrhoids are associated with bright red rectal bleeding after defaecation, pain and pruritus ani.

Clinical classification

There are three degrees of haemorrhoid:

1. First degree—present in the lumen but does not prolapse; these tend to bleed.
2. Second degree—prolapses on defaecation but returns spontaneously.
3. Third degree—remains prolapsed but can be digitally replaced.

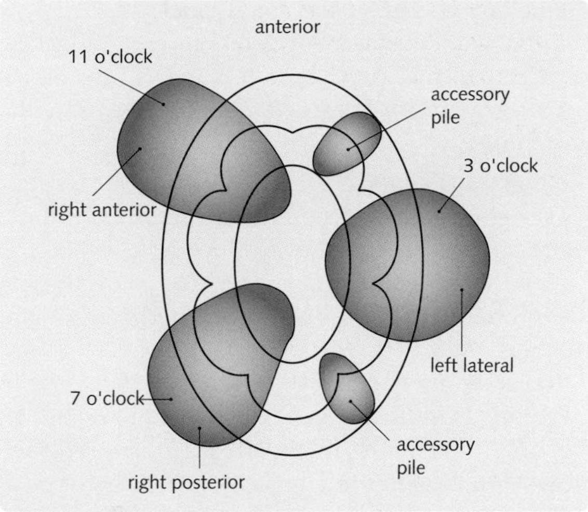

Fig. 8.40 Diagram to illustrate the 3, 7, 11 distribution of haemorrhoids around the anus. (Adapted with permission from Surgery of the Anus, Rectum and Colon, 5th edn, by J Goligher, Baillière Tindall, 1984.)

Diagnosis is by proctoscopy (to visualise the haemorrhoids) or by sigmoidoscopy (to exclude coexisting rectal pathology).

Treatment involves reducing constipation and straining with a high fibre diet, or direct therapy to the haemorrhoid with injection sclerotherapy or band ligation. Surgical removal of the haemorrhoid (haemorrhoidectomy) is rarely required.

Neoplastic disease of the intestine

Primary tumours of the small intestine are rare; those that do arise are outlined in Fig. 8.41. In contrast, tumours of the large bowel are extremely common. The colon and rectum are frequently affected by both benign and malignant tumours.

Classification of intestinal tumours

Intestinal tumours can be classified according to Fig. 8.41.

Fig. 8.41 Types of intestinal tumours

	Small intestine	Large bowel
Non-neoplastic polyps	Hamartomas Juvenile polyps Adenomatous polyps (in familial adenomatous polyposis and Gardner's syndrome) Inflammatory fibroid polyps	Hyperplastic polyps: small, flat, pale lesions typically 5 mm in size, which occur most commonly in the rectum and sigmoid colon Hamartomatous polyps: typically occur in childhood and in adolescence,eg. Peutz-Jeghers syndrome (autosomal dominant), sporadic juvenile polyps Inflammatory 'pseudopolyps' (of ulcerative colitis)

Neoplastic epithelial lesions	Adenocarcinomas	Pre-malignant:
		• Adenomas (dysplastic):
		  Tubular adenoma
		  Villous adenoma
		  Tubulovillous adenoma
		• Familial adenomatous polyposis
		Malignant:
		• Colorectal carcinoma

Mesenchymal lesions	Benign: lipoma, neurogenic tumours, leiomyoma and haemangioma Malignant: some smooth muscle tumours (leiomyosaracomas)	Rare; usually incidental findings or at post-mortem; seldom responsible for symptoms; lipomas, leiomyomas, haemangiomas, neurofibromas
Lymphoma	Common site for primary lymphoma of the GI tract; coeliac disease is a major predisposing factor	Very uncommon in large bowel
Carcinoid tumours (neuroendocrine tumours)	Most common site for carcinoid tumours (especially appendix); lesions typically scattered singly throughout GI tract; may secrete gut hormones, e.g. somatostatin, cholecystokinin, pancreatic polypeptide and VIP	Rare; do not usually produce functioning hormones

Note: GI, gastrointestinal; VIP, vasoactive intestinal polypeptide

Fig. 8.41 Types of intestinal tumours.

Neoplastic epithelial lesions

Adenomas

These premalignant tumours are derived from the glandular epithelium of the large bowel. Common in older subjects, they are present in up to 50% of persons aged over 60, males more than females by 2 : 1.

Aetiology is probably multifactorial. Both genetic and environmental (dietary) factors have been implicated.

There are three types:

1. Tubular—rounded lesions (0.5–2 cm in size). Often pedunculated (i.e. have a stalk of normal mucosa). Microscopically composed of tube-shaped glands.
2. Villous—frond-like lesions about 0.6 cm thick, which occupy a broad area of mucosa (1–5 cm in diameter). Microscopically composed of finger-like epithelial projections.
3. Tubulovillous—raised lesions (1–4 cm in size). Pedunculated but composed of both tube-shaped glands and finger-like epithelial projections.

Epithelium of all three types shows dysplastic features, which can be subjectively graded as mild, moderate or severe.

Progression from adenoma to carcinoma

Most carcinomas of the colon develop from previous adenomas. Progression from adenoma to carcinoma is the well-established basis of the polyp–cancer sequence for development of carcinoma of the colon (see Fig. 3.6).

Risk of malignant change is greatest where adenomas show the following features:

- Large—less than 1 cm (1% malignant); 1–2 cm (12% malignant); more than 2 cm (30% malignant).
- Villous—villous adenomas are more likely to undergo malignant transformation.
- Severe dysplasia.

Familial adenomatous polyposis

Familial adenomatous polyposis (FAP) is a rare autosomal dominant condition caused by a mutation in the FAP gene located on the long arm of chromosome 5. It is characterised by the presence of innumerable adenomata of the large bowel from about the age of 25. There is a 90% risk of developing a carcinoma of the colon by the age of 45.

Hereditary non-polyposis colon cancer

This is an inherited form of colon cancer, without adenomas, which is due to mutation in DNA mismatch repair genes. This is associated with microsatellite instability.

Colorectal carcinoma

This adenocarcinoma is derived from the glandular epithelium of the large bowel mucosa.

It is the second most common cause of death from neoplasia, with a peak incidence between 60 and 70 years of age; it is rare under the age of 40.

It is rare in Africa but there is a high incidence in developed countries. 55 per 100 000 males and 35 per 100 000 females in the UK are diagnosed each year, with a higher incidence in Scotland for both sexes. Environmental factors are thought to play a large role in the aetiology of colorectal cancer. Risk factors are:

- High-fat, high-protein, low-fibre diets (effects on bowel transit time, bacterial flora and levels of cellulose, amino acids and bile acids in the bowel contents).
- Presence of multiple sporadic adenomatous polyps.
- Long-standing and extensive ulcerative colitis.
- Familial adenomatous polyposis.
- Previous pelvic radiotherapy.

Macroscopically, the most common sites for colorectal carcinomas are illustrated in Fig. 8.42.

Types of colorectal carcinomas are:

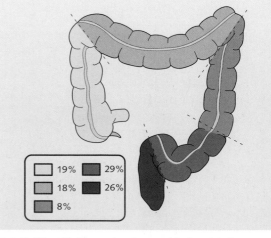

19%	29%
18%	26%
8%	

Fig. 8.42 Site and incidence of carcinomas of the large intestine.

- Polypoid—cauliflower-like growth.
- Annular—small, circumferential carcinomas that may cause stenosis.
- Ulcerated—tumours that present mainly with bleeding.
- Diffusely infiltrative—rare, but virtually identical to that seen in stomach. Often associated with carcinoma that develops in association with inflammatory bowel disease.

Right-sided carcinomas (ascending colon):

- Type of growth—polypoid.
- Pathogenesis—faecal material is soft in ascending colon, and so lesions grow to large size before causing obstruction.
- Presentation—later than for left-sided carcinomas.

Left-sided carcinomas (descending colon):

- Type of growth—annular, ulcerating.
- Pathogenesis—lesions develop where faecal material is more solid.
- Presentation—earlier due to mechanical obstruction to passage of faeces.

Microscopic features—98% of all cancers in the large intestine are adenocarcinomas; the majority of colorectal carcinomas are therefore moderately or well-differentiated adenocarcinomas forming recognisable glandular structures.

Poorly differentiated carcinomas have a poorer prognosis. Overall, 5-year survival is around 50%.

Spread of colorectal carcinoma:
- Local—adjacent bowel wall and adherent structures (e.g. bladder).
- Lymphatic—draining nodes.
- Blood—to liver and then elsewhere.
- Transcaelomic—along peritoneal cavity.

Prognosis relates to stage, which is assessed by the modified Dukes system (Fig. 8.43). Five-year survival is over 90% in Dukes A cancer but less than 5% in Dukes D. Dukes C and D cancers (common presentations) require adjuvant chemotherapy and/or radiotherapy after surgical resection.

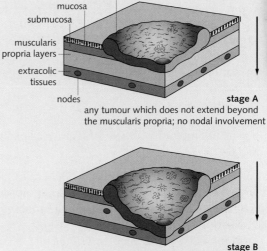

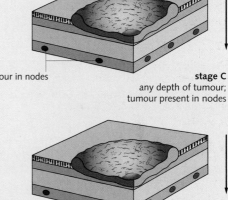

Fig. 8.43 Staging of carcinoma of the colon using the Dukes system.

DISORDERS OF THE PERITONEUM

Inflammation: peritonitis
Peritoneal infection

This can either be of primary or secondary infection. Primary infection (less common) is seen in patients with nephrotic syndrome (peritoneal dialysis), cirrhosis with ascites or abdominal trauma.

Secondary infection (most common) is typically an extension of inflammatory processes from the abdominal cavity. For example:

- Appendicitis.
- Ruptured ulcers—peptic, ulcerative colitis, typhoid ulcers, ulcerated neoplasms.
- Cholecystitis, pancreatitis, salpingitis.
- Diverticulitis.
- Chlamydial infection—a complication of female pelvic inflammatory disease that is increasing in incidence.
- Strangulated bowel.

Organisms involved are typically a mixture of normal gut commensals with a predominance of anaerobic bacteria and coliforms.

Irritation of the peritoneum by leaking bile, gastric juice, pancreatic enzymes or urine produces an exudate that is initially sterile but which usually becomes infected within 6–12 hours.

As peritonitis develops, inflammation of visceral and parietal peritoneum produces a purulent exudate; the intestine becomes flaccid, dilated, and covered with fibrinous plaques that form adhesions between bowel loops.

Clinical features are:

- Tenderness, guarding, and rebound tenderness.
- Board-like abdominal rigidity.
- Absent bowel sounds (paralytic ileus).
- Increased pulse and temperature.

Complications and management

Complications are:

- Hypovolaemic shock.
- Severe toxaemia from absorbed bacterial products.
- Paralytic ileus—paralysis of gut motility as a result of inflammation of the serosa of the small bowel.
- Fibrous adhesions as a result of organization of fibrinous adhesion by granulation tissue.
- Abscesses, particularly in the paracolic gutters and beneath the diaphragm (subphrenic recesses).
- Portal pyophlebitis—spread via the portal vein to the liver.

Diagnosis is by clinical examination and erect abdominal X-ray, which may show air under the diaphragm from perforated viscus. Blood cultures may reveal the organism responsible.

Management is by:

- Treatment of shock.
- Antibiotic therapy.
- Surgery—removal of contaminating source, e.g. appendicitis or perforated bowel.
- Peritoneal toilet and lavage.

See Fig. 8.44 for a summary of peritoneal infection.

Fig. 8.44 Summary of peritoneal infection.

Fig. 8.44 Summary of peritoneal infection	
Aetiology	Primary infection (less common): nephrotic syndrome, peritoneal dialysis, cirrhosis with ascites, abdominal trauma Secondary infection (most common): typically an extension of inflammatory processes from abdominal cavity, e.g. appendicitis, ruptured ulcers (peptic, ulcerative colitis, typhoid ulcers, ulcerated neoplasms), cholecystitis, pancreatitis, salpingitis, diverticulitis, strangulated bowel
Organisms involved	Normal gut commensals with anaerobic bacteria and coliforms predominating
Pathogenesis	Leaking bile, gastric juice, pancreatic enzymes or urine cause irritation and inflammation of peritoneum producing an exudate that typically becomes infected; intestine becomes flaccid, dilated and covered with fibrinous plaques forming adhesions between bowel loops
Clinical features	Guarding and rebound tenderness Board-like abdominal rigidity Absent bowel sounds (paralytic ileus) Increased pulse and temperature
Complications	Local: ileus, fibrinous adhesions, abscesses, portal pyophlebitis Systemic: hypovolaemic shock, severe toxaemia

Sclerosis retroperitonitis

This dense progressive fibrosis of the peritoneum particularly affects the visceral peritoneum of the small intestine. In most cases no cause is found, although there are rare associations with some medications (practolol and methysergide). It is also seen in patients undergoing long-term continuous ambulatory peritoneal dialysis.

Mesenteric cysts

These are cysts found within the mesenteries of the abdominal cavity, or attached to the peritoneal lining.

Sequestered lymphatic channels (cystic lymphangiomas)

These cystic developmental abnormalities of lymphoid type are typically asymptomatic and discovered incidentally at laparotomy or autopsy.

Pinched-off enteric diverticula (enterogenous cysts)

These common lesions are found either incorporated in the bowel wall or in mesentery detached and separated from the tract.

Urogenital ridge derivations

These developmental cysts are of urogenital origin.

'Walled-off' infections

This localised peritonitis is due to the capacity of omentum to wall-off infection (pseudocysts).

Neoplasms

Primary mesothelioma

A rare condition, this is associated with exposure to asbestos. It corresponds to the much more common pleural mesothelioma (see Chapter 7).

The peritoneal cavity is a common site of metastases; malignancy of any organ within the peritoneal cavity may lead to peritonitis.

Secondary

The most common tumours to metastasise to the peritoneal cavity are of the stomach, ovary, pancreas and colon.

Metastases result in the effusion of protein-rich fluid into the cavity (i.e. an exudate) containing neoplastic cells, which also grow as tiny white nodules on the mesothelial surface of the cavity. Nodules eventually coalesce to form tumour sheets over the surface of the viscera.

Pathology of the kidney and urinary tract

9

Objectives

In this chapter, you will learn to:

- Describe abnormalities of kidney structure, notably the common cystic diseases.
- Understand the patterns of glomerular disease and common mechanisms of injury.
- Describe common glomerular diseases and how pathology relates to clinical presentation.
- Recognise that glomerular lesions occur in systemic diseases, giving common examples.
- Recall the pathology of renal tubular and interstitial diseases.
- Describe disorders of renal blood vessels.
- Understand the neoplasms commonly encountered within the kidney and urinary tract.
- Describe disorders of the urinary tract, focusing on causes of obstruction.

ABNORMALITIES OF KIDNEY STRUCTURE

Congenital abnormalities of the kidney

Congenital anomalies of kidneys are common, affecting 3–4% of newborn infants.

Agenesis of the kidney

Unilateral

Unilateral agenesis occurs in 1 in 1000 births. It may occur alongside other congenital disease such as spina bifida. The solitary kidney undergoes marked hypertrophy and is susceptible to infections, trauma and progressive glomerulosclerosis. It affects males more than females by 2 : 1; the left kidney is usually the absent one.

Bilateral

Occurrence of bilateral agenesis is 1 in 3000 births, as part of Potter's syndrome. Affected infants have abnormal facies, and they often have abnormalities of the lower urinary tract, lungs and nervous system.

Characteristically, there is oligohydramnios in pregnancy as the kidneys are not present to contribute to amniotic fluid (absence of fetal urine). The disorder is not compatible with postnatal life.

Hypoplasia

Kidneys fail to reach the normal adult size either as a result of a congenital maldevelopment or due to shrinkage, which may have occurred as a result of chronic infection in early life.

Ectopic kidneys

One or both kidneys may be in an abnormal position: most commonly the pelvis, but some lie in the inferior part of the abdomen.

Pancake kidney

Here, there is fusion of the pelvic kidneys to form a round discoid mass.

Unilateral fused kidney

The kidneys fuse together in the pelvis, then, as one kidney ascends to the 'normal' position, the other is carried with it so that both kidneys end up on the same side.

Horseshoe kidney

The poles of the kidneys are fused, usually inferiorly, to form a large U-shaped (horseshoe) kidney. This affects about 1 in 500 people, but it is typically asymptomatic as the collecting system develops normally. However, Wilms' tumours are 2 to 8 times more frequent in children with horseshoe kidneys than in the general population (see page 199).

Cystic diseases of the kidney

Overview of cystic kidney disease

This heterogeneous group of diseases comprises:

- Hereditary disorders.
- Developmental (but not hereditary) disorders.
- Acquired disorders.

Each disease is distinguished by a characteristic distribution of cysts, illustrated in Fig. 9.1.

Figure 9.2 provides a summary of cystic diseases of the kidney.

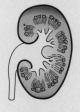
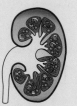
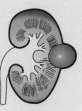
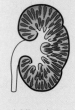
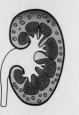
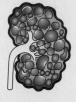

| uraemic medullary cystic disease complex | medullary sponge disease | solitary cyst |
| childhood cystic disease | congenital nephrotic syndrome | adult polycystic disease |

Fig. 9.1 Macroscopic features of cystic diseases of the kidney.

Accurate diagnosis of cystic diseases is important for two reasons:
1. Appropriate patient management to delay onset of renal failure.
2. Appropriate genetic counselling to patients/relatives in the case of hereditary cystic diseases.

Cystic renal dysplasia

The failure of differentiation of metanephric tissues affects the whole or just one segment of a kidney, either unilaterally or bilaterally. Affected areas are replaced by solid or cystic masses, in which cartilage is usually prominent.

The condition often presents in childhood as an abdominal mass and it requires surgical excision to exclude a malignant tumour (e.g. nephroblastoma). Prognosis is good for unilateral lesions.

Adult polycystic kidney disease

Adult polycystic kidney disease (APKD) is a hereditary disease. Both kidneys are progressively replaced by fluid-filled cysts, which develop and enlarge over a period of years.

Fig. 9.2 Summary of cystic diseases of the kidney	
Type of cystic disease	**Clinical features**
Hereditary	
Adult polycystic disease (autosomal dominant) Infantile polycystic disease (autosomal recessive)	Chronic renal failure and hypertension
Medullary cystic disease (autosomal dominant) Juvenile nephronophthisis (autosomal recessive)	Early-onset chronic renal failure
Medullary sponge kidney (occasionally familial)	Renal stones predispose to renal colic and infection
Developmental	
Cystic renal dysplasia	Typically asymptomatic
Acquired	
Simple renal cysts Dialysis-associated cystic disease	Typically asymptomatic

Fig. 9.2 Summary of cystic diseases of the kidney.

Incidence is 1 per 1250 live births, accounting for 8% of all end-stage renal disease, with the sexes equally affected.

It is inherited as an autosomal dominant disorder; 85% of cases are linked to the α-globin cluster located on the small arm of chromosome 16 (autosomal dominant polycystic kidney disease-1; ADPKD-1). ADPKD-2 gene mutations (15% of cases) have a slower disease onset. Both mutations are associated with berry aneurysms of the cerebral arteries and with cysts of the liver, pancreas and lung.

The condition is asymptomatic at first but—eventually—replacement and compression of the functioning renal parenchyma by the enlarging cysts leads to slowly progressive impairment of renal function.

Macroscopically, in fully developed APKD, the kidneys are asymmetrically enlarged and are composed of numerous large cysts (each up to 5 cm in diameter). Haemorrhage into the cysts is common, leading to bloodstained contents.

Microscopically, the cysts are lined by flattened cuboidal epithelium and communicate both with calyces and with each other. Surrounding parenchyma often shows extensive fibrosis and arteriosclerosis.

Complications are as follows:

- Chronic renal failure and uraemia.
- Hypertension—often preceding development of cardiac failure.
- Subarachnoid haemorrhage (10% of cases)—predisposed by the combination of berry aneurysms and hypertension.

APKD typically presents in the fourth decade or later, often with a large lobulated abdominal mass, pain, or haematuria.

Diagnosis is by ultrasound, which shows multiple bilateral cysts. Screening susceptible 18-year-olds has a 95% successful diagnosis rate. Genetic analysis is sometimes used to exclude disease.

Management is by:
- Blood pressure control—uncontrolled hypertension accelerates renal failure.
- Treating urinary infections and cardiac failure.
- Eventual dialysis or transplantation.

Infantile (childhood) polycystic disease

This is a less common autosomal recessive disorder, in which there is cystic replacement of both kidneys present at birth. Cysts are composed of dilated tubules and collecting ducts.

This is a rare condition (at 1 per 10 000 live births), and is associated with cysts of the liver, pancreas, and lungs.

It presents in stillborn or neonates with enlarged kidneys (12–16 times normal size) containing a radiating cystic pattern in the medulla and cortex ('sunburst' pattern; see Fig. 9.1). Rarely, it may present in childhood with renal insufficiency.

Prognosis—affected infants often die within the first 2 months of life; those that survive tend to develop a form of hepatic fibrosis.

Cystic diseases of the renal medulla

Medullary sponge kidney (tubular ectasia)

Multiple cysts develop in renal papillae, with an incidence of 1 in 20 000. Renal function is not usually impaired and the main clinical problem is the development of renal stones that predispose to renal colic and infection.

Nephronophthisis complex (uraemic medullary cystic disease complex)

This describes a group of hereditary diseases characterised by development of cysts at the corticomedullary junction of the kidney. These diseases are associated with tubular atrophy and interstitial fibrosis. Important examples are:

- Juvenile nephronophthisis—autosomal recessive disease presenting at about 11 years of age.
- Medullary cystic disease—autosomal dominant trait presenting at about 20 years of age.

Clinically, these conditions are characterised by thirst (polydipsia) and polyuria (due to nephrogenic diabetes insipidus; see Chapter 10) and eventually result in early-onset chronic renal failure. Together, they account for about 20–25% of cases of end-stage renal failure in the first three decades of life.

Acquired dialysis-associated cystic disease

This is seen in kidneys left *in situ* when patients are treated by dialysis or transplantation for chronic renal failure.

Simple cysts

These common lesions occur as solitary or occasionally multiple cystic spaces in otherwise normal kidneys. Incidence increases with age.

The abnormality is widely believed to be acquired, but the cause is unknown.

Macroscopically, cysts are of variable size (generally smaller than 5cm), and they contain clear watery fluid.

Microscopically, they are lined by flattened cuboidal epithelium and surrounded by a thin fibrous capsule. Clinically, cysts may cause renal enlargement, but they have no effect on renal function. However, they require clinical differentiation from tumours and other cystic disorders.

DISEASES OF THE GLOMERULUS

Overview of glomerular disease

Glomerular diseases are typically caused by disturbances of structure. Four significant components of the glomerulus may be damaged:

1. Endothelial cells lining the capillary.
2. Glomerular basement membrane.
3. Mesangium, i.e. the supporting mesentery to the capillary, which comprises mesangial cells (phagocytic support cells) and associated extracellular material (mesangial matrix).
4. Epithelial cells or podocytes, which form an outer coating to the capillary. These cells are in contact with the outer surface of the basement membrane via a series of foot processes.

Patterns of glomerular disease

Although a small number of diseases affect all glomeruli in a uniform manner, most affect different glomeruli to varying degrees. There are two patterns of disease at the glomerular level:

1. Global—affecting the whole glomerulus uniformly.
2. Segmental—affecting one glomerular segment while sparing the others within that glomerulus.

A further two terms are used to describe the extent of disease within the renal system:

1. Diffuse—affecting all glomeruli in both kidneys.
2. Focal—affecting a proportion of glomeruli, sparing others.

Thus a glomerular disease may be described as one of 'diffuse global', 'diffuse segmental', 'focal global' or 'focal segmental'. The vast majority are either 'diffuse global' or 'focal segmental'.

This explains how some glomerular diseases cause sudden acute renal failure (diffuse global diseases),

whereas others cause a selective partial renal failure (focal segmental diseases).

Aetiology of glomerular diseases

Glomerular diseases may be classified as (Fig. 9.3):

- Primary (majority)—disease process appears to start within the glomerulus. These are further classified into four main histological types: proliferative (majority), membranous, glomerulosclerotic and minimal change lesions.
- Secondary—disease process is secondary to systemic disease, which can be immune-complex-mediated, metabolic or vascular conditions. These are covered on page 191.
- Hereditary—Alport's syndrome, Fabry's syndrome and congenital nephrotic syndrome.

Clinical manifestations of glomerular disease

Glomerular pathology produces a spectrum of presentations from pure proteinuria (reflects injury to podocytes and architecture) to pure haematuria (inflammatory proliferative changes). Many diseases lie somewhere along this spectrum with a mixture of proteinuria and haematuria to differing degrees.

Five key syndromes cover most presentations. These are described below.

1. Asymptomatic haematuria

This is haematuria without significant proteinuria, which may be continuous or intermittent, varying in severity from macroscopic to microscopic. Most cases are not renal in origin (e.g. urinary tract infection, bladder cancer) and those that do originate in the kidney rarely cause rapid renal deterioration but may warn of increased future risk.

2. Asymptomatic proteinuria

This proteinuria (> 0.3 g every 24 hours) without haematuria may be continuous, orthostatic (postural) or transient. It is typically detected at a routine medical examination.

3. Acute nephritic syndrome

This presents with a sudden onset of haematuria, proteinuria (often with urinary casts) and hypertension. Loin pain and headache may be present and the patient will often feel unwell. In children there is often generalised oedema, especially around the eyes.

Fig. 9.3 Aetiology of glomerular disorders

Aetiology	Example
Primary disorders	
Antiglomerular basement membrane disease: proliferative	Goodpasture's syndrome
Immune complex-mediated lesions	
Proliferative	Diffuse proliferative glomerulonephritis Focal proliferative glomerulonephritis Membranoproliferative glomerulonephritis Crescentic glomerulonephritis
Membranous	Membranous glomerulopathy
Glomerulosclerosis	Focal segmental glomerulosclerosis
Minimal change	Minimal change disease
Secondary disorders	
Immune complex-mediated conditions	Systemic lupus erythematosus Henoch–Schönlein purpura Infective endocarditis
Metabolic conditions	Diabetes mellitus Renal amyloidosis Multiple myeloma
Vascular conditions	Polyarteritis nodosa Wegener's granulomatosis Haemolytic uraemic syndrome Idiopathic thrombocytopenic purpura Disseminated intravascular coagulation
Hereditary disorders	
	Alport's and Fabry's syndromes

Fig. 9.3 Aetiology of glomerular disorders.

It is associated with conditions such as Goodpasture's syndrome.

4. Nephrotic syndrome

Here, there is proteinuria (usually > 3.5 g every 24 hours) with hypoproteinemia and oedema. There is also hypercholesterolaemia, an increased tendency to clotting and greater risk of infection. It may be due to primary or secondary glomerular disease.

5. Chronic renal failure

This is an irreversible deterioration in renal function caused by the destruction of more and more individual nephrons over a long period of time. Impairment of excretory, metabolic and endocrine functions of the kidney leads to the clinical syndrome of uraemia.

Figure 9.4 lists the symptoms and signs of renal failure.

Management—excretory function of the kidney can be partially replaced by dialysis. However, replace-

Fig. 9.4 Symptoms and signs of renal failure

Symptoms	Signs
General malaise	Uraemia
Breathlessness on exertion	Anaemia
Nausea and vomiting	Metabolic bone disease (renal osteodystrophy)
Disordered gastrointestinal motility	Hypertension
Headaches	Acidosis
Pruritus	Neuropathy
Pigmentation	Generalised myopathy
	Endocrine abnormalities

Fig. 9.4 Symptoms and signs of renal failure.

ment of the endocrine and metabolic functions can only be achieved by successful renal transplantation.

Unless some form of supportive therapy—such as dialysis or transplantation—is available, chronic renal failure is eventually fatal.

Steps in diagnoses of glomerular lesions

Clinical presentation

This is to identify the type of urinary abnormality.

Histological identification

This is required to identify the pattern of glomerular response to injury. Percutaneous needle biopsy of the kidney allows histological examination of the glomeruli and tubules to identify structural abnormalities and to characterise patterns of damage.

Immunological investigation

This is for the detection of immune complex deposition and serological changes (see below).

Summary

Many of the diseases causing the above clinical syndromes are listed in Fig. 9.5.

However, there is considerable overlap—several diseases may give rise to the same clinical picture and, conversely, many conditions fall into more than one clinical group.

The mechanism of glomerular injury

Many glomerular diseases are caused by immune-mediated damage (listed below). Different patterns of immune-mediated damage point to different diagnoses. It is therefore important to identify the site, type and pattern of immune complexes and complement within the glomerulus by immunohistochemistry and electron microscopy.

The five main mechanisms of immune-mediated damage are as follows:

1. Circulating immune complex nephritis

This is the most common pattern of immunological disease.

Mechanism

Antigen–antibody complexes circulating in the blood are trapped at the basement membrane, the mesangium or both. Complexes activate the complement cascade via the classical pathway (see Fig. 2.6). Activated components of complement bring about the characteristic acute inflammation of glomerulonephritis by attracting neutrophil polymorphs, increasing vascular permeability and causing membrane damage (see Fig. 2.7). Damage to the basement membrane results in alteration of its properties, leading to some of the urinary abnormalities observed clinically.

Example

Poststreptococcal glomerulonephritis.

2. In-situ immune complex formation

Mechanism

Circulating antigens become 'planted' or trapped in the glomerulus, where they are targeted by circulating antibodies such that immune complexes are formed within the glomerulus. This in-situ formation explains why, unlike circulating immune complex nephritis described above, there is little complement and no inflammatory or proliferative responses.

Example

This is believed to occur in certain cases of systemic lupus erythematosus (SLE) when free DNA in the blood is trapped in the glomerular basement membrane, subsequently binding to anti-DNA antibodies.

3. Cytotoxic antibodies

Mechanism

Autoantibodies are directed to a component of the glomerular basement membrane (anti-GBM antibodies). This is an uncommon form of immune-mediated damage.

Example

This is the basis of Goodpasture's syndrome, in which autoantibodies cause direct damage to the glomerular basement membrane. The Goodpasture antigen (which is the target of the anti-GBM antibodies) has been identified as a domain on the $\alpha3$ type IV collagen chain. These antibodies may cross-react with collagen of the lung, producing simultaneous lung and kidney disease.

4. Activation of the alternative complement pathway

Mechanism

The alternative complement pathway is normally activated by the presence of bacterial cell walls, and it is independent of immune complex formation (see Fig. 2.6). However, in certain disease conditions, the

Fig. 9.5 Clinical manifestations of glomerular disease and the conditions that cause them

Clinical manifestations	Causative renal disease
Asymptomatic haematuria	Exercise haematuria IgA nephropathy Henloch–Schönlein purpura Bacterial endocarditis Systemic lupus erythematosus Polyarteritis nodosa
Asymptomatic proteinuria	Primary: • Focal segmental glomerulosclerosis • Membranoproliferative glomerulonephritis Secondary: • Henloch–Schönlein purpura • Systemic lupus erythematosus • Polyarteritis nodosa • Bacterial endocarditis
Acute nephritic syndrome	Primary: • Poststreptococcal glomerulonephritis • Rapidly progressive glomerulonephritis • Goodpasture's syndrome Secondary: • Systemic lupus erythematosus • Polyarteritis nodosa • Wegener's granulomatosis • Henloch–Schönlein purpura • Essential cryoglobulinaemia

Nephrotic syndrome	Primary:
	• Minimal change disease
	• Membranous glomerulopathy
	• Membranoproliferative glomerulonephritis
	• Focal proliferative glomerulonephritis
	• Focal glomerulosclerosis
	Secondary:
	• Immune complex-mediated conditions
	  Systemic lupus erythematosus
	  Henloch–Schönlein purpura
	  Infective endocarditis
	• Metabolic conditions
	  Diabetes mellitus
	  Renal amyloidosis
	• Vascular conditions
	  Polyarteritis nodosa
	  Wegener's granulomatosis
	  Haemolytic uraemic syndrome
	• Infections
	  Malaria, syphilis, hepatitis B

Chronic renal failure	All of the above except minimal change disease

Fig. 9.5 Clinical manifestations of glomerular disease and the conditions that cause them.

alternative pathway can be activated by different mechanisms.

Example

In type II membranoproliferative glomerulonephritis, a circulating autoantibody (termed 'C3 nephritic factor') activates complement via the alternative pathway by stabilising the enzyme C3-convertase. This enzyme normally activates C3 but has a very short half-life. Thus, stabilisation of C3-convertase prolongs the activation of C3.

5. Cell-mediated immunity

Cell-mediated immunological mechanisms are uncommon in the initiation of acute glomerular diseases but are thought to play a role in the progression of acute glomerulonephritis to a chronic phase.

Proliferative glomerulonephritis

This group of disorders is characterised histologically by varying degrees of proliferation of mesangial and epithelial (and sometimes endothelial) cells within the glomerulus.

The majority of cases of glomerulonephritis (over 70%) belong to this group.

Proliferative glomerulonephritis can be divided according to histological appearance into:

- Diffuse proliferative.
- Rapidly progressive.
- Focal proliferative.
- Membranoproliferative.

However, it must be emphasised that these subdivisions are not diagnoses but rather describe a pattern of reaction caused by glomerular insult.

Diffuse proliferative glomerulonephritis

Diffuse, global, acute inflammation of glomeruli is caused by the deposition of immune complexes in the glomeruli, stimulated by a preceding infection.

Aetiology is as follows:

- Poststreptococcal (most common)—onset is 1–2 weeks after a primary pharyngeal or skin infection with group A β-haemolytic streptococci.
- Non-streptococcal (less common)—a range of bacterial, viral and protozoal infections can also stimulate this pattern of disease.

Those antibodies produced to combat initial infection cross-react with cellular antigens producing immune complexes. These complexes circulate in the blood and are filtered-out in the glomerulus, producing four main histological changes:

1. Immune complex deposition—in lumps on the epithelial side of the glomerular basement membrane.
2. Neutrophil infiltration—activation of complement attracts neutrophils into the glomerulus.
3. Endothelial cell proliferation—degranulation of neutrophils damages endothelial cells, stimulating their proliferation.

4. Mild mesangial cell proliferation—mediated by factors derived from complement and platelets.

Rapidly progressive glomerulonephritis (crescentic glomerulonephritis)

Rapidly progressive glomerulonephritis (RPGN) is a manifestation of severe glomerular injury characterised by the formation of cellular crescent-shaped masses within the Bowman's space. It occurs in a small percentage of patients with poststreptococcal glomerulonephritis (see above) but it can also be associated with many other forms of glomerular damage.

If damage to the glomerular capillaries is severe, fibrin and blood leak into Bowman's space stimulating epithelial cell proliferation, and entry of inflammatory infiltrate. Crescent-shaped cellular masses composed of epithelial cells, macrophages and monocytes are formed within the Bowman's space. These crescents are associated with glomerular ischaemia and ultimately they result in permanent glomerular damage.

Focal proliferative glomerulonephritis

Here, there is an acute inflammation with cellular proliferation occurring in only a proportion of all glomeruli (focal) and usually affecting only one segment of the glomerular tufts (segmental). Therefore, the condition is more accurately described as focal segmental proliferative glomerulonephritis.

Several diseases can cause this pattern of response. These can be classified into two groups:

1. Primary—mainly mesangial IgA disease and Goodpasture's syndrome (Fig. 9.6).
2. Secondary—associated with other systemic diseases including infective endocarditis, vasculitis and connective tissue diseases.

Immunohistochemistry and electron microscopy are required to distinguish them.

Membranoproliferative glomerulonephritis

Membranoproliferative glomerulonephritis (MPGN) is a diffuse, global pattern of glomerulonephritis with features of both proliferation and membrane thickening (hence the name). It is also known as mesangiocapillary glomerulonephritis.

Diseases causing MPGN can be classified into two groups:

1. Primary (majority)—idiopathic. Subdivided according to clinical and pathological features

Fig. 9.6 Proliferative glomerulonephritis

Condition	Features
Mesangial IgA disease	A focal proliferative glomerulonephritis Serum IgA levels are raised and IgA is deposited in the mesangium and basement membrane
Goodpasture's syndrome	A focal proliferative glomerulonephritis. The Goodpasture antigen is a domain of type IV collagen in the basement membrane; this is a target for the autoantibodies
Type I MPGN	An immune complex disease thought to involve a disorder of complement, characterised by subendothelial deposits There is a persistently low serum C3
Type II MPGN	An autoimmune-mediated abnormality of complement. There is marked thickening of the capillary walls due to deposition of C3 (dense deposit disease)

Fig. 9.6 Examples of proliferative glomerulonephritic disease. (MPGN, membranoproliferative glomerulonephritis.)

into type I (90% of cases) and type II (10% of cases) (see Fig. 9.6).

2. Secondary—a few are secondary to systemic disorders such as SLE, infective endocarditis, malaria and infected ventricular cerebrospinal fluid (CSF) shunts.

Membranous nephropathy

There is a pattern of reaction in which the glomerular capillary basement membrane is uniformly thickened, partly due to immunoglobulin-based deposits. Unlike the proliferative types of glomerulonephritis, membranous nephropathy has no associated inflammation or endothelial/epithelial proliferation, although the mesangial cell population may be slightly increased.

It affects all age groups, but the highest incidence is between fifth and seventh decades. Males are affected more than females.

Aetiology is as follows:

- Primary—80–90% of cases have no apparent reason for development of immune complexes, and are classed as primary or idiopathic membranous nephropathy.
- Secondary—membranous nephropathy is found in association with a number of conditions which are listed in Fig. 9.7.

There are four pathological stages:

1. In-situ formation of immune complexes on the epithelial side of the basement membrane (diffuse, global pattern).
2. Mild mesangial increase.
3. New basement membrane is deposited around immune complex deposits.
4. Immune complex deposits disappear, leaving thickened 'lacy' basement membrane.

Over many years, the abnormal glomeruli develop increased mesangial matrix produced by the mesangial cells. This, together with membrane thickening, causes

Fig. 9.7 Conditions associated with membranous nephropathy

Type	Example
Infections	Malaria Syphilis Hepatitis B
Malignancy	Carcinoma (lung, breast, gastrointestinal tract) Lymphoma
Drugs	Gold, mercury, penicillamine, captopril
Systemic disease	Systemic lupus erythematosus (10% of renal involvement is of the membranous pattern)

Fig. 9.7 Conditions associated with membranous nephropathy.

gradual hyalinisation of the glomeruli (glomerulosclerosis) and death of individual nephrons.

Abnormality of the basement membrane renders it unusually permeable resulting in heavy proteinuria.

> Membranous nephropathy is the most common cause of nephrotic syndrome in adults.
>
> Prognosis is variable and related to cause but in crude figures: a third of patients undergo spontaneous remission without treatment, a third are stabilised with persisting proteinuria and a third progress to develop chronic renal failure.
>
> Long-term prognosis may be improved by treatment with high-dose corticosteroids and alkylating agents (e.g. cyclophosphamide), although there are significant side effects.

Minimal change disease (lipoid nephrosis)

The characteristic feature in this neuropathy (and the reason for the name) is that no significant abnormalities can be detected by light microscopy.

It mainly affects children under the age of 6 years, and it is less common in adults, but still accounts for 10–25% of cases of nephrotic syndrome. It is the most common cause of nephrotic syndrome in children. Males are affected more than females.

Aetiology is unknown, although in some cases an association with respiratory infection has been noted.

Pathogenesis is postulated to be immunologically related (cell-mediated damage to the basement membrane) because of the near universal response to corticosteroid therapy. Ultimately, polyanionic charges of the glomerular basement membrane are depleted, leading to failure of protein retention.

Morphological features—with electron microscopy, there is a diagnostic loss of epithelial foot processes. Tubules may show accumulation of lipid in lining cells, giving rise to the alternative name of 'lipoid nephrosis'.

Prognosis in children is good, with no permanent renal damage. In adults, the outlook is variable.

Focal segmental glomerulosclerosis

The glomerulus is partially replaced by hyaline material, which, in most cases, is excess mesangial matrix.

Aetiology is variable and related to age:

- Primary (most common)—idiopathic disease affecting children and young adults (more common in black populations).

- Secondary—in later adult life the condition is usually secondary to other disorders, especially previous focal proliferative glomerulonephritis.

Pathogenesis is unknown, but it is probably immune mediated.

Focal glomerulosclerosis initially affects the juxtamedullary glomeruli, causing an increase in mesangial matrix, which gradually expands to destroy the surrounding lobule, until global sclerosis occurs. In time, similar lesions appear in glomeruli throughout the cortex.

The patient presents with nephrotic syndrome. Later, haematuria, hypertension and renal failure are common.

Prognosis is poor with progression of disease over many years leading to chronic renal failure.

> It is useful to remember that the clinical syndromes of glomerulonephritis broadly relate to histological findings:
>
> - Asymptomatic proteinuria and nephrotic syndrome are associated with basement membrane thickening as a result of either structural change or deposition of excessive mesangial matrix, e.g. membranous nephropathy, glomerulosclerosis.
> - Asymptomatic haematuria and nephritic syndrome are associated with proliferation of the endothelial or mesangial cells, e.g. diffuse, global glomerulonephritis.
> - Mixed nephritic/nephrotic syndrome is associated with combined damage to the basement membrane and cell proliferation, e.g. membranoproliferative glomerulonephritis.

Hereditary glomerulonephritis
Alport's syndrome

This syndrome is characterised by the clinical triad of deafness, glomerulonephritis and ocular lesions. Inheritance is complex; it is X-linked in most families (a mutation of the *COLIVα5* gene), with an autosomal recessive pattern in the rest. Both types of disease are clinically indistinguishable. The genes affected encode basement membrane collagens that are found in the glomerulus and elsewhere in the body, e.g. the cochlea.

The clinical features are:

- Glomerulonephritis—usually presents as microscopic haematuria and proteinuria in childhood. There is subsequent development of nephrotic syndrome with progression to renal failure, occurring by the second decade in males, but often not until the fifth decade in females, as they are only carriers of the disease in the X-linked form.
- Ocular disease—occurs in only severely affected patients.
- Deafness—only for high-pitched sounds; this may be difficult to demonstrate.

Thin glomerular basement membrane disease

This inherited disease produces asymptomatic haematuria and may be associated with an increased long-term risk of more severe renal disease. The thinning of the glomerular basement membrane is only visible on electron microscopy. Some individuals with this disease are thought to heterozygote carriers of the autosomal recessive form of Alport's syndrome.

Fabry's syndrome

A rare, X-linked recessive syndrome of glycosphingolipid metabolism resulting in painful extremities, red hyperkeratotic papules on skin, proteinuria and renal failure.

Congenital nephrotic syndrome

A rare disorder characterised by nephrotic syndrome occurring at or shortly after birth. It is often associated with a bulky placenta, congenital heart disease and raised α-fetoprotein levels in maternal amniotic fluid. Aetiology is an autosomal recessive pattern of inheritance.

Chronic glomerulonephritis

Chronic renal failure associated with small, contracted kidneys, in which all the glomeruli are hyalinised (end-stage kidneys). It may be caused by many diseases, particularly proliferative types of acute glomerulonephritis.

In patients who present for the first time with chronic glomerulonephritis, it is often not possible to ascertain the cause because of diffuse global glomerular destruction. However, it is likely that many patients presenting for the first time have had IgA nephropathy.

Macroscopically, affected kidneys are small and there is granularity of the external surface, reflecting fine scarring due to nephron hyalinisation. However, the pelvicalyceal system is normal, an important distinction from cases of end-stage kidney disease due to chronic pyelonephritis.

Microscopically, there is hyalinisation of the glomeruli, tubular atrophy and interstitial fibrosis.

> Transplantation is the only method of fully correcting the loss of renal function in chronic renal failure. Renal replacement therapy (e.g. haemodialysis) maintains low levels of blood purification, but cannot fully replace the metabolic functions of a kidney. It is also time consuming, so affecting quality of life. Renal transplantation has become increasingly successful, with three year graft survival now reaching 80% due to better matching of donors (ABO and HLA matching) and improved post-transplantation immunosuppression.

GLOMERULAR LESIONS IN SYSTEMIC DISEASE

Systemic lupus erythematosus

Around half of all SLE patients will display renal involvement within 5 years of diagnosis. The majority of these cases are glomerular lesions, which may be of numerous histological patterns. Clinically, there is a potential spectrum from minor abnormalities such as asymptomatic proteinuria to severe glomerular disease leading to renal failure.

The basis of glomerular damage is immune-complex deposition in the basement membrane (leading to basement membrane thickening) or in the mesangium (leading to mesangial expansion).

Patterns of glomerular damage that may occur include:

- Diffuse MPGN—associated with a mixed nephritic/nephrotic syndrome and rapid progression to renal failure.
- Focal segmental proliferative glomerulonephritis—associated with haematuria, proteinuria and slow progression.

- Diffuse membranous nephropathy—associated with nephrotic syndrome and slow progression to chronic renal failure.

Immune complexes

The immune complexes of SLE are characterised by the presence of IgG, IgA, IgM, C3 and C1q (known as a 'full-house' of deposits). The detection of this pattern of immunoglobulins and complement factors, together with the particular location of the immune complexes in relation to the glomerular basement membrane, is an important factor in distinguishing lupus glomerulonephritis from non-lupus patterns.

Note that although glomerular lesions are the main abnormalities of renal involvement in SLE, there may also be extraglomerular vascular abnormalities and tubular damage, particularly interstitial nephritis.

Henoch–Schönlein purpura

This immune complex-mediated systemic vasculitis affects small arteries in the skin, joints, intestine, and kidneys (see Chapters 6 and 13). Light microscopy reveals mesangial IgA deposits.

Significant renal damage occurs in over one third of cases, ranging from proteinuria, possibly with nephrotic syndrome, to RPGN.

Bacterial endocarditis

Renal lesions in infective endocarditis are caused by two mechanisms:

1. Immune complex nephritis—immune complexes (formed with antigens of infecting organisms) are deposited in the glomerulus causing a focal segmental proliferative glomerulonephritis or a diffuse proliferative glomerulonephritis.
2. Embolism-mediated infarction—embolic vegetations from heart valves cause multiple renal infarcts.

Renal lesions typically subside when the bacterial source of the antigen is removed by intensive antibiotic therapy.

Diabetic glomerulosclerosis

Diabetic glomerular damage causes an increase in the permeability of the glomerular capillary basement membrane, leading to proteinuria and occasionally nephrotic syndrome.

The pathogenesis of basement membrane changes is probably related to the persistent insulin deficiency and/or hyperglycaemia of the diabetic state. This stimulates biochemical alterations in the composition of the basement membrane, most notably a deficiency of proteoglycans with an excess of collagen IV and fibronectin. Glomerular hypertrophy may occur in response to hyperfiltration (increased glomerular blood flow in diabetes). It is likely that the increased glycosylation of proteins also contributes to glomerular damage.

Histologically, three types of glomerular lesion occur, representing a continuous spectrum of increasing severity:

1. Capillary wall thickening—diabetic microangiopathy occurring in renal blood vessels to produce a mild proteinuria.
2. Diffuse glomerulosclerosis—excess mesangial matrix formation in an even pattern throughout the glomerulus combined with capillary thickening eventually encroaches on the capillaries.
3. Nodular glomerulosclerosis (Kimmelstiel–Wilson nodules)—nodular expansion of the mesangium at the tips of the glomerular lobules is very characteristic of diabetes.

Diabetic sclerosis causes progressive hyalinisation of glomeruli with obliteration of capillary loops and death of individual nephrons. Over a period of years this leads to chronic renal failure.

Prognosis—approximately 10% of all diabetics die in renal failure. This rises to 50% if patients developing diabetes in childhood are considered separately.

Amyloidosis

This is a condition in which amyloid—an extracellular fibrillar protein—is deposited in a variety of tissues (see Chapter 13). Amyloidosis is an important cause of the nephrotic syndrome in adults.

Amyloid is deposited as fibrils in the glomerular basement membrane and in the mesangium of the kidney, resulting in membrane thickening and increased mesangial matrix formation. The net result is the development of:

- Proteinuria—membrane thickening leads to an increase in membrane permeability.
- Nephrotic syndrome—increased deposition of amyloid causes progression of protein loss.
- Chronic renal failure—combined effect of amyloid deposition and increased mesangial

matrix formation eventually leads to expansion of the mesangium causing compression of the glomerular capillary system and transition into chronic renal failure.

Amyloid is also deposited in the walls of intrarenal vessels, particularly the afferent arterioles.

Polyarteritis nodosa

Polyarteritis nodosa is a systemic disease characterised by inflammatory necrosis of the walls of small and medium-sized arteries (see Chapter 6). Necrosis of medium-sized arteries causes small infarcts in the kidney; necrosis of arterioles and the glomerular tuft produces infarction of entire glomeruli or segments. This is visible as fibrinoid necrosis.

Wegener's granulomatosis

This immune complex-mediated systemic necrotising vasculitis primarily affects the nose, upper respiratory tract and kidneys. Renal involvement is of variable severity causing one of the following:

- Focal segmental glomerulonephritis (asymptomatic haematuria or nephritic syndrome).
- Rapidly progressive glomerulonephritis (rapidly progressive acute renal failure).

This condition usually responds to immunosuppressive therapy.

DISEASES OF THE TUBULES AND INTERSTITIUM

Acute tubular necrosis

This acute, but usually reversible, renal failure is caused by necrosis of renal tubular epithelial cells resulting from ischaemic, metabolic or toxic disturbances. The causes of acute tubular necrosis (ATN) are shown in Fig. 9.8.

The aetiology is:

- Ischaemic (most common)—caused by failure of renal perfusion, typically the result of hypotension and hypovolaemia in shock.
- Toxic—uncommon (heavy metals, organic solvents).

There are three phases to ATN (oliguric, polyuric and recovery) as follows:

1. Oliguric phase—necrosis of renal tubular cells and interstitial oedema causes tubule blockage and reduced glomerular blood flow and filtration.
2. Polyuric phase—tubules slowly open as phagocytic cells begin to remove necrotic material. Polyuria is caused by the temporary loss of the medullary concentration gradient. Regenerated renal tubule cells are undifferentiated.
3. Recovery phase—differentiated tubular cells restore renal function.

The morphologic features are:

- Ischaemic ATN—kidneys are pale and swollen. Histology reveals flattened, vacuolated epithelial cells along the entire length of the tubules.
- Necrotic ATN—kidneys are red and swollen. Histology reveals flattened, vacuolated epithelial cells restricted to proximal tubular cells, those of the distal tubule being spared.

Clinical features are oliguria (less than 500 mL urine output per day) with features of renal failure (see Fig. 9.4). As mentioned, some patients develop polyuria during recovery.

A knowledge of the aetiology (ischaemic versus toxic) and an understanding of the pathogenesis (oliguric and polyuric phases) of ATN make the morphological and clinical features easy to remember.

Treatment:

- Oliguric phase—supportive measures to prevent hyperkalaemia and fluid overload.
- Polyuric phase—replacement of fluid and electrolytes to compensate for excessive loss from urine.

The prognosis depends on the speed and efficiency with which corrective measures are put into operation, and the severity of the causal disorder.

Tubulointerstitial nephritis
Acute pyelonephritis

This is acute suppurative inflammation of the tubules and interstitium caused by bacterial infection. There are three age peaks: childhood, pregnancy and in the elderly.

Fig. 9.8 Causes of acute tubular necrosis.

Fig. 9.8 Causes of acute tubular necrosis

Type of ATN	Causes
Ischaemic	Major surgery Extensive acute blood loss Severe burns Haemorrhage
Toxic	Endogenous products: haemoglobinuria and myoglobinuria Heavy metals: lead, mercury Organic solvents: chloroform, carbon tetrachloride Drugs: antibiotics, NSAIDs, ciclosporin Others: paraquat, phenol, ethylene glycol, poisonous fungi

Most cases of infection are caused by enterobacteria from the patient's faecal flora (e.g. *Escherichia coli*, *Proteus* and *Klebsiella* species) or by staphylococci from skin (perineal) flora. The organism may enter the kidney by one of two routes: ascending infection from the lower urinary tract (promoted by pregnancy, glycosuria in diabetes, stasis of urine) or via the blood in bacteraemia/septicaemia.

Macroscopically, the condition is characterised by numerous abscesses throughout the kidney:

- Cortical abscesses—small, yellowish-white abscesses, usually spherical, less than 2 mm in diameter and sometimes surrounded by a zone of hyperaemia. Most prominent on subcapsular surface.
- Medullary abscesses—yellowish-white linear streaks that converge on the papilla. Pelvicalyceal mucosa is hyperaemic or covered with a fibrinopurulent exudate.

Microscopically, there is focal inflammation with infiltration of tubules by neutrophils, interstitial oedema and tubular necrosis.

Clinical features are fever, rigors and pain in the back. This condition is often associated with dysuria and urgency of micturition—signs of a lower urinary tract infection.

Acute pyelonephritis may resolve with or without scarring or chronic infection. In severe cases, pyonephrosis (pus-filled kidney associated with obstruction), renal papillary necrosis, perinephric abscess or death may occur.

Diagnosis is by examination of midstream urine, especially cultured to demonstrate responsible organisms:

- Significant bacteriuria is defined as $> 10^5$ culture-forming units per mL (to eliminate cases of extraneous bacterial contamination).
- Significant pyuria is defined as > 10 neutrophil polymorphs per high power field.

Treatment is by oral antibiotic therapy (e.g. trimethoprim, ampicillin or amoxicillin, which are active against *Escherichia coli*). Intravenous antibiotic therapy is used for more severe or septicaemic cases.

Untreated, infection may spread to cause Gram-negative septicaemia with shock.

Chronic pyelonephritis

Chronic inflammation of the tubules and interstitium is associated with nephron destruction and coarse scarring of the kidneys. The two forms—obstructive and reflux-associated—are described below.

Obstructive chronic pyelonephritis

Obstruction of pelvicalyceal drainage causes recurrent episodes of infection (discussed in more detail on page 200).

Reflux-associated chronic pyelonephritis

Reflux of urine from the bladder into the ureter predisposes to recurrent bouts of inflammation. It is most common in childhood and early adult life, with males affected more than females.

Normally, the ureter enters the bladder obliquely so that contraction of the bladder wall during micturition closes the ureteric orifice. In patients with vesicoureteric reflux, the terminal portion of the ureter is short and oriented at approximately 90° to the mucosal surface. Contraction of the bladder tends to hold the ureteric orifice open, thus facilitating reflux of urine, enabling organisms to gain access to the kidney from the bladder.

Macroscopically, the kidneys have irregular areas of scarring seen as depressed areas, 1–2 cm in size, most commonly sited in the renal calyces at the poles of the kidney but often associated with fibrous scarring of the renal papilla. Involvement may be either bilateral or unilateral.

Microscopically, kidneys have irregular areas of interstitial fibrosis with chronic inflammatory cell infiltration (chronic interstitial nephritis). Tubules are atrophic, or they may be dilated and contain proteinaceous casts. Glomeruli show periglomerular fibrosis and many demonstrate complete hyalinisation.

Clinical features are symptoms of urinary tract infection and of uraemia.

Diagnosis is by:

- Intravenous urography—reveals reduction in kidney size and focal scarring associated with clubbing of the adjacent calyces.
- Urine culture—for identification of infecting organism.

Treatment is by antibiotic therapy, control of hypertension, and removal of the source of obstruction.

Prognosis—the course is usually long and punctuated by acute exacerbations.

Other diseases of the tubules and interstitium are illustrated in Fig. 9.9.

DISEASES OF THE RENAL BLOOD VESSELS

Benign nephrosclerosis

This hyaline sclerosis of the arterioles and small arteries of the kidney is associated with benign hypertension and worsened by diabetes mellitus.

The condition is an important complication of long-standing benign hypertension (see page 72), chronic renal failure being one of its major sequelae.

This is the most common form of nephropathy, found in approximately 75% of autopsies over the age of 60 years.

The causes of hypertension are listed in Fig. 6.12.

In long-standing benign hypertension, there is reduced flow of blood to the glomeruli caused by vascular changes that affect:

- Branches of the renal artery—thickening of arterial walls due to fibroelastic intimal proliferation, elastic lamina reduplication and muscular hypertrophy of the media. Results in focal areas of ischaemia with scarring.
- Afferent arterioles—undergo hyalinisation (arteriolosclerosis), their muscular walls being replaced by a rigid and inelastic amorphous material.

A progressive reduction in blood flow to the nephrons leads to chronic ischaemia with slow conversion of

Fig. 9.9 Diseases of the tubules and interstitium

Condition	Features
Toxic and drug induced	Inflammation of the renal interstitium and tubules (tubulointerstitial nephritis) due to exposure to toxic agents. Two types: acute and chronic
Urate nephrophathy	Affects a small group of patients with hyperuricaemia
Hypercalcaemia and nephrocalcinosis	Hypercalcaemia causes calcification of the renal parenchyma and tubular damage
Multiple myeloma	Some types of myeloma are characterised by proliferating plasma cells, which produce monoclonal free light chains (Bence Jones proteins). These cause physical obstruction and damage to the tubules

Fig. 9.9 Diseases of the tubules and interstitium.

individual glomeruli into a mass of hyaline tissue devoid of capillary lumina (Fig. 9.10).

Blood supply to the tubules is also derived from glomerular blood flow. There is therefore eventual ischaemic destruction of the associated tubule.

The process gradually destroys individual nephrons over a period of many years.

Clinical features—no clinical symptoms initially, although a gradual increase in blood levels of urea and a reduction in glomerular filtration rate occur.

Eventually, critical numbers of nephrons become dysfunctional and the patient develops manifestations of chronic renal failure.

Prognosis—less than 5% of patients with well-developed benign nephrosclerosis die from renal failure. Death in the great majority of cases of benign hypertension occurs from congestive heart failure, coronary insufficiency, cerebrovascular accidents, or the development of malignant hypertension.

Malignant nephrosclerosis

Renal disease is associated with malignant, accelerated hypertension. This form of hypertension usually develops in individuals with pre-existing benign hypertension.

Pathogenesis—in accelerated hypertension, the rise in blood pressure is very rapid, causing a pattern of renal damage that differs from that seen in benign hypertension:

- Larger muscular vessels undergo fibroelastic proliferation of the intima, but no muscular hypertrophy. This is stimulated by factors such as platelet-derived growth factor.
- Afferent arterioles frequently undergo necrosis, often with fibrin in their damaged walls (fibrinoid necrosis) following exposure to the sudden high pressures.
- Glomerular capillary network—segmental fibrinoid necrosis of glomerular tuft.

The patient develops acute renal failure when sufficient nephrons are rendered non-functional. Afferent arteriole necrosis stimulates the renin–angiotensin system, which contributes to ischaemia by promoting intrarenal vasoconstriction.

The renal changes seen in benign and accelerated hypertensive nephrosclerosis are summarised in Fig. 9.10.

Untreated accelerated hypertension causes death from renal failure in 90% of cases, usually with marked rapidity. However, if hypertension is treated adequately, before there is evidence of impairment of renal function by a raised blood urea, then prognosis is good and subsequent renal failure unusual.

Renal artery stenosis

This narrowing of the renal arteries is typically caused by generalised atherosclerosis but rarely by arterial fibromuscular dysplasia.

Atherosclerotic occlusion of the renal artery is usually most severe at its origin from the aorta. Renal artery stenosis at this point can lead to two main pathological processes:

1. Chronic ischaemia of the affected kidney— reduction in function of all nephrons on that side produces an end-stage shrunken kidney. However, the contralateral kidney undergoes

renal muscular artery	glomerulus

normal

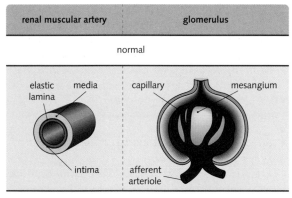

benign hypertension

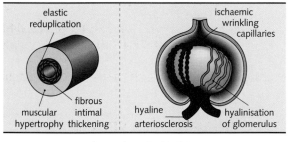

malignant hypertension

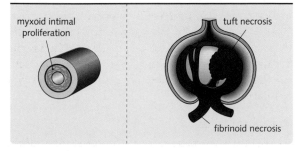

Fig. 9.10 Vascular changes associated with hypertensive renal disease.

compensatory hypertrophy so that renal function is largely unaffected.

2. Renovascular hypertension—inadequate perfusion of the kidney caused by renal artery stenosis may lead to hyper-reninism and subsequent abnormal activation of the renin–angiotensin system. This condition is important in that it is one of the rare recognised causes of hypertension that is amenable to surgical correction.

A useful diagnostic pointer for renal artery stenosis is to look for associated features of:

- Vascular disease elsewhere.
- Severe or drug-resistant hypertension.
- Abdominal bruits (over the kidneys).

Thrombotic microangiopathies

Haemolytic uraemic syndrome

Haemolytic uraemic syndrome (HUS) is a complex syndrome of disordered platelet function that is characterised by the triad of thrombocytopenia, haemolysis and acute renal failure.

There are three subtypes of HUS: childhood, adult and secondary.

Childhood HUS

This usually affects children under 4 years of age. Many cases are associated with intestinal infection by verocytotoxin-producing *Escherichia coli* (notably type 0157). The immediate prognosis is better than for adult and secondary types but future risk of renal disease is increased.

Adult HUS

This is more frequently fatal than childhood HUS and is associated with the following conditions:

- Pregnancy—occurring postpartum even several months after delivery.
- Oestrogen therapy—contraceptive pills or oestrogen therapy for men with prostatic carcinoma.
- Infections, e.g. typhoid, viruses and shigellosis.
- Chemotherapeutic and immunosuppressive therapy, e.g. ciclosporin.

Secondary HUS

This occurs as a complication of:

- Malignant hypertension.

- Progressive systemic sclerosis.
- SLE (often as a result of antiphospholipid syndrome).
- Transplant rejection.

Pathogenesis

Platelets adhere to damaged endothelium of small vessels, including the glomerular capillaries, where they undergo aggregation and trigger fibrin deposition. Reduced prostaglandin and nitric oxide production from the damaged endothelium promotes platelet aggregation. Fibrin strands form a tight mesh that deforms the erythrocytes as they are forced through the obstruction (microangiopathic haemolysis).

Morphological features are:

- Endocapillary proliferation—in response to fibrin and platelet deposition in glomerular tufts.
- Luminal narrowing—arterioles and small arteries show fibrin and erythrocytes in the walls, often with thrombosis which, when extensive, can result in cortical necrosis.

Clinical features and prognosis

Clinical features are:

- Sudden onset of oliguria with haematuria and occasionally melaena.
- Jaundice.
- Anaemia with schistocytes (fragmented erythrocytes) and thrombocytopenia.
- Hypertension in 50% of cases.

In childhood HUS, symptoms are often preceded by a prodromal episode of diarrhoea or flu-like illness lasting for 5–15 days.

Prognosis depends on the severity of attack but mortality may be as high as 40%.

Thrombotic thrombocytopenic purpura

Thrombotic thrombocytopenic purpura (TTP) and HUS are thought to represent the same disease process but with a different distribution of thrombotic lesions. In TTP, occlusive plugs lead to widespread ischaemic organ damage, often affecting the brain more than the kidney, resulting in early neurological abnormalities and progressive renal impairment.

Renal infarcts

There are two mechanisms of renal infarction: embolic infarction and diffuse cortical necrosis.

Embolic renal disease

Renal infarcts are usually due to the passage of emboli down renal arterial branches. The most common causes are:

- Embolisation of atheromatous material.
- 'Cholesterol emboli'—these are showers of cholesterol microemboli that may occur as a complication of arterial interventions (e.g. arteriography) in those with severe atheromatous disease.
- Mural thrombotic material arising from the left side of the heart, most commonly after myocardial infarction.
- Bacterial vegetation from infective endocarditis.

Resultant infarcts may be clinically silent or may result in haematuria and loin pain. Macroscopically, infarcts are pale or white and they have a characteristic wedge shape with the apex directed towards the hilum.

Diffuse cortical necrosis

This rare pattern of renal infarction is associated with conditions resulting in severe hypotension, the most common of which are hypovolaemic shock, severe sepsis and eclampsia of pregnancy.

The pathogenesis is uncertain, but diffuse spasm of renal blood vessels is thought to play a major part in precipitating ischaemic damage.

Macroscopically, necrosis is confined to the outer part of the renal cortex, which in the acute stages is pale and focally haemorrhagic.

This condition results in acute renal failure, and prognosis depends on the extent of the damage.

Sickle-cell disease nephropathy

Increased viscosity of sickle-cell blood promotes occlusion of the vasae rectae (pages 301–302), resulting in papillary necrosis and the development of haematuria and polyuria.

NEOPLASTIC DISEASE OF THE KIDNEY

Benign tumours of the kidney

These are common incidental findings at post mortem examination in about 20% of all patients; however, they rarely cause clinical problems.

Cortical adenoma

These are benign epithelial tumours derived from renal tubular epithelium.

Macroscopically, they are discrete nodules, usually less than 20 mm in diameter, situated in the cortex of the kidney.

Microscopically, appearances are similar to those of renal cell carcinomas, both being composed of well-differentiated large clear cells with small nuclei.

Difficulty in differentiating between these tumours had prompted the adoption of an arbitrary cut-off of 3 cm in size to distinguish between the smaller adenomas and the typically larger carcinomas. However, the distinction has proved unreliable and it is now considered that all adenomas should be treated.

Renal fibroma or hamartoma (renomedullary interstitial cell tumour)

This is the most common benign tumour of the kidney. It is composed of renal interstitial cells.

Macroscopically, there are firm white nodules situated in the medulla, typically 3–10 mm in size.

Microscopically, it is composed of spindle cells that surround the adjacent tubules.

These tumours are of no functional or clinical significance and do not undergo malignant transformation.

Angiomyolipoma

This hamartoma is composed of a mixture of smooth muscle, blood vessels and fat. It is situated either in the cortex or in the medulla. It is mainly seen in association with tuberose sclerosis.

Oncocytoma

This benign epithelial tumour is composed of large cells with granular, eosinophilic cytoplasm filled with mitochondria. It is a variant of the renal adenomas and can attain a considerable size, resulting in confusion with renal cell carcinoma.

Malignant tumours of the kidney

Renal cell carcinoma (renal adenocarcinoma; hypernephroma)

An adenocarcinoma derived from the renal tubular epithelium in adults, this tumour accounts for about 3% of all carcinomas and about 90% of primary malignant renal tumours. It is usually seen after the age of 50 years. Males are more often affected than females by 3 : 1.

There is an increased incidence in those who smoke tobacco (double the relative risk of non-smokers) and also in patients with von Hippel–Lindau syndrome, a rare hereditary condition (this suggests a genetic predisposition).

Associations—paraneoplastic syndromes of hypercalcaemia, hypertension and polycythaemia.

Macroscopically, tumours occur most commonly at the upper pole of a kidney. They are usually rounded masses, with a yellowish cut surface marked with areas of haemorrhage and necrosis.

Microscopically, they are composed of either clear or granular cell types. The most common is the 'clear cell pattern', in which tumour cells have clear cytoplasm because of the high content of glycogen and lipid. Granular cell types are derived from tubular and papillary carcinomas.

Route of spread is:

- Local—eroding through renal capsule into perinephric fat.
- Lymphatic—to para-aortic and other nodes.
- Blood-borne metastasis—involving the lungs, bone, brain and other sites as a result of tumour invasion of the renal vein. A characteristic feature is that large tumours may grow as a solid core along the main renal vein even entering the inferior vena cava.

Clinical features are:

- Common presenting symptoms—haematuria (60%), loin pain (40%), loin mass (25%).
- Occasional presenting symptoms—bone metastasis, brain metastasis or polycythaemia.

Prognosis depends on the stage at presentation. If the tumour is confined within a renal capsule there is a 75% 5-year survival. However, prognosis is very poor if metastases are present at diagnosis.

Differential diagnosis of unilateral enlargement of the kidney is:
- Hydronephrosis.
- Tumour.
- Renal vein thrombosis.
- Postcontralateral nephrectomy.
- Contralateral kidney failure.

Urothelial carcinoma of the renal pelvis

This malignant tumour of the renal pelvis is derived from the transitional cells of the urothelium, and it is histologically identical to transitional cell carcinoma of the bladder (see page 203). Indeed, coexistence with bladder cancer occurs in half of cases. It is associated with analgesic abuse and exposure to aniline dyes used in the dye, rubber, and plastics industries. Some cases have also been reported to develop many years after the use of 'Thorotrast', an α-particle-emitting contrast agent used in retrograde pyelography.

Tumours generally present early with haematuria or obstruction.

Wilms' tumour (nephroblastoma)

This malignant embryonal tumour is derived from the primitive metanephros. It is the most common childhood urological malignancy, with a peak incidence between the ages of 1 and 4 years. Males and females are equally affected.

At least three different types of genes are important in the formation of Wilm's tumour. The most characterised of these is the tumour suppressor gene WT1, located on chromosome 11.

Macroscopically, large amounts of kidney are replaced by rounded masses of solid, fleshy, white lesions with frequent areas of necrosis. The tumour is aggressive and grows rapidly; extension beyond the capsule into perinephric fat and even into the root of mesentery is frequent. Spread to lungs occurs early and is identified in a high proportion of cases at the time of diagnosis.

Microscopically, it is composed of up to four elements:

1. Primitive, small cell, blastaematous tissue—resembles developing metanephric blastaema.
2. Immature-looking glomerular structures.
3. Epithelial tubules.
4. Stroma composed of spindle cells and striated muscle.

Clinical presentation—large abdominal mass, abdominal pain, haematuria and hypertension are all recognised presentations.

Prognosis is related to the spread of the tumour at diagnosis. Treatment is by surgical nephrectomy with adjuvant chemotherapy (and potentially radiotherapy). Survival rates 5 years after diagnosis have increased to 80%.

DISORDERS OF THE URINARY TRACT

Congenital abnormalities of the urinary tract

Ureteric abnormalities

These occur in up to 3% of people, although they have no clinical significance in most cases.

Double and bifid ureters

The most common ureteric abnormality. These often occur in association with the duplication of the renal pelvis. They may be associated with vesicoureteric reflux and are predisposed to recurrent infections.

Ureteropelvic junction obstruction

This is most commonly caused by a stricture that may be either intrinsic (within the wall of the ureter) or extrinsic (associated with external factors such as an aberrant vessel). This appears to provide a barrier to the conduction of a wave of contraction of the ureter, and is the most common cause of hydronephrosis in children.

Diverticulum

This is a rare outpouching of the ureter.

Megaloureter

In this common congenital anomaly, retention of urine within the enlarged ureter results in hydroureter. The condition predisposes to reflux and recurrent infections.

Bladder abnormalities

Diverticula

Congenital diverticula are rare and are more often acquired as a result of bladder outlet obstruction. Symptoms are due to stasis and the resultant infection.

Urethral abnormalities

Hypospadias

The urethra opens on to the underside of the penis, either on the glans (glandular hypospadias), at the junction of the glans with the shaft (coronal hypospadias) or on the shaft itself (penile hypospadias).

Epispadias

The urethra opens on to the dorsal (upper) surface of the penis.

All varieties can be corrected surgically.

Urinary tract obstruction

This is obstruction of urine drainage from the kidney occurring at any level within the urinary tract. Obstruction may be caused by either a structural lesion (majority) or congenital neuromuscular defects that prevent contraction waves, and thus the flow of urine.

Structural lesions can be classified into:

- Intrinsic lesions—within the urinary tract, e.g. stones, caseous or necrotic debris, fibrosis following trauma or infection, tumour.
- Extrinsic lesions—cause pressure from without, e.g. tumours of the rectum, prostate, and the bladder, aberrant renal arteries, retroperitoneal fibrosis, pregnancy.

Causes vary according to the site of the obstruction (Fig. 9.11). In the list below, * indicates the most common sites of obstruction:

- Renal pelvis—calculi, tumours.
- Pelviureteric junction*—stricture, calculi, extrinsic compression.

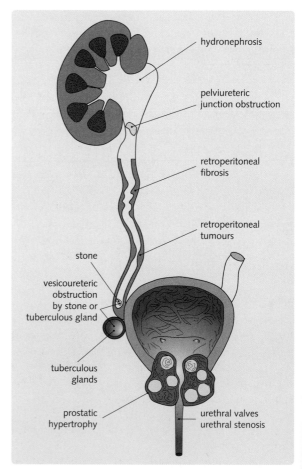

Fig. 9.11 Urinary tract showing common sites of obstruction

- Ureter—calculi, extrinsic compression (pregnancy, tumour, fibrosis).
- Bladder neck*—tumour, calculi.
- Urethra*—prostatic hyperplasia or carcinoma, urethral valves, urethral stricture.

Pathogenesis—obstruction at any point in the urinary tract causes increased pressure superior to the blockage, with dilatation of the renal pelvis and calyces (hydronephrosis):

- Obstruction at the pelviureteric junction → hydronephrosis.
- Obstruction of the ureter → hydroureter with subsequent development of hydronephrosis.
- Obstruction of the bladder neck or urethra → bladder distension with hypertrophy of its muscle (seen on cystoscopic examination as trabeculation). Subsequently leads to hydroureter and hydronephrosis.

Hydronephrosis

Hydronephrosis may be:

- Unilateral—caused by unilateral obstruction anywhere above the bladder. It is typically detected late, because renal function is maintained by the non-obstructed kidney. Renal parenchyma becomes severely atrophic and renal function is permanently impaired (end-stage hydronephrosis).
- Bilateral—caused by obstruction at the level of the bladder or urethra. Obstruction is typically detected at an earlier stage, as renal failure develops before severe atrophy of both kidneys.

In both forms, urinary tract obstruction predisposes to infection of the bladder (cystitis) and kidney (pyelonephritis or pyonephrosis) as well as stone formation.

Effects of hydronephrosis

The net result of hydronephrosis is that fluid entering the collecting ducts cannot empty into the renal pelvis, and intrarenal resorption of fluid occurs.

If the obstruction is removed at this stage then renal function returns to normal. However, persistence of obstruction leads to atrophy of the renal tubules and promotes interstitial inflammation, which leads to glomerular hyalinisation and fibrosis.

Clinical features depend on the cause and site of the lesion.

Obstruction above the bladder will cause either an acute onset of renal colic or a gradual onset of aching pain in the loins, sometimes aggravated by drinking.

The clinical feature of obstruction below the bladder is difficulty in micturition, occasionally with distension of the bladder; it may progress to bilateral loin pain.

Superimposed infection causes malaise, fever, dysuria and sometimes septicaemia.

Management is by removal of the obstruction and treatment of the infection.

Urolithiasis (urinary calculi)

This is the formation of stones in the urinary tract. It affects 1–5% of the population in the UK and onset is typically after 30 years of age, with males affected more than females.

Stones can form anywhere in the urinary tract but the most common site is within the renal pelvis.

Composition of stones:

- Calcium oxalate (70–75%).
- Triple phosphates (15%)—magnesium ammonium phosphate stones.
- Uric acid (5–10%).
- Calculi in cystinuria and oxalosis.

Aetiology is:

- Acquired—as a result of obstruction, persistent infection, or reduced urine volume.
- Inherited—primary metabolic disturbances, e.g. cystinuria.

The mechanism of stone formation is not well understood, but it is thought to involve an excess of solute in the urine (due to either a primary increase in metabolite or to stasis) or reduced solubility of solute in the urine (due to persistently abnormal urinary pH).

Calculi vary greatly in size, from sand-like particles to large round stones.

The condition may present with:

- Renal colic often with nausea and vomiting—caused by the passage of small stones along the ureter.
- Dull ache in the loins—due to the presence of stones in the kidney.
- Recurrent and intractable urinary tract infection, haematuria or renal failure.

Occasionally, the condition is asymptomatic and discovered only during radiological examination for another disease.

Management is by bed rest, application of warmth to the site of pain and administration of analgesia.

Small stones (< 0.5 cm) in diameter are usually passed naturally. Larger stones may require lithotripsy or endoscopic surgery.

Inflammation of the urinary tract

Cystitis

This is inflammation of the bladder and it is extremely common—most women will have one or more episodes of cystitis. Females are affected more often than males because they have a shorter urethra (i.e. less travelling distance for bacteria).

Aetiology

The condition is most commonly due to infection but it is occasionally caused by physical agents, e.g. radiation or mechanical irritants.

Infective causes:

- Bacterial infection (most common)—usually Gram-negative coliform bacilli, e.g. *Escherichia coli* and *Proteus* species, but *Streptococcus faecalis*, *Pseudomonas aeruginosa* and staphylococci are also common.
- Viral infection—adenovirus may cause haemorrhagic cystitis in children.
- Parasites—*Schistosoma haematobium*, which is common in Africa.
- Fungi—*Candida*.

Risk factors are:

- Urinary retention—due to obstruction, bladder paralysis, diverticula, calculi, foreign bodies, tumours, uterine prolapse.
- Infection of adjacent structures, e.g. prostatitis, urethritis and diverticular disease of the colon.
- Diabetes mellitus—glycosuria favours infection.
- Pregnancy.
- Trauma, e.g. catheterisation.

Infection normally ascends from the urethra but may descend from the kidney in some cases of renal infection (e.g. renal tuberculosis). Direct spread from adjacent organs (e.g. diverticulitis) may occur but haematogenous and lymphatic spread are rare.

Macroscopically, there is acute inflammation with oedema, erythema and later ulceration of bladder mucosa.

Microscopically, there is infiltration of mucosa with acute inflammatory cells.

Clinical features—the classic triad of increased urinary frequency, lower abdominal pain and dysuria are common. Systemic effects of inflammation (e.g. fever) may also occur.

Investigation, treatment and sequelae

Investigations—examination of midstream urine.

Treatment is with antibiotics (e.g. trimethoprim), high fluid intake and addressing underlying causes such as obstruction.

Sequelae:

- Resolution (common).
- Chronicity if the underlying cause is untreatable.
- Development of pyelonephritis and associated complications.

Interstitial cystitis (Hunner's ulcer)

This is a condition of unknown aetiology. The bladder is inflamed, fibrotic and of small capacity but the urine is sterile. It is characterised clinically by suprapubic pain and increased frequency.

Macroscopically, there is linear ulceration and erythema.

Microscopically, there is fibrosis and lymphocytic infiltration through the full thickness of the bladder wall.

Malakoplakia

A rare variant of cystitis, the bladder mucosa develops yellow plaques composed of a mixture of chronic inflammatory cells including characteristic granule-containing macrophages. Granules (known as Michaelis–Gutmann bodies) are composed of calcified bacterial debris. They are thought to reflect defective macrophage functions.

Ureteritis

This inflammation of the ureter is usually due to an ascending urinary tract infection.

Causative organisms are the same as for cystitis; an acute bacterial cystitis may lead to an ascending ureteritis.

Complications—organisms may gain access to the renal parenchyma to produce acute pyelonephritis, with the formation of abscesses in the renal medulla and cortex.

Ureteritis follicularis

This ureteritis presents with large aggregates of lymphoid cells.

Ureteritis cystica

This is a complication of chronic ureteritis in which thin-walled cysts develop in the mucosa.

Neoplastic disease of the urinary tract

Tumours of the ureter

Tumours of the ureter are extremely rare and they are almost always epithelial.

Fibro-epithelial polyps

These are benign papillary tumours.

Malignant urothelial tumours

These tumours arise from the transitional cell epithelium of the ureter. They are mainly caused by environmental agents (see below) and are identical to those seen in the bladder.

Bladder metaplasia

Glandular metaplasia (cystitis glandularis)

These small, rounded collections of urothelial cells are found just below the urothelial surface (Brunn's nests). They develop a central lumen surrounded by cuboidal or columnar cells. They are quite common and often seen in the normal bladder.

Occasionally, there is metaplasia to an intestinal variant of cystitis glandularis, lined by colonic, mucin-secreting epithelium.

Adenomatous metaplasia (nephrogenic adenoma)

This benign condition is characterised by metaplasia of the urothelium to cuboidal epithelium. Metaplastic areas resemble collecting tubules of the kidney. It is associated with chronic infections, e.g. tuberculosis.

Squamous metaplasia

There are two types:

1. Keratinising squamous metaplasia (leucoplakia)—the bladder mucosa develops white plaques, which are often secondary to chronic irritation, e.g. calculi. A significant proportion progresses to squamous carcinoma of the bladder.
2. Non-keratinising squamous metaplasia (vaginal metaplasia)—white plaques are seen on the trigone. This only occurs in women and it has no pathological significance.

Tumours of the bladder

Transitional cell papilloma

These are rare, benign tumours of the bladder that may represent the first stage of transitional cell carcinoma. A fibrovascular stalk attaches their branched structure to the mucosa.

Transitional cell carcinoma

These are tumours of the urothelium, affecting 1 in 5000 in the UK and accounting for 3% of all cancer deaths. They are most commonly found in those aged 60–70 years, with males affected more than females by 3 : 1. Cigarette smoking is an important cause.

Aetiology is as follows:

- Chemicals—exposure to environmental agents excreted in high concentrations in the urine. Known carcinogens are associated with cigarette smoking, aniline dyes and the rubber industry.
- Leucoplakia (see above)—associated with bladder stones.
- Bladder diverticula—about 3% are complicated with tumour.

Most tumours are at the base of trigone and around the ureteric orifices.

Morphological types:

- Papillary (most common)—warty masses projecting into the lumen with little or no invasion of the bladder wall. Only a small percentage evolves into invasive carcinoma.
- Solid—tumours grow directly into the bladder wall and are often ulcerated or encrusted. Most are invasive from the outset.
- Mixed papillary and solid.
- Flat in-situ carcinoma—reddened mucosal surface due to underlying telangiectatic blood vessels. May become invasive.

The majority of urothelial cancers are caused by exposure to environmental agents. Therefore, bladder tumours are usually multiple, and they are often found in conjunction with urothelial tumours at other sites of the lower urinary tract, e.g. renal pelvis, ureters or urethra.

Other tumours of the bladder

Only a small proportion of bladder cancers are of squamous origin (squamous cell carcinoma). They are most often associated with schistosomiasis infection. Adenocarcinomas and mesenchymal tumours are rare. Secondary tumours usually occur following direct invasion from the cervix, prostate or rectum.

Grading and staging of bladder carcinomas

The degree of differentiation (grade) and extent of spread (stage) are important indicators for prognosis.

Transitional cell carcinomas are graded I–III:

- Grade I (well differentiated)—vast majority are papillary growths with no evidence of invasion.
- Grade II (moderately well differentiated)— usually papillary but many are either invasive at presentation or become so. Cells show significant atypicality and an increase in mitotic figures.
- Grade III (poorly differentiated)—mainly solid lesions which are extensively invasive. Cells are pleomorphic with numerous mitoses.

TNM staging follows the same principles as other cancers (see Fig. 7.13).

Spread is as follows:

- Local—to pelvic structures.
- Lymphatic—to iliac and para-aortic lymph nodes.
- Haematogenous—to liver and lung.

Clinically, the disease classically presents with painless haematuria, but symptoms of recurrent urinary tract infections may occur. Rarely, it may present with hydronephrosis (from ureteric obstruction), pneumaturia from vesicocolic fistula, or incontinence from vesicovaginal fistula.

Treatment usually involves transurethral resection of tumour, with the potential for intravesical chemotherapy in multiple tumours. Radical cystectomy may be considered for patients with invasive disease.

Prognosis depends on the histological type of the tumour and extent of spread. Papillary, non-invasive tumours have an excellent prognosis, whereas solid, invasive, urothelial tumours have an overall 5-year survival rate of only 35%.

Pathology of the endocrine system

Objectives

In this chapter, you will learn to:
- Describe disorders of the pituitary gland leading to hyperpituitarism and hypopituitarism.
- Describe the causes and patterns of thyroid dysfunction.
- Describe the causes and patterns of parathyroid dysfunction.
- Understand Cushing's syndrome and other disorders of adrenal hyperfunction.
- Understand the importance of adrenal hypofunction and crisis.
- Recall the pathology and complications associated with diabetes mellitus.
- Briefly describe endocrine tumours including the important multiple endocrine neoplasia syndromes.

DISORDERS OF THE PITUITARY

The pituitary (hypophysis) is a small (500–1000 mg), bean-shaped gland lying in the sella turcica in the base of the skull. It is composed of two parts:

1. Anterior lobe (adenohypophysis)—synthesises and secretes a number of hormones (Fig. 10.1), most of which act on other endocrine glands.
2. Posterior lobe (neurohypophysis)—stores and secretes two hormones synthesised in the hypothalamus: antidiuretic hormone (ADH; vasopressin) and oxytocin. This lobe is in direct continuity with the hypothalamus, to which it is connected via the pituitary stalk.

Secretion of the pituitary hormones is regulated by neural and chemical stimuli from the hypothalamus, diseases of which cause secondary abnormalities in pituitary function.

This cooperation between the nervous system and endocrine apparatus is referred to as neuroendocrine signalling. Figure 10.2 shows the integration of signals between the hypothalamus, pituitary and thyroid gland in the release of thyroid hormones, with feed-back loops acting at each level.

Neuroendocrine cells are defined as those that release a hormone in response to a neural stimulus. Important examples include:

- Neurons of the supra-optic nucleus (projecting into the posterior pituitary), which release ADH.
- Chromaffin cells of the adrenal medulla, which release epinephrine (adrenaline).

The anterior pituitary: hyperpituitarism

Hyperpituitarism is defined as excessive secretion of one or more of the pituitary hormones. Its most common causes are functioning (hormone-secreting) adenomas of the anterior lobe.

Anterior lobe adenomas

Anterior lobe adenomas comprise about 10% of all intracranial tumours (posterior lobe adenomas do not occur). These tumours do not usually metastasise, but they are often life threatening because of their position and ability to secrete excess hormone.

Effects of pituitary adenomas

Pituitary adenomas cause problems because of a combination of endocrine effects (excessive secretion of a particular hormone) and compressive effects, caused by an increase in local pressure of the following:

- Remainder of the pituitary → hypopituitarism.
- Optic chiasm → visual field defects, notably bitemporal haemianopia.

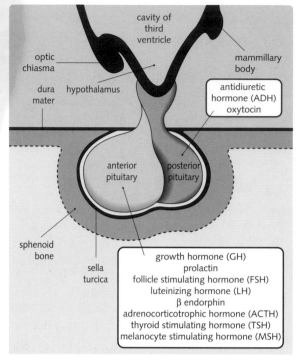

Fig. 10.1 Pituitary and hypothalamus, with the hormones released.

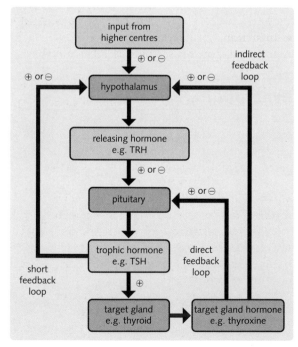

Fig. 10.2 Schematic representation of the integration between the higher centre, hypothalamus, pituitary and target organ signalling. The example is for thyroid function, highlighting the feedback loops that control hormone release at each level. (TRH, thyrotrophin releasing hormone, TSH, thyroid stimulating hormone). (Adapted with permission from Essential Endocrinology, 4th edn, by Brook and Marshall, Blackwell Publishing, 2001).

- Brain (large tumours) → distortion of the midbrain with raised intracranial pressure and hydrocephalus.
- Dura → headaches.
- Cavernous sinus → CN III, IV or VI nerve palsies.

The endocrine effects depend on which hormone is being excessively secreted (see below).

Investigations:

- Imaging—plain X-ray (can detect enlargement of sella turcica and erosion of the clinoid processes) and MRI (for visualisation and sizing of the tumour; this is superior to CT scanning).
- Hormone assays (e.g. growth hormone, prolactin).
- Functional testing of the pituitary–adrenal axis, e.g. ACTH stimulation test in which a dose of adrenocorticotrophic hormone (ACTH) is given and the plasma cortisol response measured.
- Visual field assessment.

Types of functioning adenomas

Functioning adenomas may produce any of the anterior lobe (adenophyseal) hormones but the majority produce prolactin (prolactinomas–lactotroph adenomas), growth hormone (somatotroph adenomas) or ACTH (corticotroph adenomas).

Prolactinomas

Abnormally raised serum prolactin levels are associated with menstrual irregularity and infertility in women, and with ejaculatory failure or impotence in men. Mild prolactin increases are seen with compression of the hypothalamus by any pituitary adenoma (the 'stalk effect').

Galactorrhoea is present in about 30% of affected women, but it is rare in men because oestrogen priming is required for lactation.

Somatotroph adenoma

This results in hypersecretion of growth hormone, the effects of which depend on the developmental stage of the affected individual:

- Pre-epiphyseal union (prepubertal) leads to gigantism (giantism), i.e. excessive growth in a regular and initially well-proportioned manner. Most giants also show some features of acromegaly with disproportionate enlargement, e.g. of the hands and jaw.

- Postepiphyseal union (adults) leads to acromegaly, which is characterised by enlargement of the hands, feet, and head. They may also present with secondary diabetes (growth hormone is an insulin antagonist) or cardiovascular effects (Fig. 10.3).

There are three types of treatment:

- Surgery—hypophysectomy (transfrontal or transphenoidal), especially where there are signs of compression of adjacent structures. This usually only debulks the tumour, with further (usually drug) therapy required.
- Radiotherapy—fewer complications than surgery but less successful.
- Drug therapy—bromocriptine (dopamine agonist) and octreotide (somatostatin analogue) can lower growth hormone levels in uncomplicated acromegaly.

Corticotrophin adenoma

Overproduction of ACTH by the pituitary gland (Cushing's disease) causes adrenal hyperplasia, resulting in the excessive secretion of glucocorticoids causing Cushing's syndrome, the effects of which are described later (see page 219).

Other functioning adenomas

Other endocrine secreting adenomas, e.g. of thyroid-stimulating hormone (TSH), luteinizing hormone (LH) and follicle-stimulating hormone (FSH), are extremely rare.

The anterior pituitary: hypopituitarism

Hypopituitarism is defined as insufficient secretion of the pituitary hormones. The clinical features depend on the patient's age and on the type and severity of the hormone deficiencies (Fig. 10.4).

Hypopituitarism can be caused by either hypothalamic lesions or pituitary lesions.

Hypothalamic lesions are:

- Idiopathic deficiency of one or more of the releasing factors, e.g. gonadotrophin-releasing hormone (GnRH; Kallmann's syndrome), growth-hormone releasing factor (GHRH) or, more rarely, thyrotrophin-releasing hormone (TRH) or corticotrophin-releasing factor (CRF).
- Infarction.
- Inflammation, e.g. sarcoidosis, tuberculous meningitis.
- Suprasellar tumours, e.g. craniopharyngioma or, more rarely, pinealoma, teratoma or a secondary tumour from another site.

Pituitary lesions are:

- Idiopathic deficiency of one or more of the pituitary hormones.
- Non-functioning chromophobe pituitary adenomas—adenomas of the anterior pituitary (usually derived from non-hormone-secreting chromophobe cells), which may cause hypopituitarism by compression or obliteration of normal pituitary tissue.
- Sheehan's syndrome—ischaemic necrosis of the anterior pituitary due to hypotensive shock occurring as a result of obstetric haemorrhage.
- Empty sella syndrome—an enlarged, empty sella turcica that is not filled with pituitary tissue. This may be a primary anatomical variant or it may follow spontaneous infarction, surgery, or radiotherapy of a tumour.

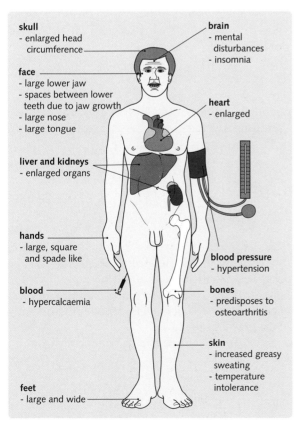

skull
- enlarged head circumference

face
- large lower jaw
- spaces between lower teeth due to jaw growth
- large nose
- large tongue

liver and kidneys
- enlarged organs

hands
- large, square and spade like

blood
- hypercalcaemia

feet
- large and wide

brain
- mental disturbances
- insomnia

heart
- enlarged

blood pressure
- hypertension

bones
- predisposes to osteoarthritis

skin
- increased greasy sweating
- temperature intolerance

Fig. 10.3 Features of acromegaly.

Fig. 10.4 Clinical features associated with specific forms of hypopituitarism.

Fig. 10.4 Clinical features associated with specific forms of hypopituitarism

Hormone deficiency	Clinical features	Tests to exclude hypofunction of anterior pituitary
Gonadotrophin deficiency	Prepubertal: • Failure to enter puberty • Undescended testes • Obesity • Eunuchoidism Postpubertal: • Infertility • Amenorrhoea • Oligospermia • Progressive loss of secondary sex characteristics (hypogonadism) • Osteoporotic collapse of spine→ loss of stature	LH reserves adequate if: • Males have a normal testosterone • Females are ovulating FSH reserves adequate if: • Males have a normal spermatogenesis • Females are ovulating
GH deficiency	Children: failure of longitudinal growth Adults: tendency to hypoglycaemia	GH reserves adequate if: random plasma level >20 mU/L stress or otherwise elevated GH peak >20 mU/L
TSH deficiency	Fetus or newborn: cretinism Adults: hypothyroidism	TSH reserves adequate if serum thyroxine within normal range
ACTH deficiency	Features of primary hypoadrenalism but with decreased pigmentation (rather than an increase)	ACTH reserves adequate if: random plasma cortisol >550 nmol/L stress-induced cortisol rise >550 nmol/L

Note: ACTH, adrenocorticotrophic hormone; FSH, follicle-stimulating hormone; GH, growth hormone; LH, luteinizing hormone; TSH, thyroid-stimulating hormone.

• Trauma, including surgery and radiotherapy.
• Granulomatous lesions—sarcoidosis, tuberculosis, histiocytosis.

Management

Management is by substitution therapy according to the deficiencies demonstrated, e.g. cortisol replacement for ACTH deficiency, thyroid hormone replacement for TSH deficiency.

The posterior pituitary

Diseases of the posterior pituitary are much less common than those of the anterior pituitary and are usually the result of damage to the hypothalamus by tumour invasion or infarction. Posterior pituitary diseases typically cause disorders of abnormal ADH secretion. There are no known effects of abnormal oxytocin secretion.

Diabetes insipidus

Diabetes insipidus (DI) is a rare condition characterised by the persistent excretion of excessive quantities of dilute urine (polyuria) and by constant thirst (polydipsia).

There are two types (Fig. 10.5):

1. Cranial DI—caused by the failure of ADH production.
2. Nephrogenic DI—distal tubules are refractory to the water reabsorptive action of ADH.

Clinical features—irrespective of aetiology, reabsorption of water from the glomerular filtrate in the renal collecting ducts does not occur, resulting in polyuria (up to 20 L per day is possible) and high risk of body water depletion. DI is potentially lethal without appropriate therapy.

Investigations—there is high clinical suspicion if a patient has a high plasma osmolality, with low or immeasurable plasma ADH, and a non-maximally concentrated urine. A water deprivation test is run for 8 hours or until 3% of the body weight is lost. Demonstration of continued polyuria and increased haemoconcentration indicates DI. This test serves to

	Cause	Features
Cranial DI	Hypothalamic or pituitary stalk damage	Surgical damage, usually in the course of tumour removal Head injury, usually transient Hypothalamic tumour (either primary or secondary) Hypothalamic inflammatory lesions, e.g. sarcoidosis, encephalitis, meningitis
	Genetic defect	Dominant Recessive: DIDMOAD syndrome-association of DI with diabetes mellitus (DM), optic atrophy (OA) and deafness (D)
	Idiopathic	About 30% of cases have no known cause
Nephrogenic DI	Hereditary	Abnormal ADH receptors
	Metabolic abnormalities	Hypokalaemia Hypercalcaemia
	Drug therapy	Lithium Demethylchlortetracycline
	Poisoning	Heavy metals

Fig. 10.5 Causes of cranial and nephrogenic diabetes insipidus (DI)

Note: ADH, antidiuretic hormone.

Fig. 10.5 Causes of cranial and nephrogenic diabetes insipidus (DI).

differentiate DI from psychogenic polydipsia. The test is then followed by ADH administration to differentiate between cranial DI (kidneys are responsive to ADH) or nephrogenic DI (kidneys are unresponsive to ADH).

Treatment of mild DI—the effects of dehydration can be counteracted by greatly increasing water intake (polydipsia).

Treatment of moderate to severe DI

- Cranial DI—treatment with desmopressin (ADH analogue but without vasoactive effects).
- Nephrogenic DI—treatment with thiazide diuretics, producing a decrease in urine volume by approximately 50%.

Diabetes insipidus and diabetes mellitus are two distinct conditions that both feature polyuria.

Syndrome of inappropriate antidiuretic hormone secretion

Increased secretion of ADH occurs as a complication of other diseases (primary hypersecretion of ADH is not recognised). The condition is characterised by water retention with haemodilution and by inappropriately concentrated urine. In severe cases, cerebral oedema supervenes with impaired consciousness, but body oedema is not usually seen as free water is evenly distributed to all body compartments.

The causes are:

- Idiopathic.
- Tumours—ectopic secretion of ADH, especially by small cell carcinomas of the lung and some other neuroendocrine tumours.
- Trauma—skull fracture, head injury or surgery may produce transiently increased secretion of ADH.
- Intracranial inflammation—meningitis, tuberculosis, syphilis.
- Non-neoplastic lung disease (e.g. pneumonia, pulmonary embolus) probably due to involvement of intrathoracic baroreceptors.

Figure 10.6 shows a comparison table of features of DI with those of inappropriate ADH secretion.

Disorders of the pineal gland

The pineal gland is located above the third ventricle and it secretes the hormone melatonin. Melatonin is thought to function in circadian rhythm control and gonadal maturation.

Pinealomas (germinomas)

These tumours of young adults and children are often called germinomas. They are thought to originate from primitive germ cells and, histologically, they resemble testicular seminomas and/or teratomas:

- Pressure on the midbrain may produce Parinaud's syndrome (paralysis of the conjugate upward gaze without paralysis of convergence).
- Pressure on the hypothalamus can produce symptoms of DI, emaciation or precocious puberty.

THYROID DISORDERS

Congenital disorders of the thyroid

Development of the thyroid

The thyroid gland develops from an endodermal thickening in the floor of the primitive pharynx at a point later indicated by the foramen caecum of the tongue (Fig. 10.7). As the embryo grows, the thyroid descends into the neck, passing anterior to the hyoid and laryngeal cartilages. During migration, the gland remains connected to the tongue by a narrow canal, the thyroglossal duct, which later becomes solid and finally disappears.

Thyroglossal cysts

Cystic remnants of parts of the thyroglossal duct are known as thyroglossal cysts (Fig. 10.7). These cysts may form anywhere along the course of descent but are always located near or in the midline of the neck, most commonly just inferior to the hyoid bone. Cysts usually develop as painless, progressively enlarging and movable masses. Infection of cysts may result in the formation of sinuses that open through the skin.

Thyrotoxicosis (hyperthyroidism)

This syndrome is caused by the excessive secretion of thyroid hormones—typically both thyroxine (T_4) and tri-iodothyronine (T_3)—in the bloodstream. Symptoms include tachycardia, sweating, tremor, anxiety, increased appetite, loss of weight and intolerance of heat.

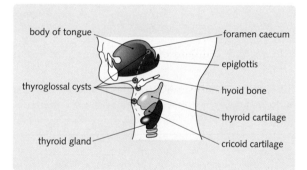

Fig. 10.7 Path of descent of thyroid gland (broken line) and localisation of thyroglossal cysts.

Fig. 10.6 Comparison of features of diabetes insipidus with those of inappropriate ADH secretion

Condition	Imbalance	Urinary and plasma osmolality	Symptoms
Diabetes insipidus	↓ ADH	Low urinary osmolality High plasma osmolality	Polyuria (5–20 L/day) Thirst Polydipsia (may lead to severe dehydration, exhaustion, coma)
Syndrome of inappropriate ADH secretion	↑ ADH	High urinary osmolality Low plasma osmolality (dilutional hyponatraemia)	Oliguria Water intoxication (may lead to confusion, neurological disturbances, coma)

Note: ADH, antidiuretic hormone.

Fig. 10.6 Comparison of features of diabetes insipidus with those of inappropriate antidiuretic hormone (ADH) secretion.

Hyperthyroidism can be classified on the basis of aetiology into:

- Primary hyperthyroidism (↑ thyroid hormones, ↓ TSH)—hypersecretion of thyroid hormones, which is not secondary to increased levels of TSH (the rise in thyroid hormones actually suppresses TSH).
- Secondary hyperthyroidism (↑ thyroid hormones, ↑ TSH)—overstimulation of the thyroid gland caused by excess TSH produced by a tumour in the pituitary or elsewhere (rare).

Primary hyperthyroidism is caused by:

- Graves' disease (exophthalmic goitre)—the most common cause of thyrotoxicosis, characterised by a diffusely enlarged thyroid gland that is stimulated to produce excess hormone by an IgG autoantibody.
- Toxic multinodular goitre (Plummer's disease)—second most common cause of hyperthyroidism.
- Toxic adenoma—solitary thyroid nodule producing excess hormone with remainder of the thyroid gland being suppressed.
- Thyroiditis—inflammation of the thyroid causing hyperthyroidism (e.g. De Quervain's thyroiditis). Note that thyroiditis is more commonly associated with hypothyroidism (see below).
- Drugs—either direct ingestion of large doses of thyroid hormone (thyrotoxicosis factitia) or through iodide-inducing drugs (e.g. amiodarone).

Effects of thyrotoxicosis

Signs and symptoms of thyrotoxicosis are a consequence of an increase in the body's metabolism, which occurs as a direct result of increased concentrations of the thyroid hormones.

The most important symptoms diagnostically are:

- Heat intolerance and excessive sweating (hyperhidrosis).
- Nervousness and irritability.
- Weight loss with normal or increased appetite.
- Goitre (an enlargement of the thyroid gland).

Other symptoms are summarised in Fig. 10.8.

Investigations—hyperthyroidism is confirmed by raised serum thyroxine and/or lowered serum TSH.

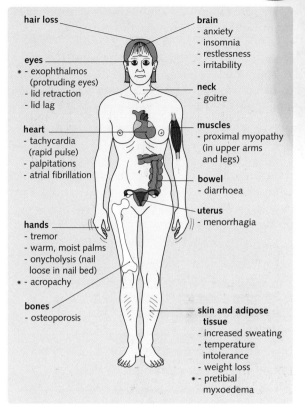

Fig. 10.8 Summary diagram illustrating features of thyrotoxicosis. (∗ = additional features seen only in Graves' disease.)

Management—options in thyrotoxicosis are:

- Surgery—reduces the amount of functioning thyroid tissue.
- Radioactive iodine—to destroy part of the gland.
- Drugs (such as carbimazole or propylthiouracil)—interfere with the production of thyroid hormones.

Graves' disease

Graves' disease is an organ-specific autoimmune disorder that results in thyrotoxicosis due to overstimulation of the thyroid gland by autoantibodies. It is the most common form of thyrotoxicosis, females being affected more than males by 8 : 1. It is usually associated with a diffuse enlargement of the thyroid.

Pathogenesis—IgG-type immunoglobulins bind to TSH membrane receptors and cause prolonged stimulation of the thyroid, lasting for as long as 12 hours (cf. 1 hour for TSH). The autoantibody binds at a site different to the hormone-binding locus and is termed the TSH-receptor autoantibody (TRAb); 95% of Graves' disease patients are positive for TRAbs.

Histologically, the gland shows diffuse hypertrophy and hyperplasia of acinar epithelium, reduction of stored colloid and local accumulations of lymphocytes with lymphoid follicle formation.

The clinical features of Graves' disease are similar to those of general thyrotoxicosis but with some additional features (see Fig. 10.8), namely:

- Exophthalmos (protrusion of the eyeballs in their sockets)—due to the infiltration of orbital tissues by fat, mucopolysaccharides and lymphocytes. May cause compression of the optic nerve, hence blindness. However, only about 5% of Graves' patients show signs of exophthalmos.
- Thyroid acropachy—enlargement of fingernails.
- Pretibial myxoedema—accumulation of mucoproteins in the deep dermis of the skin.

Treatment is as for thyrotoxicosis.

Hypothyroidism

Decreased activity of the thyroid gland results in decreased production of thyroid hormones. There are two forms:

1. Hypothyroidism present at birth → cretinism or congenital hypothyroidism.
2. Hypothyroidism in adults → myxoedema.

Cretinism (congenital hypothyroidism)

This condition occurs as a result of extreme hypothyroidism during fetal life, infancy or childhood. It has the following types and aetiology:

- Endemic cretinism—occurs in iodine-deficient countries where goitre is common. The mother almost always has a goitre and the thyroid of the affected infant is usually enlarged and nodular.
- Sporadic cretinism—caused by congenital hypoplasia or absence of the thyroid gland and often associated with deaf mutism.
- Dyshormonogenesis—a congenital familial recessive enzyme defect causing an inability to complete the formation of thyroid hormones. TSH is increased, and the thyroid gland is enlarged and shows epithelial hyperplasia.

The clinical features of cretinism are:

- Mental retardation.
- Retarded growth—skeletal growth is inhibited more than soft tissue growth, resulting in an obese, stocky, short child.
- Coarse, dry skin.
- Lack of hair and teeth.
- Pot belly (often with umbilical hernia).
- Protruding tongue.

Management is by early detection and treatment with thyroxine, which can prevent an irreversible mental defect and cerebellar damage. Many countries now have screening programs to measure serum TSH and/or thyroxine levels on heel-prick blood samples taken on the fourth or fifth day of life.

Hypothyroidism in adults (myxoedema)

This common clinical condition is associated with decreased function of the thyroid gland and a decrease in the circulating level of thyroid hormones. It affects 1% of people in the UK, with females more than males by 6 : 1. It can present at any age but most commonly between 30 and 50 years of age.

Note that, strictly speaking, myxoedema describes a non-pitting, oedematous reaction characteristic of hypothyroidism caused by the deposition of a mucoid substance (*myxa*-is a Greek prefix denoting mucus) in the skin and elsewhere in the body. However, the terms 'myxoedema' and 'hypothyroidism of adults' are now frequently used interchangeably.

Hypothyroidism can be classified according to aetiology:

- Primary ($\downarrow$ thyroid hormones, $\uparrow$ TSH)—failure of the thyroid gland itself. This is much more common than secondary hypothyroidism. Note that subclinical hypothyroidism describes an increase in TSH but with normal thyroid hormone levels, and is increasingly being treated with the aim of reducing progression to full disease.
- Secondary ($\downarrow$ thyroid hormones, $\downarrow$TSH)—failure of TSH production due to pituitary disease.

The causes of primary hypothyroidism are:

- Autoimmune thyroiditis—atrophic form, e.g. primary atrophic thyroiditis and goitrous form (such as Hashimoto's thyroiditis).
- Graves' disease—approximately 5% of patients with thyrotoxicosis develop hypothyroidism in later years, unrelated to treatment. Probably caused by a spectrum of antithyroid antibodies, some of which stimulate TSH receptor and some of which are destructive.
- Treatment of hyperthyroidism—surgical ablation, radioiodine or drug treatment.

- Severe iodine deficiency (rare in the UK)—iodine must be virtually absent from the diet before myxoedema develops.

The effects of hypothyroidism are shown in Fig.10.9.

Signs and symptoms of hypothyroidism are both widespread (due to reduced body metabolism) and localised (myxoedema due to the accumulation of mucoproteins). The most important symptoms diagnostically are:
- Mental and physical slowness.
- Tiredness.
- Cold intolerance.
- Dryness of skin and hair.

Investigations are:
- Serum thyroxine concentration (decreased).
- Serum TSH concentration (reduced in secondary hypothyroidism but increased in primary hypothyroidism).

The treatment is oral thyroxine daily for life.

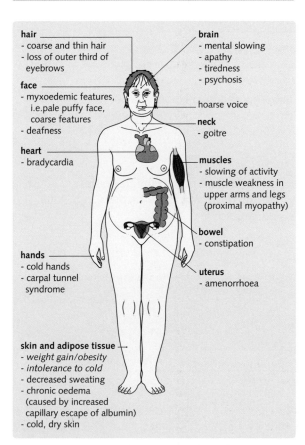

hair
- coarse and thin hair
- loss of outer third of eyebrows

face
- myxoedemic features, i.e. pale puffy face, coarse features
- deafness

heart
- bradycardia

hands
- cold hands
- carpal tunnel syndrome

skin and adipose tissue
- *weight gain/obesity*
- *intolerance to cold*
- *decreased sweating*
- *chronic oedema (caused by increased capillary escape of albumin)*
- cold, dry skin

brain
- mental slowing
- apathy
- tiredness
- psychosis

hoarse voice

neck
- goitre

muscles
- slowing of activity
- muscle weakness in upper arms and legs (proximal myopathy)

bowel
- constipation

uterus
- amenorrhoea

Fig. 10.9 Summary diagram illustrating features of hypothyroidism in the adult (myxoedema).

Thyroiditis

This inflammation of the thyroid gland can have a viral or autoimmune aetiology.

Hashimoto's thyroiditis (most common cause of hypothyroidism)

This organ-specific autoimmune disease results in destructive thyroiditis. It can occur at any age, but typically affects the middle-aged, and females more than males by $12:1$.

Thyroid peroxidase antibodies are most commonly found in the serum of affected individuals (90% of cases). The disease is associated with the HLA-DR5 and HLA-B8 haplotypes, and patients with Hashimoto's disease (and Graves' disease) show a high incidence of other autoimmune diseases.

Macroscopically, the thyroid gland is usually:

- Diffusely enlarged (typically 2–5 times normal size).
- Firm in consistency.
- White or grey on a cut surface as a result of the disappearance of brown (iodine-rich) colloid (thyroglobulin), and its replacement by lymphocytes.

Microscopically, the thyroid gland shows:

- Small thyroid follicles infiltrated by lymphocytes and plasma cells.
- Lymphoid follicle formation and increased fibrous tissue stroma.
- Acini lined with abnormal, highly eosinophilic epithelial cells (proliferation of mitochondria) known as Askanazy or Hürthle cells.
- Reduced colloid content of disrupted acini.

The condition may present due to goitre formation or because of the symptoms of hypothyroidism. The hypothyroid state tends to develop slowly. However, damage to thyroid follicles may lead to the release of thyroglobulin into the circulation causing transient thyrotoxicosis. Some cases proceed to primary atrophic thyroiditis. Furthermore, there is an increased incidence of non-Hodgkin's lymphoma originating in the thyroid of patients with Hashimoto's thyroiditis.

Treatment is by oral thyroxine, which overcomes hypothyroidism and reduces the size of the goitre.

De Quervain's thyroiditis

A rare, viral thyroiditis seen in young and middle-aged women as a slightly diffuse tender swelling of the thyroid; this is also known as subacute, giant cell or granulomatous thyroiditis. The condition usually occurs in association with a transient febrile illness, often during various viral epidemics.

The most commonly associated viruses are Coxsackie, mumps and adenovirus.

Characteristic features are:

- Painful enlargement of the thyroid (about twice normal size; normal weight is 20–30 g).
- History of usually short duration.
- Preceding general malaise, pyrexia or upper respiratory infection.

Histological examination shows:

- Inflammation with a giant cell granulomatous reaction engulfing leaked colloid (hence the synonyms giant cell or granulomatous thyroiditis).
- Degeneration of follicles with inflammatory cell infiltration (neutrophils, plasma cells, lymphocytes and histiocytes).
- Fibrous scarring (late).

The illness is usually self-limiting and settles in a few weeks. Transient hyperthyroidism can result from the release of thyroglobulin and excessive amounts of thyroid hormone.

Severe thyroiditis may be fatal in the elderly and debilitated.

Subacute lymphocytic thyroiditis

This form of autoimmune thyroiditis is characterised by focal lymphocytic infiltration of the thyroid (also known as focal lymphocytic thyroiditis).

Histological changes are similar to those in Hashimoto's thyroiditis but they are focal rather than diffuse. The disease is less severe than Hashimoto's thyroiditis, and it is often asymptomatic. It may also present with the symptoms of hyperthyroidism.

Note that some degree of progressive lymphocytic infiltration of the thyroid is seen in 5–10% of thyroid autopsies, and these are thought to be a normal ageing change. However, in subacute lymphocytic thyroiditis, lymphocytic infiltration is in excess of what would normally be expected for age-related change.

A comparison of the main types of thyroiditis is provided in Fig. 10.10.

Thyroid goitres
Definitions

A goitre is any enlargement of part or whole of the thyroid gland. There are two types:

1. Toxic goitre, i.e. goitre associated with thyrotoxicosis.
2. Non-toxic goitre, i.e. goitre associated with normal or reduced levels of thyroid hormones.

Toxic goitre
Graves' disease

This is the most common cause of toxic goitre (described above).

Toxic multinodular goitre

This results from the development of hyperthyroidism in a multinodular goitre (see below).

Non-toxic goitres
Diffuse non-toxic goitre (simple goitre)

This diffuse enlargement of the thyroid gland is classified into:

Fig. 10.10 Summary of features of thyroiditis.

Fig. 10.10 Summary of features of thyroiditis

	Hashimoto's thyroiditis	De Quervain's thyroiditis	Subacute lymphocytic thyroiditis
Aetiology	Autoimmune	Viral	Autoimmune
Histological features	Diffuse lymphocytic infiltration of thyroid	Giant cell granulomatous inflammatory reaction	Focal lymphocytic infiltration of thyroid
Hypothyroidism	Common	Rare	Rare

- Endemic goitre—due to iodine deficiency. Rare in the UK but may occur in certain geographical areas remote from the sea.
- Sporadic goitre—caused by goitrogenic agents (substances that induce goitre formation) or familial in origin. Examples of goitrogenic agents include certain cabbage species, because of their thiourea content, and specific drugs or chemicals, such as iodide, paraminosalicylic acid and drugs used in the treatment of thyrotoxicosis. Familial cases show inherited autosomal recessive traits, which interfere with hormone synthesis via various enzyme pathways (these are dyshormonogenic goitres).
- Physiological goitre—enlargement of the thyroid gland in females during puberty or pregnancy; the reason is unclear.

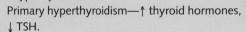

A reminder of the differences between primary and secondary hyperthyroidism and hypothyroidism:
- Primary hyperthyroidism—↑ thyroid hormones, ↓ TSH.
- Secondary hyperthyroidism—↑ thyroid hormones, ↑ TSH (excess TSH production due to pituitary tumour).
- Primary hypothyroidism—↓ thyroid hormones, ↑ TSH.
- Secondary hypothyroidism—↓ thyroid hormones, ↓ TSH (failure of TSH production due to pituitary disease).

Multinodular goitre

This is the most common cause of thyroid enlargement and is seen particularly in the elderly (nearly all simple goitres eventually become multinodular). The exact aetiology is uncertain but it may represent an uneven responsiveness of various parts of the thyroid to fluctuating TSH levels over a period of many years.

Morphological features are:

- Irregular hyperplastic enlargement of the entire thyroid gland due to the development of well-circumscribed nodules of varying size.
- Larger nodules filled with brown, gelatinous colloid; consequently, it is often termed multinodular colloid goitres.

Most patients have normal thyroid function and generally seek treatment for cosmetic reasons (an unsightly swelling in the neck) or compression symptoms, e.g. pressure on the trachea producing stridor or pressure on the recurrent laryngeal nerve producing hoarseness.

However, toxic changes occasionally occur in a multinodular goitre resulting in hyperthyroidism, when it is termed a toxic multinodular goitre.

Neoplasms of the thyroid

Tumours of the thyroid are generally benign. Carcinomas are rare and lymphomas are rarer still.

Benign tumours

Thyroid adenomas

These are solitary, or multiple, encapsulated solid nodules. Compression of the adjacent gland is a common feature, and the centre may show areas of haemorrhage and cystic changes. The most common type is follicular adenoma, which consists of colloid-containing microfollicles and columns of larger cells of alveolar arrangement.

Rarely, follicular adenomas may synthesise excess thyroid hormones ('toxic adenomas'), causing thyrotoxicosis.

Malignant tumours

These rare tumours account for less than 1% of total cancer deaths in the UK, with females affected more than males by 3 : 1. Although the aetiology of thyroid cancer is unknown in the majority, it is likely that childhood radiation exposure is involved in some cases (there is an increased incidence in those exposed to the Chernobyl fallout). Types of malignant thyroid tumours and their basic features are outlined in Fig. 10.11.

Papillary adenocarcinoma

This well-differentiated tumour is most commonly found in younger patients. It presents as a non-encapsulated infiltrative mass. It is a slow growing tumour with an excellent prognosis.

Histologically, it consists of epithelial papillary projections between which calcified spherules may be present. Epithelial cell nuclei are characteristically large with optically clear areas centrally (described as 'Orphan Annie nuclei').

Follicular adenocarcinoma

This well-differentiated, single, encapsulated lesion is histologically similar to follicular adenoma but can

Fig. 10.11 Types and features of malignant thyroid tumours

	Tumour type	Origin of tumour	Frequency (%)	Typical age range (years)	Spread	Prognosis (% for 10-year survival)
Differentiated carcinoma	Papillary	Follicular cells	70	20–40	Lymph nodes	95
	Follicular	Follicular cells	10	40–60	Bloodstream	60
Undifferentiated carcinoma	Anaplastic	Follicular cells	5	>60	Aggressive local invasion; bloodstream	1
Medullary carcinoma	—	Parafollicular C cells	5–10	>40	Local, lymphatic and blood	50 (but very variable)
Lymphoma	—	Lymphocytes	5–10	>60	Lymphatic	10

Fig. 10.11 Types and features of malignant thyroid tumours.

be differentiated by its invasion of the capsule and/or blood vessels. Spread is usually to bones, lungs and brain via the bloodstream.

Many of these tumours retain the ability to take up radioactive iodine (^{131}I), which may be used as a highly effective targeted form of radiotherapy, usually after surgical thyroidectomy. The prognosis, therefore, is good.

Anaplastic carcinoma

This highly malignant, poorly differentiated adenocarcinoma usually presents in the elderly as a diffusely infiltrative mass. In about half of cases there is a history of multinodular goitre.

Histologically, the dominant features are those of a spindle cell tumour with or without giant cell areas, or a small cell pattern.

The prognosis is very poor due to the rapid local invasion of structures such as the trachea, producing respiratory obstruction.

Medullary carcinoma

This rare neuroendocrine tumour arises from parafollicular C cells, which commonly synthesise and secrete calcitonin but which may also secrete 5-hydroxytryptamine (serotonin), various peptides of the tachykinin family, ACTH and prostaglandins.

High levels of serum calcitonin are useful diagnostically but produce no clinical effects.

Although medullary carcinoma is most common in the elderly, it also occurs in younger individuals, where it is commonly associated with other endocrine tumours, such as phaeochromocytoma as part of the multiple endocrine neoplasia (MEN) syndromes IIa and IIb (see pages 227–228).

Lymphomas

Most thyroid lymphomas are regarded as tumours of mucosa-associated lymphoma tissue. Interestingly, non-Hodgkin's B cell lymphomas occasionally arise in long-standing, autoimmune thyroiditis, especially Hashimoto's disease.

PARATHYROID DISORDERS

Parathyroid hormone

Parathyroid hormone (PTH) is a polypeptide (84 amino acid residues) secreted by the chief cells of the parathyroid glands (four glands: two in each of the superior and inferior lobes of the thyroid; total weight 120 mg).

The main action of PTH is to increase serum calcium and decrease serum phosphate. Its actions are mediated by the bones and kidneys as described below.

In bone, PTH stimulates osteoclastic bone resorption and inhibits osteoblastic bone deposition. The net effect is the release of calcium from bone.

In the kidney, PTH has the following effects:

- Increases calcium reabsorption.
- Decreases phosphate reabsorption.
- Increases 1-hydroxylation of 25-hydroxyvitamin D (i.e. activates vitamin D).

PTH also increases gastrointestinal calcium absorption.

Hyperparathyroidism

Hyperparathyroidism is defined as an elevated secretion of PTH, of which there are three main types:

1. Primary—hypersecretion of PTH by adenoma or hyperplasia of the gland.
2. Secondary—physiological increase in PTH secretions in response to hypocalcaemia of any cause.
3. Tertiary—supervention of an autonomous hypersecreting adenoma in long-standing secondary hyperparathyroidism.

> Understanding the physiological functions of PTH is essential to an understanding of the clinical effects produced by its hypo- or hypersecretion.

Primary hyperparathyroidism

This is the most common of the parathyroid disorders, with a prevalence of about 1 per 800 in the UK. It is an important cause of hypercalcaemia. More than 90% of patients are over 50 years of age and the condition affects females more than males by nearly 3 : 1. The aetiology of primary hyperparathyroidism is outlined in Fig. 10.12.

Fig. 10.12 Aetiology of primary hyperparathyroidism

Type	Frequency	Features
Adenoma	75%	Orange–brown, well-encapsulated tumour of various size but seldom > 1 cm diameter. Tumours are usually solitary, affecting only one of the parathyroids, the others often showing atrophy; they are deep seated and rarely palpable
Primary hyperplasia	20%	Diffuse enlargement of all the parathyroid glands
Parathyroid carcinoma	5%	Usually resembles adenoma but is poorly encapsulated and invasive locally

Fig. 10.12 Aetiology of primary hyperparathyroidism.

Effects of hyperparathyroidism

The clinical effects are the result of hypercalcaemia and bone resorption.

Effects of hypercalcaemia:

- Renal stones due to hypercalcuria.
- Excessive calcification of blood vessels.
- Corneal calcification.
- General muscle weakness and tiredness.
- Exacerbation of hypertension and potential shortening of the QT interval.
- Thirst and polyuria (may be dehydrated due to impaired concentrating ability of kidney).
- Anorexia and constipation.

Effects of bone resorption:

- Osteitis fibrosa—increased bone resorption with fibrous replacement in the lacunae.
- 'Brown tumours'—haemorrhagic and cystic tumour-like areas in the bone, containing large masses of giant osteoclastic cells.
- Osteitis fibrosa cystica (von Recklinghausen disease of bone)—multiple brown tumours combined with osteitis fibrosa.
- Changes may present clinically as bone pain, fracture or deformity.

However, about 50% of patients with biochemical evidence of primary hyperparathyroidism are asymptomatic.

Investigations are:

- Biochemical—increased PTH and Ca^{2+}, and decreased PO_4^{3-}.
- Radiological—90% normal; 10% show evidence of bone resorption, particularly phalangeal erosions.

Management is by rehydration, medical reduction in plasma calcium using bisphosphonates and eventual surgical removal of abnormal parathyroid glands.

Secondary hyperparathyroidism

This is compensatory hyperplasia of the parathyroid glands, occurring in response to diseases of chronic low serum calcium or increased serum phosphate.

Its causes are:

- Chronic renal failure and some renal tubular disorders (most common cause).
- Steatorrhoea and other malabsorption syndromes.
- Osteomalacia and rickets.
- Pregnancy and lactation.

Fig. 10.13 Pathogenesis of renal osteodystrophy.

Renal disease →
$$\downarrow \text{vit. D activation} \\ + \\ \downarrow Ca^{2+} \text{ reabsorption}$$
→ ↓ serum Ca^{2+} →↑ PTH → ↓ bone absorption

Morphological changes of the parathyroid glands are:

- Hyperplastic enlargement of all parathyroid glands, but to a lesser degree than in primary hyperplasia.
- Increase in 'water clear' cells and chief cells of the parathyroid glands, with loss of stromal fat cells.

Clinical manifestations—symptoms of bone resorption are dominant.

Renal osteodystrophy

Skeletal abnormalities, arising as a result of raised PTH secondary to chronic renal disease, are known as renal osteodystrophy.

The pathogenesis of renal osteodystrophy is shown in Fig. 10.13.

Abnormalities vary widely according to the nature of the renal lesion, its duration and the age of the patient, but include:

- Osteitis fibrosa (see above).
- Rickets or osteomalacia due to reduced activation of vitamin D.
- Osteosclerosis—increased radiodensity of certain bones, particularly the parts of vertebrae adjacent to the intervertebral discs.

Note that the symptoms of hypercalcaemia are not a feature of secondary hyperparathyroidism; calcium levels are likely to be decreased as this is driving the compensatory PTH secretion.

The investigations are both biochemical (raised PTH and normal or lowered Ca^{2+}) and radiological (bone changes).

Management is by treatment of the underlying disease and oral calcium supplements to correct hypocalcaemia.

Tertiary hyperparathyroidism

This condition, resulting from chronic overstimulation of the parathyroid glands in renal failure, causes one or more of the glands to become an autonomous hypersecreting adenoma with resultant hypercalcaemia.

Figure 10.14 gives a comparison of primary, secondary and tertiary hyperparathyroidism.

Hypoparathyroidism

Hypoparathyroidism is a condition of reduced or absent PTH secretion, resulting in hypocalcaemia and hyperphosphataemia. It is far less common than hyperparathyroidism.

The causes of hypoparathyroidism are:

- Removal or damage of the parathyroid glands during thyroidectomy—most common cause of

Fig. 10.14 Comparison of primary, secondary and tertiary hyperparathyroidism.

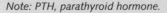

Fig. 10.14 Comparison of primary, secondary and tertiary hyperparathyroidism

	Primary	**Secondary**	**Tertiary**
Serum PTH and Ca^{2+}	↑PTH; ↑Ca^{2+}	↑PTH; normal or ↑Ca^{2+}	↑PTH; ↑Ca^{2+}
Aetiology	Adenoma Hyperplasia Carcinoma	Chronic renal failure Malabsorption Osteomalacia and rickets Pregnancy and lactation	Adenoma resulting from overstimulation of glands in secondary hyperparathyroidism
Predominant effects	Hyper-calcaemia	Increased bone absorption	Hypercalcaemia and increased bone resorption

Note: PTH, parathyroid hormone.

hypoparathyroidism resulting from inadvertent damage or removal.

- Autoimmune parathyroid disease—usually occurs in patients who have another autoimmune endocrine disease, e.g. Addison's disease (autoimmune endocrine syndrome type 1).
- Congenital deficiency (DiGeorge syndrome)— rare, congenital disorder caused by arrested development of the third and fourth branchial arches, resulting in an almost complete absence of the thymus (see Chapter 13) and parathyroid gland.

The effects of hypoparathyroidism are:

- ↓ release of Ca^{2+} from bones.
- ↓ Ca^{2+} reabsorption but ↑ PO_4^{3-} re absorption by kidney.
- ↓ 1-hydroxylation of 25-hydroxyvitamin D by kidney.

Most symptoms of hypoparathyroidism are those of hypocalcaemia:

- Tetany—muscular spasm provoked by lowered plasma Ca^{2+}.
- Convulsions.
- Paraesthesiae.
- Psychiatric disturbances, e.g. depression, confusional state and even psychosis.
- Rarely—cataracts, parkinsonian-like movement disorders, alopecia, brittle nails.

Management is by treatment with large doses of oral vitamin D; the acute phase requires intravenous calcium and calcitriol (1,25-dihydroxycholecalciferol, i.e. activated vitamin D).

DISORDERS OF THE ADRENAL GLAND

Hormones of the adrenal gland

The adrenal gland has two structurally and functionally distinct endocrine components derived from different embryonic tissue: the cortex and the medulla.

Cortex

This is the outer part of the gland, which is derived from the mesoderm. It synthesises, stores, and secretes various cholesterol-derived hormones, namely:

- Glucocorticoid hormones, e.g. cortisol— primarily from the zona fasciculata.
- Mineralocorticoid hormones, e.g. aldosterone— from the zona glomerulosa.
- Sex steroids, i.e. oestrogens and androgens—from the zona reticularis.

Medulla

This is the inner part of the gland, which is derived from the neuroectoderm, forming part of the sympathetic nervous system. Chromaffin cells synthesise and secrete the vasoactive amines epinephrine (adrenaline) and norepinephrine (noradrenaline).

Hyperfunction of the adrenal cortex

Cushing's syndrome

The symptoms and signs of Cushing's syndrome are associated with prolonged inappropriate elevation of free corticosteroid levels (Fig. 10.15).

Clinical features—the main effects of sustained elevation of glucocorticoid secretion are:

- Central obesity and moon face.
- Plethora and acne.
- Menstrual irregularity.
- Hirsutism and hair thinning.
- Hypertension.
- Diabetes.
- Osteoporosis—may cause collapse of vertebrae, rib fractures.
- Muscle wasting and weakness.
- Atrophy of skin and dermis—paper thin skin with bruising tendency, purple striae.

Aetiopathogenesis—patients with Cushing's syndrome can be classified into two groups on the basis of whether the aetiology of the condition is ACTH-dependent or independent (Fig. 10.16).

ACTH-dependent aetiology:

- Pituitary hypersecretion of ACTH (Cushing's disease)—bilateral adrenal hyperplasia secondary to excessive secretion of ACTH by a corticotroph adenoma of the pituitary gland (see page 207).
- Production of ectopic ACTH or corticotrophin-releasing hormone (CRH) by non-endocrine neoplasm, e.g. small cell lung cancer and some carcinoid tumours. In cases of malignant bronchial tumour, the patient rarely survives long enough to develop any physical features of Cushing's syndrome.

Fig. 10.15 Systemic effects of Cushing's syndrome.

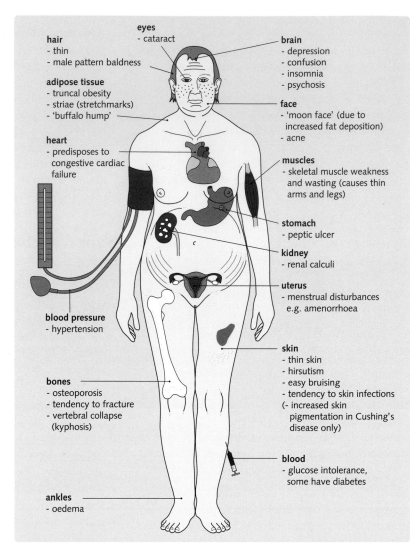

eyes
- cataract

hair
- thin
- male pattern baldness

adipose tissue
- truncal obesity
- striae (stretchmarks)
- 'buffalo hump'

heart
- predisposes to
  congestive cardiac
  failure

blood pressure
- hypertension

bones
- osteoporosis
- tendency to fracture
- vertebral collapse
  (kyphosis)

ankles
- oedema

brain
- depression
- confusion
- insomnia
- psychosis

face
- 'moon face' (due to
  increased fat deposition)
- acne

muscles
- skeletal muscle weakness
  and wasting (causes thin
  arms and legs)

stomach
- peptic ulcer

kidney
- renal calculi

uterus
- menstrual disturbances
  e.g. amenorrhoea

skin
- thin skin
- hirsutism
- easy bruising
- tendency to skin infections
(- increased skin
   pigmentation in Cushing's
   disease only)

blood
- glucose intolerance,
  some have diabetes

Non-ACTH-dependent aetiology:

- Iatrogenic steroid therapy—most common cause of Cushing's syndrome.
- Adrenal cortical adenoma—well-circumscribed yellow tumour usually 2–5 cm in diameter. Extremely common as an incidental finding in up to 30% of all post-mortem examinations. The yellow colour is due to stored lipid (mainly cholesterol) from which the hormones are synthesised. The vast majority have no clinical effects (i.e. they are non-functioning adenomas), with only a small percentage producing Cushing's syndrome.

Fig. 10.16 Classification of Cushing's syndrome	
Type	**Cause**
ACTH dependent	Iatrogenic (ACTH therapy) Pituitary hypersecretion of ACTH Ectopic ACTH syndrome (benign or malignant non-endocrine tumour)
Non-ACTH dependent	Iatrogenic, e.g. prednisolone Adrenal cortical adenoma Adrenal cortical carcinoma

Fig. 10.16 Classification of Cushing's syndrome.

- Adrenal cortical carcinoma—rare and almost always associated with the overproduction of hormones, usually glucocorticoids and sex steroids. Patients usually have features of Cushing's syndrome mixed with androgenic effects which are particularly noticeable in women. Tumours are usually large and yellowish-white in colour. Local invasion and metastatic spread are common.

The therapeutic administration of glucocorticosteroids (e.g. prednisolone) is a common cause of the features of Cushing's syndrome. Avoid confusing the disease and the syndrome. *Remember*: Cushing's disease is used specifically to describe Cushing's syndrome secondary to excessive pituitary ACTH secretion.

Irrespective of the aetiology, the diagnosis is based on clinical features and the demonstration of a raised plasma cortisol level.

The aetiology of the disorder is elucidated through:

- Raised urinary cortisol in the first instance, but further testing is required.
- Low-dose dexamethasone suppression test (suppression of cortisol levels in Cushing's disease due to suppression of pituitary ACTH secretion, but a lack of suppression suggests ACTH-independent Cushing's syndrome).
- MRI and CT scan visualisation of pituitary and adrenal glands.
- Analysis of blood ACTH (high = pituitary adenoma or ectopic ACTH source; low = primary adrenal tumour due to feedback suppression).

Treatment of the underlying cause is essential as untreated Cushing's syndrome has a 50% 5-year mortality rate.

Hyperaldosteronism

Excessive production of aldosterone by the zona glomerulosa of the adrenal cortex results in increased Na^+ retention and increased K^+ loss.

The aetiology is as follows:

- Primary hyperaldosteronism—autonomous hypersecretion of aldosterone, which is almost

invariably caused by adrenal cortical adenoma (Conn's syndrome).
- Secondary hyperaldosteronism—hypersecretion of aldosterone secondary to an increased production of angiotensin II following activation of the renin–angiotensin system. May be precipitated by congestive cardiac failure, cirrhosis, pregnancy, nephrotic syndrome or decreased renal perfusion. This is more common than the primary form of the disorder.

The effects of hyperaldosteronism are shown in Fig. 10.17.

Clinical features are:

- Hypertension—often the only presenting feature. Commonly occurs in the younger age group.
- Hypokalaemia—usually accompanies hypertension and may give rise to polyuria, nocturia, polydipsia, paraesthesia, cardiac arrhythmias, muscle weakness or paralysis.

Secondary hyperaldosteronism also has additional features of underlying disease.

Biochemical diagnosis:

- ↑ Na^+, ↓ K^+.
- ↑ Aldosterone.
- Plasma renin—↓ in Conn's syndrome but ↑ in secondary hyperaldosteronism.

Radiological diagnosis is by visualisation of adrenal cortical adenoma by CT scan or MRI.

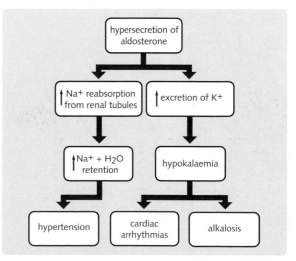

Fig. 10.17 Effects of hyperaldosteronism.

Management:

- Primary hyperaldosteronism—medical aldosterone antagonism (e.g. spironolactone) or surgical removal of the affected adrenal.
- Secondary hyperaldosteronism—treatment of the underlying cause.

Congenital adrenal hyperplasia

This rare, autosomal recessive disorder is usually caused by a deficiency of the enzyme 21-hydroxylase, required for the synthesis of both cortisol and aldosterone. 21-hydroxylase acts on 17OH-progesterone, and consequently raised levels of 17OH-progesterone are measured in the blood of affected individuals; this is routinely tested in the first week of life. Failure of cortisol production produces an increase in ACTH secretion by the pituitary and hyperplasia of the adrenal cortex.

Production of androgens by the adrenal cortex does not require 21-hydroxylase. Consequently, adrenal hyperplasia causes excessive secretion of androgens resulting in masculinisation of females and precocious puberty in males. Also, aldosterone deficiency is serious, causing a life-threatening salt loss ('salt wasting syndrome') unless replacement therapy is given.

Hypofunction of the adrenal cortex

Addison's disease

This rare condition of chronic adrenal insufficiency is due to a lack of glucocorticoids and mineralocorticoids. Its estimated prevalence in the developed world is 0.8 cases per 100 000 population.

The clinical features outlined in Fig. 10.18 are a result of glucocorticoid and mineralocorticoid insufficiency, loss of adrenal androgen production and increased ACTH secretion.

Aetiology—autoimmune destruction of the cortex of both adrenals is the most common cause of Addison's disease. It is often associated with autoimmune thyroid disease, autoimmune gastritis and other endocrine organ autoimmune diseases. Addison's disease is also a well-recognised complication of patients with acquired immune deficiency syndrome (AIDS), bilateral adrenal tuberculosis (caseous necrosis) and, more rarely, metastatic cancers, haemochromatosis and amyloidosis.

Biochemical features:

- Measurement of plasma ACTH and cortisol— ↑ ACTH, ↓ cortisol.
- ACTH stimulation test—ACTH is administered and plasma cortisol levels are monitored. Failure of cortisol levels to rise indicates Addison's disease.
- Plasma electrolytes— ↓ Na^+, normal or ↑ K^+, ↑ urea.
- Blood glucose—usually low.
- ↑ Plasma renin activity and normal or ↓ aldosterone.

Management is by glucocorticoid replacement therapy, and usually mineralocorticoid therapy.

Primary acute adrenocortical insufficiency (adrenal crisis)

This may occur as a result of:

- Iatrogenic—abrupt cessation of prolonged high-dose therapeutic corticosteroids (prolonged corticosteroid therapy produces lowered endogenous steroid production, leading to atrophy of the adrenal cortex).

Fig. 10.18 Clinical features of Addison's disease.

Fig. 10.18 Clinical features of Addison's disease	
Hormonal abnormality	**Clinical features**
Glucocorticoid insufficiency	Vomiting and loss of appetite Weight loss Lethargy and weakness Postural hypotension Hypoglycaemia
Mineralocorticoid insufficiency	↓serum Na^+, ↑serum K^+ Chronic dehydration Hypotension
Increased ACTH secretion	Brownish pigmentation of skin and buccal mucosa
Loss of adrenal androgen	Decreased body hair, especially in females

Note: ACTH, adrenocorticotrophic hormone

- Bilateral massive adrenal haemorrhage—caused by Gram-negative (usually meningococcal) septicaemia (Waterhouse–Friderichsen syndrome) producing haemorrhage and disseminated intravascular coagulation. Adrenal haemorrhage is also seen in neonates following traumatic birth.
- Complication of chronic adrenal failure—Addisonian crisis is precipitated by sudden stress requiring increased output from chronically failing adrenal glands.

> Clinical features of an adrenal crisis are:
> - Profound hypotension and cardiovascular collapse (shock).
> - Vomiting.
> - Diarrhoea.
> - Abdominal pain.
> - Pyrexia.
>
> An adrenal crisis is a medical emergency and requires intravenous hydrocortisone and fluid replacement. The precipitating cause should be sought and if possible treated.

Secondary adrenocortical insufficiency

This adrenocortical insufficiency is caused by adrenal atrophy secondary to:

- Hypothalamic or pituitary disease (tumours, infection, infarction, surgical destruction), which produces lowered ACTH, hence lowered endogenous glucocorticoids and aldosterone.
- Glucocorticoid therapy, which produces lowered ACTH (suppression), hence lowered endogenous glucocorticoids and aldosterone.

The adrenal medulla

Phaeochromocytoma

This is a rare tumour of the chromaffin cells—the cells that secrete epinephrine (adrenaline) and norepinephrine (noradrenaline) in the adrenal medulla (see page 62).

Tumours of extra-adrenal paraganglia

Neuroblastomas

These rare tumours are derived from neuroblasts. Affected sites are the adrenal medulla, the mediastinum (usually in association with the sympathetic chain) and the coeliac plexus.

Neuroblastomas are almost exclusively tumours of children, occurring very rarely over the age of 5 years. They are highly malignant and usually inoperable.

Ganglioneuroma

A benign tumour derived from sympathetic nerves. Most commonly found in the posterior mediastinum, although 10% of cases arise in the adrenal medulla.

DISORDERS OF THE ENDOCRINE PANCREAS

Diabetes mellitus

Diabetes mellitus (DM) is a multisystem disease of an abnormal metabolic state characterised by hyperglycaemia due to inadequate insulin action/production. It can be classified into primary and secondary.

Primary DM is a disorder of insulin production/action. It accounts for 95% of diabetic cases.

In 5% of cases, diabetes may be secondary to:

- Pancreatic diseases, e.g. chronic pancreatitis.
- Hypersecretion of hormones that antagonise the effects of insulin, e.g. glucocorticoids in Cushing's syndrome, growth hormone in acromegaly, epinephrine (adrenaline) in pheochromocytomas.

Primary DM is by far the most important cause of diabetes and it is further classified into:

- Type I, also known as insulin-dependent DM (IDDM) or juvenile-onset diabetes.
- Type II, also known as non-insulin-dependent DM (NIDDM) or mature-onset diabetes.

The basic features of these two types of diabetes are described in Fig. 10.19.

Type I diabetes mellitus

Aetiology and pathogenesis—type I diabetes mellitus is an organ-specific, autoimmune-induced disorder characterised by antibody-mediated destruction of the β-cell population of the islet of Langerhans.

Two main factors are thought to predispose to autoimmunity:

1. Genetic predisposition—90–95% of patients with type I diabetes are HLA-DR3 or HLA-DR4 positive, a feature that is also seen in other organ-specific autoimmune diseases. However, identical twins show a 40% concordance in the

Fig. 10.19 Table comparing type I and type II diabetes mellitus (DM).

Fig. 10.19 Table comparing type I and type II diabetes mellitus (DM)

Type I	Type II
Childhood/adolescent onset	Middle-aged/elderly onset
1/3 of primary diabetes	2/3 of primary diabetes
Females = males	Females = males
Acute/subacute onset	Gradual onset
Thin	Obese
Ketoacidosis common	Ketoacidosis rare
Plasma insulin absent or low	Plasma insulin normal or raised
Insulin sensitive	Insulin insensitive (end-organ resistance)
Autoimmune mechanism (islet cell antibodies present)	Non-autoimmune mechanism (no islet cell antibodies)
Genetic predisposition associated with HLA-DR genotype	Polygenic inheritance

development of the disease, indicating the additional importance of environmental factors.

2. Viral infection—viral infection may trigger the autoimmune reaction; viruses implicated include mumps, measles and Coxsackie B.

One postulated mechanism is that viruses induce mild structural damage to the islet cells, thereby releasing previously shielded β-cell antigens and leading to the recruitment and activation of lymphocytes in the pancreatic tissue.

Histologically, the pancreas shows lymphocytic infiltration and destruction of insulin-secreting cells of islets of Langerhans (β-cells). This results in insulin deficiency with hyperglycaemia and other secondary metabolic complications.

Type II diabetes mellitus

Aetiology and pathogenesis—the precise aetiopathogenesis of type II diabetes is unclear but the following factors are thought to be involved:

- Genetic factors—familial tendency with up to 90% concordance rate amongst identical twins. However, there are no HLA associations and inheritance is considered to be polygenic.
- Insulin resistance—tissues are unable to respond to insulin because of an impairment in the function of insulin receptors on the surface of target cells. This is associated with obesity, sedentary lifestyle and poor diet; it is increasingly being seen in younger (even adolescent) individuals.
- Relative insulin deficiency—reduced secretion compared with the amounts required, possibly related to islet cell ageing.

Diagnosis of diabetes mellitus

Irrespective of aetiology, the diagnosis of DM depends on the finding of hyperglycaemia. However, the distribution curve of blood glucose concentration for whole populations is unimodal, with no clear division between normal and abnormal values.

Diagnostic criteria (Fig. 10.20) are, therefore, arbitrary and, in general, diabetes mellitus is indicated by either:

- Fasting venous plasma glucose level of > 7.0 mmol/L.
- Random venous plasma glucose level of > 11.1 mmol/L.

A distinction is made between diabetes mellitus and impaired glucose tolerance in cases where fasting or random blood sugar level is borderline; in this case, the response to an oral load of glucose can be assessed via a glucose tolerance test.

Fig. 10.20 Diagnostic criteria for diabetes mellitus using an oral glucose tolerance test

Diagnosis	Venous plasma blood glucose	
	Fasting sample	*2 hours after 75g glucose load*
Normal	<5.6 mmol/L	<7.8 mmol/L
Impaired glucose tolerance	5.6–6.9 mmol/L	7.8–11.0 mmol/L
Diabetes mellitus	≥7.0 mmol/L	≥11.1 mmol/L

Fig. 10.20 Diagnostic criteria for diabetes mellitus using an oral glucose tolerance test.

Complications of diabetes mellitus

Acute complications

Individuals with diabetes are particularly prone to several types of coma. These result from (in decreasing order of frequency):

- Hypoglycaemia—complication of overtreatment with insulin.
- Diabetic ketoacidosis (DKA)—common in type I diabetes due to ↑ breakdown of triglycerides → ↑ production of ketone bodies → ketoacidosis → impaired consciousness.
- Hyperosmolar non-ketotic (HONK) state— ↑ plasma glucose concentration → ↑ plasma osmolarity → cerebral dehydration → coma. More common in type II diabetes.
- Lactic acidosis—increased concentrations of lactic acid (produced as an end product of glycolysis instead of pyruvate) may cause coma.

The complications of DM are important; 80% of adults with diabetes die from cardiovascular disease and patients frequently develop serious renal and retinal disease.

Chronic complications

In recent years, with the advent of insulin therapy and various oral hypoglycaemic agents, morbidity and mortality associated with DM are more commonly the result of the chronic rather than the acute complications of the disorder (Fig. 10.21).

The complications of diabetes are macrovascular (affecting large and medium-sized muscular arteries) and microvascular (small vessel microangiopathy).

Macrovascular changes involve accelerated atherosclerosis. In diabetic microangiopathy, small arterioles and capillaries show a characteristic pattern of wall thickening, which is due to a marked expansion of the basement membrane (termed hyaline arteriolosclerosis).

Therefore, the most important chronic complications of diabetes are:

- Macrovascular accelerated atherosclerosis increasing stroke and myocardial infarction risk.
- Renal disease—diabetic nephropathy (mainly microvascular).
- Eye disease—diabetic retinopathy (microvascular).
- Peripheral nerve damage—diabetic neuropathy (microvascular).
- Predisposition to infections.

Macrovascular disease

Compared with non-affected people of the same age and sex, individuals with diabetes suffer from an increased severity of atherosclerosis, probably due to the increased plasma levels of cholesterol and triglycerides.

The main clinical sequelae of this are seen in:

- Heart → ischaemic heart disease.
- Brain → cerebral ischaemia.
- Legs and feet → gangrene—ischaemia of toes and areas on the heel is a characteristic feature of diabetic gangrene.
- Kidney → chronic nephron ischaemia, an important component of the multiple renal lesions in diabetes.

Diabetic nephropathy

Diabetes is now one of the most common causes of end-stage renal failure. Associated renal disease can be divided into three forms:

- Complications of diabetic vascular disease— macrovascular atherosclerosis affecting aorta and renal arteries → ischaemia; microvascular glomerular capillary basement membrane thickening (hyaline arteriolosclerosis) → ischaemic glomerular damage. Microalbuminuria is a reliable marker of the progression of diabetic nephropathy.

Fig. 10.21 Chronic complications of diabetes mellitus.

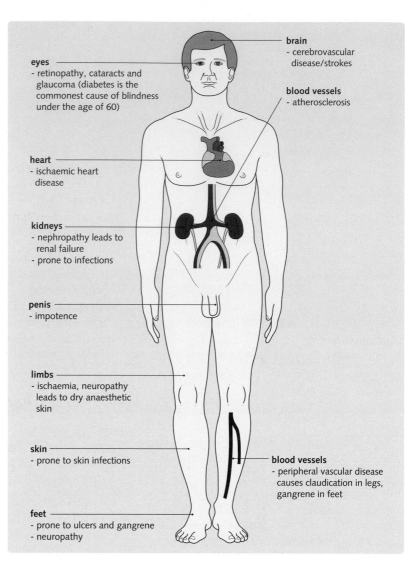

eyes
- retinopathy, cataracts and glaucoma (diabetes is the commonest cause of blindness under the age of 60)

brain
- cerebrovascular disease/strokes

blood vessels
- atherosclerosis

heart
- ischaemic heart disease

kidneys
- nephropathy leads to renal failure
- prone to infections

penis
- impotence

limbs
- ischaemia, neuropathy leads to dry anaesthetic skin

skin
- prone to skin infections

blood vessels
- peripheral vascular disease causes claudication in legs, gangrene in feet

feet
- prone to ulcers and gangrene
- neuropathy

- Diabetic glomerulosclerosis (diffuse and nodular types)—↑ leakage of plasma proteins through capillary wall into glomerular filtrate → proteinuria and progressive glomerular hyalinisation with eventual chronic renal failure.
- Increased susceptibility to infections → papillary necrosis. Acute pyelonephritis is a common complication of diabetes mellitus and occurs as a result of the relative immunosuppression of diabetes together with reduced neutrophil function.

Eye disease

Diabetes is the most common cause of acquired blindness in the Western world. It can affect the eyes in five main ways:

1. Background retinopathy—small vessel abnormalities in the retina leading to hard exudates, haemorrhages and microaneurysms. Does not usually affect acuity.
2. Proliferative retinopathy—extensive proliferation of new capillaries in the retina. Sudden deterioration in vision may result from vitreous haemorrhage as a consequence of proliferating new vessels or from the development of retinal detachment.
3. Maculopathy—caused by oedema, hard exudates or retinal ischaemia and results in a marked reduction of acuity.
4. Cataract formation—greatly increased incidence in individuals with diabetes.

5. Glaucoma—increased incidence in those with diabetes due to neovascularisation of the iris (rubeosis iridis).

Predisposition to infections

Patients with diabetes have an increased tendency to develop infections, usually of a bacterial or fungal nature. The main target organs are:

- Skin—folliculitis, erysipelas, cellulitis and superficial fungal infections.
- Oral and genital mucosae—especially with *Candida*.
- Urinary tract—increased predisposition to acute pyelonephritis, often associated with recurrent lower urinary tract infections.

Persistent glycosuria in individuals with poorly controlled diabetes predisposes to urinary and genital infection.

Diabetic neuropathy

Clinically, most cases of diabetic neuropathy affect the peripheral nervous system, although central nervous system pathology does occur. The main effects are:

- Microvascular thickening of basement membrane and microthrombi formation in small vessels supplying peripheral nerves.
- Axonal degeneration with patchy, segmental demyelination.
- Thickening of Schwann cell basal lamina.

The presentation may be of polyneuropathy (classically 'glove and stocking' sensory impairment), mononeuropathy (e.g. carpal tunnel syndrome) or autonomic neuropathy (symptoms include postural hypotension, nausea, vomiting, impotence and gustatory sweating).

Blood glucose control in diabetes lowers the incidence and progression of vascular complications. This can be achieved by:
- Diet alone—in type II patients.
- Diet and oral hypoglycaemic drugs (e.g. sulphonylureas, biguanides, thiazolidinediones)—in type II patients who fail on diet alone.
- Diet and insulin—all type I patients and some type II.

Pancreatic transplantation is curative in type I diabetes but is limited by organ availability. Islet cell transplants are a potential future therapy.

Islet cell tumours

These tumours are rare compared with those of the exocrine pancreas. They occur most commonly in individuals aged 30–50 years.

Insulinomas

The most common tumour of the islet cells. Insulinomas are derived from pancreatic β-cells:

- Produce hypoglycaemia through hypersecretion of insulin.
- May produce attacks of confusion, stupor and loss of consciousness.
- Majority are solitary, non-metastasising lesions (10% are multiple and 10% are malignant).

Zollinger–Ellison syndrome

This syndrome of gastric hypersecretion, multiple peptic ulcers and diarrhoea is caused by the gastrin-secreting tumour (gastrinoma) of the pancreatic G cells. Tumours are multiple in 50% of cases and are often malignant, with 10–20% occurring in other sites, e.g. the duodenum.

It may also be part of the MEN I syndrome, with adenomas also present in other endocrine glands (see below).

Other islet cell tumours

For a summary of islet cell tumours see Fig. 10.22.

VIPomas

These produce vasoactive intestinal polypeptide (VIP), resulting in a syndrome of watery diarrhoea, hypokalaemia and achlorhydria (WDHA).

Glucagonomas

These glucagon-secreting tumours are derived from pancreatic α-cells and cause secondary diabetes mellitus (usually mild), necrolytic migratory erythema (skin rash) and uraemia.

Somatostatinomas

These somatostatin-producing tumours derived from pancreatic δ-cells are associated with diabetes mellitus, cholelithiasis and steatorrhoea.

MULTIPLE ENDOCRINE NEOPLASIA SYNDROMES

These are syndromes in which patients develop tumours in a number of different endocrine organs.

Fig. 10.22 Summary of islet cell tumours.

Fig. 10.22 Summary of islet cell tumours		
Islet cell tumour	Occurrence	Clinical features
Insulinoma	70–75%	Hypoglycaemia
Gastrinoma	20–25%	Zollinger–Ellison syndrome: gastric hypersecretion, multiple peptic ulcers and diarrhoea
VIPoma	Rare	Water diarrhoea, hypokalaemia and achlorhydria
Glucagonoma	Rare	Secondary diabetes mellitus, necrolytic migratory erythema and uraemia
Somatostatinoma	Rare	Diabetes mellitus, cholelithiasis and steatorrhoea

Patients are younger than those who develop single sporadic tumours and usually have a strong family history of multiple endocrine tumours with autosomal dominant inheritance.

There are three main types of MEN syndrome:

1. MEN I (Werner's) syndrome.
2. MEN IIa (Sipple's) syndrome.
3. MEN IIb (sometimes called MEN III) syndrome.

MEN I (Werner's) syndrome

Patients usually show a combination of hyperparathyroidism (chief cell hyperplasia and adenomas), pituitary adenomas (usually prolactinomas) and pancreatic tumours (gastrin and insulin producing). Rarely, there may also be thyroid tumours and adrenal cortical adenomas. MEN I syndrome is caused by a germ-line mutation in the MEN-1 tumour suppressor gene.

MEN IIa (Sipple's) syndrome

Patients have a combination of phaeochromocytoma (50% bilateral) and medullary carcinoma of the thyroid (often bilateral and multinodular). Rarely, there may also be hyperparathyroidism due to parathyroid hyperplasia. MEN IIa and IIb syndromes have been linked to mutations in the *RET* oncogene, with near 100% disease penetrance

MEN IIb (MEN III) syndrome

Patients have all of the features of MEN IIa with additional features of:

- Neuromas and ganglioneuromas in the dermis and submucosal regions throughout the body.
- Marfanoid body habitus with poor muscle development.
- Skeletal abnormalities, e.g. kyphosis, pes cavus and high arch palate.

The facial appearance is characteristic with thick, bumpy lips, broad-based nose, everted eyelids and grossly abnormal dental enamel.

Genetic screening of at-risk family members in MEN II families now allows prophylactic thyroidectomy in those with RET mutations to avoid the near certainty of medullary carcinoma.

Pathology of the reproductive system

Objectives

In this chapter, you will learn to:

- Describe infection and neoplasia of the vulva, vagina and cervix, particularly cervical cancer.
- Understand inflammatory and neoplastic disease of the uterus and endometrium.
- Recall disorders of the ovary and fallopian tubes, with the focus on ovarian cancer.
- Describe ectopic pregnancies, spontaneous abortion and other disorders of the placenta and pregnancy.
- Understand the common forms of breast disease, particularly breast carcinoma.
- Briefly describe disorders of the penis.
- Recall testicular cancer and other disorders of the testis and epididymis.
- Describe benign prostatic hyperplasia and prostatic carcinoma.

DISORDERS OF THE VULVA, VAGINA AND CERVIX

Infections of the lower genital tract

Bartholin's cyst

This common, benign, mucus-secreting cyst on the vulva is derived from Bartholin's glands (mucus-secreting glands in the posterior part of the labia majora). Frequently there is superimposed infection—Bartholin's abscess.

Viral infection

Viral infections of the vulval skin are typically due to either herpes simplex virus (HSV) or human papillomavirus (HPV).

Herpes simplex virus

HSV type 2 infection of the vulva (herpes vulvitis) produces initially painless blisters, which subsequently break down to form a painful, sore, eroded area. HSV-2 infection is now a major sexually transmitted disease and is becoming more common in young women.

Human papillomavirus

This sexually transmitted disease may present with a thickening of the vulval skin and mucosa (flat condyloma) in the labia minora, or as multiple protuberant warts (condylomata acuminata) that can be either

sessile or pedunculated. There is a strong link between HPV infections of the vulva and intraepithelial neoplastic change in both the vulva (see below) and cervix.

Bacterial and protozoal infections

Gardnerella vaginalis

This Gram-negative coccobacillus is often associated with other sexually spread infections. The patient complains of a foul-smelling discharge, which is thin, greyish and sometimes shows bubbles. Examination confirms both the discharge and the odour.

Chlamydia trachomatis

One of the most common sexually transmitted diseases in the UK; 80% of women are asymptomatic, increasing the likelihood of silent spread amongst the population. Ascending infection into the upper genital tract (pelvic inflammatory disease) is increasingly common; this is an important cause of tubal infertility.

Genital infection with *Chlamydia trachomatis* may produce painful superficial groin nodes (lymphogranuloma venereum), which develop over weeks from initially painless vulval papules. Later, chronic lymphatic obstruction may lead to non-pitting oedema of the external genitalia.

Trichomonas vaginalis

This sexually transmitted flagellated protozoan is typically asymptomatic in men, but in women it often produces an intensely irritating vaginal discharge with inflammation of the vulva, vagina and cervix. The discharge is often frothy and offensive.

Treponema pallidum

Now rarely sexually transmitted, this spirochaetal bacterium is responsible for syphilis. This granulomatous disease typically involves three stages (primary, secondary and tertiary). It affects the penis in the primary stage.

- Primary—small indurated lesions (chancres) develop at the site of entry but then spontaneously heal.
- Secondary—occurs several weeks later and is characterised by multiple, moist, warty, vulvovaginal lesions (condylomata lata), with skin rashes and generalised illness (fever, malaise).
- Tertiary—develops in untreated individuals and often involves the CNS (see Chapter 5).

Fungal and yeast infection

Fungal infections are usually caused by either superficial dermatophytes or *Candida albicans*. There is usually associated fungal vaginitis, presenting with a copious vaginal discharge and vulval reddening and soreness.

Candida albicans

This is a normal commensal of the vagina but its proliferation is usually suppressed by commensal vaginal flora.

Conditions that predispose to candidal overgrowth are:

- Pregnancy/oestrogen contraceptives—high concentration of oestrogens in the blood.
- Immunosuppressive therapy, e.g. cytotoxic drugs and corticosteroids.
- Glycosuria, e.g. diabetes, pregnancy (due to lowering of the renal threshold for sugar).
- Antibiotic therapy—destruction of normal commensal bacteria.
- Chronic anaemia—iron stores are needed to maintain an adequate immune reaction.

Macroscopically, white plaques of fungal hyphae develop on inflamed vaginal mucosa. Vaginal discharge is associated with severe vulval irritation. Infections are often severe in people with diabetes.

Dermatophytes

Infection of vulval skin with dermatophytic fungi produces a similar superficial inflammation and soreness.

Treatment

Both candidal infections and dermatophytes can be treated with antifungal pessaries or systemic therapy.

Figure 11.1 shows the organisms that cause infections of the lower genital tract.

Dysplastic and neoplastic disorders of the vulva and vagina

Tumours of the vulva

Squamous cell carcinoma

This is the most common malignant tumour of the vulva, typically occurring in elderly women and often showing extensive local invasion and metastases to the inguinal lymph nodes. The majority of cases appear to arise *de novo*, but some form from dysplastic epithelium amounting to carcinoma *in situ*, known as vulval intraepithelial neoplasia.

It is also thought that squamous cell carcinoma may develop from areas of lichen sclerosus (atrophic lesions that are most common after the menopause).

Vulval intraepithelial neoplasia

This is generally seen in patients younger than those with invasive tumours. In 90% of cases there is coexistent evidence of incorporated HPV DNA (especially serotypes 16 and 18), usually with visible warty change in the affected and adjacent epithelium. Although invasive carcinoma and vulval intraepithelial neoplasia (VIN) do occasionally coexist in elderly women, it is thought that progression of VIN to invasive carcinoma is not common.

Tumours of the vagina

Dysplastic

Vaginal intraepithelial neoplasia (VAIN) is rare compared with cervical intraepithelial neoplasia (CIN).

Fig. 11.1 Organisms that cause infections of the lower genital tract

Infection	Organism
Viruses	HPV HSV
Bacteria	*Gardnerella vaginalis* *Chlamydia trachomatis* (lymphogranuloma venereum) *Treponema pallidum* (syphilis)
Protozoa	*Trichomonas vaginalis*
Fungi and yeast	Dermatophytes, *Candida albicans*

Fig. 11.1 Organisms that cause infections of the lower genital tract.

Most cases are found in women previously treated for CIN or invasive cervical cancer.

Neoplastic

Primary malignant tumours of the vagina are extremely rare, but include squamous cell carcinomas and adenocarcinomas.

Secondary tumours are more common, particularly from malignant tumours of the cervix, endometrium, and ovary. Vaginal bleeding after hysterectomy for uterine or ovarian malignancy should always be investigated and biopsied because of the frequency of metastatic tumour in the residual vaginal vault.

Inflammation of the cervix

Acute and chronic cervicitis

Acute and chronic inflammation of the cervix is particularly common in the presence of an intrauterine contraceptive device.

Acute cervicitis

There is acute inflammation of the cervix with erosion. It is occasionally seen in herpes simplex infection, typically with herpetic disease of the vulva and vagina.

Chronic cervicitis

This chronic inflammation of the cervix is typically caused by the same organisms responsible for infective vaginitis: *Trichomonas*, *Candida* and *Gardnerella* species and the gonococci. It is characterised by a heavy plasma cell and lymphocytic infiltrate.

Endocervical polyps

These common abnormalities derived from the endocervix affect up to 5% of women. Large polyps may protrude from the cervix through the external os and can cause intermenstrual bleeding from erosion and ulceration.

Macroscopically, these are smooth, rounded or pear-shaped polyps about 1–2 cm in diameter.

Microscopically, they are composed of endocervical stroma and glands. The surface of the polyp may show ulceration and inflammation, often accompanied by squamous metaplasia.

Neoplasia of the cervix

Cervical intraepithelial neoplasia

Cervical intraepithelial neoplasia (CIN) is the pre-neoplastic (dysplastic) proliferation of epithelium of the transformation zone of the cervix.

Aetiology—there is a strong association with HPV infection, particularly serotypes 16 and 18.

Risk factors are:

- Sexual intercourse—very low incidence in virgins, with increased risk in those who have had multiple sexual partners and first intercourse at an early age.
- Human papillomavirus—DNA from HPV types 16, 18, 31 or 33 has been identified in over 90% of cervical carcinomas. Proteins produced by HPV are thought to inactivate products of tumour suppressor genes thereby facilitating tumour development. For example, the viral protein E6 of HPV subtype 16 can bind and inactivate the function of the *p53* tumour suppressor protein (see Chapter 3). It is likely that new HPV vaccines targeted against serotypes 16 and 18 will reduce HPV infection and CIN development.
- Combined oral contraceptive pill—prolonged use is associated with an increased risk in those who carry HPV infection (may be linked to increased sexual risk-taking when on contraceptive pill).
- Smoking—associated with increased risk.
- Immunosuppression—predisposes to carcinoma of the cervix, e.g. HIV patients.

Classification

Three grades of severity are recognised. Grading depends on the proportion of the cervical epithelium wall that is replaced by atypical cells:

1. CIN I (mild dysplasia)—upper two-thirds of the epithelium normal, basal third atypical cells.
2. CIN II (moderate dysplasia)—upper half of the epithelium normal, atypical cells occupy the lower half.
3. CIN III (severe dysplasia)—corresponds to carcinoma *in situ*. Atypical cells extend throughout the full thickness of the epithelium with minimal differentiation and maturation on the surface.

Progression

CIN is associated with a risk of progression to an invasive carcinoma, the risk for CIN I being lowest and for CIN III being the highest.

The natural history of CIN is important as it determines how often screening is required to detect progression of the disease.

Cervical screening aims to detect preinvasive atypical cells by cytological examination of surface epithelial cells. Smears repeated every 3 years are considered adequate for population screening (from 20 to 65 years old). In the UK it is estimated that regular attendance at screening prevents up to 90% of cervical cancer. Management of CIN is by the local destruction of abnormal epithelium using cryotherapy, laser therapy or cone biopsy following histological confirmation of its nature.

Squamous cell carcinoma

The vast majority of cervical carcinomas are squamous cell carcinomas arising from the transformation zone or ectocervix.

There are around 3000 cases of cervical cancer in the UK each year, with 1300 deaths. This equates to a lifetime risk of around 1% (similar across the developed world), compared to 5% in parts of the developing world where screening programs do not exist. This type of carcinoma occurs in all ages from late teens onwards, but the average age is 45 years.

The carcinoma is preceded by the preinvasive phase of CIN (see above and Fig. 11.2). Risk factors are as for CIN.

Macroscopically, tumours demonstrate the following features (Fig. 11.2):

- Early—areas of granular irregularity of the cervical epithelium, with progressive invasion of the stroma causing abnormal hardness of the cervix.
- Late—fungating ulcerated areas, which doestroy the cervix.

Microscopically, lesions may be keratinising or non-keratinising.

The common presenting symptom is vaginal bleeding in the early stages. Advanced neglected tumours may cause urinary obstruction due to bladder involvement.

Invasive carcinomas are managed according to the degree of local invasion and survival is related to the stage of the disease (Fig. 11.3).

Early invasive carcinoma is usually managed by radical hysterectomy and/or radiotherapy, whereas advanced disease is usually only amenable to radiotherapy and/or chemotherapy. Involvement of the para-aortic lymph nodes is associated with a very poor prognosis.

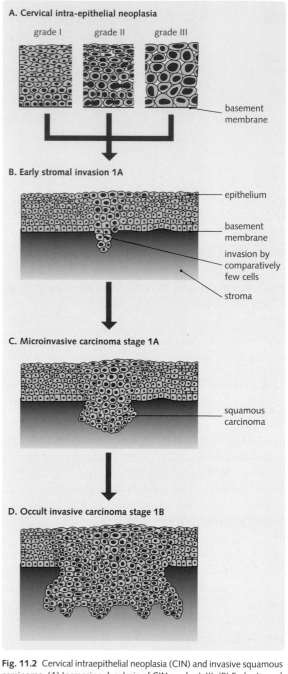

Fig. 11.2 Cervical intraepithelial neoplasia (CIN) and invasive squamous carcinoma. (A) Increasing dysplasia of CIN grades I–III. (B) Early stromal invasion of < 1 mm. (C) Micro-invasive carcinoma with invasion of < 3 mm. (D) Occult invasive carcinoma with invasion > 500 mm³. There is some risk of spread to the lymph nodes but the tumour is still clinically undetectable. (Adapted from Underwood, 2000.)

Fig. 11.3 Stages and prognosis for carcinomas of the cervix		
Stage	**5-year survival (%)**	**Degree of local invasion**
I	85–90	Confined to cervix
II	60	Invasion of upper part of vagina or adjacent parametrial tissues
III	40	Spread to pelvic side wall, lower vagina or ureters
IV	15	Invasion of rectum, bladder wall or outside pelvis

Fig. 11.3 Stages and prognosis for carcinomas of the cervix.

DISORDERS OF THE UTERUS AND ENDOMETRIUM

Inflammatory disorders

Chronic endometritis

An inflammation of the endometrium, chronic endometritis is typically associated with menstrual irregularities and is often found in women who are being investigated for infertility.

Microscopically, there is lymphoid and plasma cell infiltration of the endometrium.

Risk factors—the majority of cases are associated with a definite clinical risk factor for developing inflammation:

- Recent pregnancy, miscarriage or instrumentation (50% of cases).
- Chronic pelvic inflammatory disease, e.g. following chlamydial infection (25% of cases).
- Use of an intrauterine contraceptive device (about 20% of cases).
- Tuberculosis in developing countries (5% of cases).

Disorders of the endometrium

Adenomyosis

This is a condition in which the endometrium grows down to develop deep within the myometrium, occurring in 20% of women. This may cause enlargement of the uterus and is sometimes associated with menstrual abnormalities and dysmenorrhoea.

Macroscopically there are small, irregular, endometrial lesions—some of which are cystic—that can be seen within the affected myometrium. Involvement of the myometrium may be diffuse (more common) or focal with deep nodules of endometrium (nodular adenomyosis).

Microscopically, irregular nests of endometrial stroma are found deep within muscle but in continuity with surface endometrium.

Endometriosis

This is defined as endometrial glands or stroma occurring outside the uterus, and still capable of responding to cyclical hormonal stimulation. Phases of proliferation and breakdown are associated with the development of the fibrous adhesions and accumulation of haemosiderin pigment. This affects 1 in 15 women of reproductive age. There are numerous sites:

- Common—ovaries, fallopian tubes, round ligaments, pelvic peritoneum.
- Less common—intestinal wall, bladder, umbilicus, laparotomy scars.

Theories of origin

The aetiopathogenesis of endometriosis remains unclear but three main theories operate to various degrees:

1. Retrograde menstruation—fragments of endometrium migrate along the fallopian tubes during menstruation.
2. Metaplasia of peritoneal epithelium— differentiation of peritoneal epithelium into endometrium.
3. Metastatic spread of endometrium, via the blood or lymphatic vessels.

Macroscopically, the foci of endometriosis appear as cystic and solid masses, which are characteristically dark brown because of accumulated iron pigment from repeated bleeding.

Microscopically, solid masses of endometriosis are composed of endometrial glands and stroma, fibrosis, and macrophages containing iron pigments.

Endometriosis may present with cyclical pelvic pain, dysmenorrhoea and infertility.

The complications are:

- Infertility (about 30% of cases)—often due to adhesions and blockages affecting ovulatory pathways.

- Bowel obstruction—due to fibrous adhesions between adjacent organs.
- Chocolate cysts—the whole of the fallopian tube and ovary may be converted into a cystic mass containing brown, semi-liquid material.

Endometriosis is dependent on oestrogen for continued growth and proliferation, with the disease becoming inactive after oophorectomy or onset of the menopause. Thus, induction of the hypo-oestrogenic state by suppression of ovulation is effective in many cases (e.g. continuous progesterone therapy).

Functional endometrial disorders

Anovulatory cycle

An anovulatory cycle is one that is not associated with the development and release of the ovum from the ovary. This is normal and common at both the start and end of reproductive life. Several follicles may start to develop and for a time produce hormones. However, the attempt ends in atresia and the atretic follicle is absorbed.

It is associated with irregular menstruation, although the effects of excessive oestrogen stimulation are manifest in the endometrium as the proliferation of glands.

Other causes of anovulation are listed in Fig. 11.4.

Inadequate luteal phase

The irregular ripening of a follicle is associated with infertility. This may be caused by failure of the production of progesterone by the corpus luteum or by defective receptors for progesterone within the endometrium. Examination of the endometrium in the second half of the menstrual cycle shows inadequate or absent development of secretory changes.

Effects of contraceptives and hormone replacement therapy

Oral contraceptive pill

This causes changes in the structure of the endometrium, which is greatly reduced in bulk. Glands become small and inactive with poor development of stroma.

Intrauterine devices (IUD)

Newer versions of these contraceptive devices (e.g. Mirena coil) act locally within the uterus by slowly releasing progesterone (over several years) to prevent endometrial proliferation.

Older, copper-bearing IUDs act as a foreign body within the uterus to virtually eliminate the chance of successful implantation.

The initial insertion of IUDs is associated with a slight increase in the risk of pelvic inflammatory disease.

Hormone replacement therapy (HRT)

The menopause is the cessation of menstruation. It normally occurs between 45 and 56 years of age due to exhaustion of the supply of oocytes and because of a more refractory receptor function in the granulosa and thecal cells.

After the menopause, endometrial glands may form large cystic spaces. There is no evidence of mitotic activity, reflecting a lack of oestrogenic stimulation. The uterus becomes smaller and less supported due to atrophy of the cardinal, uterosacral and uteropubic ligaments.

HRT provides mainly oestrogenic supplementation to reduce some of the side effects of the menopause and protects against osteoporosis. However, unopposed oestrogen therapy (i.e. no progesterone) is

Fig. 11.4 Non-physiological causes of anovulation.

Fig. 11.4 Non-physiological causes of anovulation

Type	Cause	Clinical feature
Primary ovarian dysfunction	Genetic	e.g. Turner's syndrome, autoimmune
Secondary ovarian dysfunction	Disorders of gonadotrophin regulation	Hyperprolactinaemia
	Gonadotrophin deficiency	Pituitary tumour Pituitary infarction Pituitary ablation
	Functional	Weight loss Exercise
	Polycystic ovary syndrome	Associated with obesity and insulin resistance

associated with endometrial hyperplasia and carcinoma, and increased thromboembolic disease. Combined HRT (i.e. oestrogen and progesterone) increases the risk of breast cancer.

Endometrial hyperplasia

Hyperplasia of the endometrium typically occurs in the third and fourth decades of life, in response to oestrogenic stimulation. It presents with haemorrhage but the severity or frequency is not related to the degree of pathological change. Certain types of endometrial hyperplasia are associated with a degree of risk for malignant change (severe/atypical hyperplasia).

Figure 11.5 shows the different types of endometrial hyperplasia.

The importance of endometrial hyperplasia is that it is associated with an increased risk of the development of endometrial adenocarcinoma, i.e. it is thought to be preneoplastic.

Neoplastic disorders

Benign

Endometrial polyps

These localised overgrowths of endometrial glands and stroma are very common and are typically seen in the perimenopausal age range. They are caused by inappropriate proliferation of glands in response to oestrogenic stimuli.

Macroscopically, they are found in the uterine fundus projecting into the endometrial cavity; their size is variable but they are usually 1–3 cm in diameter. They have a firm, smooth, nodular appearance within the endometrial cavity but occasionally prolapse through the cervical os. They may ulcerate or undergo torsion.

Microscopically, they are cystically dilated endometrial glands in a vascular stroma.

Clinical features are associated with menstrual abnormalities and dysmenorrhoea.

Fibroids (leiomyomas)

These benign, smooth muscle tumours arise in the muscle wall of the uterus (myometrium). They are the most common of all pelvic tumours, affecting over half of all women over the age of 30, usually becoming symptomatic in the decade before the menopause. Their cause is unknown but risk factors include:

- Age—rare under 30 years.
- Race—more common in Afro-Caribbean populations.
- Parity—more common in nulliparous and women with low fertility.
- Genetic—often a family history.

Leiomyomas have the following features:

- Oestrogen sensitive.
- Fast growing in pregnancy.
- Shrink at menopause or with antigonadotrophic hormone therapy.

Fig. 11.5 Types of endometrial hyperplasia

Degree of hyperplasia	Morphological features	Progression to adenocarcinoma (%)	Time taken (years) to develop into adenocarcinoma
Mild (most common)	Cystic glandular hyperplasia with characteristic appearance of 'Swiss cheese'. (Previously known as metropathia haemorrhagica.) Cells show no cytological atypia	1	10
Moderate	Crowding of glands in a back-to-back fashion. Epithelium is stratified and mitoses are relatively frequent. Cells show no cytological atypia	5	7
Severe	Cellular atypia is prominent, glands are distorted by intraglandular polypoid formations, and mitoses are frequent	30	4

Fig. 11.5 Types of endometrial hyperplasia.

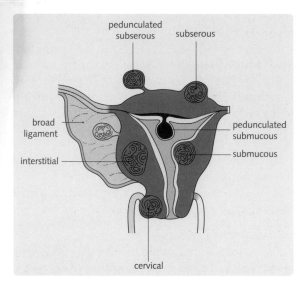

Fig. 11.6 Fibroids within the uterus.

Sites within the uterus (Fig. 11.6) are:

- Subserous—just beneath the peritoneum on the outer uterine surface.
- Interstitial (most common)—surrounded by smooth muscle.
- Submucous—lying immediately below the endometrium.

Macroscopically, they are:

- Rounded, rubbery, pale nodules with whorled appearance on cut surface.
- Well circumscribed with pseudocapsule that may become pedunculated forming polyps.
- Size is variable. Most common are 2–4 cm but they range from < 1 cm to 20–30 cm in diameter.
- Typically multiple.

Microscopically, they are seen as:

- Islands of smooth muscle cells with intervening collagenous stroma.
- Lacking cellular atypia and with very few mitoses (compared to malignant leiomyosarcomas). Malignant change in leiomyomas is considered extremely rare.

Clinical features—leiomyomas may present with abnormal menstrual bleeding, dysmenorrhoea and infertility.

Complications occur following ischaemic degeneration, pregnancy and compression.

Investigations are by ultrasound and laparoscopy.

Management is:

- Surgical—women who no longer wish to conceive usually undergo hysterectomy.
- Medical—uterine leiomyomas may be shrunk by gonadotrophin-releasing hormone (GnRH) agonists, which induce hypo-oestrogenism. This allows easier surgical removal by myomectomy.

> Remember that fibroids are not fibromas. Fibroids are benign tumours of smooth muscle (leiomyomas).

Malignant

Endometrial carcinoma

Adenocarcinomas of the endometrium are the second most common gynaecological malignancy. The mean age of presentation is 56 years, and 80% of women are postmenopausal.

Endometrial carcinoma is associated with:

- Hyperoestrogenic state—obesity, diabetes, late menopause, prolonged use of unopposed oestrogens, oestrogen-secreting tumours.
- Previous pelvic irradiation.
- Lower parity.

There are two main groups: hyperoestrogenic and non-hyperoestrogenic tumours.

Hyperoestrogenic tumours (type 1 disease)—these are associated with a generally good prognosis. They occur in patients close to the menopause, associated with an abnormal oestrogenic stimulation of the endometrium and endometrial hyperplasia. Most tumours are adenocarcinomas (60%) and are graded (I–III) according to the amount of glandular and solid pattern within the tumour. High-grade tumour is associated with a worse prognosis.

Non-hyperoestrogenic tumours (type 2 disease)—these are more often associated with a poor prognosis, occur in older postmenopausal women and are not associated with oestrogenic stimulation or endometrial hyperplasia.

Macroscopically, there are:

- Small tumours—diffuse, solid areas or polypoid lesions in the endometrium.
- Larger tumours—fill and distend the endometrial cavity with soft, white, friable tissue.

Fig. 11.7 Clinical staging of endometrial cancer

Stage	Proportion of cases (%)	Degree of invasion	5-year survival (%)
I	75	Corpus of uterus only	85
II	10	Corpus and cervix	65
III	10	Invasion confined to pelvis	40
IV	5	Invasion outside pelvis or involves bladder or rectal mucosa	10

Fig. 11.7 Clinical staging of endometrial cancer.

Microscopically, they are seen as:

- Hyperoestrogenic tumours—typically well-differentiated adenocarcinomas composed of hyperplastic endometrial glandular tissue with only superficial myometrial invasion at diagnosis.
- Non-hyperoestrogenic tumours—typically poorly differentiated with deep myometrial invasion.

The condition classically presents as postmenopausal bleeding.

The main route of spread is by local invasion to the fallopian tubes, ovaries, bladder, or rectum.

If venous and lymphatic invasion occurs, there may be involvement of the vagina and para-aortic nodes. Widespread haematogenous metastasis is uncommon except with papillary serous carcinomas and clear cell carcinomas.

The amount of direct invasion into the myometrium is closely correlated with prognosis.

The prognosis of uterine carcinoma is related to stage (Fig. 11.7).

DISORDERS OF THE OVARY AND FALLOPIAN TUBE

Inflammatory disorders and infections

Salpingitis

Inflammation of the fallopian tube(s).

Suppurative salpingitis

Aetiology—it is almost always caused by ascending infection from the uterine cavity.

Predisposing factors are:

- Following pregnancy and endometritis.
- Following insertion of an IUD.

- Sexually transmitted disease (*Mycoplasma*, *Chlamydia* and gonococci).

Macroscopically, tubes are swollen and congested, and the serosal surface appears red and granular due to vascular dilatation.

Microscopically, tubal epithelium shows neutrophil infiltration and the lumen may contain pus.

Chronic inflammation may supervene, with sequelae of fibrosis and occlusion of the tubal lumen on resolution.

Complications are:

- Infertility—fibrosis causes distortion of mucosal plicae and occlusion of tubal lumen.
- Pyosalpinx—massive distension of tubal lumen by pus.
- Hydrosalpinx—dilatation of a fallopian tube by clear watery fluid (product of the proteolysis of pus on resolution of an infection).

Tuberculous salpingitis

This is a rare tuberculous infection of the fallopian tubes caused by the spread of *Mycobacterium tuberculosis* from outside the genital tract.

Tubes develop multiple granulomas in the mucosa and wall, causing adhesions to adjacent tissues (especially ovaries). In advanced cases, tubes may develop into cavities filled with caseous necrotic material.

Pelvic inflammatory disease

Pelvic inflammatory disease (PID) is a combined infection of the fallopian tubes, ovaries and peritoneum. It is typically a result of ascending infection or, less commonly, postoperative infection. Predisposing factors are as for suppurative salpingitis (see above).

Neisseria gonorrhoeae and *Chlamydia trachomatis* are the most common responsible organisms, although anaerobic organisms are often found in pelvic abscesses.

Inflammation is initially acute and, without prompt treatment, may progress to chronic PID, which often results in tubal infertility.

Clinical features are:

- Symptoms— gradual onset of pelvic pain, irregular bleeding, vaginal discharge, fever.
- Signs—abdominal tenderness and guarding; extreme tenderness of the adnexa.

Treatment is by the removal of an IUD (if present) and the use of broad-spectrum antibiotics.

Cysts

Ovarian cysts

Ovarian cystic lesions are extremely common. They can be either neoplastic or non-neoplastic. The majority of non-neoplastic cysts arise from developing Graafian follicles; a minority is derived from surface epithelium.

Follicular cysts

These unruptured, enlarged Graafian follicles are lined by granulosa cells, with an outer coat of thecal cells. Normal ovaries commonly contain one or more small cysts (< 5 cm in diameter), which typically disappear by the resorption of fluid. However, multiple follicular cysts are found in:

- Mild endometrial (cystic) hyperplasia—also termed metropathia haemorrhagica.
- Polycystic ovary syndrome (see below).

Most cysts are clinically insignificant though some may be a cause of hyperoestrogenism.

Luteal cysts (luteinized follicular cysts)

These are similar to follicular cysts, except the thecal coat is luteinized. These occasionally rupture to cause a peritoneal reaction.

Polycystic ovary syndrome (PCOS)

This is a complex adrenal–ovarian disorder in which multiple small follicular cysts develop beneath a thickened, white ovarian capsule as a result of increased androgenic activity. This is thought to be secondary to a decrease in peripheral insulin sensitivity (promoted by obesity) causing hyperinsulinaemia.

Clinical features—patients have a persistent anovulatory state, high levels of luteinizing hormone (LH) and oestrogen, low levels of follicle-stimulating hormone (FSH) and high levels of circulating androgen.

Common presenting symptoms are:

- Menstrual irregularity.
- Infertility.

- Hirsutism.
- Acne.
- Occasional galactorrhoea.

Complications—high oestrogen levels may cause endometrial hyperplasia and increase the risk of the development of endometrial carcinoma. Cardiovascular disease, diabetes mellitus and breast cancer are also increased in this group.

Cysts of the fallopian tubes

Benign cysts of the fallopian tubes are common. There are two main types:

1. Fimbrial cysts—extremely common, small, benign cysts containing clear fluid. Unilocular and typically situated at the fimbrial end of the tube.
2. Cysts of Morgagni (paratubal cysts)—cystic lesions situated adjacent to the fimbrial ends of the fallopian tubes and thought to be derived from remnants of the Müllerian duct.

Neoplastic disorders of the ovary

Ovarian cancer is responsible for more deaths than any other gynaecological malignancy (5000 cases per year in the UK, with 3700 deaths), largely because it often presents at an advanced stage. The ovarian tumour marker CA125 is used routinely to monitor for relapse in patients who have undergone treatment. CA125, along with other markers, may be used in future screening programs for ovarian cancer.

Primary ovarian cancers account for 6% of all malignancies in women, but only 5–10% have a direct hereditary component. In these women, mutations are usually found on either the *BRCA1* or *BRCA2* tumour suppressor genes (see Chapter 3). Ninety-five per cent of ovarian cancer cases are sporadic and show complex genetic abnormalities including a high incidence of *p53* mutation (50% of cases) and amplification of the *erbB-2* (*HER-2/neu*) oncogene (30% of cases). There are several different tumour types.

A logical way of classifying ovarian tumours is according to the normal tissue constituents from which they are derived:
- Surface epithelial tumours (70% of all cases).
- Germ cell tumours (20% of all cases).
- Sex cord and stromal tumours (10% of all cases).

Surface epithelial stromal tumours

Epithelial tumours of the ovary comprise about 70% of all ovarian tumours and about 90% of malignant tumours. They are typically found in adult life.

As with all ovarian tumours, it appears that there is a decreased risk associated with pregnancy and the oral contraceptive pill. This is part of the 'incessant ovulation' hypothesis, whereby continuous monthly repair of the ovarian epithelium has been suggested as one factor in the development of ovarian cancer.

Types—epithelial tumours are derived from surface epithelium, which in turn is derived from embryonal coelomic epithelium. Tumours with this origin can differentiate along different pathways into different types of tumours: tubal differentiation (serous tumours), endometrial differentiation (endometrial and clear cell tumours), endocervical differentiation (mucinous tumours) and transitional differentiation (Brenner tumours).

Microscopically, these tumours are classified into benign, malignant and borderline (abnormal tissue architecture with atypical cells but no evidence of invasion). The majority of borderline tumours behave in a benign fashion but some appear capable of low-grade malignancy.

Serous tumours of the ovary

These ovarian cystic tumours of tubal differentiation contain a watery fluid; the majority (70%) are benign:

- Benign (serous cystadenoma)—thin-walled, unilocular cystic tumour lined by cuboidal regular epithelium.
- Malignant (serous cystadenocarcinoma)—characterised by pleomorphic cells and mitoses with invasion of the ovarian stroma. Over half of cases occur bilaterally. A frequent histological finding is concentrically laminated calcified concretions called Psammoma bodies.
- Borderline serous tumours—presence of cellular atypia but with no invasion.

Mucinous tumours of the ovary

These multilocular cystic ovarian tumours of endocervical differentiation contain gelatinous material:

- Benign (mucinous cystadenoma)—no atypical features or mitoses.
- Malignant (mucinous cystadenocarcinoma)—invasion of the ovarian stroma. Less than 10% of mucinous tumours are malignant.
- Borderline mucinous tumours—presence of cellular atypia but with no invasion.

Endometrioid tumours

These ovarian tumours show endometrial differentiation. The vast majority are malignant (endometrioid carcinomas), accounting for 20% of all ovarian carcinomas.

The clear cell carcinoma is a variant of endometrioid carcinoma, characterised by the presence of cells with clear cytoplasm and containing abundant glycogen.

Brenner tumours of the ovary (transitional cell)

Tumours composed of nests of epithelium resembling the transitional cell epithelium of the urinary tract; these are associated with a spindle-cell stroma. The epithelial component may be benign, borderline, or malignant. The majority are unilateral and benign.

Germ cell and sex-cord stromal tumours are illustrated in Fig. 11.8.

Metastatic

The ovary is a common site of tumour metastasis. This may be of Müllerian origin (e.g. uterus, fallopian tubes) or from extra-Müllerian sites (typically the breast and gastrointestinal tract).

Krukenberg's tumour

This describes bilaterally enlarged ovaries containing metastatic signet ring-cell adenocarcinoma (typically of gastric origin).

Tumours of the fallopian tubes

Tumours of the fallopian tubes are extremely rare. They can be benign or malignant.

Benign

Adenomatoid tumours

These are typically subserosal or in the mesosalpinx (part of the broad ligament).

Malignant

Malignant tumours of the fallopian tubes can be:

- Primary—adenocarcinomas, typically affecting postmenopausal women. Poor prognosis due to late presentation.
- Secondary—from the endometrium or pelvic peritoneum.

DISORDERS OF THE PLACENTA AND PREGNANCY

Ectopic pregnancies

This describes any fertilised ovum that is implanted outside the uterine cavity. Ectopics occur in about 1 in

Fig. 11.8 Germ cell and sex cord stromal ovarian tumours.

Fig. 11.8 Germ cell and sex-cord stromal ovarian tumours

Tumour	Features
Germ cell tumours	
Teratoma	
Benign cystic teratomas (dermoid cyst)	Cysts may be lined by structures such as the skin, hair, teeth, bone, or respiratory tract tissue
Solid teratomas	Composed of a variety of tissues, including cartilage, smooth muscle, or epithelium
Dysgerminoma	
	Similar to seminoma of the testis
Yolk-sac tumours	
	Cystic, solid, and haemorrhagic; secrete α-fetoprotein
Sex-cord stromal tumours	
Granulosa cell tumours	Composed of granulosa cells derived from follicles
Sertoli–Leydig cell tumours	Mixture of cell types usually seen in the testis
Gonadoblastomas	Primitive germ cells and sex-cord stromal derivatives are present
Steroid cell tumours	Composed of cortical adrenal like cells containing abundant lipid

300 pregnancies. The fallopian tube (especially in the ampulla) is by far the most common site for this; other sites of abnormal implantation are very rare but include the peritoneal cavity, the ovary and the cervix.

The aetiology is uncertain but ectopic pregnancies are possibly the result of some structural abnormality of the fallopian tube, e.g. scarring or adhesions resulting from previous episodes of salpingitis or endometriosis, or previous tubal surgery for contraceptive purposes, i.e. sterilisation. However, half of ectopic pregnancies occur without such predisposing factors.

Pathogenesis—following implantation, the proliferation of trophoblasts erodes the submucosal blood vessels, precipitating severe bleeding into the tubal lumen (haematosalpinx). The muscular wall of the fallopian tube is unable to undergo hypertrophy or distension, and so tubal pregnancy almost always results in the rupture of the fallopian tube and death of the fertilised ovum. This typically occurs in the early stages of pregnancy and often before the patient is even aware of being pregnant.

The types of rupture are:

- Into the lumen of the fallopian tube—common in ampullary pregnancy. Conceptus is extruded towards the fimbriated end of the tube. Mild haemorrhage into the peritoneal cavity occurs, which may collect as a clot in the pouch of Douglas.
- Into the peritoneal cavity—occurs most commonly from the isthmus of the tube, either spontaneously or as a result of pressure (e.g. straining at the stool, coitus or pelvic examination). Haemorrhage is likely to be severe.
- Retroperitoneal (rare)—rupture occurs into the potential space between the leaves of the broad ligament. Haemorrhage into the site is more likely to be controlled.

Clinical features of an ectopic rupture are:
- Severe lower abdominal pain—usually localised to the side of the ectopic pregnancy.
- Vaginal bleeding—occurs after fetal death, and is an effect of oestrogen withdrawal.
- Signs of anaemia—due to internal blood loss.
- Shock may occur if haemorrhage is severe and rapid, e.g. due to large vessel erosion. This is the most dangerous and dramatic consequence of tubal pregnancy.

Spontaneous abortion

Many fertilised ova fail to implant successfully. It has been estimated that around 40% of all conceptions fail to convert into recognisable pregnancies. Of those that survive this far, 15% terminate in a clinically recognised spontaneous abortion.

Aetiology—causes of spontaneous abortion differ according to the stage of pregnancy, as shown in Fig. 11.9.

Types of spontaneous abortions
Threatened
There is vaginal bleeding in an ongoing pregnancy. The cervix is closed but there may be a few painful uterine contractions. The pregnancy is likely to continue.

Inevitable
Bleeding with some cervical dilatation and often severe abdominal cramps. By definition, spontaneous abortion cannot be prevented from this point.

Incomplete
Expulsion of some, but not all, of the products of conception. Abortion is usually completed by curettage to prevent prolonged bleeding and reduce infection risk.

Complete
All the products of conception (fetus and placenta) have been passed per vaginum and the uterus is empty. There is little bleeding, the uterus is small and the cervix closed.

Missed (silent) abortion
The embryo fails to develop or dies *in utero* but the products of conception are not expelled. The whole pregnancy is gradually absorbed, and often presents gynaecologically as an unexplained amenorrhoea. After about 12 weeks, the formation of a carneous mole (lobulated mass of ovum and clotted blood) is likely and after 18 weeks a macerated fetus is usually expelled.

Recurrent
This refers to three or more consecutive spontaneous abortions.

Fig. 11.9 Causes of spontaneous abortion.

Fig. 11.9 Causes of spontaneous abortion

Time	Cause
First trimester	Abnormal chromosomal karyotypes, particularly Turner's syndrome Structural developmental abnormalities, e.g. neural tube defects Maternal SLE Transplacental infection, e.g. *Brucella*, *Listeria*, rubella, *Toxoplasma*, cytomegalovirus and herpes
Second trimester	Chorioamnionitis Rupture of membranes Placental haemorrhages Structural abnormalities of the uterus, e.g. congenital uterine malformations Large submucosal leiomyomas Incompetence of the cervix Abnormal placentation (but more common in third trimester)
Third trimester	Uncontrolled hypertension Eclampsia Placental abnormalities, e.g. placental haemorrhage, abruption and infarction
At any time	Endocrine abnormalities: diabetes, hypothyroidism, deficiency of progesterone or luteinizing hormone Trauma: surgical operation, blow to abdomen, or hypotensive shock

Note: SLE, systemic lupus erythematosus.

To remember the causes of abortion at different stages of pregnancy, learn the following rules of thumb:

- First trimester causes—majority are associated with abnormal fetuses.
- Second trimester causes—mainly due to uterine abnormalities.
- Third trimester causes—mainly the result of maternal abnormalities.

Pre-eclampsia and eclampsia

Pre-eclampsia

This is high blood pressure (> 140/90 mmHg) and proteinuria developing during pregnancy in a woman whose blood pressure was previously normal. An increase in blood pressure alone is termed gestational hypertension. Hypertensive disorders occur in about 10% of all pregnant women. The aetiology is unknown.

Risk factors are:

- First pregnancy (primigravidae)—increased risk.
- Multiple pregnancies (e.g. twins).
- Medical comorbidities—diabetes, pre-existing hypertension, systemic lupus erythaematosus (SLE).
- Extremes of maternal age—older or younger women.
- Family history.

The pathology is unclear but probably relates to inadequate placental invasion by spiral arteries, leading to placental ischaemia. This is thought to release a chemical factor that triggers vasoconstriction and endothelial damage to promote hypertension.

Endothelial cells of kidney arterioles become swollen and fibrin deposition occurs in glomeruli leading to proteinuria (Fig. 11.10).

Pre-eclampsia may be mild or severe according to the level of blood pressure derangement. Severe proteinuria leads to peripheral oedema.

Effects of pre-eclampsia

Reduced placental blood flow causes an increased risk of fetal hypoxia in late pregnancy, particularly during

Fig. 11.10 Pathogenesis of pre-eclampsia.

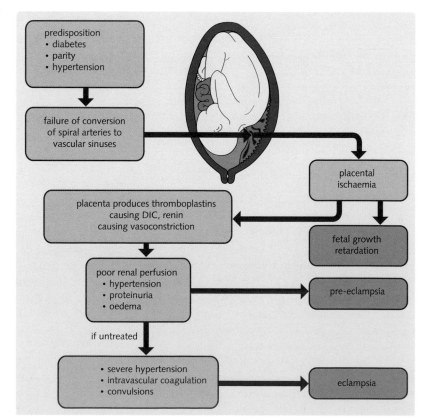

labour, with resultant perinatal mortality. The fetus may also suffer intrauterine growth retardation and have a low birth weight.

Maternal problems are less common, being largely confined to severe pre-eclampsia, which may progress into full-blown eclampsia (see below).

The disease resolves immediately after delivery.

Eclampsia

This is the occurrence of one or more convulsions not caused by other conditions such as epilepsy or cerebral haemorrhage in a woman with pre-eclampsia.

Incidence is rare; only a small proportion of patients with severe pre-eclampsia develop eclampsia.

Clinical features are severe systemic disturbance, i.e. frontal headaches, visual disturbance, rapid and sustained rise in blood pressure, severe epigastric pain, shock, anuria and fits.

There is disseminated intravascular coagulation with widespread occlusion of blood vessels, fibrinoid necrosis of vessel walls and, in fatal cases, widespread micro-infarcts in the brain, liver, kidneys and other organs.

Eclampsia is associated with a maternal mortality of 2% and a neonatal mortality of 3.5%. However, fatal eclampsia is now rare because of screening and treatment for the pre-eclamptic syndrome.

Neoplastic disorders of trophoblastic origin

Hydatidiform mole

This is the abnormal development of a gestational trophoblast leading to the formation of a benign mass of cystic vesicles derived from chorionic villi. It occurs in 1 in 2000 pregnancies in the UK and USA, but it is seen more frequently amongst some racial groups such as the Japanese population.

The disease is the result of an error in embryogenesis. There are two types:

1. Partial—a partial mole is triploid with most containing one maternal and two paternal haploid sets of chromosomes. Cystic vesicles are found in only a part of the placenta. Fetal parts and some normal placental villi are present along with the abnormal trophoblastic tissue. There is a low risk of subsequent development of a malignant tumour of the trophoblast (choriocarcinoma).
2. Complete—a complete mole is entirely of paternal origin (no maternal genetic contribution) and usually forms a bulky mass that may fill the uterine cavity. No fetal parts or normal placental villi are present. The risk of subsequent choriocarcinoma is greater than in a partial mole, occurring in about 3% of cases.

The aetiopathogenesis is unknown.

Clinical features are:

- Amenorrhoea and other symptoms of pregnancy, followed by continuous or intermittent vaginal bleeding. Many molar pregnancies spontaneously miscarry.
- Enlarged soft uterus (often larger than dates would suggest).

Diagnosis is by elevated human chorionic gonadotrophin (hCG) excretion in urine (typically much greater than in normal pregnancies) and by ultrasound for the absence of the fetus. Very high hCG levels may cause extreme morning sickness (hyperemesis gravidarum) and promote pre-eclampsia.

Treatment is by evacuation of the uterus, with a second aspiration or curettage 2–4 weeks later to ensure complete removal of the mole.

Follow-up is by regular estimations of hCG for at least a year. Detection of hCG after 1 month may suggest incomplete removal and the persistence of trophoblastic disease. Untreated, this carries a risk of subsequent choriocarcinoma.

Invasive mole (chorioadenoma destruens)

A hydatidiform mole that invades through the decidua into the myometrium and associated blood vessels. Perforation of the uterus may occur, resulting in invasion of the parametrium. True malignant transformation is rare.

Choriocarcinoma

These malignant tumours of trophoblastic tissue have a propensity for invading vessel walls, and blood-borne metastases occur early to many sites, particularly the lung and brain.

They are rare in the UK and USA (at 1 per 50 000 pregnancies) but more common in Asia, South America, and Africa.

Aetiology—about 50% develop from a hydatidiform mole and about 20% arise after a normal pregnancy with a variable time lag (a few months to many years).

The prognosis is excellent as the tumours respond well to cytotoxic chemotherapy (particularly if post-treatment monitoring of hCG levels is carried out).

Placental site trophoblastic tumour

This is a rare tumour in which the bulk of the tissue consists of chorionic epithelium but with very few villi. Typically benign, it may undergo malignant change.

DISORDERS OF THE BREAST

Inflammatory disorders and infections

Acute mastitis and breast abscess

These are uncommon and are usually complications of lactation. The most frequent organism is *Staphylococcus aureus*, which gains access through cracks and fissures of the nipple and areola. An abscess may form if drainage is inadequate.

Mammary duct ectasia

There is an abnormal progressive dilatation of the large breast ducts, which accumulate inspissated (thickened) secretions. The aetiology is unknown and it affects older women (perimenopausal age range). Patients develop a firm breast lump, but this does not mimic a carcinoma. There may also be a clear or green-coloured discharge.

Fat necrosis

This is usually caused by trauma. Histology shows necrosis with multinucleated giant cells and later fibrosis. It may cause a discrete lump mimicking a carcinoma.

Fibrocystic changes

Simple fibrocystic change

This is a generic term for a number of benign lesions that may occur together, producing lumpiness in the breast tissue. Peak incidence is around the menopause. It is thought that fibrocystic change is caused by hormonal imbalance.

The histological changes that may be present include:

- Cysts—ranging in size from microscopic to palpable lesions 1–2 cm in diameter. Diagnosis is confirmed by needle aspiration of clear fluid (blood-stained aspirate requires further investigation).
- Apocrine metaplasia—epithelial lining of hyperplastic ducts undergoes metaplasia to that of normal apocrine glands.

- Fibrosis—replacement of breast tissue by dense fibrous tissue, which can be due to cyst rupture.
- Sclerosing adenosis—marked proliferation of specialised hormone-responsive stromal tissue and myoepithelial cells, i.e. the number of acini per lobule increases. This forms localised areas of irregular stellate, collagenous sclerosis in which epithelial elements are also present. Occasionally difficult to distinguish from some patterns of invasive carcinoma.

There is no increased risk of a carcinoma unless there is accompanying epithelial hyperplasia (see below).

Epithelial hyperplasia

This describes the proliferation of epithelial cells within ducts or lobules (ductal hyperplasia and lobular hyperplasia respectively). There are two types:

1. Hyperplasia of the usual type—normal cytology and tissue architecture with no signs of malignancy.
2. Hyperplasia of atypical type—biological spectrum between some abnormalities of cytology/architecture and carcinoma *in situ*.

The risk of subsequent invasive breast carcinoma is increased in individuals with florid usual hyperplasia, further increased in subjects with atypical hyperplasia and much higher in those specifically with lobular carcinoma *in situ*.

Epithelial hyperplasia can only be diagnosed histologically.

Breast lumps are relatively common presentations. The following benign pathologies may cause discrete breast lumps or nipple discharge that mimic carcinomas:

- Fat necrosis.
- Intraduct papilloma.
- Fibroadenoma.

The best form of management is so-called 'triple assessment.' This consists of:

- History and examination (both the lump and regional nodes).
- Imaging (mammography or ultrasound)
- Tissue sampling if required (fine-needle aspiration or core biopsy).

Neoplasms of the breast

Fibroadenoma

This is the most common benign tumour of the female breast. There is proliferation of both stroma and epithelium, usually in young women (most frequently the 25–35 age group). It produces discrete but mobile breast lumps typically 1–4 cm in size, often multiple and bilateral.

Phyllodes tumour

This is a tumour composed of both stroma and epithelium, but the stroma is more cellular than in fibroadenomas. It is less common than fibroadenoma and occurs in the older age group (peak incidence being 45 years of age). Clinically, the tumour presents as a breast lump.

Macroscopically, there are rubbery white lesions consisting of a whorled pattern of slit-like spaces and solid areas.

Microscopically, there is a variable appearance, classified into benign (90% of cases), or of borderline malignant potential or definitely malignant.

There is the potential for local recurrence with increasing aggressiveness, and the tumour may eventually metastasise. Phyllodes tumours are therefore excised with a wide margin or, if necessary, are treated by mastectomy.

Intraductal papilloma

Epithelial proliferation within ducts produces papillary structures. These occur in older women and may produce a blood-stained nipple discharge. Papillomas are usually solitary with no increased risk of a carcinoma. However, a rare condition of multiple intraduct papillomas is premalignant.

Carcinoma

Incidence—this comprises 30% of all cancers in women and is the most common cause of death in 35- to 55-year-old women, increasing with age steeply to 45 years and continuing to increase less steeply thereafter. There are around 40 000 cases each year in the UK; 5-year survival is 80%.

There is a 200-fold female preponderance, with the highest rates in America, Western Europe and the Antipodes, and the lowest rates in Africa and Southeast Asia.

Predisposing factors
These include:

- Atypical epithelial proliferation—4- to 5-fold increased risk in severe atypia.

- Mutations of *BRCA1* (chromosome 17) and *BRCA2* genes (chromosome 13)—5% of cases.
- First-degree relative with breast cancer—increased risk independent of *BRCA* mutations.
- Long interval between menarche and menopause, i.e. early menarche and/or late menopause.
- Older age at first pregnancy.
- Ionizing radiation, as seen in those receiving intensive radiotherapy for Hodgkin's disease (up to 30% risk of breast cancer within 30 years of treatment).
- Obesity and dietary factors—postmenopausal obesity risk linked to higher oestrogen levels. Role of dietary fat is controversial.

Carcinoma *in situ*

All breast carcinomas are adenocarcinomas derived from epithelial cells of the terminal ductal lobules. Carcinoma *in situ* refers to neoplastic cells confined to the ducts and lobules, with no evidence of invasion through the basement membrane. Ductal carcinoma *in situ* (DCIS) is the more common form, presenting as microcalcifications on mammography. Lobular carcinoma *in situ* (LCIS) is more common in younger women and is more likely to affect both breasts. LCIS is not associated with calcifications on mammography or a mass, and is therefore often an incidental finding on biopsy.

DCIS may progress to invasive carcinoma, but is highly treatable at the *in situ* stage. LCIS may progress to invasive carcinoma, but is predominantly thought to be a strong risk marker for carcinoma in either breast.

Invasive carcinoma

Invasive carcinomas are tumours that have eroded through the basement membrane of their tissue of origin to invade surrounding structures. The most common presentation is a painless palpable mass, excluding those detected early by mammographic screening (see below). Large masses may cause skin dimpling or interfere with lymphatic drainage to produce classic skin changes (e.g. *peau d'orange*). Nipple retraction can also occur. Axillary lymph nodes may be palpable, reflecting metastasis from the primary site.

Investigation is by ultrasound, mammography, core biopsy or fine-needle aspiration cytology. Invasive carcinomas are categorised histologically:

- Invasive ductal (most common at 75%).
- Invasive lobular.
- Mucinous.

- Tubular.
- Medullary.
- Papillary.

The classification of breast cancer is summarised in Fig. 11.11.

Macroscopic features—a discrete lump with tethering to the skin or surrounding connective tissue. The macroscopic appearance of the tumour depends on the amount and type of stroma within the carcinoma.

Spread is as follows (Fig. 11.12):

- Direct—skin and muscles of the chest wall.
- Lymphatic—axillary lymph nodes, internal mammary lymph nodes.
- Blood—lungs, bone, liver, and brain.
- Transcoelomic—pleural cavities and pericardium.

Management and prognosis

The mainstay of treatment is surgical excision, often with axillary node clearance. Radiotherapy and chemotherapy are often used after surgery to reduce the risk of relapse.

Prognosis—related to tumour grade and type (tubular has the best prognosis), size of the tumour, lymph node status and oestrogen receptor status (usually responds to tamoxifen if positive). *C-erbB-2* (*HER-2*) is a proto-oncogene that is found in 15–20% of breast cancers. It is associated with poorer prognosis but this may be improved by novel monoclonal antibody therapy (Herceptin).

Figure 11.13 shows the TNM staging used for breast carcinoma.

Screening for breast carcinoma

There is no direct screening method equivalent to the cytology of the uterine cervix. The primary screening modality is mammography, which is more effective in older women with less radiodense breast tissue. Abnormalities seen on mammograms include calcification and soft tissue deformity. In the UK there is a National Health Service Breast Screening Programme

Fig. 11.11 Types of breast carcinoma

Character	Neoplasm
Non-invasive	Ductal carcinoma *in situ* Lobular carcinoma *in situ*
Invasive	Invasive ductal carcinoma (85%) Invasive lobular carcinoma (10%) Mucinous Tubular Medullary Papillary

Fig. 11.11 Types of breast carcinoma.

Fig. 11.12 Spread of breast carcinoma

Spread	Area
Direct	Skin
Lymphatic	Axillary lymph nodes Internal mammary lymph nodes Supraclavicular lymph nodes
Haematogenous	Liver Lung Opposite breast Bone Brain

Fig. 11.12 Spread of breast carcinoma.

Fig. 11.13 TNM staging of breast carcinoma.

Fig. 11.13 TNM staging of breast carcinoma

Tumour	Nodes	Metastases
T1 tumour 20 mm or less; no fixation or nipple retraction	N0 node negative	M0 no distant metastases
T2 tumour 20–50 mm, or less than 20 mm with fixation	N1 axillary nodes mobile	M1 distant metastases present
T3 tumour 50–100 mm, or less than 50 mm with fixation	N2 axillary nodes fixed	
T4 greater than 100 mm, or chest wall invasion	N3 supraclavicular nodes positive or arm oedema	

with 3-yearly mammography for all women over the age of 50 (until 70 years). Long-term studies suggest that such screening successfully reduces the mortality from breast carcinoma; it is possible that the age range screened may be extended in the future.

The male breast
Gynaecomastia
This is the benign enlargement of breast tissue.

Aetiology—hormonal influences including increased oestrogen production or receptor sensitivity. It is associated with liver cirrhosis, stilboestrol therapy for prostate carcinoma and drugs such as chlorpromazine.

Carcinoma
Less than 1% of breast carcinomas occur in men. The condition is associated with Klinefelter's syndrome and is usually of the ductal type; the lobular type is extremely rare.

DISORDERS OF THE PENIS

Inflammation and infection
Viral infection
Common viral infections of the penis include genital herpes and genital warts (condyloma acuminatum).

Genital herpes
This is an acute infection of the penile mucosa by the herpes simplex virus with the formation of typical herpetic vesicles on the glans penis. The vesicles soon burst to produce shallow painful ulcers.

The virus may remain latent for many years. Recurrent herpes infections are caused by reactivation of the virus, which may be precipitated by a febrile illness, immune suppression, emotional stress, or UV light.

Condyloma acuminatum (genital warts)
These cauliflower-like warts are seen on the penis and around the perineum. They are caused by the human papillomavirus subtypes HPV6 and HPV11, which are sexually transmitted.

Bacterial infection
Inflammation of the glans (balanitis) and prepuce (posthitis) can be caused by a variety of bacterial organisms, the most common of which are staphylococci, coliforms, gonococci and *Chlamydia*.

The appearance is that of marked congestion and oedema with exudate on the surface of the glans.

Ulceration with chronic scarring may occur if untreated; this is a common cause of phimosis.

Syphilis
This *Treponema pallidum* infection follows the same pattern as described for females (see page 230). The most common primary sites are the glans and the inner side of the prepuce, but the shaft is occasionally affected.

Lymphogranuloma venereum (lymphogranuloma inguinale)
This chronic, ulcerative venereal disease is characterised by granulomatous lesions caused by *Chlamydia trachomatis* (serotypes L1–L3).

Clinical features are:

- Small primary lesion—develops at site of inoculation, usually transient and often unnoticed.
- Unilateral lymphadenopathy (primarily inguinal)—occurs 1–2 weeks after infection. Nodes are at first discrete but later coalesce.

The disease follows a chronic course varying from weeks to months. Healing occurs with fibrosis resulting in lymphatic blockage.

Late complications are external genitalia elephantiasis or rectal strictures due to lymphatic obstruction.

Fungi
Infection with *Candida albicans* is common in men with diabetes mellitus.

Neoplastic disorders
Benign
Condyloma acuminatum
This is described above (genital warts).

Malignant
Carcinoma in situ
Penile carcinoma in situ is seen in two forms: Bowen disease (opaque plaques with shallow ulceration) affecting the shaft and scrotum, and erythroplasia of Queyrat, which is restricted to the glans, presenting with flat, red, glistening plaques. There is a spectrum of changes from dysplasia to carcinoma *in situ* grouped together as penile intraepithelial neoplasia. Many cases are associated with HPV infection (most commonly serotype 16).

Penile carcinoma *in situ* is a precancerous condition and may lead to invasive cancer unless treated vigorously with local irradiation or 5-fluorouracil cream.

Squamous cell carcinoma

This is a well-differentiated, keratinising, invasive tumour usually seen in elderly men. It occurs most commonly in uncircumcised men and is thought to be associated with a previous infection with human papillomavirus.

It presents as a warty, cauliflower-like growth that bleeds easily. It is typically slow growing but it is often neglected because of patient embarrassment.

DISORDERS OF THE TESTIS AND EPIDIDYMIS

Congenital abnormalities and regression

Cryptorchidism (undescended testis)

This is a condition caused by maldescent of the testes, affecting about 5% at birth, and 1% by the first birthday.

In the embryo, the testes develop from the genital ridge high on the posterior wall.

At about 7 months' gestation, the testes migrate down the posterior abdominal wall. They are guided by a cord (the gubernaculum) through the inguinal ring into the scrotum.

Occasionally, migration fails to occur and one (75% of cases) or both (25% of cases) testes become arrested somewhere along the route (Fig. 11.14). There are three conditions:

1. Abdominal testicle—usually found just inside the internal ring.

2. Inguinal testicle—in the inguinal canal, particularly exposed to trauma.
3. Retractile testicles (most common)—either high or low, depending on ability to be manoeuvered into correct position. Usually settles at puberty and does not need an operation.

The complications are:

- Infertility—temperature of aberrant locations is higher than in the scrotum and prevents normal germ cell development. The testis remains small and incapable of producing effective spermatozoa.
- Malignancy—more common in an undescended testis; about 1 in 10 of all testicular tumours arise in association with cryptorchidism.
- Inguinal hernia—there is nearly always a patent tunica vaginalis that predisposes to the development of an inguinal hernia.
- Torsion of the testicle (see below).

Management is by detection and correction of testicular maldescent. This is important because of the increased risk of testicular carcinoma. Some restoration of function may be achieved by 'orchidopexy' at an early stage (the testis is surgically pulled down and fixed to the scrotum).

Abnormalities of the tunica vaginalis

The tunica vaginalis and tunica albuginea (membrane sheaths surrounding the testes) are invested with mesothelial cells and may be the site of fluid accumulation, inflammation or (uncommonly) tumour formation.

Hydrocele

Fluid accumulates in the cavity bounded by the tunica vaginalis. This is the most common cause of swelling within the scrotum.

This is often idiopathic, but the aetiology may involve:

- Congenital patency of the processus vaginalis, often with continuity into the peritoneal cavity.
- Secondary to tumours, epididymitis, mumps or acute orchitis.

Haematocele

Blood accumulates in the cavity bounded by the tunica vaginalis, usually due to trauma or torsion and rarely due to tumour spread.

Chylocele

Accumulation of lymph secondary to obstructed drainage.

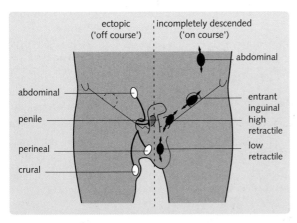

Fig. 11.14 Maldescended testes showing common sites of arrest. (Adapted with permission from Lecture Notes on Urology, 5th edn, by J Blandy, Blackwell Science, 1998.)

Hernias

Indirect inguinal hernias (described in Chapter 8) typically occur as a result of patent processus vaginalis.

Trauma and vascular disturbances

Torsion

There is twisting of a testicle on its pedicle with obstruction of venous return such that blood continues to enter the testis but cannot leave. The testis is engorged and painful, eventually becoming infarcted (venous infarction). In advanced torsion, the testis is almost black as a result of vascular congestion.

Early detection and surgical relief are required to save testicular viability. Surgical removal is necessary for advanced disease.

Varicocele

This describes variceal dilatation of the veins of the pampiniform plexus of the spermatic cord.

Neoplastic disorders

Tumours of the testis, although relatively uncommon, are important because many occur in young men; they are the most common tumour among 15- to 35-year-olds.

The exact aetiology is unknown but there are links with testicular maldescent and/or dysgenesis, possibly with some genetic susceptibility.

Clinical presentations are:

- Painless unilateral enlargement of testis (majority).
- Secondary hydrocele.
- Symptoms of metastases—especially in malignant teratoma, e.g. haemoptysis from lung deposits.
- Endocrine effects—gynaecomastia, precocious puberty (typically from Leydig or Sertoli cell tumours).

There are two main groups of testicular tumour:

1. Germ cell tumours (97% of cases)—derived from multipotential germ cells of the testis arising mainly as teratomas and seminomas.
2. Non-germ cell tumours (3% of cases)—derived from specialised and non-specialised support cells of the testis.

Germ cell tumours

Seminoma

The most common malignant testicular tumour, accounting for about 50% of all malignant germ cell tumours, with a peak age of onset between 30 and 40 years. The tumour shows spermatogenic differentiation.

Histological types of seminoma are:

- Classic seminoma (most common subtype)—characteristic feature is the presence of fibrous septa with lymphocytic infiltrate.
- Spermatocytic seminoma—larger tumour cells with some small cells resembling spermatocytes.
- Anaplastic seminoma—cells show marked pleomorphism and increased mitotic activity.

Teratoma

This tumour of germ cell origin is composed of several types of tissue representing endoderm, ectoderm, and mesoderm. The tumours retain their totipotentiality for differentiation and are more aggressive than seminomas. The peak age of onset is 20–30 years.

Teratomas are classified according to their histological pattern; two systems exist (Fig. 11.15), with the British classifications described below:

- Differentiated teratoma—a rare type of teratoma of mature and well-differentiated tissue,

Fig. 11.15 Comparison of the British and World Health Organization classifications of teratomas.

Fig. 11.15 Comparison of the British and WHO classifications of teratomas

Type of differentiation	British	WHO
Somatic	Differentiated teratoma	Mature teratoma
	Malignant teratoma intermediate	Immature teratoma or mixed teratoma and embryonal carcinoma
None	Malignant teratoma undifferentiated	Embryonal carcinoma
Extra-embryonic	Yolk sac tumour	Yolk sac tumour
	Malignant teratoma trophoblastic	Choriocarcinoma

producing a wide range of organoid structures (e.g. skin, hair, cartilage and bone). Lesions are usually seen in young children. They behave in a benign fashion.

- Malignant teratoma intermediate—partly solid and partly cystic tumour, with less maturity and areas of malignancy with cellular pleomorphism and necrosis.
- Malignant teratoma undifferentiated—completely undifferentiated tumour with marked nuclear pleomorphism and a high mitotic rate.
- Malignant teratoma trophoblastic—identical to choriocarcinoma in the placenta (see page 243), this highly malignant tumour contains areas of syncytiotrophoblast and cytotrophoblast cells. hCG and α-fetoprotein (AFP) are useful markers.
- Yolk sac tumour (orchioblastoma)—the pure form is seen in children up to 3 years old and has a good prognosis. The adult (mixed) form is more aggressive. AFP is a useful marker.

Combined germ cell tumour

Between 10 and 15% of germ cell tumours consist of a mixture of seminomatous and teratomatous elements.

Prognosis of germ cell tumours

The prognosis of testicular teratomas has improved greatly with the use of cytotoxic chemotherapy, and it is related to histological type, as well as to tumour stage. Seminomas are more likely to respond to radiotherapy. In general, germ cell tumours containing trophoblastic, yolk sac, and undifferentiated elements have the worst prognosis.

Non-germ cell tumours

Interstitial (Leydig) cell tumour

This rare tumour arises from the interstitial or Leydig cells of the testis. It may produce androgens, oestrogens or both, causing precocious development of secondary sexual characteristics in childhood or loss of libido/gynaecomastia in adults. Ninety per cent are benign.

Sertoli cell tumour (androblastoma)

This well-circumscribed tumour is composed of cells resembling normal Sertoli cells of the tubules. Most lesions are benign.

Malignant lymphomas

The non-Hodgkin's-type lymphoma is usually a poorly differentiated B cell lymphoma with a diffuse pattern. These comprise about 5% of testicular tumours with a peak incidence between 60 and 80 years of age.

Metastatic tumours

The spread of other tumours to the testis may occasionally occur, particularly in acute leukaemia.

Figure 11.16 provides a summary of testicular tumours.

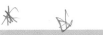

Many testicular tumours have useful cell markers:
- Trophoblastic germ cell tumours—↑ hCG.
- Yolk sac tumours—↑ α-fetoprotein.
- 90% of patients with malignant teratoma undifferentiated—↑ α-fetoprotein, ↑ hCG or both.
- 50% of patients with malignant teratoma intermediate—↑ α-fetoprotein, ↑ hCG or both.

DISORDERS OF THE PROSTATE

Benign prostatic hyperplasia

Non-neoplastic enlargement of the prostate is the most common disorder of the prostate, affecting almost all men over the age of 70. However, it is found with increasing frequency and severity from about 45 years.

Fig. 11.16 Summary of testicular tumours	
Germ cell tumours (97% of cases)	
Seminomas	Classic seminoma Spermatocytic seminoma Anaplastic seminoma Seminomas with trophoblastic giant cells
Teratomas	Differentiated teratoma Malignant teratoma intermediate Malignant teratoma undifferentiated Malignant teratoma trophoblastic Yolk sac tumour
Combined	Mixture of seminomatous and teratomatous elements
Non-germ cell tumours (3% of cases)	
Sex-cord and stromal tumours	Interstitial (Leydig) cell tumour Sertoli cell tumour
Others	Malignant lymphomas Metastatic tumours

Fig. 11.16 Summary of testicular tumours

The aetiopathogenesis is uncertain but believed to be a result of androgen–oestrogen imbalance. Central (periurethral) prostatic glands are hormone sensitive and they undergo hyperplasia. Their continuing enlargement compresses peripheral prostatic glands leading to their collapse, leaving only fibrous supporting stroma (Fig. 11.17).

Affected lobes are:

- Two lateral lobes (majority of cases).
- Posterior lobe (uncommon), causing an obstruction of the urinary outflow tract at the internal urinary meatus at the bladder neck.

Histologically:

- Nodular pattern of hyperplastic glandular acini lined with tall columnar epithelial cells and separated by fibrous stroma.
- Some nodules are cystically dilated and contain a milky fluid.
- Other nodules contain numerous calcific concretions (corpora amylacea).

Infarction causes necrotic areas with a haemorrhagic margin. There is often muscular hypertrophy particularly in the region of the bladder neck.

Clinical presentation—compression of the prostatic urethra by the enlarged prostate causes difficulties with micturition, mainly hesitation, poor stream and terminal dribbling.

Complications—prolonged prostatic obstruction can lead to several complications, which are outlined in Fig. 11.18.

Neoplastic disorders

Prostatic carcinoma

This is an adenocarcinoma of the prostate, and it is shown in Fig. 11.19. It is the second most common cause of cancer death in males and its detected incidence is increasing (30 000 per year in the UK). It is rare before 55 years of age with a peak incidence between 60 and 85 years; 5-year survival is 65%.

Its aetiology is uncertain but there is probably hormonal involvement (reduced androgens).

Unlike benign hyperplasia, carcinoma usually arises in the peripheral zone of the prostate and it is therefore often well established before the development of urinary symptoms. Indeed, some tumours

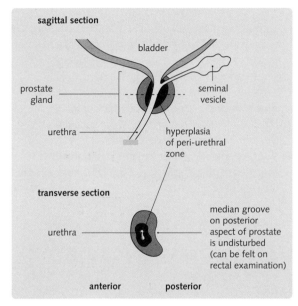

Fig. 11.17 Benign prostatic hyperplasia.

Fig. 11.18 Complications of benign prostatic hyperplasia.

Fig. 11.18 Complications of benign prostatic hyperplasia	
Bladder wall	Hypertrophy of smooth muscle Trabeculation: due to prominent bands of thickened smooth muscle Diverticula: protrude between trabeculae
Bladder size	Dilation: due to failure of bladder wall compensatory mechanisms
Ureteric changes	Dilation of ureters
Urinary infection (cystitis)	Bladder fails to empty completely after micturition, and residual urine is liable to infection
Kidney disease	Pyelonephritis: from ascending infection Impaired renal failure Hydronephrosis Calculi

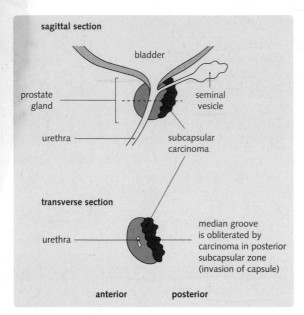

Fig. 11.19 Prostatic carcinoma.

may remain silent even in the presence of widespread metastases.

Types are divided into three groups on the basis of their behaviour:

1. Latent—small foci of well-differentiated carcinoma, frequently an incidental finding in prostatic glands of elderly men. Remain confined to the prostate for a long period.
2. Invasive—invade locally and metastasise.
3. Occult—not clinically apparent in primary site (small tumour) but present as widespread symptomatic metastatic disease.

Macroscopically, there are diffuse areas of firm, white tissue merging into fibromuscular prostatic stromal tissues. Distortion and extension outside the prostatic capsule is common, producing a firm, craggy mass that can be palpated on rectal examination.

Microscopically, the majority has a well-differentiated glandular pattern (good prognosis); a minority has poorly differentiated sheets of cells with no acinar pattern (poor prognosis).

Spread is:

- Direct—to the base of the bladder and adjacent tissues. May cause obstruction of the urethra (difficulty in micturition) and may block the ureters, causing hydronephrosis.
- Lymphatic—to pelvic and para-aortic nodes.
- Haematogenous—most commonly to bone, but also to the lungs and liver. Bone metastases are typically sclerotic with bone production (dense on radiograph) rather than lytic with bone destruction.

Diagnosis is by:

- Imaging—ultrasound, X-ray, isotope bone scan (for bony metastases).
- Needle biopsy—histological examination together with immunohistochemical detection of prostate-specific antigen (PSA) and prostate-specific acid phosphatase (PSAP) in biopsy material.
- Serology—PSA and PSAP may also be used as serum markers for disease, levels being particularly raised when there is metastatic disease. However, raised PSA alone is relatively non-specific for prostate carcinoma, meaning that screening programs are likely to have a high false-positive rate.

The clinical features of prostatic carcinoma:
- Urinary symptoms (hesitancy, poor stream, terminal dribbling).
- Hard, craggy prostate on rectal examination.
- Bone metastases: pain (especially back pain), fracture, anaemia.

Treatment—if tumour is confined to prostate, radical prostatectomy or radiotherapy may be curative. If spread has occurred, androgen suppressing drugs (e.g. luteinizing hormone releasing hormone analogues) suppress testosterone and improve survival from this slow-growing tumour. Orchidectomy is occasionally performed for the same effect.

Pathology of the musculoskeletal system

Objectives

In this chapter, you will learn to:

- Describe common disorders of bone structure, particularly osteoporosis and Paget's disease.
- Recall the infectious causes of bone disease and their manifestations.
- Describe fractures and bone healing, including the complications that may occur.
- Briefly describe the tumours of bone.
- Understand the causes of disruption to the neuromuscular junction.
- Describe inherited and acquired myopathies.
- Describe in detail osteoarthritis, rheumatoid arthritis and the wider effects of rheumatoid disease.
- Understand ankylosing spondylitis and arthritis associated with systemic disease.
- Recall the pathologies of the crystal arthropathies.
- Understand the causes and effects of septic arthritis.

DISORDERS OF BONE STRUCTURE

Achondroplasia

This hereditary disorder of endochondral ossification is the most common cause of true dwarfism, occurring in approximately 1 per 50 000 births.

Aetiology—autosomal dominant with a high incidence of spontaneous mutation accounting for the 80% of cases in which an achondroplastic child is born to unaffected parents (increased incidence with paternal age). The affected gene is for fibroblast growth factor receptor (chromosome 4).

Pathogenesis—the mutation suppresses cartilage proliferation in the growth plate, resulting in diminished lengthening of cartilage bones (e.g. long bones, base of the skull and pelvis). Periosteal bone formation is normal. Cartilage bones are, therefore, shortened but thick and strong. Membranous bone (such as the vault of the skull) is not affected.

Disorders of the bone matrix

Osteogenesis imperfecta (brittle bone disease)

This heterogeneous group of rare congenital disorders is characterised by abnormal collagen formation with unusually brittle and fragile bones.

Achondroplasia results in non-proportional dwarfism, i.e. the trunk appears too long compared to the length of the arms and legs. The head is also enlarged, with a depression at the root of the nose. Other common types of dwarfism (e.g. pituitary hormone deficiency or malnutrition) are typically proportional, with all bones being affected equally.

Aetiology—mutation of genes coding for type I collagen results in abnormal collagen formation in the osteoid. The pattern of inheritance can be either dominant or recessive, and it involves mutation at sites on chromosomes 7 and 17.

Appearance—there is a marked variation in severity but widespread weakness of bone results in multiple fractures frequently leading to severe deformity. Lax joint ligaments, blue sclera and hearing loss are also often seen, once more reflecting decreased collagen synthesis.

Osteoporosis

This slowly progressive disorder is characterised by reduced bone mass as a result of a relative increase in bone erosion. The bone structure remains qualitatively normal, but there is less of it.

Incidence—the most common metabolic bone disease. Peak bone mass is achieved in early adulthood, with bone density decreasing with age from the third or fourth decade of life. A high peak bone mass protects against future osteoporosis.

Osteoporosis is widespread in the elderly, where it is an important cause of morbidity and even mortality, as weakened bone predisposes to minimal trauma fractures. Bone loss in women is accelerated by oestrogen deficiency, making postmenopausal women a high-risk group for osteoporosis. Hormone replacement therapy is partly protective (see Chapter 11). The risk factors for osteoporosis are illustrated in Fig. 12.1.

Macroscopically—bones are lighter in weight, less dense on radiography (Fig. 12.2) and show thinning of the cortex. Lumbar vertebral bodies are more biconcave than normal, such that the intervertebral disc space appears more spherical ('fish vertebrae').

Microscopically—bone trabeculae are thinner and reduced in number, and there is a decrease in the number of osteoblasts. Mineralisation is not affected.

Complications are:

- Bone pain—especially in the back because of compression of vertebral bodies. This may reduce overall height and cause an anteroposterior bending of the spine (kyphosis).

- Pathological fractures—following minimal trauma, especially of the femur (hip fracture), neck, and at the wrist.

Osteoporosis may also develop in a localised area of bone secondary to disuse, surrounding inflammation or in conditions such as myeloma (see Chapter 13).

Diagnosis is by bone densitometry scanning at the hip and spine to show the degree of bone loss. Osteopenia describes reduced bone density that has not yet reached osteoporotic levels.

Management—emphasis is on prevention rather than treatment, namely avoidance of risk factors, with

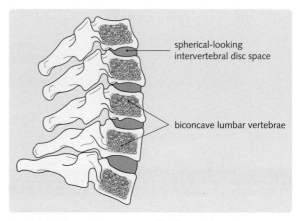

Fig. 12.2 Radiographic appearance of lumbar vertebrae in osteoporosis.

Fig. 12.1 Type and associated risk factors for osteoporosis. The mnemonic 'MASCARA' can be used to help remember the causes of secondary generalised osteoporosis.

Fig. 12.1 Type and associated risk factors for osteoporosis	
Type	**Risk factors**
Idiopathic	Female Early menopause Small stature Thin physique Family history Advanced age Nulliparity
Secondary: generalised	**M**etabolic: low calcium intake, impaired supply of protein (e.g. nephritic syndrome or cirrhosis of liver), scurvy **A**ssorted endocrine disorders: thyrotoxicosis, panhypopituitarism and Cushing's syndrome **S**teroid therapy **C**igarette smoking **A**lcohol abuse **R**educed physical activities **A**luminium antacids
Secondary: localised	Disuse atrophy: especially in neurological limb paralysis or post fracture

encouragement of physical exercise and adequate calcium intake. Bisphosphonates are highly effective drugs for reducing the rate of decline in osteoporosis.

Osteomalacia and rickets

Osteomalacia is a disease of defective bone mineralisation that is most commonly seen in the developing world. It is usually due to a lack of vitamin D or disturbances in its metabolism (e.g. conversion to active vitamin D via the liver and kidney).

Bone is incompletely calcified, with the development of wide 'seams' of osteoid. The bone is weak and prone to fracture.

Rickets—the same disorder—occurs in the growing bones of children, leading to characteristic skeletal changes, e.g. bowing of long bones.

Both disorders are potentially reversible with early dietary supplementation to correct deficiencies, or treatment of underlying disorders of vitamin D metabolism.

Mucopolysaccharidoses

This group of autosomal recessive disorders of mucopolysaccharide metabolism results in abnormal accumulation of glycosaminoglycans (e.g. dermatan sulphate) in cells of the brain and other tissues.

The main disorders are Hurler's syndrome (deficiency of α-L-iduronidase) and Hunter's syndrome (deficiency of iduronate sulphatase), both of which are associated with a wide variety of clinical features including stiff joints, malformed bones and short stature.

Disorders of osteoclast function

Osteopetrosis (marble bone disease; Albers–Schönberg disease)

This rare inherited disorder is characterised by increased density of all cartilaginous bones, especially the vertebrae, pelvic bones and ribs.

Pathogenesis—defective resorption of bone by osteoclasts produces diffuse symmetrical skeletal sclerosis.

Appearance—there is no discernible differentiation of cartilaginous bones into cortex and medulla: the cortical compact bone extends into the medulla, which is thus devoid of cancellous bone.

Effect—bones are excessively dense, yet extremely brittle and prone to fracture. There is a lack of bone marrow function predisposing to infection, and increased risk of cranial nerve compression within the base of the skull.

Paget's disease of the bone (osteitis deformans)

This chronic disease of excessive uncontrolled resorption and deposition of bone particularly affects the skull, backbone, pelvis, and long bones. It is rare before 40 years of age, but increases in incidence with age thereafter. It is relatively common in the UK, affecting 3% of those over 40, but rare in Asia, Africa and the Middle East.

Aetiology—unknown, but recent evidence suggests a paramyxovirus infection of the osteoclasts. Electron microscope studies have demonstrated probable viral inclusions in the nuclei of osteoclasts.

Pathogenesis—large, abnormal, multinucleated osteoclasts cause excessive bone erosion with destruction of trabecular and cortical bone. Each wave of bone destruction is followed by a vigorous but uncoordinated osteoblastic response, producing new osteoid to fill the defects left by the osteoclasts. However, both osteoclastic erosion and osteoblastic deposition are random, haphazard and unrelated to functional stresses on the bone, resulting in greatly distorted bone architecture.

Morphology—bone shows a characteristic woven, non-lamellar pattern indicative of rapid reparative deposition. Well marked 'cement lines' are often visible, producing the characteristic 'mosaic' or 'crazy-paving' appearance. The bone becomes increasingly sclerotic and brittle, thereby prone to fracture.

Disruption of bone architecture is followed by progressive increased vascularity in the spaces between the thickened bone trabeculae.

The effects of Paget's disease can be widespread (affecting many bones) or localised (15% of cases confined to one area in a single-bone—monostotic—Paget's disease).

Most patients present with one or both of the following features:

- Bone pain—usually localised to site of most active disease.
- Bone deformity—following extensive disease, most commonly enlargement of skull, kyphosis, or bowing of tibia.

Complications—some patients occasionally present with the complications of Paget's disease:

- Nerve compression symptoms—usually seen in association with Paget's disease of the skull, in which enlargement of the pagetic bone can lead to cranial nerve palsies (e.g. CN VIII compression results in deafness). Spinal stenosis may compress spinal nerve roots.

- Pathological fracture—bone is increased in bulk but is weaker than normal and more likely to fracture with trivial trauma.
- Cardiac hypertrophy—due to increased vascularity of bones.
- Malignant tumour (1% of cases)—usually osteosarcoma, which may develop in areas of long-standing active Paget's disease. This is the most common cause of osteosarcoma in the elderly and has a poor prognosis.

Investigations in Paget's disease are:
- Serology—normal calcium and phosphate, increased alkaline phosphatase.
- Urine—increased urinary excretion of hydroxyproline.
- Abnormal isotope bone scans.
- X-ray—localised bone enlargement, altered trabecular pattern and alternating areas of rarefaction and increased density.

Management is by analgesia for bone pain, and calcitonin or bisphosphonates for severe bone pain not controlled by analgesics. The latter inhibit bone resorption.

Hyperparathyroidism

Elevated secretion of parathyroid hormone (PTH) stimulates osteoclastic bone resorption and inhibits osteoblastic bone deposition. This is described in more detail on page 217.

INFECTIONS AND TRAUMA

Osteomyelitis

This infection of bone typically affects the cortex, medulla, and periosteum, and it is most commonly encountered in children under the age of 12 years. Adult onset is usually due to compromised host resistance (e.g. severe debilitation, immunosuppression). The most common causative organisms are *Staphylococcus aureus* (over 80% of identified cases), *Mycobacterium tuberculosis, Escherichia coli* (particularly in infants and the elderly), and *Salmonella* species (particularly in patients with sickle-cell disease).

Infective organisms gain access to the medullary cavity of the bone by two main routes:

1. Direct access through an open wound, particularly when open fractures are involved. This route is also important in postoperative orthopaedic patients (particularly those with prosthetic joint replacements).
2. Blood-borne spread: following bacteraemia from a focus of sepsis elsewhere.

Clinical features—abrupt onset of severe pain at the site of bone infection accompanied by fever and malaise.
Complications and sequelae:

- Resolution—with appropriate antibiotic therapy, ideally based on blood cultures or aspiration material.
- Pathological fracture—purulent acute inflammatory exudate formed in closed compartment of marrow cavity causes compression of vessels with necrosis of medullary bone trabeculae, resulting in increased predisposition to fractures.
- Adjacent sepsis—destruction of cortical bone may lead to discharge of pus into extraosseous connective tissue, and infection may track through to the skin surface producing a chronic discharging sinus. Spread may also occur to other bones (malignant osteomyelitis) or neighbouring joints (septic arthritis – see later).
- Chronicity—in chronic osteomyelitis, the organisms may remain viable within the marrow cavity for many years. Chronicity results in extensive bone destruction, marrow fibrosis and recurrent focal suppuration (Brodie's abscess). There is also reactive new bone formation, particularly around inflamed periosteum, leading to a thickened and abnormally shaped bone. Given that osteomyelitis is most common in children, growth disturbance may occur if the physis is damaged.
- Amyloidosis—chronic osteomyelitis is a significant cause of secondary amyloid-associated (AA) amyloidosis (see Chapter 13).

Diagnosis is by blood culture and isotope scan.
Management is by analgesia, antibiotic therapy and potential surgical drainage of abscesses.

Tuberculous osteomyelitis and Pott's disease

In tuberculous osteomyelitis the marrow cavity contains rapidly enlarging caseating granulomas, which destroy trabecular and cortical bone.

The mode of infection is usually by haematogenous spread from a lung focus, most commonly in adolescents, immunosuppressed adults, or the elderly. Vertebral bodies (Pott's disease) are the most common site (affected in 50% of cases) but long bones, fingers and joints are also involved. The disease tends to be more destructive than pyogenic osteomyelitis.

Healing occurs with antituberculous chemotherapy, firstly by fibrosis and subsequently by new bone formation.

Skeletal syphilis

Two types, both of which are now rare:

1. Congenital syphilis—causes osteochondritis and periostitis.
2. Acquired syphilis (tertiary stage)—periostitis and gummas (syphilitic growths).

Fractures

A fracture is a break in the structural continuity of bone. Note that any break, even of only one cortex, constitutes a fracture. Fractures are the most common abnormality of bone, and they are caused by physical trauma.

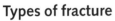

> There are several ways of classifying fractures, e.g. according to causation, according to pattern of fracture, or according to their relation to surrounding tissues. The latter is the simplest method.

Types of fracture

Fractures can be classified into two main types according to their relation to surrounding tissues:

1. Simple (closed)—without contact with external environment, i.e. skin or mucous membrane overlying bone is intact. Simple fractures are less likely to become infected.
2. Compound (open)—with direct contact between the fracture and external environment, e.g. a fracture of the tibia with laceration of overlying skin. Compound factures are more likely to become infected.

Other descriptive terms for fractures are:

- Comminuted—more than two fragments present.
- Complicated—involvement of a nerve, artery or viscus.

- Pathological—fracture occurring in abnormal bone, e.g. in osteoporosis or due to a bone tumour.
- Stress—slowly developing fracture resulting from repeated application of minor force.
- Greenstick—usually seen in children, this is where only one side of a bone is fractured, leaving it bent but intact.

Processes of healing

Bone fractures heal by granulation tissue formation with fibrous repair, followed by new bone formation in the fibrous granulation tissue (see Chapter 2 for wound healing of the skin).

The sequence of events in healing of a simple undisplaced fracture is illustrated in Fig. 12.3.

Complications of healing

Bones show great capacity for healing, but certain complications can occur:

- Malunion—poor anatomical alignment of fractures results in deformity, angulation or displacement.
- Delayed union—this is common, and it is said to have occurred when a fracture has not united in a reasonable time (defined as 25% longer than the average time).
- Non-union—if union has not occurred within 1 year then the terminology is changed from one of 'delayed union' to one of 'non-union'. The defect is typically filled with fibrous tissue/fibrous ankylosis.

Causes of complications

Efficient healing of fractures requires optimal conditions. Factors that prevent efficient healing are:

- Poor apposition of fractured bone ends—a fracture is 'reduced' to achieve the best alignment possible.
- Inadequate immobilisation—immobilisation should be achieved by splinting.
- Interposition of foreign bodies or soft tissues.
- Infection.
- Corticosteroid therapy.
- Poor general nutritional status.
- Poor blood supply.

Avascular necrosis (osteonecrosis)

Ischaemic necrosis of cortical and trabecular bone is caused by:

- Interrupted vascular supply (most important cause)—fractures, dislocations and infection. Common fractures are those affecting the femoral

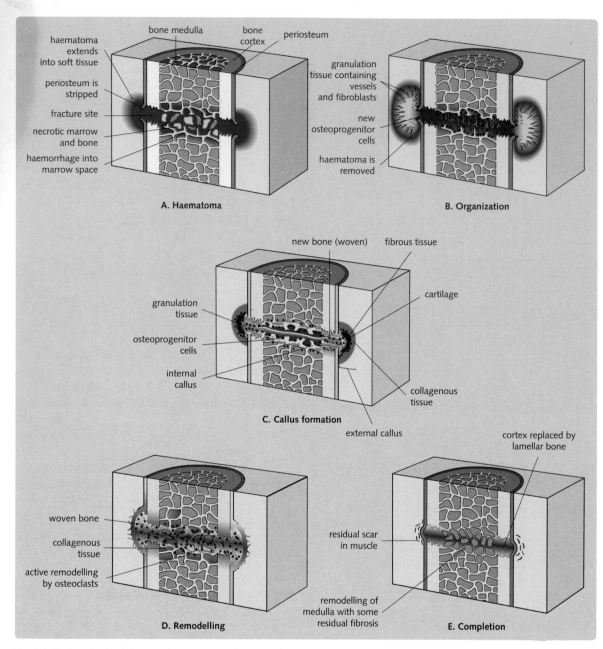

Fig. 12.3 Healing of a simple fracture. (A) Haematoma formation, due to tearing of medullary blood vessels. (B) Organization: migration of neutrophils and macrophages into fracture with organization of haematoma within about 24 hours. Capillaries and fibroblasts proliferate forming fibrovascular granulation tissue. New osteoprogenitor cells (derived from mesenchymal precursor cells) mature into osteoblasts, and they migrate into granulation tissue. (C) Callus formation: osteoblasts deposit large quantities of osteoid collagen in a haphazard way producing a woven bone pattern. Fracture is bridged on outside by external callus (may contain cartilage) and it is bridged in medullary cavity by internal callus (rarely contains cartilage). However, direct ossification may occur between fractured ends if they are closely apposed. (D) Remodelling: about 3 weeks post fracture, callus is well established and undergoes remodelling. Osteoclastic resorption and osteoblastic osteoid synthesis removes surplus calcified callus, replacing bulky, woven bone with compact, organised, lamellar bone. Process takes several months. (E) Completion: formation of new lamellar trabecular bone is complete. Bone is orientated in a direction determined by stresses to which it is exposed with mobilisation. However, even after remodelling, cortical irregularities and minor marrow space fibrosis persist at site of fracture.

head, proximal part of scaphoid and the body of talus.

- Arteriolar occlusion—vasculitis of extraosseous arteries, sickle-cell disease, fat and nitrogen emboli.
- Capillary compression—can be caused by corticosteroids (produce fatty infiltration) or alcohol abuse.
- Idiopathic—without identified cause.

Note that osteoarthritis (OA) is also associated with necrotic bone change, particularly at the hip.

Investigation is ideally by magnetic resonance imaging (MRI) as this shows the earliest changes, although isotope bone scanning with ^{99}Tc diphosphonate is also useful.

Management is by avoiding weight bearing, analgesia for pain relief and non-steroidal anti-inflammatory drugs (NSAIDs) for anti-inflammatory action.

Surgery:

- Bone decompression.
- Realignment osteotomy to reduce mechanical stresses on affected bone segments.
- Joint replacement is often required in patients with more advanced disease and secondary OA.

TUMOURS OF THE BONES

Metastatic disease of the skeleton

Most common tumours in bone are blood-borne metastases from other primary sites or are tumours of the haemopoietic cells located within the marrow spaces of bones, particularly myeloma.

Carcinomas

There are five common carcinomas that have a predilection for metastasising to bone:

1. Adenocarcinoma of the breast.
2. Carcinoma of bronchus (particularly small cell, undifferentiated carcinoma).
3. Adenocarcinoma of the kidney.
4. Adenocarcinoma of the thyroid.
5. Adenocarcinoma of the prostate.

Metastases are typically multifocal, occurring most commonly in parts of the skeleton that contain vascular marrow, especially vertebral bodies, ribs, the pelvis, and upper ends of the femur and humerus.

Osteolytic versus osteosclerotic metastases

Most metastatic tumour cells within bone marrow spaces lead to erosion of bone (osteolytic metastases), through the release of substances that promote osteoclastic resorption (e.g. prostaglandins, parathyroid-hormone-related peptide; PRHRP). However, prostatic carcinoma (and very rarely breast carcinoma) produces metastatic deposits in which there is osteoblastic stimulation of new bone formation (osteosclerotic metastases) particularly in the lumbosacral vertebrae.

Clinical features:

- Bone pain—usually localised to site of deposits.
- Pathological fractures—erosion of trabecular bone either directly, or through osteoclast-stimulated bone erosion (osteolytic metastases) → bone weakness → fracture.

Complications are:

- Leucoerythroblastic anaemia—a result of extensive replacement of bone marrow.
- Symptoms of hypercalcaemia—caused by the release of calcium from bone by osteolytic process.
- Nerve and spinal cord compression—particularly in vertebral metastases.

Haematopoietic malignancies

Haematopoietic malignancies found in bone (e.g. myelomas, lymphomas, leukaemias) are discussed in Chapter 13.

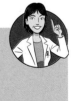

Secondary tumours of bone are more common in adults than children, whereas primary tumours of bone are generally more common in children than adults.

Bone-forming tumours

These are rare primary bone tumours, derived from cells involved in bone formation and modelling.

Osteoma

Benign, smooth, rounded bone tumour is seen on the surface of long bones or skull bone. Apart from visible or palpable swelling, there are usually no symptoms. Such tumours are slow-growing and do not undergo malignant transformation. Patients with Gardner's syndrome have multiple osteomas and intestinal polyps.

Osteoid osteoma and osteoblastoma

Osteoid osteoma

Rarely causing severe bone pain, this typically arises between the ages of 10 and 30 years. It is more common in males. Most frequently it affects long bones of the lower leg but it may occur in any bone except the skull. Tumours are composed of active osteoblasts, which deposit large, irregular masses of osteoid collagen in a haphazard manner.

Osteoid osteomas are painful; pain is usually relieved by aspirin but not by rest. Radiographs characteristically show a central dense area surrounded by a halo of translucency. Excision is usually curative and lesions do not recur.

Osteoblastoma (giant osteoid osteoma)

This large tumour with identical histological features to osteoid osteoma mainly affects the bones of the hands, feet and vertebrae. Tumours are typically more locally aggressive, generating a dull achy pain that is unresponsive to aspirin.

Osteosarcoma

This malignant tumour of osteoblasts occurs most often in adolescent children, with a second peak in the fifth decade of life linked to highly active Paget's disease. Some cases are associated with familial cancer syndromes of retinoblastoma syndrome (defect in RB1) and the Li-Fraumeni syndrome (defect in *p53*). The majority arise around the knee (lower femur or upper tibia) and a minority in other long bones such as the upper end of humerus or femur.

Symptoms are bone pain increasing gradually with tumour growth, but the tumour is often well-advanced at the time of diagnosis. A progressively enlarging bony lump may be palpable.

Spread—the tumour grows rapidly within the medullary cavity, eventually eroding through the cortical plate into soft tissue. Metastasis occurs early via the bloodstream, usually to the lung.

Prognosis has improved with the adoption of earlier surgical treatment combined with chemotherapy. However, 5-year survival is still only 50%.

Cartilage-forming tumours

Osteochondroma

This is the most common tumour of bone. It is benign, growing as an exophytic nodule from metaphyses of long bones. It is also known as a 'cartilage-capped exostosis' as it is composed of protuberant bone covered with a cap of cartilage and an outer layer of perichondrium.

Lesions are found most commonly in the humerus, femur and the upper end of the tibia. They may be solitary or multiple (typically autosomal dominant condition, hereditary multiple exostoses). Solitary lesions usually first develop in adolescence. Chondrosarcomatous change is rare in solitary lesions but more common in hereditary multiple exostoses.

Chondroma

This is a benign tumour of hyaline cartilage, composed of well circumscribed nodules of cytologically benign chondrocytes embedded in a cartilaginous matrix.

Tumours are thought to originate from residual nests of cartilage cells left behind in metaphysis as bone growth proceeds. They are found most commonly in small bones of hands and feet.

They may be single (solitary enchondroma) or multiple (enchondromatosis or Ollier's disease). The term 'enchondroma' is used to indicate that the tumour arises and grows within the medullary cavity of bone (compared to osteochondroma, which grows as a nodular exophytic lesion). A solitary chondroma rarely undergoes malignant change, but occasionally it occurs in multiple enchondromatosis.

Chondrosarcoma

This slow-growing malignant tumour often reaches a large size, eventually breaking through the periosteum into surrounding soft tissue, but usually maintaining a clearly defined border.

Macroscopically, there is a glistening white appearance, similar to that of normal cartilage.

Microscopically:

- The majority are low-grade, well-differentiated tumours that metastasise very late, and are histologically similar to benign cartilaginous tumours. Radical local surgery may be curative.
- The minority are high-grade, poorly differentiated tumours with marked pleomorphism, high mitotic activity and grow rapidly with early blood-borne metastases.

Chondroblastoma (Codman's tumour)

A rare usually benign tumour derived from chondroblasts, this typically occurs in males aged under 20 years. Typically it affects epiphyseal bone, almost always at the knee.

Microscopically, cells frequently show mitoses and osteoclast-type 'giant' cells.

Chondromyxoid fibroma

This rare, benign tumour is composed of lobules of fibrous tissue separated by myxomatous tissue containing cells in lacunae (thus mimicking the appearance of cartilage). Typically it occurs in males below the age of 30 years, arising at the epiphyseal line but sparing the epiphysis.

Fibrous and fibro-osseous tumours

Fibroma

A benign tumour, this is composed of inactive, acellular, fibrous tissue. Stroma may ossify to form an ossifying fibroma. The main complication is pathological fracture.

Fibrous dysplasia

This condition results from the disorganization of tissue differentiation and diaphyseal modelling. Shafts are usually thickened, and they may be painful. It may affect one bone (monostotic) or many (polyostotic) when deformity may be severe. Pathological fractures often occur, but they have normal healing potential.

Fibrosarcoma and malignant fibrous histiocytoma

Fibrosarcoma

This malignant tumour of fibroblasts can be classified into two types:

1. Endosteal fibrosarcoma—arises within bones and gives rise to destructive lesions as it grows out. Metastasis is associated with a poor prognosis.
2. Periosteal fibrosarcoma—seldom invades bone or metastasises to distant sites. Treatment is by local excision.

Malignant fibrous histiocytoma

This high-grade malignant bone tumour contains a mixture of spindle-shaped fibroblasts with histiocytic cells, many of which are multinucleated giant cells. Fibroblasts are characteristically arranged in a cartwheel-like formation (storiform pattern).

Other tumours

Ewing's sarcoma

A highly malignant bone tumour probably derived from primitive neuroendocrine cells, this affects children between the ages of 5 and 15 years. It has a characteristic chromosomal translocation—t(11;22) (q24;q12)—that results in the fusion of the *FLT-1* gene from chromosome 11 with the *EWS* gene on chromosome 22. The sarcoma usually arises in the diaphyses of long bones, particularly the femur.

Areas of osteolytic bone destruction surrounded by layers of new periosteal bone give the tumour a characteristic 'onion skin' appearance on X-ray. Pain, swelling and tenderness may be associated with fever and leucocytosis (thus tumours are sometimes mistaken for osteomyelitis). Effective chemotherapy, radiotherapy and surgical excision (often amputation) has increased five-year survival to 75%.

Giant cell tumour (osteoclastoma)

Osteolytic lesions arise in the epiphyses of long bones, typically in young and middle-aged adults. It only occurs in bones where the epiphyses have fused.

The tumour is composed of a mass of large multinucleated giant cells resembling large osteoclasts embedded in a supporting spindle-celled stroma. There is a gradual expansion of lesions into the metaphysis and the erosion of cortical bone; penetration of the periosteum or articular cartilage may occur.

Osteoclastoma is generally classed as benign, although a significant number become locally invasive and tend to recur after removal. About 10% of cases are truly malignant and metastasise to the lung via the bloodstream.

Figure 12.4 provides a summary of bone tumours.

DISORDERS OF THE NEUROMUSCULAR JUNCTION

Overview

Several diseases of muscle have been shown to result from disorders affecting transmission at the neuromuscular junction (NMJ).

Clinical presentation of NMJ dysfunction:

- Fatigability—primarily affecting proximal limb muscles, extraocular muscles (causing ptosis or diplopia) and muscles of mastication, speech and facial expression.
- Periodic paralysis—sudden reversible attacks of paralysis and flaccidity.

Disorders can be classified into two types, pre- and postsynaptic abnormalities, depending on which of the synaptic membranes is affected.

Fig. 12.4 Summary of bone tumours

Type	Tumour	Clinical features
Metastatic (secondary)	Carcinoma of bronchus (especially small cell) Adenocarcinomas of the breast, kidney and thyroid Prostate	Metastases occur most commonly to vertebral bodies, ribs, pelvis and upper ends of femur and humerus
Primary	Bone-forming tumours	Osteoma Osteoid osteoma Osteoblastoma Osteosarcoma
	Cartilage-forming tumours	Osteochondroma Chondroma Chondroblastoma (Codman's tumour) Chondrosarcoma Chondromyxoid fibroma
	Fibrous and fibro-osseous tumour	Fibroma Fibrous dysplasia Fibrosarcoma Malignant fibrous histiocytoma
	Others	Ewing's sarcoma Giant cell tumour (osteoclastoma)

Fig. 12.4 Summary of bone tumours.

Presynaptic abnormalities

Botulism

This rare form of food poisoning is caused by ingestion of a toxin produced by the bacterium *Clostridium botulinum*, found in imperfectly treated tinned food or preserved fish contaminated with the microbe.

Pathogenesis—the toxin binds irreversibly to those presynaptic nerve terminals of axons whose impulse transmission is acetylcholine (ACh) mediated. These include the NMJ, autonomic ganglia and parasympathetic nerve terminals. Binding of the toxin prevents fusion of ACh vesicles with the neuronal membrane, thereby preventing ACh release.

Clinical symptoms are chiefly vomiting and paresis of skeletal, ocular, pharyngeal and respiratory muscles. Antitoxin is available, but it has no effect once the toxin is bound. Recovery of transmission is achieved by terminal axonal sprouting and the formation of new synaptic contacts. Mortality can be high.

Lambert–Eaton myasthenic syndrome

This autoimmune disorder is characterised by abnormal fatigability and is often found in patients with lung cancer (when it is considered a paraneoplastic syndrome). Autoantibodies are thought to bind to presynaptic voltage-dependent calcium channels at motor nerve terminals to cause functional loss. This in turn causes the reduced release of ACh in response to nerve stimulation. Small cell lung carcinoma cells express calcium channels, suggesting that cross-reactive autoantibody production is triggered by these tumour antigens.

Postsynaptic abnormalities

Myasthenia gravis

This autoimmune disease is characterised by a progressive failure to sustain a maintained or repeated contraction of striated muscle. Prevalence is about 1 in 30 000. The disease usually appears between the ages of 15 and 50 years, and females are more often affected than males.

Aetiology—autoantibodies against the post-synaptic acetylcholine receptor are produced by B lymphocytes that are defectively controlled by T lymphocytes as a result of a disorder of the thymus gland. As a result of this interaction, receptors are degraded via a complement reaction, or blocked to activation by acetylcholine. This severely hampers neurotransmission. About 15% of cases have a thymoma (see Chapter 13) and 65% of patients have thymic gland hyperplasia.

There is a strong link to other autoimmune diseases, including thyrotoxicosis (Graves' disease), diabetes mellitus, rheumatoid arthritis (RA), and systemic lupus erythaematosus (SLE). There is linkage with various human leucocyte antigens (HLA), such as A1, B7 and DRw3.

Presentation:

- Early symptoms—intermittent ptosis or diplopia, weakness of chewing, swallowing, speaking or of moving the limbs. Movement is initially strong, but it rapidly weakens by the end of the day or after exercise.
- Later symptoms—respiratory muscles may be involved and respiratory failure is not an uncommon cause of death. Asphyxia occurs readily as the cough may be too weak to clear foreign bodies from the airways. Muscle atrophy may occur in long-standing cases.

The disease runs a remitting/relapsing course, and relapses may be precipitated by emotional disturbances, infections, pregnancy, or severe muscular effort.

The prognosis is variable. If the disorder is confined to eye muscles, then the prognosis for life is normal and disability slight. A prognosis of myasthenia associated with thymoma is markedly worse.

Investigations in myasthenia gravis:
- Tensilon test—short-acting, anticholinesterase drug trial increases acetylcholine (ACh) concentrations in the synaptic cleft and transiently relieves symptoms.
- Autoantibody screen—elevated ACh receptor antibody in 80% of cases.
- Electromyography (EMG)—characteristic decremental response.
- CT thorax scan— identify thymomas.
- Autoimmune screening—especially for thyroid diseases.
Management:
- Medical—anticholinesterase drugs (prevent ACh breakdown); immunological treatment: plasma exchange (removes autoantibody), intravenous immunoglobulin, immunosuppressant treatment.
- Surgical—thymectomy.

MYOPATHIES

Definition

Myopathy is any condition that primarily affects muscle physiology, structure or biochemistry.

Inherited myopathies
X-linked muscular dystrophy

Muscular dystrophy is the term used to describe inherited degenerative muscle diseases.

X-linked muscular dystrophy is characterised by the progressive degeneration of single muscle cells over a prolonged period of time. It results in muscle fibre destruction with the development of fibrosis.

Duchenne muscular dystrophy

The pattern of inheritance is X-linked recessive (p21 region); hence the disorder is almost exclusively seen in males. This is the most common form of muscular dystrophy in childhood, affecting 1 in 3500 male births.

The disorder is due to a mutation of the gene coding for dystrophin, a protein that normally anchors the actin cytoskeleton of muscle fibres to the basement membrane via a membrane glycoprotein complex (Fig. 12.5). Dystrophin helps to transmit the forces of contraction, meaning that muscle fibres in Duchenne patients are liable to tearing with repeated contraction.

Different degrees of severity of Duchenne dystrophy result from different mutations within the dystrophin gene:

- Severe Duchenne dystrophy—complete failure to produce dystrophin as a result of mutations causing gene frameshifts.

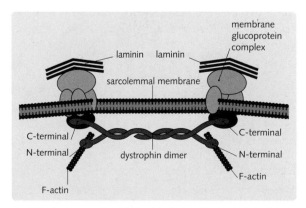

Fig. 12.5 Anchorage role of dystrophin. Dystrophin molecule is a long, rod-shaped protein, one end binding to membrane glycoprotein, the other to actin, with middle rod region.

- Moderate to severe forms of Duchenne dystrophy—dystrophin is produced but anchorage is inefficient because of mutations in binding sites for either membrane glycoprotein complex or actin cytoskeleton.
- Mild form of Duchenne dystrophy (Becker's dystrophy)—mutation in the middle rod region produces an abnormally weighted dystrophin protein which is still capable of anchoring muscle to basement membrane. Becker's dystrophy has a later onset than Duchenne.

Morphological features—muscle changes associated with Duchenne are illustrated in Fig. 12.6.

Clinical features—childhood onset of muscle weakness is associated with a high serum creatine phosphokinase level (caused by muscle necrosis) and calf hypertrophy due to fatty replacement of muscle (pseudohypertrophy; Fig. 12.6). Cardiac muscle is also affected leading to cardiomyopathy (see Chapter 6).

The prognosis depends on the degree of severity. For severe Duchenne it is very poor; most affected individuals are wheelchair dependent in their early teens and dead by their early twenties.

Myotonic disorders

Myotonic disorders are diseases in which there is a continuing contraction of muscle after voluntary contraction has ceased.

Myotonic muscular dystrophy

This autosomal dominant disorder is characterised by muscle weakness, myotonia (inability to relax muscles) and several non-muscle features including cataracts, frontal baldness in males, gonadal atrophy, cardiomyopathy and (in some cases) dementia.

This is the most common inherited muscle disease of adults, affecting 1 in 8000.

The genetic abnormality is an unstable CTG repeat sequence in a cAMP-dependent protein kinase located on chromosome 19. The disease shows anticipation, meaning that it appears at a younger age in each succeeding generation. The mechanism by which this mutation causes myotonia is unknown.

Microscopically, affected muscles show abnormalities of fibre size with fibre necrosis, abundant internal nuclei, and replacement by fibrofatty tissue.

The disorder usually becomes apparent in adolescence or early adulthood with facial weakness and disturbed gait.

Prognosis—death is commonly due to involvement of respiratory muscles in middle-age.

Acquired myopathies

Idiopathic inflammatory myopathies

There is primary inflammation of muscle with resulting fibre necrosis. The inflammatory infiltrate is mainly composed of T lymphocytes and monocytes as part of an abnormal autoimmune response. There are three main types of inflammatory myopathies, any of which may occur as part of an immune-mediated systemic disease such as systemic sclerosis.

Polymyositis

This inflammatory muscle disorder is characterised by weakness, pain, and swelling of proximal limb muscles and facial muscles, often with ptosis and dysphagia. It is the most common inflammatory muscle disorder, though still relatively rare. It occurs most frequently in adults, with females affected more than males by 3 : 1.

Aetiology—cytotoxic T cells and other lymphoid cells are found within the endomysium suggesting autoimmune injury of myocytes, but the mechanism of sensitisation is unknown.

Associations:

- Increased predisposition in people with HLA-B8/DR3.
- Connective tissue diseases such as SLE, RA or scleroderma.

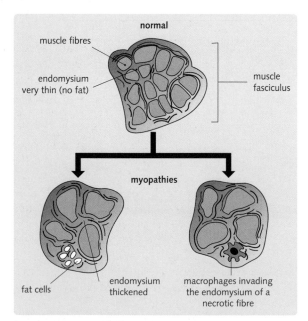

Fig. 12.6 Changes in muscle associated with Duchenne muscular dystrophy.

- Dermatomyositis—see below.
- Malignancy—particularly in association with non-Hodgkin's lymphoma, lung and bladder cancer.

Microscopically, there is a lymphocytic infiltration of muscle with fibre necrosis.

Clinical features—an insidious onset in the third to fifth decade of life, with symmetrical proximal muscle weakness initially affecting the lower limbs. Progression is typically slow but it may eventually involve pharyngeal, laryngeal and respiratory muscles leading to dysphagia, dysphonia and respiratory failures.

Investigations—blood: increased muscle enzymes (e.g. creatine kinase); tests for rheumatoid factor and antinuclear factor are often positive. Electromyography: useful for demonstrating myopathy without neuropathy. Muscle biopsy: muscle necrosis and regeneration in association with inflammatory cell infiltrate. Magnetic resonance imaging: non-invasive detection of active myositis.

Treatment—it may respond to immunosuppressive treatment such as corticosteroids and azathioprine.

Dermatomyositis

This has the muscle components of polymyositis accompanied by periorbital oedema and a characteristic purple 'heliotrope' rash on the upper eyelids. Often, there is also an erythaematous, scaling rash on the face, shoulders, upper arms and chest with red patches over the knuckles, elbows and knees. Arthralgia, weight loss and fever sometimes occur.

Dermatomyositis has an even stronger association with malignancy than polymyositis, especially affecting the ovary, pancreas, colon, lung and stomach.

Inclusion body myositis

This slowly progressive inflammatory muscle disorder is similar to polymyositis, but typically affects distal muscles in an asymmetric pattern. It also occurs mainly in the elderly. By light microscopy, histological features also appear similar to polymyositis, but with electron microscopy vacuoles containing filamentous inclusion bodies can be seen within fibres.

Endocrine myopathies

There is a weakness and wasting of muscle associated with endocrine disease. The main causes are:

- Corticosteroid-induced myopathy—either therapeutic or in Cushing's disease. Corticosteroids are associated with type 2 muscle fibre atrophy.

- Myopathies of thyroid dysfunction—associated with both hyperthyroidism and hypothyroidism.
- Myopathy of osteomalacia—painful myopathy often without much wasting or weakness.

Changes are usually reversible with appropriate therapy.

Toxic myopathies

Muscle damage may by incurred by a wide variety of drugs, the most common of which is alcohol. Damage to muscle is usually reversible on withdrawal of the toxic agent.

Ethanol

This may cause a spectrum of muscle diseases varying from mild, proximal weakness to severe muscle necrosis. Biopsy shows selective atrophy of type 2b fibres, which is reversible in the early stages.

Chloroquine

This drug is used principally in the treatment of malaria, and may produce a proximal myopathy and mild peripheral neuropathy. Damage is reversible on drug withdrawal but recovery is slow.

L-tryptophan

Eosinophilic myalgia has been reported with tryptophan-containing products.

ARTHROPATHIES

Osteoarthritis

Osteoarthritis (OA) is a degenerative disease of articular cartilage. It is associated with secondary changes in underlying bone resulting in pain and impaired function of the affected joint. Although the name suggests that primary OA is an inflammatory process, its main effects on the erosion of cartilage are independent of acute or chronic inflammation, even though inflammatory cells may be present in the affected joint.

It is extremely common—80% of the elderly population show radiographic evidence of OA, although only around 25% of these are symptomatic.

Females are affected more than males, except at the hip where both genders are equally prone to OA. It is increasingly common above 60 years of age but it may also occur in younger age groups following any form of mechanical derangement.

OA affects joints that are constantly exposed to wear and tear, typically large weight-bearing joints (e.g. those of the hip and knee) but also small joints in the hands, particularly the base of the thumb.

The aetiology is as follows:

- Primary—no obvious causes or predisposing factors (majority of cases).
- Secondary—arising as a complication of other joint disorders, mainly inflammatory joint disease, congenital joint deformities, trauma to joints, avascular necrosis of bone.

Secondary OA is also an important component of occupational joint disease, e.g. OA of the fingers in typists and of the knee in professional footballers.

Risk factors for the development of OA are:

- Fixed—ageing, genetic predisposition, female gender (except hip OA), abnormal joint structure.
- Modifiable—abnormal load on joints, repetitive loading, trauma.

Pathological changes

Pathological changes involve cartilage, bone, synovium and joint capsule with secondary effects on muscle (Fig. 12.7).

Early stage:

- Erosion and destruction of articular cartilage— degenerate superficial cartilage splits along lines of fibres to produce fronds (fibrillation). Narrowing of the joint space can be seen on radiography.
- Inflammation and thickening of the joint capsule and synovium.

Later stages:

- Sclerosis of subarticular bone—caused by constant friction of naked bone surfaces which now articulate in the absence of cartilage (bone eburnation).
- Osteophytes form around the periphery of the joint by irregular outgrowth of bone. Some may break off to form loose bodies within the joint. In distal interphalangeal joints of the fingers, osteophytes appear as small nodules (Heberden's nodes); in proximal interphalangeal joints, they are called Bouchard's nodes.
- Small cysts may develop in areas where the bone is not thickened as a result of synovial fluid accumulation in underlying bone.
- Reactive thickening of synovium and joint capsule due to inflammation caused by bone and cartilage debris.

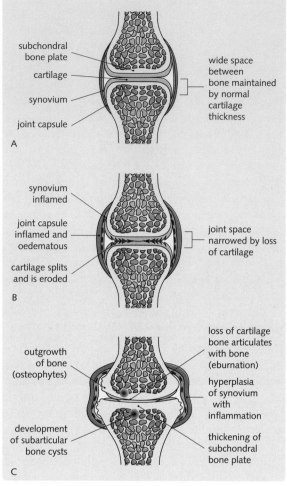

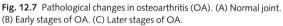

Fig. 12.7 Pathological changes in osteoarthritis (OA). (A) Normal joint. (B) Early stages of OA. (C) Later stages of OA.

- Disuse atrophy of muscle due to immobility of the diseased joint.

OA can be classified according to the main presenting features as follows:

- Primary generalised OA—usually associated with development of Heberden's nodes on fingers. It is most common in postmenopausal women.
- Erosive inflammatory OA—form of OA in which there is severe inflammation and erosion of cartilage, with rapid progression.
- Hypertrophic OA—florid osteophyte formation and bone sclerosis, but with slow progression and a relatively good prognosis.

Clinical features

The main symptoms of OA are pain and limitation in the movement of the affected joint, which often leads to functional impairment (e.g. difficulty walking in hip OA). Sometimes OA is associated with visible swelling around the joint margins (usually as an effect of osteophytes).

In OA of the cervical vertebrae (cervical spondylosis), osteophytes compressing emerging spinal nerves are responsible for much of the symptomatology.

OA diagnosis is largely clinical, although there are four classic X-ray signs (of which one or more may be seen):

1. Narrowed joint space.
2. Osteophytes (at bone margins).
3. Cysts.
4. Sclerosis.

Treatment:

- Lifestyle—reduce pressure across joint (e.g. weight loss, walking stick) and encourage strengthening exercises.
- Medical—analgesics and NSAIDs for pain relief; intra-articular or periarticular corticosteroid injections if severe pain (especially knee OA).
- Surgical—joint replacement for advanced hip or knee disease.

Rheumatoid arthritis

Rheumatoid arthritis (RA) is a chronic inflammatory joint disease caused by a multisystem connective tissue autoimmune disorder, rheumatoid disease (see below). It affects about 1% of the UK population, females more than males by about 3 : 1. Onset is typically between 35 and 45 years of age but it follows a normal distribution curve and no age group is exempt.

RA mainly affects peripheral synovial joints such as the fingers and wrists, but it can also affect the knees and more proximal joints. The most common presentations are symmetrical.

The aetiology is autoimmune, and there is an association with HLA-DR4 haplotype in most ethnic groups. The condition is characterised by autoimmune-mediated activation of CD4+ T cells within affected joints. The antigen for this reaction is unknown, but once it has been triggered, the release of proinflammatory cytokines drives the destruction of the joint.

Many RA patients have a circulating autoantibody directed against the Fc portion of native immunoglobulins (rheumatoid factor). The presence of rheumatoid factor (seropositive arthritis) helps to distinguish RA from several other inflammatory joint diseases (seronegative arthritis), but not all RA patients are rheumatoid factor positive. The exact role and underlying stimulus of rheumatoid factor is uncertain. However, immunological techniques have demonstrated it in plasma cells located in the synovium of affected joints. There is increasing evidence to suggest that RA is a disease of both cellular and humoral immune mechanisms.

Pathological changes

There are three main pathological changes (Fig. 12.8):

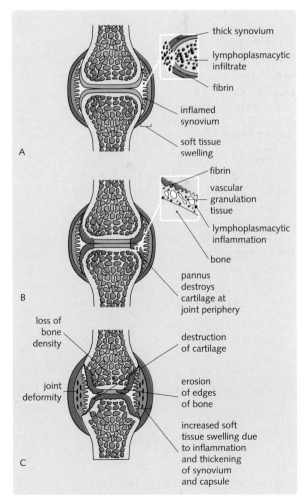

Fig. 12.8 Pathological changes in rheumatoid arthritis (RA). (A) Rheumatoid synovitis. (B) Articular cartilage destruction. (C) Focal destruction of bone.

1. Rheumatoid synovitis.
2. Articular cartilage destruction.
3. Focal destruction of bone.

Rheumatoid synovitis

The synovium becomes swollen and shows a villous pattern. Chronic inflammatory cells (mainly lymphocytes and plasma cells) increase in number within the synovial stroma, often forming an exudate that effuses into the joint space. Fibrin is deposited on the surface of the synovium, which undergoes hypertrophy. Soft tissue swelling from synovial inflammation may be marked.

Articular cartilage destruction

Inflammatory granulation tissue grows across the surface of the cartilage (pannus) from the edges of the joint. The articular surface shows the loss of cartilage beneath the extending pannus, most marked at joint margins.

Focal destruction of bone

Osteolytic destruction of bone occurs at the edges of the joint. Bone 'erosions' can be seen on radiography and are associated with joint deformity. There is also increased soft tissue swelling due to inflammation and thickening of the synovium and capsule.

Clinical features

Symmetrical polyarthritis

The insidious onset of arthritis first attacks finger joints (mainly metacarpophalangeal and proximal interphalangeal joints) followed by metatarsophalangeal joints and joints of the ankles, wrists, knees, shoulders, elbows and hips (in decreasing order of frequency). RA can also affect synovial joints of the spine (particularly cervical). Affected joints become swollen, painful and warm, often with redness of overlying skin. Stiffness tends to be worse in the mornings or following inactivity.

In the hands, rheumatoid arthritis tends to affect metacarpophalangeal (MCP) and proximal interphalangeal (PIP) joints whereas OA tends to affect PIP and distal interphalangeal (DIP) joints.

Joint deformities

As the disease progresses, muscle atrophy and joint destruction result in limitation of joint motion, joint instability, subluxation and deformities. Subluxation is the partial dislocation of a joint such that the bone ends still make contact, but are misaligned. There are also flexion contractures of small joints of the hands and feet, knees, hips and elbows.

Of the hands:

- Anterior subluxation of the metacarpophalangeal (MCP) joints with ulnar deviation of the fingers.
- 'Swan neck' deformity—hyperextension of proximal interphalangeal (PIP) joint with fixed flexion at distal interphalangeal (DIP) joints.
- Boutonnière (buttonhole) deformity—fixed flexion of proximal interphalangeal joint and extension of the terminal interphalangeal joint.
- Z deformity of the thumbs—fixed flexion at metacarpophalangeal joint and hyperextension at interphalangeal joint.

In the wrists there is often a fixed flexion deformity with a prominent, tender ulnar styloid process and pain on pronation/supination.

In the knees, Baker's cyst (cystic swelling in the popliteal fossa) is seen.

In the cervical spine, there is atlantoaxial subluxation.

Deformities are initially correctable but permanent contractures eventually develop such that joints become completely disorganized.

Rheumatoid nodules

Joint changes are often associated with development of subcutaneous rheumatoid nodules, usually located over the extensor aspect of the forearm but occasionally found overlying other bony prominences. Nodules are composed of extensive areas of fibrinoid material surrounded by a giant cell granulomatous reaction. They occur elsewhere in the body as part of the rheumatoid disease (see below).

Complications

- Secondary OA as a result of loss of articular surface, particularly in weight-bearing joints such as the knee.
- Septic arthritis—infection of the joint secondary to invasion from an ulcerated nodule or infected skin lesion.
- Amyloidosis—found in 25–30% of RA patients at autopsy.
- Carpal tunnel syndrome.
- Ruptured extensor tendons of the hand.

Investigations and diagnosis

Investigations

- Radiography—periarticular osteopenia, loss of articular cartilage (joint space), erosions, subluxation and ankylosis.
- Serology—rheumatoid factors (IgG- or IgM-type immunoglobulins that react with the Fc portion of IgG). This is present in 60–80% of those with RA and in 10% of people without RA.
- Measuring acute phase response—usually present in widespread RA as measured by, e.g. erythrocyte sedimentation rate (ESR), C-reactive protein (CRP).

Diagnosis

Diagnosis of RA can be made with four or more of the following criteria (which have been taken from the American Rheumatism Association, 1988 revision):

- Morning stiffness (> 1 hour), of at least 6 weeks duration.
- Arthritis of three or more joint areas, of at least 6 weeks duration.
- Arthritis of hand joints, of at least 6 weeks duration.
- Symmetrical arthritis, of at least 6 weeks duration.
- Rheumatoid nodules.
- Rheumatoid factor.
- Radiological changes.

RA treatment involves:
- Symptom management—analgesics, NSAIDs, intra-articular steroid injections.
- Disease-modifying anti-rheumatic drugs (DMARDs)—improve symptoms and reduce radiological progression, e.g. sulfasalazine, methotrexate. Newer anti-TNFα monoclonal antibody agents are used in refractory disease.
- Surgery—for advanced painful joint disease.

RA is associated with increased mortality, reducing lifespan by an average of 8–15 years. Worse prognosis is associated with being female, being positive for rheumatoid factor and having MTP joint or systemic involvement.

Extra-articular features (rheumatoid disease)

Lungs

Pulmonary involvement causes interstitial pneumonitis and fibrosing alveolitis, which eventually leads to a pattern of interstitial pulmonary fibrosis. Also, patients may develop lesions similar to the subcutaneous rheumatoid nodule, both within the lungs and on the pleural surfaces. These rheumatoid granulomas are particularly common in patients who already have industrial lung disease caused by inhaling various types of silica; the association of coalworker's lung with rheumatoid granulomas in seropositive miners is called Caplan's syndrome. Pleural effusions, bronchitis and bronchiectasis are all more common in rheumatoid patients.

Blood vessels

There may be development of vasculitis which is either:

- Acute neutrophilic vasculitis, presenting with purpura and occasional foci of ulceration.
- Lymphocytic vasculitis, producing a more low-key erythaematous patchy rash.

Eyes

Dry eye syndrome (keratoconjunctivitis sicca) is caused by lymphocytic inflammation of both lacrimal and mucous glands (secondary Sjögren's syndrome, present in 15% of all RA patients). Lack of tears leads to secondary inflammation of the cornea. In addition, sight-threatening scleritis may occur because of degeneration of collagenous tissue in the eye.

Haemopoietic and lymphoreticular systems

Anaemia of chronic disease is common in rheumatoid patients, and a minority develops hypersplenism or lymphadenopathy. The risk of lymphoma is also increased in longstanding rheumatoid disease. Felty's syndrome describes splenomegaly, lymphadenopathy, anaemia and leucopenia with RA. Sepsis is an important and common cause of death in these patients.

Neurological system

Hypertrophied synovium and joint deformities increase the likelihood of peripheral compression neuropathies. Bilateral carpal tunnel syndrome is a relatively common early manifestation of RA. Spinal nerve compression also occurs; severe and potentially fatal cord compression may follow atlantoaxial subluxation.

Heart

About a third of RA patients develop asymptomatic pericarditis, which occasionally becomes complicated by a pericardial effusion. Rheumatoid nodules may cause heart block, cardiomyopathy and ischaemia (by coronary artery compression).

A summary of the effects of rheumatoid disease is provided in Fig. 12.9.

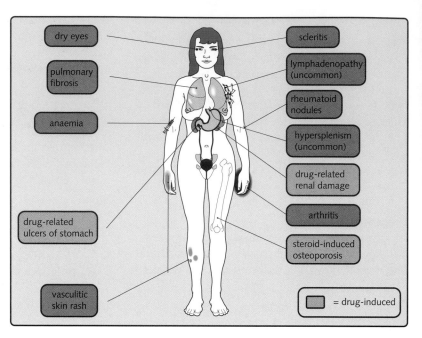

Fig. 12.9 Clinical features of rheumatoid disease.

dry eyes

pulmonary fibrosis

anaemia

drug-related ulcers of stomach

vasculitic skin rash

scleritis

lymphadenopathy (uncommon)

rheumatoid nodules

hypersplenism (uncommon)

drug-related renal damage

arthritis

steroid-induced osteoporosis

☐ = drug-induced

Juvenile rheumatoid arthritis

This accounts for approximately 15% of cases of juvenile chronic arthritis. By definition, it begins before 16 years of age. Clinical features are similar to those of adults but smaller joints tend to be spared, rheumatoid nodules are usually absent and rheumatoid factor is often negative. Systemic manifestations are more common and prognosis is considered worse than for adults.

Ankylosing spondylitis

This is an example of a seronegative arthritis (rheumatoid factor negative). It is an inflammatory arthritic disorder characterised by a rigid spine due to ossification of the spinal joints and ligaments. The condition begins in the lumbar vertebral spine and sacroiliac joints, extending upwards to involve thoracic and cervical vertebrae over a period of months or years. There may also be involvement of peripheral joints, mainly the hips and knees.

It affects 0.5% of the population in the UK, typically presenting in late adolescence and young adults (age 15–30 years of age), and in males more than females by 3 : 1.

The aetiology is unknown but more than 90% of individuals with ankylosing spondylitis have the HLA-B27 antigen (less than 10% of the normal population have this antigen), which suggests an autoimmune disorder. HLA-B27 positivity is a common feature of the seronegative arthritides.

Morphological changes—chronic inflammation of vertebral ligaments slowly heals by dense fibrosis and ossification ('bony ankylosis') to form a rigid shell that links the periphery of the vertebral bodies. Eventually the vertebral column becomes fused, inflexible and rigid ('bamboo spine').

There is typically an insidious onset of recurring episodes of low back pain and stiffness, sometimes radiating to the buttocks or thighs. Symptoms are characteristically worse in early morning and after inactivity.

Systemic manifestations include aortic valve incompetence (as a result of rheumatoid aortitis), anterior uveitis and amyloidosis.

On investigation, ESR and CRP are usually raised but may be normal, serology is negative for rheumatoid factor and X-rays may show sacroiliitis and bridging syndesmophytes between vertebrae.

The disease progresses slowly but unremittingly. Management is by:

- Lifestyle—regular physiotherapy and exercise (e.g. non-weight-bearing sports like swimming) to maintain as full mobility as possible and prevent deformity.
- Medical—mainly NSAIDs for symptomatic relief.
- Surgery for associated hip disease, including hip replacement.

75% of individuals with ankylosing spondylitis maintain a good quality of life with minimal disability.

A comparison of joint diseases is provided in Fig. 12.10.

Arthritis in association with other systemic disease

Reiter's syndrome

This inflammatory syndrome is characterised by the triad of arthritis, urethritis and conjunctivitis. It complicates 0.8% of urethral infection in males and 0.2% of cases of dysentery. It occurs in males more than females by 15 : 1 and the usual age of onset is 20–40 years of age. More than 80% of patients are HLA-B27 positive.

Classification is on the basis of aetiology:

- Genital type—usually follows non-specific (nongonococcal) urethritis or, less commonly, cystitis or prostatitis.
- Intestinal or postdysenteric type—in some parts of the world it may follow dysentery or occasionally non-specific diarrhoea, occurring 10–30 days after intestinal manifestations.

The underlying pathological mechanism is unknown but is probably autoimmune, triggered by the prior infection.

Clinical features are:

- Arthritis, usually affecting knee or ankle, and developing within weeks of the infectious episode. Clinically and histologically, arthritis resembles rheumatoid arthritis with chronic inflammatory synovitis.
- Dysuria and penile (or vaginal) discharge.
- Conjunctivitis (in 30% of cases).

Prognosis—the first attack typically resolves spontaneously within 6 months. However, 50% of patients relapse and some have continued relapsing chronic arthritis, causing disability but seldom deformity. In a minority of cases, there is development of severe spondylitis and features very similar to ankylosing spondylitis.

Psoriatic arthritis

About 5% of psoriasis patients develop arthropathy, which characteristically involves the distal interphalangeal joints (see Chapter 14).

Fig. 12.10 Comparison of joint diseases

	Osteoarthritis	Rheumatoid disease	Ankylosing spondylitis
Affected age group	Elderly	Any age	Onset usually before 30 years
Rheumatoid factor	Negative	Positive	Usually negative
Sex	Females > males	Females > males	Males > females
HLA association	None known	HLA-DR4	HLA-B27
Hands	Heberden's nodes (DIP) Bouchard's nodes (PIP)	Ulnar deviation of MCP joints Swan neck deformity Boutonnière deformity Z deformity of thumbs Prominent ulnar styloid process	—
Affected joints	Mainly hip, knees and spine. Usually asymmetrical.	Any Usually symmetrical	Mainly spine
Joint pathology	Erosion of cartilage Osteophytes	Destruction of joints	Bony ankylosis
Synovial pathology	Slight synovial hyperplasia	Florid synovial hyperplasia; pannus	—
Associated diseases	—	Rheumatoid disease Sjögren's syndrome Interstitial lung fibrosis	Aortic valve incompetence Uveitis Amyloidosis

Note: DIP, distal interphalangeal; MCP, metacarpophalangeal; PIP, proximal interphalangeal

Fig. 12.10 Comparison of joint diseases. (DIP, distal interphalangeal; MCP, metacarpophalangeal; PIP, proximal interphalangeal.)

Arthritis associated with gastrointestinal disease

Bacterial gastroenteritis

Like Reiter's syndrome, this is a reactive arthritis, occurring after infection with *Salmonella*, *Yersinia* or *Campylobacter* species. HLA-B27 antigen is again present in 80% of affected patients.

Inflammatory bowel disease

Enteropathic arthritis is seen at some stage in up to 20% of patients with ulcerative colitis and Crohn's disease. Typically it involves knee joints, but occasionally also ankles, elbows and small digital joints. Sacroiliitis and ankylosing spondylitis are also much more frequent in patients with inflammatory bowel disease.

Others

Neuropathic (Charcot's) joint disease

This joint disease occurs secondary to the loss of pain and position sense within the joint, which is swollen and deformed but not painful. Possible causes of loss of joint sensation include diabetic neuropathy, tabes dorsalis, syringomyelia, leprosy and cauda equina lesions (e.g. myelomeningocele).

Sarcoid arthritis

Arthritis occurs in 10% of patients with sarcoidosis, with onset typically in the first year of the disease. It may be of two types:

1. Early acute transient type—polyarticular symmetrical arthritis typically affecting knees and ankles, and usually associated with erythema nodosum. Arthritis is typically self-limiting.
2. Chronic persistent type—polyarticular associated with chronic sarcoidosis.

Chronic haemodialysis

There is an increased predisposition to septic arthritis (see below).

Crystal arthropathies

These diseases are characterised by deposition of crystals in joints and soft tissues. Affected patients usually present with an episode of acute arthritis, inflammation being caused by the deposition of the crystals, sometimes called a 'chemical arthritis'. With time, inflammatory changes lead to the development of chronic arthritis with features of OA (secondary OA).

Nomenclature

The term 'gout' is used as a clinical description of joints affected by crystal deposition. This term is then refined by demonstrating the type of crystal involved. There are two main types of crystal arthropathies: urate gout ('true gout' or simply 'gout') and calcium pyrophosphate gout ('pseudogout'). A comparison of the two types is shown in Fig. 12.11.

Gout

This acute inflammatory crystal arthropathy is caused by the deposition of urate crystal in joints and soft tissues as a result of hyperuricaemia. Prevalence is about 1% of the UK population and it is largely confined to men (90%), although some women develop the condition postmenopausally. It can present at any time above the age of 20.

Aetiology—uric acid is normally derived from the breakdown of purines and is excreted in the urine. Increased concentrations of serum uric acid (hyperuricaemia) can result in gout.

There are two main causes of hyperuricaemia:

1. Underexcretion of uric acid (most common)—of uncertain origin but clinically associated with hyperlipidaemia, renal failure, lactic acidosis (alcohol, exercise, starvation, vomiting) and thiazide diuretics.
2. Overproduction of uric acid (least common)—a result of either high cell turnover (e.g. leukaemia,

Fig. 12.11 Comparison of true gout and pseudogout.

Fig. 12.11 Comparison of true gout and pseudogout		
	True gout	**Pseudogout**
Crystal type	Urate	Calcium pyrophosphate
Underlying process	Hyperuricaemia	Chondrocalcinosis
Joints affected	Small	Large
Pain	Severe	Moderate

chemotherapy, severe psoriasis) or rare congenital enzyme defects of purine metabolism.

However, it should be noted that the majority of patients who have a raised blood uric acid level will never develop gout or any of its complications. The condition has a familial tendency, and it is believed to be polygenically inherited.

Pathogenesis

Gout affects the joints, soft tissues and kidney, as discussed below.

Joints—supersaturation of urate in synovial fluid results in the precipitation of urate crystals in certain joints, forming white powdery deposits on the surface of articular cartilage, beneath which degenerative changes can be seen. Crystal release into the synovial fluid stimulates an acute inflammatory reaction leading to the excruciating pain, oedema and the redness seen in acutely inflamed joints. Microscopically, neutrophil polymorphs can be seen to phagocytose urate crystal in the joint fluid. Repeated acute attacks eventually produce chronic arthritis and large urate crystal aggregations (tophi).

Soft tissues—uric acid crystals are also deposited in the soft tissues around joints, where their presence excites a foreign body, giant cell reaction. These soft tissue masses may also enlarge to produce tophi, especially around the pinna of the ear.

Kidney—in 10% of patients, urate crystals deposited in the kidney may lead to an interstitial nephritis and to renal calculi composed of uric acid. Crystals may also cause urinary obstruction, increasing the likelihood of complications such as pyelonephritis.

Clinical features

Characteristics of gout are:

- Intermittent attacks of excruciating pain, oedema and redness (acute gouty arthritis).
- Monoarthropathy (90%); polyarthropathy (two or more affected joints) 10%.
- Metatarsophalangeal joint of the big toe is most commonly affected (podagra, 75% of cases), but gout occasionally affects the ankle and, less commonly, the knee and hip.

Recurrent attacks affecting the same joint eventually lead to articular cartilage destruction, chronic synovial thickening and secondary OA-chronic gouty arthritis.

Diagnosis:

- Clinical features (as above).
- Raised serum urate level.

- Presence of crystals of sodium urate in aspirated synovial fluid from joint (detected with polarising light).

Management—analgesia for acute attacks: NSAIDs (e.g. indometacin) and colchicine. Preventative measures in recurrent disease:

- Allopurinol—suppresses uric acid synthesis by inhibiting xanthine oxidase.
- Uricosuric agents—e.g. probenecid.
- Diet—excessive purine intake and overindulgence in alcohol should be avoided.

Prognosis—some patients have only a single attack or suffer another only after an interval of many years. More often there is a tendency towards recurrent attacks that increase in frequency and duration so that, eventually, attacks merge and the patient remains in a prolonged state of subacute gout.

Pseudogout

This acute inflammatory crystal arthropathy is caused by deposition of calcium pyrophosphate crystals in articular cartilage of joints (chondrocalcinosis). It is most common in the elderly and affects males more than females.

The aetiology can be sporadic, metabolic or familial:

- Sporadic—in the vast majority of cases, the cause of pyrophosphate deposition is unknown but it is probably an age-related phenomenon.
- Metabolic—in patients under the age of 60 years, the disease is often associated with hyperparathyroidism, haemochromatosis or other less common metabolic or endocrine disorders.
- Familial—in a minority of patients, the disease is inherited as an autosomal dominant disorder.

Pathogenesis

Chondrocalcinosis is often asymptomatic. However, if crystals are shed into the joint space, patients develop an acute arthritis similar to that seen in urate gout. This shedding of crystals may be precipitated by trauma or intercurrent illness, or it may be spontaneous.

With time, damage to cartilage leads to the development of secondary OA.

Clinical features—as with gout, the affected joint becomes suddenly painful, warm, swollen, and tender. However, the most commonly affected joint is the knee (> 50% of cases), followed by the wrist, shoulder and ankle. The duration of the attack can vary from days to weeks and recurrent attacks are uncommon.

Diagnosis is by X-ray – cartilaginous calcification is usually obvious on X-ray – and by the presence of calcium pyrophosphate dihydrate crystals in aspirated synovial fluid from the joint (detected with polarising light).

Intra-articular aspiration and corticosteroids are the most effective treatment for acute pseudogout (anti-inflammatory drugs and colchicine also work but are often avoided in the elderly).

Infective (septic) arthritis

This inflammation of a joint is caused by infection—typically bacterial. This may affect any age group but children and young adults are the most commonly affected. It is a medical emergency, with a mortality rate of 10%. In older adults, most cases are associated with penetrating injury. Males are affected more often than females by 2 : 1. The knee and hip are the most common sites.

Aetiology—a wide range of bacteria may be responsible, but *Staphylococcus aureus*, streptococci and *Haemophilus* species are the most important. Patients who have developed septic arthritis always have bacteraemia.

Risk factors are diabetes, RA, joint puncture, surgery and immunosuppressive treatment.

Bacteria gain access to a joint via:

- Local trauma—well-recognised complication of penetrating injury such as open fractures, insertion of surgical prosthesis and non-sterile, intra-articular injection of steroids for established autoimmune arthritis.
- Spread from adjacent infective foci—especially in neonates with epiphyseal osteomyelitis.
- Haematogenous spread—most common route, usually from the skin or upper respiratory tract. Intravenous drug users are particularly likely to develop septic arthritis associated with Gram-negative bacteraemia.

Clinical features—there is an abrupt onset of severe pain, tenderness, swelling and erythema. The majority of cases affect a single joint only but some cases of gonococcal arthritis and arthritis in intravenous drug abusers may affect more joints.

Complications—untreated, it proceeds rapidly to joint destruction often with osteomyelitis, sinus formation, ankylosis and dislocation of the hip.

Septic arthritis is one of a group of conditions that may cause gait abnormalities in children (the 'limping child'). Trauma and septic arthritis occur throughout childhood, but other disorders are relatively age-specific:

- 1–5 years—developmental dysplasia of the hip (DDH): unstable hip joints more common in girls.
- 5–10 years—Perthes' disease: avascular necrosis of the femoral head.
- 10–15 years—slipped upper femoral epiphysis (SUFE): displaced femoral head, most commonly in pubertal boys.

Diagnosis—radiographs are normal at first but useful to exclude fractures or other bony injury. Later in the course of the disease, features of periarticular osteoporosis, joint space narrowing, periostitis and articular erosions may become apparent. Examination and culture of aspirated joint space fluid is essential for identification of the causative organism.

Treatment is by antibiotic therapy (intravenous or intramuscular).

The prognosis for recovery without joint damage is directly related to the speed with which antibiotic therapy is instituted.

Other types of infective arthritis
Tuberculous arthritis
Now rare, this is the result of bloodstream spread from pulmonary tuberculosis (TB). It produces a persistent monoarticular arthritis with typical caseating granulomatous lesions. The hip and knee are most commonly involved in children, whereas in adults the vertebral column is most often affected.

Infective arthritis in syphilis and brucellosis is now rare.

Lyme disease
This arthritis is due to the spirochaete *Borrelia burgdorferi*. It occurs in outbreaks in the USA and Europe (see Chapter 14).

Virus-associated arthritis
Many different viral infections are associated with a transient arthritis or at least distinct pain within joints. Examples include rubella, viral hepatitis and infectious mononucleosis (Epstein–Barr virus).

Objectives

In this chapter, you will learn to:

- Describe the patterns of common autoimmune diseases.
- Discuss the causes of primary and secondary immunodeficiency.
- Understand amyloidosis and its widespread effects.
- Recall the causes of increased and decreased numbers of white blood cells.
- Discuss neoplasms of white blood cells, focusing on lymphomas, leukaemias and myelomas.
- Describe disorders of the spleen and thymus.
- Logically describe the causes for the common clinical presentation of anaemia.
- Recall the mechanisms that produce polycythaemia.
- Discuss common disorders of haemostasis affecting blood vessel walls, platelets and clotting factors.

AUTOIMMUNE DISEASE

Autoimmune diseases that cause damage in many tissues and organs, involving a number of systems, are termed 'multisystem' or 'systemic' autoimmune diseases (Fig. 13.1).

Systemic lupus erythematosus

This inflammatory disorder of connective tissues is associated with autoantibodies to DNA and other nuclear components. Many tissues are affected but synovial joints, skin, kidneys and the brain are the major target organs (Fig. 13.2).

Systemic lupus erythematosus (SLE) affects 30 per 100 000 of the UK population, and it presents most commonly in the young and middle-aged with a peak incidence between 20 and 30 years of age. Females are more affected than males by about 8:1.

Incidence is higher in Black people and Asians than in Caucasians.

The aetiology is unknown but there is a strong familial tendency. Drugs (hydralazine, phenytoin, procainamide), chemicals and unidentified viral infections have all been postulated as the sensitising stimulus to autoantibody production.

Pathogenesis—SLE appears to be a disorder of the mechanisms that control self-tolerance, as patients develop autoantibodies to a wide array of self-antigens.

Antibodies are produced against components of both nucleic acids and cytoplasmic phospholipids:

- Anti-dsDNA—antibody against double-stranded DNA (most frequently detected).
- Anti-ssDNA—antibody against single-stranded DNA.
- Anti-DNA histone—antibody to a protein (histone) packaged with DNA in chromosomes.
- Antibodies to other nuclear components— anti-Ro, anti-La and anti-Sm.
- Antiphospholipid (cardiolipin)—causes thrombotic tendency, recurrent abortions and false-positive test for syphilis.
- Red cell antibodies—cause autoimmune haemolytic anaemia.
- Rheumatoid factors—antibodies directed against self-IgG antibodies.
- Cell- or organelle-specific antibodies (mitochondrial, smooth muscle, gastric parietal cell, etc.).

None of these antibodies is specific for SLE, and most have been detected in other connective tissue disorders or in diseases with an immunological basis.

Microscopically, fibrinoid necrosis is typically seen in vessels of affected organs, especially small arteries, arterioles and capillaries. In chronic SLE, fibrous thickening of vessels may lead to luminal narrowing.

The disease commonly presents with malaise, weight loss, fever, marked musculoskeletal symptoms

Fig. 13.1 Summary of systemic autoimmune diseases

Disorder	Sex ratio	Type of autoimmunity	Clinical features
SLE	8F : 1M	Antibodies directed against components of nucleic acids and cytoplasmic phospholipids	Skin rashes, neurological disorders, glomerulonephritis, haematological disorders, etc
Rheumatoid disease	3F : 1M	Rheumatoid factors: autoantibodies directed against native IgG	Chronic polyarthritis, subcutaneous nodules, vasculitis, interstitial pulmonary fibrosis, splenomegaly, etc.
Polymyositis and dermatositis	3F : 1M	Cell-mediated autoimmunity	Weakness, pain and swelling of proximal limb muscles and facial muscles Ptosis and dysphagia Dermatomyositis (= additional features of erythematous, scaling rash)

Fig. 13.1 Summary of systemic autoimmune diseases.

Fig. 13.2 Multisystem manifestations of systemic lupus erythematosus (SLE).

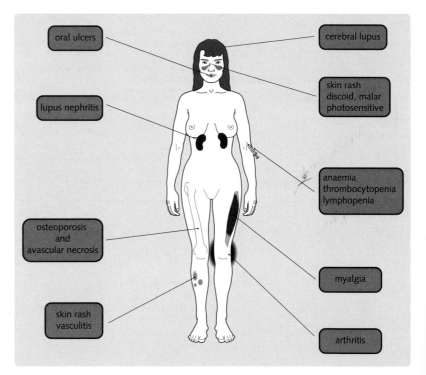

and a rash. However, the range of features that may occur is vast as demonstrated in the list below.

The American Rheumatism Association's list of diagnostic criteria for SLE

The criteria are listed in order of specificity:

- Discoid skin rash—round ('discoid'), red, scaly, telangiectatic plaques, usually on the face and scalp and less commonly on the hands.
- Neurological disorder—most common feature is non-organic psychiatric disorder, thought to be due to vasculitides in the brain. Vessel occlusion due to the prothrombotic action of antiphospholipid antibody on platelets can cause infarction and neuronal loss; this may present with symptoms such as seizure or even psychosis.

- Malar skin rash—symmetrical erythematous rash on the cheeks and the bridge of the nose (butterfly rash).
- Skin photosensitivity—malar or discoid rash on sun-exposed areas. Caused by immune complex deposits on the dermal side of the basement membrane.
- Oral ulceration—red erosions closely resembling oral lichen planus.
- Renal abnormality (lupus nephritis)—variable pattern from asymptomatic proteinuria to severe glomerular disease leading to renal failure (see Chapter 9).
- Evidence of immunological disorder—presence of autoantibodies, particularly of the antinuclear type.
- Haematological disorders—normocytic hypochromic anaemia, autoimmune haemolytic anaemia, leucopenia (usually due to lymphopenia), thrombocytopenia (sometimes associated with antiplatelet antibodies), predisposition to thrombosis (especially if antiphospholipid antibody positive).
- Serosal inflammation—pleurisy, pericarditis.
- Arthritis, bone disease and/or myalgia—often misdiagnosed as rheumatoid arthritis, SLE arthritis is non-erosive and involves two or more peripheral joints. Myalgia in the form of skeletal muscle pain is common, and it is thought to be caused by a lymphocytic vasculitis.

Clinical features

Diagnosis is based on a combination of clinical features and the result of laboratory investigation, primarily the identification of autoantibodies, especially those directed against nuclear DNA. The condition is frequently underdiagnosed.

Treatment is by systemic corticosteroid therapy for acute and life-threatening manifestations of SLE. Immunosuppressive drugs are often used to aid maintenance with less exposure to severe steroid side effects. Lifelong warfarin is needed in antiphospholipid syndrome to reduce the risk of thrombosis.

The disorder follows a protracted course of relapses and remissions. Renal, CNS and cardiac lesions are the most important prognostically. With treatment, in excess of 90% of patients can be anticipated to survive for 10 years.

Rheumatoid disease

Rheumatoid disease is a common and important autoimmune presentation with widespread effects on the musculoskeletal, cardiovascular, respiratory, haematological, ocular and neurological systems. It is covered in detail in Chapter 12 (see page 269).

Organ-specific or cell-type specific disease

Autoimmune diseases involving a single organ or cell-type are known as organ-specific or cell-type specific autoimmune diseases. Fig. 13.3 is an overview of these conditions, providing page references to the detailed discussions of each condition elsewhere.

> Although organ-specific autoimmune diseases specifically affect one organ, they frequently occur together, e.g. Addison's disease is often associated with autoimmune gastritis.

Hashimoto's thyroiditis

Causes hypothyroidism as a result of antibody-mediated destruction of the thyroid gland.

Graves' disease

Causes thyrotoxicosis due to overstimulation of thyroid-stimulating hormone (TSH) receptors by autoantibodies. This condition is discussed in more detail in Chapter 10.

Type I diabetes mellitus

Type I (insulin-dependent) diabetes mellitus is characterised by hyperglycaemia, which is responsive to insulin. The disorder is caused by antibody-mediated destruction of the insulin-secreting β-cell population of the pancreas.

As well as being an organ-specific disease (of the pancreas), the resultant hyperglycaemia has effects on many other systems. Consequently, diabetes mellitus is also classified as a multisystem disease.

Addison's disease

This rare condition of chronic adrenal insufficiency is most commonly caused by the autoimmune-mediated destruction of the adrenal cortex. It is often associated with other autoimmune endocrine disease, e.g. of the thyroid.

Fig. 13.3 Organ-specific autoimmune diseases.

Fig. 13.3 Organ-specific autoimmune diseases.

Disease	Associated autoantibody	Comment	Full discussion
Graves' disease	Anti-TSH receptor antibody (TRAb)	Hyperthyroidism	p. 211
Hashimoto's disease	Anti-thyroid hormones	Hypothyroidism	p. 213
Type I diabetes mellitus	Anti-islet β-cell antibody	Insulin-responsive hyperglycaemia	p. 223
Addison's disease	Antiadrenal antibodies	Hypoadrenocorticalism	p. 222
Autoimmune gastritis	Antiparietal cell and/or anti-intrinsic factor antibodies	Pernicious anaemia	p. 135
Vitiligo	—	Hypopigmentation	p. 332
Myasthenia gravis	Anti-acetylcholine receptor antibody	Muscle fatigue	p. 262

Note: *TSH, thyroid-stimulating hormone.*

Autoimmune gastritis

Chronic inflammation of the gastric mucosa caused by the autoimmune destruction of gastric parietal cells, with or without intrinsic factor autoantibodies (cause pernicious anaemia).

Vitiligo

The autoimmune destruction of melanocytes causes patchy loss of pigmentation.

Myasthenia gravis

The autoimmune destruction of acetylcholine receptors occurs at the neuromuscular junction.

DISEASES OF IMMUNODEFICIENCY

Immunodeficiency can be defined as the occurrence of, or increased susceptibility to, severe and prolonged infection caused by a specific defect in the immune system. Primary immunodeficiencies are a rare group of diseases, which usually result from genetic defects in one or more of the effector components of the immune system. Symptoms commonly develop in infancy, after the initial protection of maternal antibodies has ended (Fig. 13.4). More than 95 inherited immunodeficiency disorders have now been identified. Secondary immunodeficiencies are acquired disorders that result from extrinsic or environmental causes. There are many origins of secondary immunodeficiencies.

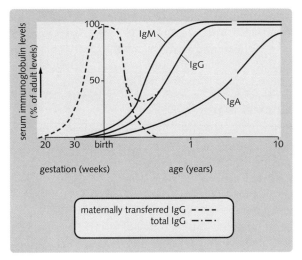

Fig. 13.4 Serum immunoglobulin levels in the neonate. (Adapted with permission from Introduction to Clinical Immunology, by M Haeny, Butterworths, London, 1985).

The type of infection associated with diseases of immune deficiency depends on the category of immune disorder:
- B cell deficiencies (defective antibody response)—increased susceptibility to opportunistic infections caused by extracellular organisms.
- T cell deficiencies (defective cell-mediated immunity)—increased susceptibility to opportunistic infections caused by intracellular organisms.
- Mixed B and T cell deficiencies (defective antibody response and cell-mediated immunity)—increased susceptibility to most infections.

Primary immunodeficiencies

Transient physiological agammaglobulinaemia of the neonate

This natural transient trough in antibody levels usually occurs between 3 and 6 months of age. It is caused by falling levels of maternally derived IgG prior to the appearance of the infant's own antibody (IgM followed by IgG and IgA; see Fig. 13.4). It can be more prolonged and more severe in premature infants.

X-linked agammaglobulinaemia of Bruton

In this X-linked recessive disorder, affected males present with recurrent infections from between 4 months and 2 years of age (maternal IgG protects against earlier infection). Pre-B cells are unable to differentiate into mature B cells because of a lack of an enzyme called Bruton's tyrosine kinase (located on chromosome Xq22). This kinase normally transduces maturation signals from the antigen receptor of a pre-B cell. The disease is characterised by:

- Deficiency of B cells and plasma cells.
- Negligible levels of immunoglobulins.
- Small lymph nodes and absent tonsils.

T cell numbers and functions are normal and infections are therefore primarily bacterial. Recurrent bacterial infections of the upper respiratory tract (e.g. by *Streptococcus pneumoniae*) are a common first presentation.

Treatment is with long-term prophylactic immunoglobulin replacement therapy and the rigorous use of antibacterial agents.

Common variable immunodeficiency

This is a heterogeneous group of conditions, many of which are inherited although sporadic cases do occur. No single pattern of inheritance is seen in the familial forms of disease. The common feature is agammaglobulinaemia, characterised by an increased susceptibility to infections, especially bacterial, and presenting most often in late childhood or adolescence. Both sexes are affected equally. It is also known as late-onset hypogammaglobulinaemia.

Pathogenesis is variable, although most cases appear to affect the differentiation of mature B cells into plasma cells. This may be due to a defect in T cell signalling.

The disease is more common and more variable than the X-linked form (hence the name); however, the pattern of infection is similar, chiefly affecting the lungs, sinuses, and gastrointestinal (GI) tract. In contrast to X-linked disease, lymphoid tissue becomes hyperplastic, highlighting that mature B cells exist in this condition. The risk of autoimmune disease is also increased in these patients.

Treatment is as for X-linked deficiency.

Isolated IgA deficiency

The most common form of immunodeficiency, this affects 1 in 700 Caucasians (but it is very rare in other ethnic groups). The condition may be familial or acquired secondary to infection (toxoplasmosis and measles have been described).

Circulating B cells bearing surface IgA are immature and fail to differentiate into IgA-secreting plasma cells.

Patients are prone to sinopulmonary infections and bowel colonisation with *Giardia*, *Salmonella* and other enteric pathogens.

It is associated with an increased incidence of autoimmune diseases and allergies.

DiGeorge syndrome (thymic hypoplasia)

This rare, congenital disorder is caused by the arrested development of the third and fourth branchial arches, resulting in an almost complete absence of the thymus and parathyroid gland. The genetic defect has been mapped to chromosome 22q11.

Immunoglobulin levels are normal, but affected individuals have decreased circulating levels of T lymphocytes, resulting in impaired cell-mediated immunity.

Patients typically develop a triad of infections: candidiasis, pneumocystis pneumonia and persistent diarrhoea.

The syndrome is also characterised by tetany from hypocalcaemia (due to hypoparathyroidism) and is associated with abnormalities of the great vessels (e.g. transposition or Fallot's tetralogy).

Treatment requires transplantation of thymic tissue.

Severe combined immunodeficiency (SCID)

This inherited deficiency of lymphocytic stem cells is characterised by:

- Deficiency of both T and B cells.
- Negligible circulating immunoglobulins.
- Greatly reduced cell-mediated immunity.
- Hypoplastic thymus.

The condition can be X-linked (gamma chain of interleukin-2 receptor at Xq13-21.1) or an autosomal recessive disorder. It presents during the first few months of life with a failure to thrive and persistent infections. In addition infants are at risk from graft-versus-host disease. One example of this occurs when maternal T cells cross the placenta; another involves T cells in non-irradiated blood products.

Death usually occurs within the first 2 years of life from multiple infections, although a bone marrow transplant can be an effective cure in some cases. X-linked SCID has become the first human disease to be successfully corrected by gene therapy, although work is continuing on a possible increased risk of leukaemia following such procedures.

Secondary immunodeficiencies

Secondary immunodeficiencies are those that result from extrinsic or environmental causes, as listed in Fig. 13.8 (see page 282). The pathologies of most of these diseases are covered in other chapters.

Acquired immunodeficiency syndrome

Acquired immunodeficiency syndrome (AIDS) is caused by infection with the human immunodeficiency virus (HIV). It is characterised by a profound defect in cell-mediated immunity with lymphopenia and diminished T lymphocyte responses.

The usual cause is HIV-1 (Fig. 13.5), although another strain of the virus (HIV-2) has also been associated with AIDS in Africa.

Routes of transmission are threefold: sexual contact, blood-borne (transfusions or contaminated needles) and maternal (placental or via breast milk). It is estimated that 39 million people worldwide are now infected with HIV.

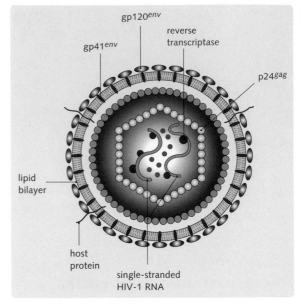

Fig. 13.5 Structure of the human immunodeficiency virus (HIV)-1.

Pathogenesis

HIV is an enveloped RNA retrovirus that binds to CD4 receptors present on T helper cells and various cells of the monocyte/macrophage system via its cell surface heterodimer of glycoproteins, gp120/gp41.

- Following cell entry, the virus loses its coat and utilises its enzyme, reverse transcriptase, to make viral DNA, which is inserted into the host chromosome.
- Viral replication is initially repressed by intracellular factors and by cell-mediated immunity mediated by CD8+ cytotoxic T cells, and so the virus can remain latent (i.e. dormant) for months or even years.
- Activation of latently infected T cells triggers viral replication, and infectious virus particles are released, resulting in the infection of more CD4+ cells.

Eventually, there is depletion of T helper cells, which results in a severely impaired cell-mediated immunity, with a high risk of multiple opportunistic infections.

There is a correlation between the fall in the CD4 cell count and increasing viral antigen levels (Fig. 13.6).

Clinical features

The clinical outcome of HIV infection has been classified into four stages (Fig. 13.7).

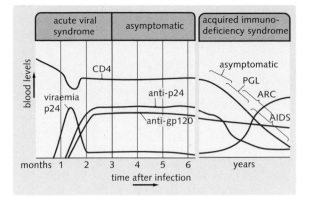

Fig. 13.6 CD4 count, viral antigen (p24) and antibody levels following HIV infection. (AIDS, acquired immunodeficiency syndrome; ARC, AIDS-related complex; p24, nucleocapsid protein; PGL, persistent generalised lymphadenopathy.)

The duration of each stage is highly variable – some patients pass directly through stages II and III to AIDS-related conditions or even to fully developed ('full blown') AIDS, whereas others remain in the earlier stages for months or years. Opportunistic infections tend to develop when the CD4 count drops below 200 cells/mm^3. A small proportion of HIV-infected patients do not develop clinical AIDS.

The reasons for these variations in the course of the disease are poorly understood and the factors that determine progression from one stage into the next remain unclear.

Prognosis and treatment

The prognosis for HIV patients with access to highly active anti-retroviral therapy (HAART) is improving. HAART is a combination of three drugs, including a reverse transcriptase and a protease inhibitor. In addition, antimicrobial therapy is given with the aim of preventing or treating infection (prophylactic antibiotics or antifungals).

In the initial stages of HIV infection, viral load and CD4 cell counts are monitored only; HAART treatment is generally delayed to avoid the development of drug resistance. Unfortunately, many AIDS patients in developing countries have a very poor prognosis because these expensive therapies are unavailable.

Figure 13.8 provides a summary of immune deficiencies.

Fig. 13.7 Classification of HIV infection.

Fig. 13.7 Classification of HIV infection	
Stage I	Initial infection; can be either: • Symptomatic seroconversion: mononucleosis-like syndrome, mild meningoencephalitis • Asymptomatic seroconversion
Stage II	Chronic asymptomatic infection: laboratory tests typically normal but may have anaemia, neutropenia, thrombocytopenia, low CD4 lymphocytes, lymphopenia and hypergammaglobulinaemia
Stage III	Persistent generalised lymphadenopathy: with or without laboratory test abnormalities as in stage II
Stage IV	AIDS-related complex: generalised lymphadenopathy with persistent fever, weight loss, unexplained diarrhoea, CNS manifestations and haematological abnormalities including thrombocytopenia, leucopenia and anaemia Fully developed AIDS: • Wide spectrum of opportunistic infections including *Pneumocystis carinii*, toxoplasmosis, *Cryptococcus*, cryptosporidiosis, atypical mycobacteria, herpes simplex or zoster, oral hairy leucoplakia, histoplasmosis, candidiasis, cytomegalovirus, *Salmonella* • Secondary cancers, e.g. Kaposi's sarcoma, non-Hodgkin's lymphoma, squamous carcinoma of the mouth or rectum

Fig. 13.8 Summary of immune deficiencies.

Category	Deficiency	Example
Primary	B cell (antibody deficiency)	Transient hypogammaglobulinaemia of infancy X-linked agammaglobulinaemia Acquired common variable hypogammaglobulinaemia Selective IgA or IgG subclass deficiencies
	T cell	Thymic hypoplasia (DiGeorge syndrome)
	Mixed B and T cell	Severe combined immune deficiency
Secondary	B cell (antibody deficiency)	Myeloma Protein deficiency
	T cell	AIDS Hodgkin's disease Non-Hodgkin's lymphoma Drugs, e.g. steroids, ciclosporin, azathioprine
	Mixed B and T cell	Chronic lymphocytic leukaemia Post-bone marrow transplantation Post-chemotherapy/radiotherapy Chronic renal failure Splenectomy

Fig. 13.8 Summary of immune deficiencies

AMYLOIDOSIS

Definition and chemical nature of amyloid

Amyloidosis is the pathological deposition of abnormal extracellular fibrillar protein, amyloid, in different tissues. Amyloid is composed of a meshwork of rigid, straight fibrils formed from precursor peptides (immunoglobulin light chains, serum amyloid protein A, peptide hormones) lined up in a cross-β-pleated sheet structure. The β-pleated sheet structure is important because enzymes in the body are incapable of digesting such large molecules in this form. It is detected histologically as a bright pink hyaline material that readily takes up Congo red stain, which is used in diagnosis.

It is important to note that it is the physical arrangement of the constituent amino acids that make a protein an amyloid rather than any specific amino acid sequence.

There are many different types of amyloid, each being formed from different precursor amino acids with the precursors themselves often being fragments of larger proteins.

Amyloid formation

Fifteen distinct forms of amyloid have been described, but three predominate:

1. AA (amyloid associated)—synthesised in liver (non-immunoglobulin).
2. AL (amyloid light chain)—immunoglobulin light chains derived from plasma cells.
3. Aβ amyloid—forms the cerebral lesion of Alzheimer's disease.

Amyloid formation occurs because of the production of either:

- Abnormal amounts of normal precursor peptide (common), e.g. immunoglobulin light chains in multiple myeloma or serum amyloid A protein in acute-phase response. It may be a result of overproduction, reduced degradation or reduced excretion of protein.
- Normal amounts of abnormal (amyloidogenic) peptide (rare), e.g. due to transthyretin or gelsolin polymorphisms, which make these proteins more prone to misfolding and aggregation.

Normally, misfolded proteins would be degraded by proteosomes within a cell or by macrophages extracellularly. In amyloidosis, however, the macrophage control mechanisms appear to fail and the misfolded proteins aggregate extracellularly.

Amyloid also contains a serum glycoprotein called serum amyloid P protein (pentraxin family), which is thought to assist in its polymerisation.

Classification of amyloidosis

Clinically, amyloidosis presents with organ involvement that is either:

- Systemic—may involve many tissues as it is particularly deposited in the blood vessel walls and basement membranes. Usually fatal, death generally occurring from renal or cardiac disease.
- Localised—affects only one organ or tissue. Rarely, it may be found without any obvious predisposing cause. The skin, lungs and urinary tract are the most frequent sites.

In both cases, the progressive accumulation of amyloid leads to cellular dysfunction by preventing the normal processes of diffusion through extracellular tissues and by physical compression of functioning parenchymal cells.

Systemic amyloidosis

Reactive systemic amyloidosis

This amyloid is composed of protein A and is termed the AA type. It is derived from serum amyloid A (SAA) protein, which is an acute-phase reactant synthesised in the liver. SAA increases are seen in response to a variety of diseases, invariably featuring chronic inflammation:

- Rheumatoid arthritis (most common cause): in up to 3% of rheumatoid patients.
- Chronic infections (e.g. tuberculosis).
- Hodgkin's disease.
- Inflammatory bowel disease.
- Bronchiectasis.
- Chronic osteomyelitis.

Such reactive disease in response to chronic inflammatory disorders tends to produce more severe systemic involvement when compared to other forms of amyloidosis. AA-type amyloid is deposited in many organs but it has a predilection for the liver, spleen and kidney. It results in hepatosplenomegaly with or without renal vein thrombosis and nephrotic syndrome.

AL amyloidosis

This amyloid is composed of immunoglobulin light chains (and/or parts of their variable regions) and is termed AL type. Immunoglobulin light chains are formed by proliferating plasma cells usually in association with:

- Multiple myeloma—occurs in up to 15% of patients with this condition.
- Waldenström's macroglobulinaemia.
- Heavy-chain disease.
- Primary amyloidosis.

Primary amyloidosis is a myeloma-associated amyloidosis that occurs in the absence of any clinically obvious myeloma. It is caused by a clinically occult plasma cell tumour, which is revealed only by serum electrophoresis showing the presence of a monoclonal immunoglobulin band. It is also known as benign monoclonal gammopathy.

AL-type amyloid is deposited in many organs, including the tongue, skin, heart, nerves, kidneys, liver and spleen. It has a predilection for connective tissue within these organs.

A common presentation of advanced AL amyloidosis is nephrotic syndrome and biventricular cardiac failure. Macroglossia (enlarged tongue), peripheral neuropathy, carpal tunnel syndrome and overt renal failure are also seen.

Haemodialysis-associated amyloidosis

This amyloidosis is associated with long-term haemodialysis for chronic renal failure. Amyloid material deposited in the affected tissues appears to be β_2-microglobulin, which is ineffectively filtered out of the blood by haemodialysis. The amyloidosis is termed AH type (H for haemodialysis).

Clinical features include arthropathy and carpal tunnel syndrome.

Hereditary amyloidosis

Hereditary forms of amyloidosis are rare, and they include familial Mediterranean fever (AA type) and familial neuropathic forms (pre-albumin, AF type).

Localised amyloidosis

Alzheimer's disease

The most common example of amyloid deposition occurs in the nervous system, in both Alzheimer's disease (see Chapter 5) and in normal ageing (cerebral angiopathy). The amyloid (Aβ) is composed of peptide fragments termed β-protein or A4 protein, both of which are derived from a normal, neuronal membrane protein—amyloid precursor protein (APP).

Endocrine amyloidosis

Amyloid material is often found in the stroma of peptide hormone-producing tumours. It is particularly characteristic of medullary carcinoma of the thyroid, a tumour of the calcitonin-producing parafollicular C cells (see Chapter 10). In this instance, the amyloid contains calcitonin precursor molecules arranged in a β-pleated sheet configuration.

In type II diabetes, the excessive secretion of amylin by the β-cells of the pancreas is associated with its deposition as islet amyloid.

Senile amyloidosis

Minute deposits of amyloid usually derived from serum transthyretin (pre-albumin) are found in the heart and in the walls of blood vessels in many organs of elderly people. However, cardiomyopathy and/or arrhythmias occur in only a few cases.

DISORDERS OF WHITE BLOOD CELLS

Leucopenia

Leucopenia is defined as a reduction in circulating leucocytes. The classification of leucocytes is shown in Fig. 13.9.

Neutropenia

Neutropenia, a deficiency of neutrophil granulocytes, is the most important form of leucopenia. The lower limit of normal neutrophil count is $2.5 \times 10^9/L$ (except in Black people and in the Middle East, where it is $1.5 \times 10^9/L$). Levels of less than these values are classified as neutropenia.

Neutropenia may be selective or part of a general pancytopenia. The causes of both types are listed in Fig. 13.10.

Clinical features depend on the degree of neutropenia:

- Mild—usually asymptomatic.

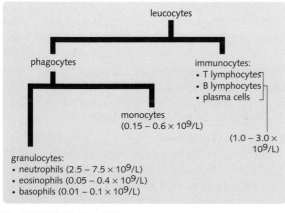

Fig. 13.9 Classification of leucocytes.

- Moderate to severe ($< 0.5 \times 10^9/L$)—associated with a progressive increase in risk and severity of infection.
- Levels of $< 0.2 \times 10^9/L$ are associated with a high mortality from overwhelming infection.

Severe neutropenia is termed agranulocytosis. Infections are predominantly bacterial and are usually opportunistic, most commonly Gram-positive skin organisms (e.g. *Staphylococcus* and *Streptococcus* species) or Gram-negative gut bacteria (e.g. *Pseudomonas*, *Escherichia coli*, *Proteus*, etc.).

They can be either localised (e.g. of the mouth, throat, skin or anus) or generalised (neutropenic sepsis). The latter may be rapidly fatal.

Treatment is of the underlying cause and with antimicrobial therapy.

Leucocytosis

Leucocytosis is defined as an increase in numbers of circulating white blood cells.

Types of leucocytosis

Each type of leucocyte (see Fig. 13.9) may be increased in number (neutrophilia, eosinophilia, etc.). Monocytosis and lymphocytosis are the terms used for increases in monocytes and lymphocytes, respectively.

Neutrophilia is the most common cause of leucocytosis, produced by common events such as acute bacterial infection or acute inflammation.

Leucocytosis can be:

- Primary—caused by bone marrow disease, e.g. leukaemias, lymphomas (described later).
- Secondary—caused by the normal response of bone marrow to abnormal conditions, e.g. infection. Also known as reactive leucocytosis (Fig. 13.11).

Lymphadenitis

This inflammation of lymph nodes is usually caused by infection and is characterised by a painful swelling of the affected nodes as a result of:

- Increased blood flow.
- Macrophage activation and increased cell number.
- Lymphocyte activation and increased cell number. Histologically, lymphoid follicles with large germinal centers become prominent within the node.

Additional changes depend on the type of lymphadenitis:

Fig. 13.10 Causes of neutropenia.

Fig. 13.10 Causes of neutropenia

Type	Cause	Clinical features
Selective neutropenia	Reduced granulopoiesis	Congenital: Kostmann's syndrome—autosomal recessive disease presenting in the first year of life with life-threatening infections Cyclical: rare syndrome characterised by recurrent severe but temporary neutropenia with a periodicity of 3–4 weeks Nutritional: vitamin B_{12} or folate deficiency Racial: African races
	Accelerated granulocyte removal	Immune: • autoimmune • systemic lupus erythematosus • Felty's syndrome • hypersensitivity and anaphylaxis Infectious: • viral, e.g. hepatitis, influenza, HIV • fulminant bacterial, e.g. typhoid, miliary tuberculosis
	Drug-induced neutropenia	Drug-induced damage of either neutrophils or precursor marrow cells can occur via direct toxicity or immune-mediated mechanisms in susceptible individuals; examples of such drugs include: • anticancer chemotherapy agents: chlorambucil, methotrexate • anti-inflammatory: phenylbutazone, cyclophosphamide • antibacterial: chloramphenicol, cotrimoxazole, sulfasalazine • anticonvulsants: phenytoin • antithyroid: carbimazole • hypoglycaemic: tolbutamide • phenothiazines: chlorpromazine, thioridazine • psychotropics and antidepressants: clozapine, imipramine • miscellaneous: gold, penicillamine
Part of general pancytopenia	Reduced granulopoiesis	Bone marrow failure, megaloblastic anaemia
	Accelerated granulocyte removal	Splenomegaly

- Acute non-specific lymphadenitis—typically caused by acute infections (e.g. infectious mononucleosis, rubella, pertussis, mumps). Bacterial infection commonly involves infiltration of a node by neutrophils. Most commonly affected are cervical lymph nodes (in the neck) associated with tonsillitis.
- Chronic non-specific lymphadenitis—typically caused by chronic infections (e.g. brucellosis, tuberculosis, syphilis, hepatitis). Additional changes include increased plasma cells and granuloma formation.

Malignant lymphomas

In this group of lymphoproliferative diseases, normal lymphoid tissue is replaced by abnormal cells of lymphoid origin, forming solid malignant tumours of the lymph nodes. The majority of lymphomas are of B cell origin. All lymphomas are broadly classified as either Hodgkin's disease or non-Hodgkin's lymphomas.

Fig. 13.11 Causes of reactive leucocytosis

Cause	Clinical features
Neutrophilia ($> 7.5 \times 10^9$/L)	Acute infections Haemorrhage/hemolysis Inflammation and tissue necrosis Metabolic disorders Myeloproliferative diseases Neoplasia Steroid therapy Strenuous exercise
Monocytosis ($> 0.8 \times 10^9$/L)	Chronic infections, e.g. tuberculosis Rickettsiosis and malaria Inflammatory disorders, e.g. rheumatoid disease, SLE, Crohn's disease
Eosinophilia ($> 0.44 \times 10^9$/L)	Allergy, e.g. asthma Parasites, e.g. tapeworms Skin disease, e.g. eczema, psoriasis Neoplasia, especially Hodgkin's disease Miscellaneous, e.g. polyarteritis nodosa, sarcoidosis
Basophilia ($> 0.1 \times 10^9$/L)	Myxoedema Chickenpox Myeloproliferative disorders
Lymphocytosis ($> 3.5 \times 10^9$/L)	Acute infections, e.g. infectious mononucleosis Chronic infections, e.g. tuberculosis, brucellosis, hepatitis

Note: SLE, systemic lupus erythematosus

Fig. 13.11 Causes of reactive leucocytosis.

Hodgkin's disease

Hodgkin's disease is characterised by the painless enlargement of one or more groups of lymph nodes (painless lymphadenopathy) and the presence of large binucleate cells (Reed–Sternberg cells) within them.

It affects 4 per 100 000 in the UK, with a slight male excess. It can occur at any age but there are two peaks of incidence: one in young adults (20–30 years old) and the other in late middle age (50–70 years old).

The aetiology of Hodgkin's disease is obscure, as is the origin of the malignant Reed–Sternberg (RS) cells. Although no causal link has been established with Epstein–Barr virus (EBV), Hodgkin's disease sufferers are three times more likely to have had glandular fever in the past.

RS cells form only a small percentage of the total population of the affected node, the majority being composed of reactive lymphocytes, plasma cells, histiocytes and eosinophils.

Hodgkin's disease often presents clinically as the enlargement of accessible nodes, most often in the upper half of the body (e.g. cervical or axillary). The disease is initially localised to a single peripheral lymph node region but it spreads in a fairly consistent pattern to adjacent nodes via the lymphatics and then, following splenic involvement, to other organs via the bloodstream.

One-third of patients have systemic symptoms, notably weight loss and pyrexia (so-called 'B symptoms'). These are due to:

- Lymph node enlargement—producing mediastinal compression and lymphoedema.
- Haematology—normochromic–normocytic anaemia, neutrophilia, eosinophilia, lymphopenia (advanced disease), raised erythrocyte sedimentation rate (ESR).
- Immunology—depression of T cell function and susceptibility to infection.

The stage (extent of spread) of Hodgkin's disease is determined by the Ann Arbor staging system (Fig. 13.12). A clinical addition is the presence of 'B symptoms'—systemic features associated with poorer prognosis, namely weight loss, night sweats and unexplained fever.

Treatment depends on the stage: either localised (radiotherapy) or generalised (systemic chemotherapy). Five-year survival is approximately 75%, but long-term survivors of chemotherapy and/or radiotherapy are at increased risk of second cancers.

Diagnosis of Hodgkin's disease can only be made on examination of biopsied lymph nodes:

- Macroscopically—affected lymph nodes are enlarged, with a smooth surface, and the lymph node capsule is rarely breached (cf. non-Hodgkin's lymphomas).
- Microscopically—four subtypes of Hodgkin's disease are recognised and classified according to the Rye classification system (Fig. 13.13).

Non-Hodgkin's lymphomas

Non-Hodgkin's lymphomas (NHLs) include all lymphomas other than Hodgkin's disease. They are predominantly diseases of middle and later life, with males slightly more affected than females.

Fig. 13.12 Ann Arbor staging system of Hodgkin's disease

Stage	Comment
I	Involvement of single lymph node region (I) or of single extralymphatic organ or site (hence Ie)
II	Involvement of two or more lymph node regions, with all lesions confined to the same side of the diaphragm (II), or localised involvement of an extralymphatic site and one or more lymph node regions confined to one side of the diaphragm (IIe)
III	Involvement of lymph node regions on both sides of the diaphragm (III) which may also involve the spleen (IIIs), localised extralymphatic sites (IIIe) or both (IIIse)
IV	Widespread involvement of extralymphoid sites such as the liver, lung and bone marrow with or without lymph node involvement

Fig. 13.12 Ann Arbor staging system of Hodgkin's disease. Suffix A indicates the absence of systemic symptoms; suffix B indicates the presence of systemic symptoms. For example, stage IIIeB denotes involvement of lymph nodes on both sides of the diaphragm accompanied by localised involvement of an extralymphatic site with systemic symptoms.

Fig. 13.13 Rye classification of Hodgkin's disease

Type	Characteristics
Nodular sclerosis (60–70%)	Thick bands of collagen encircle abnormal tissue; lacunar cells (variants of RS cell) are often numerous; good prognosis Most common presentation in young females
Mixed cellularity (15%)	Numerous RS cells and intermediate numbers of lymphocytes, plasma cells and eosinophils; poor prognosis Most common presentation in elderly patients
Lymphocyte predominant (10%)	Numerous lymphocytes, few RS cells and a scattering of unusual Hodgkin's cells: 'popcorn' cells (so named due to their excessively lobulated nuclei); increased risk of development on non-Hodgkin's B cell lymphoma; otherwise good prognosis
Lymphocyte depleted (2%)	Dominance of RS cells but sparse lymphocytes with or without diffuse fibrosis; worst prognosis

Note: RS, Reed–Sternberg

Fig. 13.13 Rye classification of Hodgkin's disease.

The aetiology of NHLs is poorly understood but several factors have been implicated:

- Immunosuppression—increased incidence in primary immunosuppressive diseases, e.g. X-linked agammaglobulinaemia, and in secondary immunosuppression, e.g. drug induced after transplantation.
- Viral infection—with lymphotropic viruses, e.g. EBV, human T-lymphotropic virus (HTLV-1), HIV.
- Bacterial infection—*Helicobacter pylori* infection linked to gastric lymphoma.
- Radiation.

Chromosomal translocations are a feature of many types of lymphoma, for example:

- Burkitt's lymphoma—translocation 8:14. Also associated with EBV infection.
- Follicular B cell lymphoma—translocation 14:18.
- Small or large cell diffuse lymphomas—associated with translocation 11:14.

These translocations cause a neoplastic transformation as a result of the transfer of an oncogene or oncogene–regulatory gene to an abnormal site. This causes the increased expression of these oncogenes, e.g. *bcl-2* in follicular lymphoma, which inhibits apoptotic cell death.

In malignant lymphomas, the tumour represents a clone of cells whose maturation is fixed at a particular stage of development.

The majority (70%) of NHLs are B-cell lymphomas, which are derived from follicle centre cells. These tumours have either follicular or diffuse architecture.

Recognising the normal development of lymphocytes (Fig. 13.14) is essential to understanding lymphomas and other neoplastic proliferations of white blood cells.

Clinical features

The clinical manifestations of NHLs are similar to those of Hodgkin's disease but they are more varied because of their heterogeneous nature. The majority

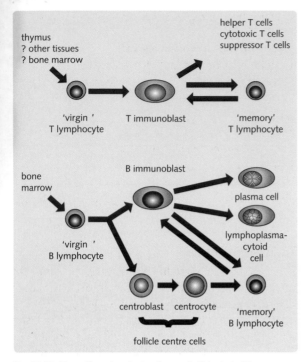

thymus
? other tissues
? bone marrow

helper T cells
cytotoxic T cells
suppressor T cells

'virgin'
T lymphocyte

T immunoblast

'memory'
T lymphocyte

bone
marrow

B immunoblast

plasma cell

'virgin'
B lymphocyte

lymphoplasma-
cytoid
cell

centroblast   centrocyte

'memory'
B lymphocyte

follicle centre cells

Fig. 13.14 Normal lymphocyte development. (Adapted with permission from Essential Hematology, 3rd edn, by V Hoffbrand and J Pettit, Blackwell Science, 1993.)

Common primary extranodal sites include the orbit, nasopharynx, tonsil, GI tract, skin and bone. Compression syndromes may also occur, e.g. gut obstruction, superior vena cava obstruction.

Systemic symptoms are often prominent in extensive disease, along with hepatosplenomegaly.

Classification and management

Several classification systems are used for NHLs.

One relatively simple classification is based on the Kiel system (Fig. 13.15), which considers the following:

- Degree of malignancy—low grade (well differentiated, relatively inactive cell types; progress over years); high grade (primitive actively proliferating cells; progress over weeks or months).
- Tumour architecture—follicular or diffuse.
- Functional cell type—either T cell or B cell.
- Specific cell type or size, e.g. centroblastic or immunoblastic, large or small cell.

A similar staging system to that used in Hodgkin's disease may be used but the clinical grade is better related to the prognosis.

Treatment is by single or combination chemotherapy with which some patients show long-term remission if not cure. Bone marrow transplantation is under evaluation.

The prognosis depends on the type of lymphoma and varies widely from highly proliferative and rapidly fatal diseases (e.g. immunoblastic lymphoma) to indolent and well-tolerated malignancies with a mean survival of about 7 years (e.g. follicular centrocytic lymphoma).

of cases present with asymmetric, painless enlargement of lymph nodes in one or more peripheral lymph node regions. However, extranodal presentation is more frequent than in Hodgkin's disease, with 20% of all NHLs originating within extranodal sites.

Fig. 13.15 Classification of non-Hodgkin's lymphomas (NHLs) based on the Kiel system.

Fig. 13.15 Classification of NHLs based on the Kiel system

Grade	B cell	T cell
Low-grade malignancy	Follicular: • Centrocytic • Centroblastic-centrocytic Diffuse: • Lymphocytic: chronic lymphocytic and hairy cell leukaemia • Lymphoplasmacytoid • Plasmacytic: multiple myeloma • Centrocytic • Centroblastic-centrocytic	Lymphocytic Small cerebriform cell: • Mycosis fungoides • Sézary's syndrome Lymphoepithelioid Angioimmunoblastic T zone Pleomorphic small cell
High-grade malignancy	Diffuse: • Centroblastic • Immunoblastic • Anaplastic • Lymphoblastic • 'Burkitt-type': small, non-cleaved cell	Pleomorphic medium or large cell (HTLV-1) Immunoblastic Anaplastic Lymphoblastic

Leukaemias

Leukaemias are neoplastic proliferations of white blood cell precursors in the bone marrow.

Classification—leukaemias are classified into two broad groups according to the ability of the leukaemic cells to differentiate. The ability to differentiate also reflects the rate of disease progression:

1. Acute—characterised by numerous immature 'blast' cells (leucocyte precursors) and rapid disease progression.
2. Chronic—characterised by large numbers of precursor cells that are more differentiated than blast cells, and associated with slower disease progression.

These groups are then further classified into two main groups depending on neoplastic cell types:

1. Myeloid leukaemia (cells of granulocytic series).
2. Lymphocytic leukaemia (cells of the lymphoid series).

Aetiology—in the majority of cases, the cause of leukaemia is unknown. However, certain factors are known to initiate leukaemic transformation:

- Genetics—slight familial tendency (high concordance in monozygotic twins); chromosome abnormalities (both quantitative and qualitative) are present in about 50% of patients; increased incidence in Down syndrome.
- Ionising radiation—excessive exposure in therapy, e.g. for ankylosing spondylitis, malignant disease; nuclear explosions/accidents as at Hiroshima and Chernobyl.
- Drugs—prolonged chemotherapy, e.g. with alkylating agents (cause myeloid leukaemia).
- Immune status—increased incidence in immunosuppressed individuals.
- Viruses—e.g. HTLV-I causes adult T cell leukaemia/lymphoma; HTLV-II is associated with hairy cell leukaemia.
- Industrial benzene exposure.

Common features of leukaemias

The common features of leukaemias are bone marrow failure, gout and metastasis.

Bone marrow failure

Overproduction of leucocyte precursor cells causes the suppression of normal blood cell production, thus:

- Deficiency of red cell production → anaemia.
- Deficiency of platelet production (thrombocytopenia) → haemorrhage.
- Deficiency of normal leucocyte production (granulocytes and lymphocytes) → failure to control infection.

Gout

Increased cell turnover leads to increased uric acid synthesis, which may result in gout.

Metastasis

There is infiltration of organs such as the liver, spleen, lymph nodes, meninges and gonads by the leukaemic cells.

Acute leukaemia

Acute leukaemia is a failure of maturation, leading to the rapid and uncontrolled proliferation of immature blast cells (lymphoblasts or myeloblasts).

There are two main types: acute lymphoblastic leukaemia (ALL) and acute myeloblastic leukaemia (AML). These are further subclassified according to cytological features of the blast cells. There are three subtypes for ALL (L_1–L_3) based on the degree of uniformity of cell size and vacuolation. There are eight subtypes for AML (M_0–M_7) based on the degree of cytoplasmic granularity.

Figure 13.16 outlines the features of ALL and AML.

The clinical features of both AML and ALL are similar. They commonly present with symptoms of anaemia (e.g. tiredness, malaise, breathlessness, angina) and their course is typified by a series of overwhelming infections and mucosal haemorrhage.

Onset is frequently rapid and progression to death from anaemia, haemorrhage or infection occurs within weeks if no treatment is given.

The clinical course is less catastrophic in childhood ALL.

Haematological investigations reveal:

- Anaemia—normocytic, normochromic.
- Leucocytosis—although leucopenia may be an occasional feature, despite massive marrow infiltration with blast cells.
- Neutropenia—susceptibility to overt infections.
- Thrombocytopenia—petechiae, purpura, epistaxis, bleeding gums, GI haemorrhage, cerebral haemorrhage.
- Blood film—this shows blast cells and can be diagnostic. If not clear from blood film, diagnosis is sought from bone marrow biopsy. This shows a

Fig. 13.16 Features of acute lymphoblastic and acute myeloblastic leukaemia.

Fig. 13.16 Features of acute lymphoblastic and acute myeloblastic leukaemia

Type	Acute lymphoblastic leukaemia (ALL)	Acute myeloblastic leukaemia (AML)
Epidemiology	Mainly (>90%) affects children of <14 years with highest incidence at 3–4 years Second increase in incidence occurs around middle-age	Occurs at all ages and is the commonest form of acute leukaemia in adults
Proliferating cell type	Neoplastic lymphoblasts (lymphocyte precursor cells)	Neoplastic myeloblast (granulocyte/monocyte precursor cell)
Degree of differentiation	Blast cells show no differentiation	Blast cells usually show some evidence of differentiation to granulocytes
Prognosis	Children aged 2–9 years: 50–75% cure rate Adults: 35% cure rate with chemotherapy; 50% with allogeneic bone marrow transplant	20–25% cure rate with standard chemotherapy 50% with allogeneic bone marrow transplant

hypercellular marrow with normal elements replaced by blast cells. If Auer rods are present in the cytoplasm of these cells, the pattern is AML. Cytogenetics and immunological staining can help diagnosis.

Involvement of other organs:

- Skeleton (bone pain, especially in children)—probably caused by osteolytic lesions.
- Lymphadenopathy.
- Symptoms and signs secondary to CNS infiltration.

Management:

- Supportive therapy—this actually increases survival and involves correction of anaemia, thrombocytopenia (i.e. blood product transfusions) and treatment of infections.
- Repeated courses of combination chemotherapy to induce remission.
- Bone marrow transplantation—usually reserved for those in relapsing chemotherapy-induced remission. Encouraging results in younger patients but largely depends on availability of suitable tissue matched donor.

For the prognosis, see Fig. 13.16.

Chronic leukaemias

Chronic myeloid leukaemia

Chronic myeloid leukaemia (CML) is a disorder of proliferation, with excessive and uncontrolled neoplastic proliferation of an abnormal myeloid clone of leucocyte precursors in the bone marrow.

About 90% of cases are characterised by the presence of a specific karyotypic abnormality—the Philadelphia chromosome—within the haemopoietic stem cells. This involves reciprocal translocation of part of the long arm (q) of chromosome 22 with the long arm of chromosome 9. This creates a chimeric gene (*BCR-abl*), which produces a tyrosine kinase thought to be involved in the pathogenesis of CML.

CML occurs in all age groups but most frequently between the ages of 40 and 60 years. The disease has three recognised stages:

1. Chronic phase—characterised by anaemia and splenomegaly; responsive to chemotherapy.
2. Accelerated phase—due to the emergence and dominance of a more malignant clone of myeloid cells. Disease becomes harder to control.
3. Blast crisis phase—transformation to an acute leukaemia (usually AML), often rapidly fatal. Progression from chronic phase is unpredictable and may occur at any time.

Haematological investigation reveals leucocytosis and normocytic anaemia. Note that in contrast to acute leukaemias, neutropenia, lymphopenia and thrombocytopenia are not common in the chronic phase, and that infection and bleeding are not typical.

There is sometimes massive splenomegaly (10% of cases), and often hepatomegaly.

Treatment of Philadelphia-chromosome-positive CML has recently been transformed by the drug imatinib. This novel tyrosine kinase inhibitor blocks the product of the chimeric *BCR-abl* gene and appears to offer long-term remission as long as the patient remains on the drug.

Chronic lymphocytic leukaemia

This chronic lymphoproliferative disorder is characterised by the proliferation of an abnormal lymphoid clone of leucocyte precursors in the bone marrow.

Chronic lymphocytic leukaemia (CCL) is the most common leukaemia of adults, comprising about 30% of all leukaemias, with males affected more than females by 2 : 1. It is a disease predominantly of the elderly, with peak incidence at 65 years old.

This disease is much less aggressive than other leukaemias, following a predictable course over a period of years.

Haematological changes are:

- Leucocytosis—small, non-functional lymphocytes of B cell origin.
- Anaemia and thrombocytopenia are late developments.
- Secondary autoimmune haemolytic anaemia develops in 10% of cases.

The lymph nodes, liver and spleen are characteristically involved, and normal architecture may become completely effaced by the infiltrating cells.

The staging of CLL is summarised in Fig. 13.17. Clinical features are similar to a low-grade lymphoma, but with the eventual development of bone marrow failure (anaemia, thrombocytopenia, infection).

Treatment is often reserved for the later stages, comprising combined chemotherapy and occasionally splenectomy.

Survival for more than 10 years from diagnosis is common, and where CLL affects the elderly, death is often from an unrelated cause. CLL in younger individuals tends to be more aggressive.

Fig. 13.17 Clinical features and staging of chronic lymphocytic leukaemia according to the RAI classification

Stage	Features
0	Lymphocytosis of blood and marrow
I	Lymphocytosis and enlarged nodes
II	Lymphocytosis and enlarged liver or spleen
III	Haemoglobin < 11 g/dL, with features of stages 0, I or II
IV	Platelet count < 100 × 10^9/L, with features of stages, I, II or III

Fig. 13.17 Clinical features and staging of chronic lymphocytic leukaemia (CLL) according to the RAI classification.

Myelodysplastic syndromes

This group of acquired neoplastic disorders of the bone marrow is characterised by increasing bone marrow failure with quantitative and qualitative abnormalities of all three myeloid cell lines (red cell, granulocyte/monocyte and platelets) due to a defect of stem cells. They are also known as refractory anaemias.

In most cases, the disease arises *de novo* and the aetiology is likely to be as for the leukaemias. The disorders are seen as steps in the progression to leukaemia (preleukaemic) and AML develops in many instances, often after many years. However, in a significant proportion of cases, the disease is secondary to treatment with chemotherapy (with or without radiotherapy) for a previous neoplastic disease.

The hallmark of the disease is ineffective haemopoiesis resulting in pancytopenia despite a marrow of either normal or increased cellularity.

Bone marrow contains morphologically abnormal cells including ring sideroblasts and hypogranular white cells, often with abnormal chromosomes.

Clinical features—more than half the patients are over 70 years old and more than 75% are over 50; males are affected more often than females. Symptoms are generally sequelae of the variable cytopenia, and include anaemia, infection and haemorrhage.

Diseases are subclassified depending on the presence of ring sideroblasts and the proportion of leukaemic-type blast cells in the bone marrow (Fig. 13.18).

Treatment is largely supportive, by blood transfusion and treatment of infection.

Morbidity and deaths are largely attributable to the refractory cytopenias either directly (e.g. from haemorrhage) or indirectly (e.g. from transfusion-related haemosiderosis).

Fig. 13.18 Classification of myelodysplastic syndromes (MDS).

Fig. 13.18 Classification of myelodysplastic syndromes (MDS)

Type of MDS	Peripheral blood	Bone marrow	Medial survival (months)
Refractory anaemia (RA)	Blasts < 1%	Blasts < 5%	50
RA with ring sideroblasts (RARS)	Blasts < 1%	Blasts < 5% Ring sideroblasts > 15% of total erythroblasts	50
RA with excess blasts (RAEB)	Blasts < 5%	Blasts 5–20%	10
RAEB in transformation (RAEB-t)	Blasts < 5%	Blasts 20–30% or Auer rods present	5
Chronic myelomonocytic leukaemia (CMML)	Blasts < 1% Monocytes > 1.0 × 10^9/L	Blasts 5–20% Promonocytes	10

Hairy cell leukaemia

This rare, B cell leukaemia is characterised by variable numbers of 'hairy' cells in the blood, bone marrow, liver, and other organs. Hairy cells are so named because of their characteristic irregular outline caused by cytoplasmic projections or 'hairs'.

The disease has a peak incidence at 40–60 years old, affecting males more than females by 6 : 1.

It is characterised clinically by features of pancytopenia (mainly recurrent infections) and splenomegaly.

The disorder typically runs a chronic course and remission is common with chemotherapy or interferon treatment. Splenectomy is also useful in management.

Myeloproliferative disorders

These are autonomous proliferations of one or more myeloid cells (erythroid, granulocytic, megakaryocytic) with differentiation to mature forms (Fig. 13.19).

Progression from one disorder to another within the group is common.

Polycythaemia rubra vera

This idiopathic condition is characterised by an above normal increase in red cell concentration, usually with concomitant increases in haemoglobin concentration and haematocrit. Red cell mass is greatly increased.

The disorder has a prevalence of 1 per 100 000 in the UK. It typically affects the middle-aged, and males more so than females.

Progression of this disease is chronic but about 20% of cases evolve into myelofibrosis, and another 5–10% into acute leukaemia.

Onset is usually insidious and non-specific, e.g. malaise, fatigue, headache and dizziness. The principle symptoms are caused by vascular engorgement, increased haematocrit and thrombosis, with or without haemorrhage. Diagnosis requires raised red cell mass without another cause and palpable splenomegaly.

Treatment is by venesection or myelosuppression using chemotherapy or radioactive ^{32}P. Treated patients have a mean survival of about 13 years, with increased morbidity and mortality from coronary and cerebral disease related to the raised haematocrit.

Note that most cases of polycythaemia are not due to polycythaemia rubra vera but they are secondary to conditions resulting in chronic hypoxia (see page 104). Splenomegaly and pancytosis are not features of these conditions.

Myelofibrosis

This condition is characterised by a proliferation of fibroblasts in the bone marrow and obliterative marrow fibrosis, with a corresponding massive extramedullary haemopoiesis in the liver and spleen.

Fig. 13.19 Myeloproliferative disorders and their basic features

Disorder	Principal proliferations	Bone marrow morphology	Clinical features
Polycythaemia rubra vera	Erythroblasts	Increased cellularity, especially erythroid	Erythrocytosis with increased Hb and PCV Often neutrophilia and thrombocytosis Pruritus (relating to basophilia) Thrombosis or haemorrhage Splenomegaly
Myelofibrosis	Fibroblasts	Increased deposition of collagen/reticulin; bone marrow difficult to aspirate	Leucoerythroblastic blood picture Anaemia with tear-drop poikilocytes Hepatosplenomegaly
Chronic granulocytic leukaemia	Myeloblasts	Increased cellularity, especially myeloid	Leucoerythroblastic blood picture Anaemia, neutrophilia, basophilia Splenomegaly
Essential thrombocythaemia	Megakaryoblasts	Increased megakaryocytes	Thrombocytosis Thrombosis or haemorrhage Occasional splenomegaly

Fig. 13.19 Myeloproliferative disorders and their basic features. (Hb, hemoglobin; PCV, packed cell volume).

The condition is a chronic disorder of late and middle age. It may arise *de novo* (with unknown aetiology) or as an end-stage of other myeloproliferative disorders (e.g. polycythaemia rubra vera). In these cases, it is thought that neoplastic megakaryocytes release fibrogenic factors to stimulate bone marrow fibrosis.

The disease is usually slowly progressive, with a median survival of 4 years. Acute leukaemic transformation sometimes occurs.

Clinical features are:

- Blood film—typically leucoerythroblastic; erythropoiesis is ineffective leading to anaemia with marked anisocytosis (unequal sized blood cells) and tear-drop poikilocytes (tear-drop shaped red cells).
- Splenomegaly is invariable.
- Hepatomegaly is common.
- Increased bone density due to sclerosis (myelosclerosis is an alternative name for myelofibrosis).

Symptoms are usually caused by anaemia and massive splenomegaly. Systemic symptoms (e.g. fever, weight loss) are usually late features.

Primary (essential/idiopathic) thrombocythaemia

This condition is characterised by increased platelet production due to a clonal proliferation of megakaryocytes. It is most commonly seen in patients over 50 years of age. Its features are:

- Large, atypical platelets with increased platelet count, often $> 1000 \times 10^9$/L.
- Combined pathological haemorrhages and thromboembolic episodes.
- Iron-deficiency anaemia due to chronic blood loss is an occasional feature.
- Spleen may be enlarged but it is usually normal or reduced in size because of thromboembolic infarction.

Treatment with chemotherapy and antiplatelet drugs (e.g. aspirin) is effective and median survival with treatment is 8–10 years.

Myeloma

This describes the malignant, monoclonal proliferation of plasma cells in the marrow. Most cases affect multiple sites (multiple myeloma), although solitary myeloma does occur (see below).

Multiple myeloma

This typically affects the elderly, with almost all cases occurring after the age of 40. There is a male predominance and the disease is more common in people of Afro-Caribbean ancestry than in other races.

Pathogenesis—normal plasma cells produce polyclonal immunoglobulins. In myeloma, only monoclonal immunoglobulins or light chains are produced; these are referred to as the 'M component' or paraprotein (*Note*: the 'M' stands for myeloma not IgM).

The M component is usually IgG (> 60%) but may be IgA (20%) or just the immunoglobulin light chain [κ (kappa) being more frequent than λ (lambda)].

IgD and IgE are unusual, and IgM-producing plasma cells are a feature of a different type of plasma cell neoplasm: Waldenström's macroglobulinaemia.

The presence of a single type of immunoglobulin is reflected in the electrophoretic pattern which shows normal levels of α- and β-globulins but a dramatic increase in the levels of γ-globulins (Fig. 13.20).

Diagnosis of myeloma requires two out of the following three findings:

- Marrow plasmacytosis.
- Serum or urinary paraprotein (M component).
- Skeletal lesions (see below).

Renal impairment

Whole immunoglobulins are too large to pass through the glomerular filter but in two-thirds of cases of IgG and IgA myelomas, monoclonal free light chains are also produced, which are small enough to enter the urine, where they are called Bence-Jones proteins.

During passage through the tubules, the protein precipitates as 'casts', causing damage to the tubular epithelial cells, with concomitant formation of surrounding giant cells: 'Bence-Jones or myeloma kidney'.

Light chains that pass through capillaries are incorporated into amyloid (systemic amyloidosis; see page 283) by mechanisms not yet fully elucidated, causing damage to many organs including the kidneys.

Raised blood uric acid (from increased cell turnover) worsens renal impairment (urate nephropathy, treated with allopurinol), as does increased blood calcium from bone osteolysis (hypercalcaemia, treated with bisphosphonates).

Bone changes

These are characteristic of myeloma:

- Hypercellular marrow with a large proportion of abnormal plasma cells, especially in the skull, ribs, vertebrae and pelvis.
- Osteolysis of medullary and cortical bone due to increased numbers of bone-resorbing osteoclasts: thought to be stimulated by cytokines (e.g. interleukins) produced by the malignant plasma cells.
- Osteolytic lesions are seen as 'punched out' defects in the bones, the skull showing this appearance particularly well ('pepper-pot skull').
- Generalised osteoporosis may result in pathological fractures or vertebral compression.

Haematological findings

These are as follows:

- Anaemia—usually normochromic, normocytic.
- Marked rouleaux formation—red cells pile together adhering by their rims forming cylinders.
- Raised blood viscosity—depending on the type of immunoglobulin.
- Reduced concentration of unaffected immunoglobulins— 'immune paresis'.
- Abnormal plasma cells—occasionally seen in peripheral blood, but most are in the marrow.
- Neutropenia and thrombocytopenia—common features of bone marrow failure in late stages.

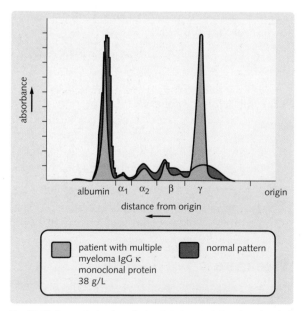

Fig. 13.20 Serum electrophoresis showing characteristic gamma band of multiple myeloma. (Adapted with permission from Essential Hematology, 3rd edn, by V Hoffbrand and J Pettit, Blackwell Science, 1993.)

Clinical features of myeloma:
- Bone pain—especially backache and pathological fractures.
- Anaemia—lethargy, breathlessness, tachycardia, etc.
- Repeated infections—deficient antibody levels and bone marrow failure.
- Abnormal bleeding tendency—M component may interfere with platelet function and coagulation factors; thrombocytopenia in advanced disease.
- Features of renal failure and/or hypercalcaemia.

Treatment involves chemotherapy and radiotherapy but median survival is only 3 years with treatment. Allogeneic bone marrow transplant may benefit some patients.

Solitary myeloma

This rare disease is characterised by discrete solitary tumours of proliferating monoclonal plasma cells, usually in the bone.

Proliferation does not occur in parts of the skeleton beyond the primary lesion, and marrow aspirates distant from the primary tumour are usually normal.

The associated M component usually disappears following radiotherapy to the primary lesion. However, a minority of cases progress to multiple myeloma.

DISORDERS OF THE SPLEEN AND THYMUS

Splenomegaly

The spleen serves as the site of filtration and phagocytosis of the following:

- Effete cells and cell debris, especially red cells.
- Microorganisms.
- Abnormal or excess material derived from metabolic processes.

Splenomegaly (enlargement of the spleen) is a common physical sign. It can have many causes, the main types of which are summarised in Fig. 13.21.

Fig. 13.21 Causes of splenomegaly

Cause	Comments
Infections	Bacterial, e.g. typhoid, tuberculosis, brucellosis, infective endocarditis Viral: infectious mononucleosis Protozoal: malaria, leishmaniasis, trypanosomiasis, toxoplasmosis
Congestion	Due to persistent elevation of splenic venous blood pressure, the cause of which may be: • Prehepatic: thrombosis of hepatic, splenic or portal vein • Hepatic: long-standing portal hypertension associated with cirrhosis • Posthepatic: raised venous pressure of inferior vena cava, e.g. due to right-sided heart failure, which is transmitted to the spleen via the portal system
Storage disease	Heritable enzyme deficiencies, which result in storage of material in splenic macrophagic cells, e.g. Gaucher's disease, Niemann–Pick disease and Tay–Sachs disease
Neoplasia	Primary: rare Secondary: • Lymphomas: Hodgkin's disease and non-Hodgkin's lymphomas • Leukaemias: especially chronic leukaemias • Metastases: splenic metastases from solid tumours, e.g. carcinomas or sarcomas, are rare • Extramedullary haemopoiesis, e.g. in myeloproliferative diseases and diseases with diffuse marrow replacement by tumour
Haematological disorders	Haematological anaemias, e.g. hereditary spherocytosis, β-thalassaemia, autoimmune haemolysis Autoimmune thrombocytopenia: destruction of antibody-coated platelets in spleen results in accumulation of foamy histiocytes in sinuses
Immune disorders	Felty's syndrome: follicular hyperplasia in spleen associated with hypersplenism and rheumatoid disease, Sarcoidosis: spleen infiltrated by granulomas Amyloidosis: spleen infiltrated with amyloid

Fig. 13.21 Causes of splenomegaly.

A palpable spleen is at least twice its normal size, and it is vulnerable to traumatic rupture, e.g. in glandular fever or malaria.

Effect of splenomegaly

Irrespective of the cause, enlargement of the spleen may result in the development of hypersplenism, i.e. a decrease in the circulating numbers of erythrocytes, leucocytes and platelets (pancytopenia), resulting from the destruction or pooling of these cells by the enlarged spleen.

Hypersplenism is often accompanied by a compensatory response—hyperplasia of the bone marrow.

Splenectomy leads to clinical and haematological improvement.

Congestive splenomegaly

This is enlargement of the spleen caused by any condition that leads to a persistent elevation of splenic venous blood pressure. Causes of raised splenic venous pressure are outlined in Fig. 13.22.

Morphological features—sinusoids of the spleen are initially distended with red cells. Fibrosis of both the spleen and capsule eventually occurs and sinusoids then appear ectatic and empty.

The cut surface of the spleen has a purple–red colour with an inconspicuous white pulp and it is often flecked with firm, brown nodules (called Gamna–Gandy nodules) that represent foci of fibrosis.

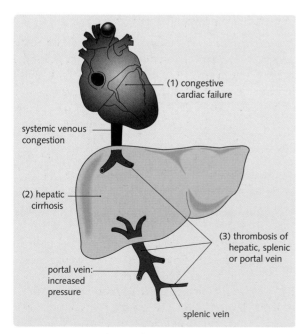

Fig. 13.22 Causes of raised splenic venous pressure.

296

Foci of extramedullary haemopoiesis are an occasional feature and are thought to be secondary to local hypoxia.

> A quick revision of splenic venous anatomy is helpful in understanding the causes of raised splenic venous pressure (Fig. 13.22). These are heart failure, cirrhosis and venous thrombosis.

Splenic infarcts

Splenic infarction follows occlusion of the splenic artery or its branches and it may be caused by:

- Emboli that arise in the heart (most common). May be septic if associated with infective endocarditis.
- Local thrombosis, e.g. in sickle-cell diseases, myeloproliferative disorders and malignant infiltrates.

Infarcts may be single or multiple and are generally wedge shaped and pale.

Rupture of the spleen

Rupture of a normal spleen usually occurs following a considerable abdominal trauma, particularly as occurs in some automobile accidents.

Spontaneous rupture of an abnormal enlarged spleen may occur, particularly in infectious mononucleosis, malaria, or splenic haemopoietic proliferations such as myelofibrosis.

A massive intraperitoneal haemorrhage usually follows splenic rupture, necessitating emergency splenectomy.

Disorders of the thymus

The thymus is composed of lymphoid cells and specialised epithelial cells; it is known as the 'primary' lymphoid organ. It is concerned with the development and processing of the long-lived T lymphocytes prior to their distribution to lymphoid tissues and to a circulating pool of T lymphocytes.

Thymic activity is maximal in fetal and childhood stages; regression is rapid after puberty.

Developmental disorders

Thymic hypoplasia and aplasia
These occur due to the developmental failure of either:

- Epithelial tissue—thymus is completely absent or is represented by a fibrous streak, e.g. DiGeorge syndrome (see page 279) and Nezelof's syndrome.
- Lymphoid tissue—severe combined immunodeficiency syndromes, ataxia, telangiectasia and reticular dysgenesis.

Both types of developmental disorder result in T-cell deficiency associated with a disordered, cell-mediated immune response.

Thymic cysts
These rare cysts are lined with thymic tissue. They occur in the neck or anterior mediastinum. Usually congenital, they may be acquired due to degeneration within the thymus gland or within thymic neoplasms.

Thymic hyperplasia
This is a rare condition in which lymphoid follicles (germinal centers) composed of B cells develop in the thymic medulla. It is often accompanied by an increase in the size of the thymus and is associated with autoimmune disease, especially myasthaenia gravis. In some cases autoantibodies are thought to be produced by the lymphoid tissue.

Thymomas
These rare tumours are derived from thymic epithelial cells; they can be benign or malignant. Most arise within the thymus but ectopic thymomas occasionally arise in the soft tissues of the neck, the hilum of the lung and other sites within the mediastinum or rarely the thyroid.

Histologically, thymomas are composed of uniform epithelial cells variably mixed with reactive lymphoid cells.

They are associated with a variety of disorders including myasthaenia gravis and non-organ-specific autoimmune diseases.

Benign thymomas
The majority (80–90%) of thymomas are benign, well-circumscribed, encapsulated, lobulated tumours. Most are asymptomatic but some present with local disease caused by the compression of adjacent mediastinal structures:

- Respiratory passages—dyspnoea and cough.
- Oesophagus—dysphagia.
- Great veins—cyanosis and suffusion of the face.

The remainder present with autoimmune disease. Complete surgical excision is curative.

Malignant thymomas
Around 10–20% of thymomas are malignant and invade the local tissues. There are two types:

1. Type 1—appears cytologically benign but invades local tissues, e.g. pericardium, lungs, pleura. Rarely spread outside the thorax.
2. Type 2 (thymic carcinoma)—rare malignant thymomas appearing cytologically malignant. Most are squamous cell carcinomas with a poor prognosis.

DISORDERS OF RED BLOOD CELLS

Abnormalities of red cell size and shape
Many haematological and systemic disorders are associated with specific abnormalities of red cell size (anisocytosis) and/or abnormal red-cell shape (poikilocytosis).

A diagrammatic representation of some of the variations in red cell size and shape, and the disorders that cause them, is given in Fig. 13.23.

Anaemia classifications
Anaemia can be defined as a state in which the blood haemoglobin level is below the normal range for the patient's age and sex. The normal haemoglobin range in males is 13.0–18.0 g/dL (130–180 g/L) and in females is 11.5–16.5 g/dL (115–165 g/L). Anaemia can be classified by the underlying mechanism for reduced haemoglobin, as shown in Fig. 13.24.

It is worth noting that, in clinical practice, anaemias are usually classified by the mean cell volume (MCV) of red cells—this can be increased (macrocytic anaemia), normal (normocytic) or reduced (microcytic). In general terms:

- Macrocytic—megaloblastic anaemias (vitamin B_{12} or folate deficiency) or haemolytic anaemias (new immature red blood cells are large in size).
- Normocytic—anaemia of chronic disease or hypoplastic anaemias (bone marrow suppression).
- Microcytic—iron-deficiency anaemia (most common cause of anaemia) or thalassaemia.

A	Anisocytosis
Type	**Clinical features**
normocyte	
microcyte	• iron deficiency • thalassaemia
round macrocyte	• liver disease • alcohol abuse • hypothyroidism
oval macrocyte	• megaloblastic anaemia

B	Poikilocytosis
Type	**Clinical features**
pencil cell	• iron deficiency
target cell	• iron deficiency • megaloblastic anaemia • haemoglobinopathy • liver disease • hyposplenism
microspherocyte	• hereditary spherocytosis • immune haemolytic anaemia • burns
sickle cells	• homozygous sickle cell disease
tear-drop cell	• myelofibrosis • marrow infiltration
schistocyte	• microangiopathic haemolytic anaemia

Fig. 13.23 Diagrammatic representation of (A) abnormalities in red cell size (anisocytosis) and (B) abnormalities in red cell shape (poikilocytosis). (Adapted from Underwood, 2000.)

Fig. 13.24 Causes of anaemia

Cause	Clinical features
Increased red cell loss, lysis or pooling	Blood loss Haemolysis: • Intrinsic abnormalities of red cells: hereditary (membrane defects, enzyme defects, haemoglobinopathies) and acquired (paroxysmal nocturnal haemoglobinuria) • Extrinsic abnormalities of red cells: antibody-mediated red cell destruction and mechanical trauma to red cells Hypersplenism
Impaired red cell production	Deficiency of haematinics: • Megaloblastic anaemias: lack of vitamin B_{12} or folate • Iron-deficiency anaemia Dyserythropoiesis (production of defective cells): • Anaemia of chronic disorders • Myelodysplasia • Sideroblastic anaemia Hypoplasia of marrow (failure to produce cells): • Aplastic anaemia • Red cell aplasia Invasion of marrow by malignant cells: • Leukaemias • Myeloproliferative diseases • Non-haematological malignancies

Fig. 13.24 Causes of anaemia.

The colour (quantity of haemoglobin) of a red cell is also described with the terms hypochromic (low), normochromic (normal) and hyperchromic (high).

The sections that follow describe the mechanisms that cause these anaemias.

Anaemia from blood loss

Acute blood loss

Following acute blood loss, a state of cardiovascular collapse may occur. The shock syndrome is often the predominant feature.

On cessation of haemorrhage, the plasma volume begins to be restored from the interstitial fluid compartment; this results in haemodilution and anaemia becomes apparent.

The blood picture is:

• Normocytic and normochromic anaemia.

- Polychromatic erythrocytes and reticulocytes (immature red blood cells), reflecting increased haemopoiesis.
- Transient leucocytosis and thrombocytosis.
- Plasma proteins and other biochemical constituents are restored rapidly (in 2–3 days). Full red cell restoration may take up to 6 weeks.

Chronic blood loss

Chronic blood loss is the most common cause of iron-deficiency anaemia, causing a hypochromic microcytic blood picture. The main causes of chronic haemorrhage are:

- Diseases of the gastrointestinal tract—particularly peptic ulceration, carcinoma (colourectal, stomach).
- Menorrhagia.
- Lesions in the urinary tract.

Patients with unexplained iron-deficiency anaemia require careful screening for an occult cause of blood loss.

Haemolytic anaemias

The basic pathological change in all haemolytic anaemias is a reduction in the lifespan of the red cells due to an increased rate of destruction; this is termed haemolysis. The effects of increased haemolysis are:

- Anaemia—commonly macrocytic due to increased reticulocytes (large cells) in the blood but may be normocytic.
- Erythroid hyperplasia of bone marrow.
- Splenomegaly.
- Unconjugated hyperbilirubinaemia due to red cell breakdown, which may lead to the development of pigment gall stones and jaundice (kernicterus in neonates).
- Haemoglobinuria—leading to tubular damage in the kidney.

The aetiology of haemolytic anaemias can be broadly classified into:

- Intrinsic abnormalities of red cells—hereditary defects, acquired defects.
- Extrinsic abnormalities of red cells—antibody-mediated red-cell destruction, mechanical trauma to red cells.

Hereditary defects of the red cell can be classified into:

- Cell membrane defects—hereditary spherocytosis and hereditary elliptocytosis.

- Enzyme deficiencies—deficiency of glycolytic enzymes or hexose monophosphate shunt enzymes.
- Haemoglobinopathies—e.g. thalassaemias and sickle-cell disease.

Hereditary spherocytosis and hereditary elliptocytosis

Hereditary spherocytosis is the most common cause of hereditary haemolytic anaemia in the UK. It is usually an autosomal dominant condition caused by an abnormality of spectrin, the cytoskeletal-associated membrane protein.

The cells are spherical, of reduced deformability and abnormally fragile.

Reduced deformability of the spherical red cells causes their retention in the splenic microcirculation where they undergo metabolic stress caused by a lack of glucose and acidosis. Increased fragility of metabolically stressed cells causes spontaneous lysis or premature phagocytosis by the splenic macrophages.

Blood film shows:

- Increased microspherocytes, which are more deeply stained with loss of the central pallor of normal erythrocytes.
- Increased polychromatic cells and reticulocytes.

The general clinical features are anaemia, splenomegaly (splenectomy usually performed) and jaundice.

Hereditary elliptocytosis is similar to spherocytosis but the red cells are elliptical. This is caused by abnormalities of the cytoskeletal-associated membrane proteins ankyrin, spectrin or band 42 protein.

This condition is not as severe as hereditary spherocytosis and does not usually cause anaemia or jaundice.

Enzyme deficiencies

In erythrocytes, 90% of glucose is metabolised anaerobically to lactate via the Embden–Meyerhof glycolytic pathway (pathway is similar to regular glycolysis except that the end product is lactate not pyruvate); 10% of glucose is used in the hexose monophosphate shunt (also known as the pentose phosphate pathway) to increase the levels of NADPH to those required for the reduction of glutathione. Reduced glutathione is essential for maintaining haemoglobin (Hb) in the reduced (ferrous) state (Fig. 13.25).

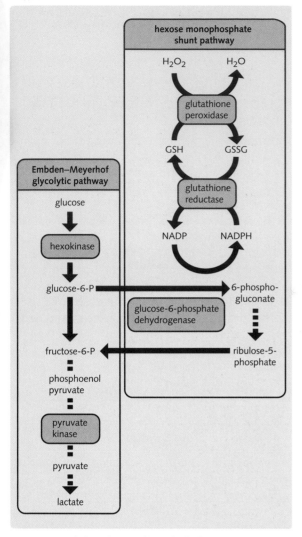

Fig. 13.25 Metabolic pathways of the red cell. (fructose-6-P, fructose-6-phosphate; glucose-6-P, glucose-6-phosphate; GSH, GSSG, reduced and oxidised glutathione; H_2O_2, hydrogen peroxide; NADP, NADPH, oxidised and reduced nicotinamide–adenine dinucleotide phosphate).

Deficiencies of glycolytic enzymes

Pyruvate kinase deficiency is a rare, autosomal recessive defect that results in congenital chronic haemolytic anaemia. Red cells become rigid due to reduced ATP formation, and they are removed by the spleen.

This is characterised by mild anaemia, jaundice and gallstones. The blood film shows raised poikilocytosis and distorted 'prickle cells'.

Many other enzymopathies of glycolytic enzymes exist but they are extremely rare, e.g. deficiencies of hexokinase, glucose phosphate isomerase and phosphofructokinase. The effects are similar to pyruvate kinase deficiency.

Deficiencies of hexose monophosphate shunt enzymes

The most common deficiencies are glucose-6-phosphate dehydrogenase (G6PD) deficiency, and glutathione synthetase deficiency.

G6PD deficiency is an X-linked recessive condition that is especially common among Black races. It results in a decreased ratio of NADPH/NADP, which impairs reduction of glutathione, and so increases susceptibility to oxidative stress.

Spontaneous anaemia is rare but haemolytic crises are frequently precipitated by infections, certain foods (e.g. fava (broad) beans), or certain drugs (quinine, phenacetin).

Blood film during haemolytic crises shows raised poikilocytosis with bite-shaped defects ('bite' cells) or surface blebs ('blister' cells) and Heinz bodies (red cells containing oxidized, denatured haemoglobin). The blood picture is normal between haemolytic episodes.

Female heterozygotes have the advantage of being resistant to falciparum malaria.

A deficiency of glutathione synthetase leads to defective synthesis of glutathione causing a similar syndrome to G6PD deficiency.

Haemoglobin abnormalities (haemoglobinopathies)

Haemoglobinopathies are caused by either:

- Decreased α- or β-globin synthesis—the α- and β-thalassaemias.
- Synthesis of abnormal haemoglobin—e.g. sickle-cell disease, unstable haemoglobins.

Anaemias are usually a combined result of both dyshaemopoiesis and haemolysis.

Thalassaemias

Normal adult haemoglobin (HbA) is composed of two α-globin chains and two β-globin chains ($α_2β_2$). The anaemia of thalassaemias is hypochromic, with excessive production of the non-affected haemoglobin chain often producing insoluble red cell inclusions, which affect the marrow (ineffective erythropoiesis) and cause premature cell death (haemolysis).

The disease is inherited and many different causative mutations have been identified. It is common in the Mediterranean, the Middle and Far East and South-East Asia, where carrier rates of 10–15% are found.

α-thalassaemia—mainly caused by deletion (rather than mutation) of parts of the α-globin genes. Normal individuals have four copies of the α-globin gene, two copies on each chromosome 16. There are, therefore, four possible degrees of α-thalassaemia, depending on how many genes are abnormal (Fig. 13.26). Haemolysis is less severe than in β-thalassaemia.

β-thalassaemia—caused by a mutation of the β-globin gene(s) leading to either reduced (β^+) or absent (β^0) synthesis of the β-globin chain. Normal individuals have two copies of each β-globin gene (one on each chromosome 11). There are, therefore, two possible degrees of β-thalassaemia:

1. Thalassaemia minor—heterozygous trait associated with mild anaemia.

2. Thalassaemia major—homozygous syndrome associated with severe haemolytic anaemia.

Sickle-cell disease

This is caused by an abnormal form of haemoglobin—HbS ($\alpha_2\beta_2^S$)—which is caused by a point mutation (resulting in the substitution of valine for glutamate) in the gene coding for the β-globin chain.

The disease is common in west and central Africa, the Mediterranean and the Middle East. In areas of Africa where malaria is endemic, up to 30% of the population is heterozygous. This is thought to be because carriage of the gene confers some protection against falciparum malaria.

Fig. 13.26 Thalassaemia disorders

Types of thalassaemia		Globin chains present	Clinicopathological features
β-thalassaemia	Thalassaemia minor	Heterozygous $\beta^0\beta$	Moderate reduction in HbA
		Heterozygous $\beta^+\beta$	Compensatory increase in HbA$_2$($\alpha_2\delta_2$)
			Mild anaemia with hypochromic cells
	Thalassaemia major	Heterozygous $\beta^0\beta^0$	Hypochromic microcytic anaemia
		Heterozygous $\beta^+\beta^+$	Severe haemolysis with hepatosplenomegaly
		or occasionally $\beta^+\beta^0$	Marrow hyperplasia causing skeletal deformities
			Iron overload from repeated transfusions
α-thalassaemia	Silent carrier	$-\alpha/\alpha\alpha$	Asymptomatic with normal haematology or slightly reduced MCV
	α-thalassaemia trait	$--/\alpha\alpha$ or $\alpha-/\alpha-$	Asymptomatic but mild haemolytic anaemia with some microcytic cells
	Haemoglobin H disease	$--/\alpha-$	Excess β-chains form tetramers: HbH
			Moderate haemolytic anaemia with hypochromia and microcytosis
			Splenomegaly
	Hydrops fetalis	$--/--$	Death *in utero*

Note: Hb, haemoglobin; MCV, mean cell volume.

Fig. 13.26 Summary of the thalassaemia disorders.

HbS polymerises at low oxygen saturations, causing an abnormal rigidity and deformity of red cells, which assume a sickle shape (Fig. 13.27). As a result, deoxygenated red cells undergo aggregation (causing vascular occlusion of small vessels) and haemolysis (due to increased fragility).

Heterozygous versus homozygous state

- Heterozygous condition—sickle-cell trait in which only 30% of the haemoglobin is HbS, resulting in no significant clinical abnormality.
- Homozygous condition—sickle-cell disease in which more than 80% of the haemoglobin is HbS, the rest being HbF (fetal haemoglobin) and HbA. It is associated with serious clinicopathological features.

Fig. 13.28 shows the pathogenesis and clinical features of sickle-cell disease.

'Crises' of sickle-cell disease

In addition to the effects of aggregation and haemolysis, sickle-cell disease is characterised by various 'crises' that occur after the age of 1 or 2 years, when HbF levels have fallen and the proportion of HbS has increased. HbF inhibits HbS polymerisation, initially preventing these crises. There are three main patterns:

1. Sequestration crises—sudden pooling of red cells in the spleen, which can lead to death from a rapid fall in haemoglobin.
2. Infarctive crises—blood vessel occlusion in bone (especially femoral head), spleen (leading to splenic atrophy) and skin (leg ulcers).

Fig. 13.28 Pathogenesis and clinical features of sickle-cell disease

Pathogenesis	Clinical features
Vascular occlusion	Cerebral infarction Retinopathy → blindness Pulmonary infarction → acute respiratory distress Cor pulmonale Haematuria and polyuria Splenic atrophy → hyposplenism → infections Bone necrosis → osteomyelitis Leg ulcers
Chronic haemolysis	Anaemia Jaundice and gall stones Haemochromatosis (due to iron overload in transfused patients)

Fig. 13.28 Pathogenesis and clinical features of sickle-cell disease.

3. Aplastic crises—splenic infarction predisposes to infection leading to depression of red cell production and exacerbation of pre-existing anaemia.

Treatment is by the avoidance of factors known to precipitate crises, especially hypoxia. Blood transfusions are necessary during crises.

Mean survival figures are variable reflecting differing standards of medical care. However, death in infancy or childhood is usual in underdeveloped countries.

Unstable haemoglobins

Hereditary abnormalities in globin chains result in the decreased stability of the haemoglobin molecule with haemolytic anaemia of variable severity. Examples are haemoglobins Köln and Zurich.

Acquired defects of the red cell

Paroxysmal nocturnal haemoglobinuria

This rare disorder of young adults is caused by a clonal abnormality of erythrocytes, which renders them abnormally sensitive to lysis by complement. The cells lack the enzyme required for the synthesis of phosphatidyl inositol, which usually anchors several proteins to the red cell membrane. This may arise *de novo* or follow an episode of aplastic anaemia. Venous thrombosis is a frequent complication.

Haemosiderinuria is common and can cause iron deficiency. However, nocturnal haemolysis is present in only about 25% of cases. Chronic haemolysis is more usual.

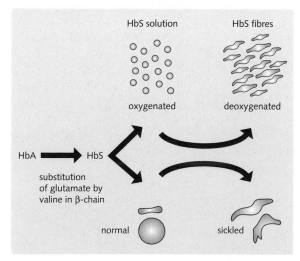

Fig. 13.27 Aggregation of sickle-cell haemoglobin in conditions of low oxygen.

Isoimmune antibody-mediated haemolytic anaemia

Incompatible ABO blood transfusion

This classic example of red cell haemolysis is caused by iso-antibodies (Fig. 13.29).

For example, if donor blood is group A (cells contain A antigen) and recipient blood is group O (plasma contains both anti-A and anti-B antibodies), then anti-A antibodies of the recipient will cause agglutination and haemolysis of donor red blood cells.

> The clinical effects of an ABO incompatible transfusion:
> - Massive intravascular haemolysis leading to collapse, hypotension and lumbar pain.
> - Haemoglobinuria is common and renal failure may ensue.
> - Disseminated intravascular coagulation may be triggered by red cell lysis.
>
> The effects may be precipitated with only a few milliliters of incompatible red cells.
>
> Transfusion-induced haemolysis due to incompatibility of the rhesus system is generally milder, since antibodies to the rhesus system are not complement fixing.

Haemolytic disease of the newborn (HDN)

This haemolysis of red blood cells in rhesus (Rh)-positive fetuses is caused by the placental passage of maternal anti-rhesus IgG antibodies from rhesus-negative mothers. It is particularly associated with D antigen of the rhesus blood group.

The pathogenesis is as follows:

- First pregnancy—Rh-positive fetus in Rh-negative mother with no antibodies: healthy baby.

Fig. 13.29 ABO blood group system

Genotype	Phenotype	Antibodies	Frequency of phenotype in UK
OO	O	Anti-A, Anti-B	Most common
AA or AO	A	Anti-B	Common
BB or BO	B	Anti-A	Rare
AB	AB	None	Rarest

Fig. 13.29 The ABO blood group system.

However, if fetal red blood cells enter maternal circulation during breach of placental barrier (e.g. at birth or miscarriage), then isoimmunization of mother will occur.
- Subsequent pregnancies—anti-Rh antibodies acquired by mother during previous pregnancy cause HDN in Rh-positive fetuses.

Incidence is now reduced by prophylactic anti-D injection in Rh-negative mothers before isoimmunization can occur.

HDN is categorised into three groups according to severity.

1. Congenital haemolytic anaemia—mild anaemia and jaundice, usually self limiting.
2. Icterus gravis neonatorum—rapidly developing severe anaemia and jaundice. May result in brain damage due to kernicterus (effect of unconjugated bilirubin), hepatosplenomegaly due to extramedullary haemopoiesis or death from severe anoxia.
3. Hydrops fetalis—death *in utero* associated with severe anoxia and cardiac failure.

Autoimmune haemolytic anaemia

This is the most common type of haemolytic anaemia, caused by the immune destruction of red blood cells by the host's own antibodies. It may be idiopathic, secondary to other diseases or drug related.

It is divided into two main groups according to the temperature at which haemolytic reactions occur.

1. 'Warm' antibody type

The more common form, with IgG autoantibody most reactive at 37°C leading to chronic anaemia with microspherocytes. Red cell destruction occurs in the spleen.

Clinical features are those of haemolytic anaemia: pallor, jaundice, and splenomegaly (Fig. 13.30).

2. 'Cold' antibody type

Autoantibody is IgM and is most reactive at 4°C but it can still bind complement and agglutinate red cells at 30°C, the temperature of peripheral tissues (hands, feet, nose and ears). There is destruction of red cells by Kupffer cells of the liver.

Clinical features are of anaemia and of blueness and coldness of the extremities, occasionally progressing to ischaemia and ulceration. Disorder is chronic and usually mild (Fig. 13.31).

Figure 13.32 summarises the antibody-mediated haemolytic anaemias.

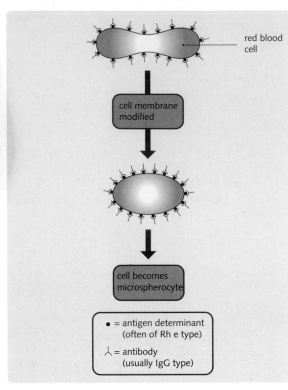

Fig. 13.30 'Warm' antibody-type haemolysis. The red cell membrane is modified and becomes a microspherocyte with consequences similar to hereditary spherocytosis: early sequestration in the spleen, etc. (Adapted with permission from Pathology Illustrated, 4th edn, by A Govan, P Macfarlane and R Callander, Churchill Livingstone, 1995.)

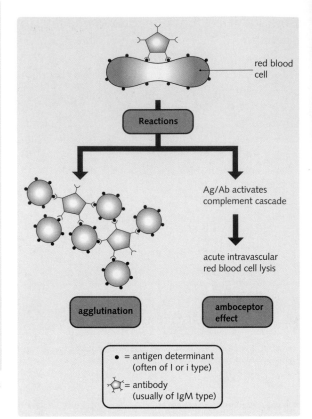

Fig. 13.31 'Cold' antibody-type haemolysis. The antibody combines with red blood cells, resulting in agglutination (clinically presenting as painful hands and feet) or the amboceptor effect (clinically presenting as paroxysmal cold haemoglobinuria–haemoglobinemia and haemoglobinuria). (Adapted with permission from Pathology Illustrated, 4th edn, by A Govan, P Macfarlane and R Callander, Churchill Livingstone, 1995.)

Mechanical trauma to red cells

Mechanical damage to red cells may lead to reduced lifespan and haemolysis.

There are several groups of mechanical haemolysis, as described below.

Microangiopathic haemolytic anaemia

Haemolysis is caused by physical trauma to erythrocytes as they are forced through narrow areas in the vasculature. It is commonly present in:

- Disseminated intravascular coagulation (see later)—red blood cells are damaged in fibrin-narrowed small blood vessels.
- Haemolytic uraemic syndrome.
- Thrombotic thrombocytopenic purpura (TTP).

Blood film shows the presence of schistocytes, helmet cells and echinocytes.

Macroangiopathic haemolytic anaemia

This is caused by physical trauma to erythrocytes as they are forced through prosthetic (usually mechanical) heart valves. Blood film is as above.

Splenic sequestration

Splenic sequestration of red cells causes their premature haemolysis resulting in hypersplenism (see below).

Malaria

Haemolysis is common in malaria. *Plasmodium* species enter the erythrocytes where they multiply and mature to form schizonts, which eventually escape by rupturing the erythrocytes. Extreme splenomegaly is often present.

Chemical

Snake bites, spider bites, scorpion stings and chemicals are occasionally causes of haemolysis.

Hypersplenism

There is a decrease in the numbers of circulating erythrocytes, leucocytes and platelets (pancytopenia) as a direct result of their destruction or pooling by an enlarged spleen (see page 295).

Fig. 13.32 Summary of antibody-mediated haemolytic anaemias

Isoimmune	Autoimmune	
	'Warm' antibody type (auto antibody is IgG class)	**'Cold' antibody type** (auto antibody is IgM class)
Transfusion reactions Haemolytic disease of the newborn	Idiopathic (50%) Secondary: • chronic lymphocytic leukaemia • lymphoma related • systemic lupus erythematosus and other autoimmune disorders • viral infections • drug related, e.g. methyl-dopa, penicillin, quinidine	Idiopathic Secondary: • lymphoma related • infectious mononucleosis • mycoplasma pneumonia

Fig. 13.32 Summary of antibody-mediated haemolytic anaemias.

Haematinic deficiency

There is a deficiency of those dietary factors required for either haemoglobin synthesis or erythrocyte production.

Megaloblastic anaemia

This type of anaemia is the result of impaired DNA synthesis in marrow precursor cells, and it is caused by a deficiency of vitamin B_{12} or folic acid (folate).

In the marrow, lack of vitamin B_{12} or folate causes the development of abnormally large red cell precursors (megaloblasts), which develop into abnormally large red cells (macrocytes):

- Macrocytic anaemia, neutropenia and thrombocytopenia—bone marrow becomes hypercellular with megaloblasts.
- Haemolytic anaemia—defective cells are prematurely destroyed.

Note that the effects of B_{12} and folate deficiency occur in most organs of the body and are prominent where cell turnover is rapid, e.g. in the marrow and mucous membranes of the alimentary tract and genitalia.

Vitamin B_{12} (cobalamin)

The source is animal products, e.g. meat and eggs.

Requirements are 1 µg per day but up to several years' supply are stored in the liver.

Absorption—vitamin B_{12} is normally absorbed in the terminal ileum, via binding to intrinsic factor (IF), which is secreted by gastric parietal cells. The causes of vitamin B_{12} deficiency are as follows:

- Pernicious anaemia—most common cause of vitamin B_{12} deficiency, and in females more than males. Caused by autoimmune atrophic gastritis resulting in lack of production of IF and malabsorption of vitamin B_{12}. Corrected by injections of vitamin B_{12}.
- Congenital—lack of IF.
- Surgical gastrectomy—results in loss of IF.
- Surgical removal of the terminal ileum—loss of vitamin B_{12} absorption site.
- Disease of terminal ileum (e.g. Crohn's disease)—loss of vitamin B_{12} absorption site.
- Bacterial overgrowth—compete for vitamin B_{12}.
- Malnutrition—rare given liver stores but occasionally seen in veganism.

The effects of vitamin B_{12} deficiency are as follows:

- Megaloblastic anaemia—with associated neutropenia and thrombocytopenia.
- Lesions of the nervous system—myelin degeneration of posterior and lateral columns of spinal cord—subacute combined degeneration of the cord (see Chapter 5).
- Malabsorption—due to mucosal changes—weight loss.

Treatment is by correction of the underlying cause (if possible), and/or injections of vitamin B_{12}.

Folic acid

Sources are vegetables, cereals, meat and eggs.

Requirements are up to 200 µg per day and only 50–100 days supply is stored in the liver.

Absorption—folic acid is normally absorbed from the diet in the jejunum. The causes of folate deficiency are as follows:

- Malnutrition, e.g. from anorexia, alcoholism, poor diet, overcooking of food. This is the most common cause of deficiency and occurs more rapidly than vitamin B_{12} deficiency because of the smaller body stores.
- Malabsorption, e.g. coeliac disease, dermatitis herpetiformis, Crohn's disease.
- Increased requirements, e.g. pregnancy and lactation, haemolysis, malignancy, extensive psoriasis or dermatitis.
- Drugs may cause malabsorption (e.g. anticonvulsants) or may block utilisation, e.g. methotrexate.

The effects of folate deficiency—blood and bone marrow changes are identical to those in vitamin B_{12} deficiency. However, deficiency of folate is not associated with the neurological features of vitamin B_{12} deficiency (Fig. 13.33).

Treatment is by oral folic acid supplements, resulting in a complete reversal of the pathological features, even in malabsorption states.

Iron-deficiency anaemia

Iron deficiency is the most common cause of anaemia.

Iron is abundant in meat, vegetables, eggs and dairy foods.

Requirements are:

- In men and postmenopausal women—1 mg per day.
- In menstruating women—2 mg per day.
- In pregnancy—3 mg per day.
- In children—1.5 mg per day.

Absorption is via the duodenum and upper jejunum in the ferrous (Fe^{2+}) form.

The causes of iron deficiency are:

- Chronic blood loss—most common cause (e.g. diseases of the GI tract, menorrhagia, lesions of the urinary tract).
- Increased requirements, e.g. in childhood and pregnancy.
- Malabsorption due to gastrectomy, coeliac disease.
- Malnutrition.

The effects of iron deficiency on the blood film are:

- Hypochromic microcytic erythrocytes.
- Low numbers of reticulocytes for the degree of anaemia.
- Poikilocytosis (especially 'pencil' cells).
- Anisocytosis.

Laboratory findings are as follows: reduced total serum iron, reduced serum ferritin (iron storage protein), and reduced transferrin saturation (iron carrying protein), but with a greatly increased total iron binding capacity.

Fig. 13.33 Comparison of vitamin B_{12} and folate deficiency.

Fig. 13.33 Comparison of vitamin B_{12} and folate deficiency

	Vitamin B_{12} deficiency	Folate deficiency
Source	Animal produce	Most foods
Requirements	1 µg/day (heat stable, body stores = several years)	Minimally 50 µg/day (heat labile, body stores = months)
Nutritional deficiency	Uncommon (only in vegans)	Common
Time of onset	Slow (years)	Over several weeks
Area of absorption	Absorbed in terminal ileum and requires intrinsic factor	Absorbed in jejunum (and duodenum)
Disease causing deficiency	Gastric or terminal ileal disease may cause deficiency	Jejunal disease may cause deficiency
Drug involvement	No	May be drug related (anticonvulsants or antimetabolites)
Neurological involvement	Neurological lesions frequent	No

Treatment is of the underlying cause and iron supplementation (ferrous sulphate).

Clinical features of iron-deficiency anaemia are:
- Anaemia—lethargy, dyspnoea, headache, palpitations.
- Angular cheilitis—fissures at angles of mouth.
- Atrophic glossitis (smooth tongue).
- Oesophageal webs.
- Hypochlorhydria.
- Koilonychia (spoon-shaped nails)—seen in severe cases only.
- Brittle nails.
- Pica (indiscriminate eating of non-nutritious substances such as grass, stones or clothing).

Dyserythropoiesis

This group of disorders is characterised by the production of defective red cells. The pathogenesis of associated dyserythropoiesis is poorly understood.

Anaemia of chronic disorders

Chronic disorders are a common cause of anaemia, being second only to iron-deficiency.

It may develop in patients with:

- Non-organ-specific autoimmune diseases, e.g. rheumatoid disease and SLE.
- Chronic infective diseases, e.g. tuberculosis, malaria and schistosomiasis.
- Neoplasia: lymphoma and some carcinomas.

Blood film—mainly normocytic and normochromic but a mild degree of microcytic, hypochromic anaemia.

Laboratory findings—a reduced serum iron and reduced serum iron-binding capacity, but the iron stores (ferritin) are normal or increased (cf. iron-deficiency anaemia).

Erythropoietin (EPO, the hormone that stimulates erythropoiesis) is reduced, possibly due to cytokines produced by chronic disease processes. EPO injections in rheumatoid arthritis improve the anaemia.

Myelodysplasia

This acquired neoplastic disorder is caused by a defect of the stem cells. It is characterised by progressive bone marrow failure with quantitative and qualitative abnormalities of all three myeloid cell lines (red cell, granulocyte/monocyte and platelets) (see page 291).

Sideroblastic anaemia

This anaemia, caused by defective haem synthesis, results in the accumulation of excess iron in the cytoplasm of red blood cell progenitors in the form of haemosiderin, forming cells termed ring sideroblasts.

There are two groups of the disease:

1. Primary sideroblastic anaemia—one of the myelodysplastic syndromes.
2. Secondary sideroblastic anaemia—drug-, toxin- and neoplasia-related.

Hypoplasia

This anaemia is due to the failure or suppression of red cell production in the bone marrow.

Aplastic anaemia

A severe life-threatening disease caused by failing bone marrow stem cells, this is characterised by pancytopenia. The marrow is hypocellular, and it is replaced by fat.

It may be idiopathic or secondary to:

- Whole body irradiation—therapeutically (e.g. haematological neoplasms) or in nuclear accidents (e.g. Chernobyl).
- Antineoplastic chemotherapy—vincristine, busulfan.
- Drugs—chloramphenicol, streptomycin, chlorpromazine.
- Toxins—benzene.
- Viruses—papovavirus, HIV-1.
- Fanconi's anaemia—rare autosomal recessive disorder of DNA repair.

Red cell aplasia

This anaemia is caused by the suppression of red cell progenitor cells only. In contrast to aplastic anaemia, other blood cells are not affected. There are three main types:

1. Self-limited red cell aplasia—occurs after parvovirus infection or exposure to certain toxins.
2. Chronic acquired red cell aplasia—autoimmune and it may be associated with thymomas (see page 297).
3. Chronic constitutional red cell aplasia—due to a hereditary defect in progenitor cells.

Marrow infiltration

Extensive infiltration of the bone marrow may cause the obliteration of normal haemopoietic elements. It is caused by:

- Leukaemias.
- Myelofibrosis.
- Disseminated carcinomas.
- Disseminated lymphomas.

Patients develop leucoerythroblastic anaemia characterised by circulating erythroblasts and primitive white cells. Extramedullary haemopoiesis commonly develops.

Polycythaemia

Polycythaemia (erythrocytosis) is essentially the opposite of anaemia, defined as a sustained increase in red cell numbers, usually with a corresponding increase in haemoglobin concentration and haematocrit.

Relative polycythaemia

This occurs when the haematocrit reading is raised due to a decrease in plasma volume, usually as a result of fluid loss (haemoconcentration). This is not 'true' (absolute) polycythaemia.

Absolute polycythaemia

Primary

Primary polycythaemia occurs in a rare condition termed polycythaemia rubra vera, which is one of the myeloproliferative disorders (see page 292).

Secondary

Most cases of polycythaemia are secondary to conditions resulting in:

- Chronic hypoxia (common)—'appropriate' polycythaemia, e.g. high altitude, cyanotic heart disease, respiratory disease (such as chronic bronchitis, emphysema), smoking, haemoglobinopathies (resulting in defective release of O_2 to tissues).
- Renal tumours and ischaemia (rare)— 'inappropriate' polycythaemia, e.g. renal carcinomas or cysts, renal artery stenosis.

Both chronic hypoxia and renal tumours/ischaemia result in increased erythropoietin hormone production, which stimulates the bone marrow production of red cells.

Figure 13.34 compares the main features of primary and secondary polycythaemia.

DISORDERS OF HAEMOSTASIS

Definitions

Purpura

This skin rash results from bleeding into the skin from capillaries. It is caused either by defects in capillaries or by defects or deficiencies of blood platelets. Individual small purple spots of the rash are called petechiae.

Ecchymosis

This is a bruise, presenting as a bluish-black mark on the skin resulting from the release of blood into the tissues either through injury or through the spontaneous leaking of blood from the vessels.

Fig. 13.34 Comparison of the main features of primary and secondary polycythaemia.

Fig. 13.34 Comparison of main features of primary and secondary polycythaemia

	Primary	Secondary
Prevalence	Rare	Common
Cause	Unknown	Hypoxia Renal tumours/ischaemia
Erythropoietin	Normal or decreased	Increased
Blood film	↑ RBCs (may be hypochromic) ↑ leucocytes ↑ megakaryocytes	↑ RBCs (normochromic)
Splenomegaly	Common	None

Note: RBC, red blood cell

Haematoma

This accumulation of blood within the tissues clots to form a solid swelling.

Abnormalities of the vessel walls

This heterogeneous group of conditions (the 'non-thrombocytopenic purpuras') is characterised by easy bruising and spontaneous bleeding from small vessels. The underlying lesions are of two main types:

1. Abnormal perivascular connective tissue which leads to inadequate vessel support.
2. Intrinsically abnormal or damaged vessel wall.

Haemorrhages are mainly in the skin, causing petechiae, ecchymoses or both. In some disorders there is also bleeding from the mucous membranes. Bleeding is not usually serious.

Infections

Some bacterial and viral infections cause purpura as a result of either vascular damage (vasculitis) by the organism or through disseminated intravascular coagulation (DIC), e.g. measles, meningococcal septicaemia.

Drug reactions

A variety of drugs may sometimes cause vasculitic reactions, often through stimulating immune-complex deposition which triggers hypersensitivity vasculitis.

Scurvy and Ehlers–Danlos syndrome

Vitamin C is required for the hydroxylation of proline as a step in collagen synthesis. In both Ehlers–Danlos syndrome (an inherited disorder of collagen synthesis) and scurvy (vitamin C deficiency) capillaries are fragile because of defective collagen synthesis.

Perifollicular petechiae, bruising, and mucosal haemorrhages are common.

Steroid purpura

Long-term steroid therapy or Cushing's syndrome results in purpura caused by loss of vascular supportive tissue.

Henoch–Schönlein purpura

This immune complex (type III) hypersensitivity reaction is usually found in children and often follows an acute infection. It is characterised by red wheals and a purple rash on the buttocks and lower legs due to bleeding into the skin from inflamed capillaries and venules.

Arthritis, acute glomerulonephritis, haematuria and GI symptoms may also occur.

It is a self-limiting condition but occasionally patients develop renal failure.

Osler–Weber–Rendu syndrome (hereditary haemorrhagic telangiectasia)

This rare, autosomal dominant disorder is characterised by multiple dilatations of small vessels (telangiectasia) that appear during childhood and become more numerous in adult life.

Telangiectasia develops in the skin, mucous membranes and internal organs. It frequently bleeds spontaneously or following relatively mild trauma.

Reduced platelet count (thrombocytopenia)

Decreased production

This is the most common cause of thrombocytopenia (normal platelet count $150–350 \times 10^9/L$).

Generalised disease of bone marrow

Seen in aplastic anaemia (see page 307) and marrow infiltration (e.g. haematological malignancies) that obliterates normal haemopoietic elements.

Specific impairment of platelet production

Selective megakaryocyte depression may result from either drug toxicity (alcohol, cytotoxics) or viral infections (measles, HIV).

Ineffective megakaryopoiesis

- Megaloblastic anaemia (folate or vitamin B_{12} deficiency)—is characterised by decreased numbers of platelets or increased numbers of megakaryocytes.
- Paroxysmal nocturnal haemoglobinuria—may cause ineffective megakaryopoiesis.

Decreased platelet survival

Immune destruction: autoimmune thrombocytopenic purpura

The destruction of antibody-coated platelets by the reticuloendothelial system, especially the spleen, increases the likelihood of haemorrhage:

- Skin—petechiae and ecchymoses.
- Mucous membranes—e.g. epistaxis, bleeding gums, menorrhagia, haematuria, melaena.
- CNS—may be fatal.

This is often associated with anaemia (secondary to blood loss).

Clinical types are:

- Acute—often in children and usually self-limiting with spontaneous resolution. May be post-infective, e.g. measles.
- Chronic—usually in adults, mainly idiopathic but occasionally related to chronic lymphocytic leukaemia (CLL) or lymphoma. Or it may occur in association with another autoimmune disease, e.g. rheumatoid arthritis, SLE.
- Drug induced—e.g. quinine, heparin, sulphonamides.

Non-immune destruction

This is mainly through thrombotic thrombocytopenic purpura (TTP) and haemolytic–uraemic syndrome (HUS).

HUS and TTP are thought to represent the same disease process but with different distributions of thrombotic lesions.

Thrombocytopenia occurs due to abnormal platelet activation and consumption. Platelets adhere to the endothelium of capillaries and precapillary arterioles where they undergo aggregation, with fibrin deposition, which results in microvascular occlusive platelet plugs and microangiopathic haemolytic anaemia (see page 197).

Aetiology—the underlying cause of the disorder is obscure but the following pathogenic factors have been implicated:

- Immune-mediated vessel damage.
- Platelet hyperaggregation due to deficiency of an IgG inhibitor of platelet-agglutinating factor in normal plasma.
- Diminished production of prostaglandin by vessel walls.
- Excess of high-molecular-weight multimers of von Willebrand's factor, which interact with platelet agglutinating factor, causing platelet adhesion to vascular endothelium.

In TTP, occlusive plugs lead to widespread ischaemic organ damage, especially of the brain and kidney, resulting in neurological abnormalities and progressive renal impairment. In HUS, organ damage is limited to the kidney. Children tend to develop HUS rather than TTP.

Disseminated intravascular coagulation can also cause widespread consumption of platelets, resulting in simultaneous thrombosis and haemorrhage (see page 313).

Splenic sequestration

Thrombocytopenia is common in hypersplenism due to platelet 'pooling' by the spleen. Unlike red cells, platelets tolerate splenic stasis without injury and so platelet lifespan is unaffected.

Dilutional thrombocytopenia

Platelets are unstable at 4°C and so blood transfusions contain few viable platelets. Therefore transfusion with massive amounts of stored blood may cause thrombocytopenia. The effect can be minimised by replacement with specific screened products, e.g. fresh frozen plasma and platelet concentrates.

Figure 13.35 summarises the causes of thrombocytopenia.

Defects of platelet function
Congenital
Defective adhesion (Bernard–Soulier syndrome)

This rare disease causes life-threatening haemorrhages. The platelets are deficient in glycoprotein receptors (glycoprotein Ib/IX complex), which are essential for the binding of von Willebrand's factor. The platelets are larger than normal and there is defective adherence to exposed subendothelial connective tissues and defective platelet aggregation. There is also a variable degree of thrombocytopenia.

Defective aggregation: thromboesthaenia (Glanzmann's disease)

This failure of primary platelet aggregation is due to a deficiency of membrane receptors (glycoprotein IIb–IIIa complex) for fibrinogen binding.

Defective secretion (storage pool disease)

A common, mild defect of platelet function. It causes easy bruising and bleeding after trauma. It is caused by a deficiency of 'dense granules' within the platelets, which normally store ADP. The decreased storage pool of ADP prevents complex platelet functions such as thromboxane release.

Acquired
Aspirin

Aspirin therapy is the most common cause of defective platelet function, and it produces an abnormal bleeding time.

Aspirin irreversibly inhibits cyclooxygenase, causing impairment in thromboxane A_2 synthesis, which is necessary for the platelet release reaction and aggregation. After a single dose the effects last 7–10 days.

Fig. 13.35 Causes of thrombocytopenia.

Fig. 13.35 Causes of thrombocytopenia

Cause	Clinical features
Decreased platelet production	Generalised disease of bone marrow: • aplastic anaemia, marrow infiltration Specific impairment of platelet production: • drugs: alcohol, thiazides, cytotoxics • infections: measles, HIV Ineffective megakaryopoiesis: • megaloblastic anaemia and paroxysmal nocturnal haemoglobinuria
Decreased platelet survival	Immune destruction: • autoimmune thrombocytopenic purpura Non-immune destruction: • thrombotic thrombocytopenic purpura/haemolytic-uraemic syndrome • disseminated intravascular coagulation
Splenic sequestration	—
Dilutional thrombocytopenia	—

Bleeding tendency is mild, with increased skin bruising and bleeding after surgery. The use of aspirin may contribute to GI haemorrhage associated with acute mucosal erosions. It can be life threatening.

Uraemia

In uraemia, defects may be caused by an abnormal arachidonate metabolism with reduced synthesis of thromboxane. Platelet interactions with the subendothelium are abnormal and bleeding may be severe.

Clotting factor abnormalities

Hereditary factor abnormalities

Von Willebrand's disease

This is the most common of the hereditary coagulation disorders. It is usually an autosomal dominant disorder of abnormal platelet adhesion associated with low factor VIII activity. The primary defect is the reduced production of von Willebrand's factor, a protein synthesised by platelets and endothelial cells which has two main functions:

1. Promotes platelet adhesion.
2. Carrier molecule for factor VIII, protecting it from premature destruction.

The severity of presentation is variable; most cases are very mild and of little significance but some individuals have virtually no detectable von Willebrand's factor.

The disease is characterised by operative and post-traumatic haemorrhage, mucous membrane bleeding (e.g. epistaxis, menorrhagia) and excessive blood loss from superficial cuts and abrasions.

Severe bleeding episodes are treated with intermediate-purity factor VIII concentrates that contain both von Willebrand's factor and factor VIII.

Haemophilia A (factor VIII deficiency)

A common hereditary disorder of blood coagulation. It is characterised by the absence or low levels of plasma factor VIII.

Inheritance is X-linked but 33% of patients have no family history and the disorder presumably results from spontaneous mutation; it affects 1 per 10 000 in the UK.

Blood clotting time is prolonged and, in severe disease, the blood is incoagulable.

Operative and post-traumatic haemorrhage is life threatening, both in severely and mildly affected patients.

Mild, moderate and severe forms of the disease are recognised, depending on the residual clotting factor activity (Fig. 13.36). Haemophilia A 'breeds true' in that the same severity of disease is seen in all affected members of a family.

Treatment—control can be achieved by intravenous clotting factor replacement, although antibodies against the factor VIII develop in some cases. Note

Fig. 13.36 Classification of haemophilias.

Fig. 13.36 Classification of haemophilias

Category	Frequency	Coagulation factor activity (% of normal)	Clinical features
Severe	40%	<2%	Frequent spontaneous bleeding episodes from birth Degenerative joint disease
Moderate	10%	2–10%	Post-traumatic bleeding Occasional spontaneous episodes Bruising
Mild	50%	10–50%	Post-traumatic bleeding may be subclinical

that the transmission of hepatitis C and HIV occurred in many haemophiliacs prior to full donor screenings.

Haemophilia A is characterised by frequent episodes of spontaneous haemorrhage into a major joint, especially knees, hips, elbows and ankles. Without factor replacement therapy, bleeding continues until the intra-articular pressure rises sufficiently to prevent further haemorrhage (tamponade).

Resolution of acute haemarthrosis occurs slowly with recurrent bleeds producing massive synovial hypertrophy, erosion of joint cartilage and bone, and changes of severe osteoarthritis.

Bleeding into muscles, retroperitoneal tissues, urinary tract and epistaxis occur.

Haemophilia B (factor IX deficiency)

Inheritance, clinical features and treatment principles of factor IX deficiency are identical to those of haemophilia A. However, factor IX deficiency is less common, the incidence being only about one-fifth of that of haemophilia A. This is also known as Christmas disease.

The features of the most common hereditary clotting factor deficiencies are summarised in Fig. 13.37.

Other deficiencies

Hereditary deficiencies of most of the other coagulation factors have also been described, but they are extremely rare.

Acquired factor abnormalities

Acquired disorders of coagulation are far more common than the inherited disorders, and multiple clotting factor deficiencies are usual.

Vitamin K deficiency

Vitamin K is essential for the γ-carboxylation and hence activation of factors II, VII, IX and X, as well as proteins C and S (inhibitors). The deficiency is associated with decreased activity of these proteins, leading to coagulopathies. This may present in the newborn or in later life.

Fig. 13.37 Common hereditary clotting factor abnormalities

	Haemophilia A	Factor IX deficiency	Von Willebrand's disease
Deficiency	Factor VIII	Factor IX	Von Willebrand factor→ factor VIII deficiency
Inheritance	X-linked	X-linked	Dominant
Prevalence in the UK	1 in 10 000	1 in 50 000	1 in 5000
Main sites of haemorrhage	Muscle, joints: post trauma or post surgery	Muscle, joints: post trauma or post surgery	Mucous membranes, post trauma and operation

Fig. 13.37 Common hereditary clotting factor abnormalities.

Vitamin K is obtained from green vegetables and bacterial synthesis in the gut. It is a fat-soluble vitamin and requires bile for its absorption.

Causes of vitamin K deficiency:

- Inadequate diet.
- Malabsorption—e.g. obstructive jaundice (reduced bile), coeliac disease.
- Drugs—warfarin (a vitamin K antagonist). A very commonly used drug requiring regular monitoring of blood clotting (via the international normalised ratio; INR). In emergency life-threatening bleeds, vitamin K supplementation is used.

Neonates are particularly susceptible to vitamin K deficiency because of their lack of gut bacteria and low concentrations of the vitamin in breast milk. A life-threatening disease called haemorrhagic disease of the newborn occurs in affected neonates. Vitamin K can be prophylactically supplemented at birth in at-risk babies.

Liver disease

This is commonly associated with coagulation defects due to:

- Impaired absorption of vitamin K caused by biliary obstruction, producing decreased activation of factors II, VII, IX and X and proteins C and S.
- Reduced synthesis of clotting factors and of fibrinogen, and increased amounts of plasminogen activator in severe hepatocellular disease and cirrhosis.
- Thrombocytopenia from hypersplenism associated with portal hypertension.

- Dysfibrinogenemia: functional abnormality of fibrinogen found in many patients with liver disease.
- Qualitative platelet disorders.

Disseminated intravascular coagulation

DIC is characterised by increased coagulation, which leads not only to widespread thrombosis but also to haemorrhage due to consumption of platelets and coagulation factors. Thus both thrombosis and haemorrhage are features of this disorder.

The disorder may cause a severe haemorrhagic syndrome with high mortality or may run a milder, more chronic course.

Aetiology—this is shown in Fig. 13.38.

Pathogenesis—the causes listed in Fig. 13.38 activate the coagulation system in small vessels throughout the body via:

- Release of procoagulant material into circulation, e.g. obstetric disorders, certain malignancies, liver disease, severe falciparum malaria and haemolytic transfusion reactions.
- Widespread endothelial damage, e.g. septicaemia, certain viral infections, severe burns or hypothermia.
- Platelet aggregation: some bacteria, viruses and immune complexes may have a direct effect on platelets.

The main effects of DIC are:

- Thrombosis causes ischaemic organ damage and microangiopathic haemolysis.
- Consumption of platelets, clotting factors and fibrinogen causes haemorrhage.

Fig. 13.38 Causes of disseminated intravascular coagulation

Problem	Cause
Infections	Septicaemia, viral infections (purpura fulminans), malaria
Malignancy	Carcinomas of pancreas, lung and prostate Acute promyelocytic leukaemia
Obstetric complications	Amniotic fluid embolism, placental abruption, retained dead fetus
Hypersensitivity reactions	Anaphylaxis, incompatible blood transfusion
Widespread tissue damage	Burns, major accidental trauma, major surgery, shock, intravascular haemolysis, dissecting aortic aneurysm
Liver disease	Various causes

Fig. 13.38 Causes of disseminated intravascular coagulation.

DIC is a very important condition. Remember that it causes both thrombosis and haemorrhage. It may be triggered by a wide variety of conditions (Fig. 13.38) and can be rapidly fatal if not recognised quickly.

- Activation of fibrinolytic system results in increased fibrin degradation products (e.g. D-dimer, which is measurable). These products may themselves have anticoagulant effects causing further haemorrhage.

Treatment is of the underlying cause, with clotting factor and platelet replacement.

Thrombosis

Thrombosis is the formation of a solid mass of blood constituents—a thrombus—within the vascular system during life. It is not to be confused with a clot, which occurs in non-flowing blood.

Thrombosis can affect both arteries and veins. It is considered in detail in Chapter 6 (see page 76).

Pathology of the skin

Objectives

In this chapter, you will learn to:

- Use the correct terms for macroscopic and microscopic appearances in dermatology.
- Understand psoriasis and dermatitis (eczema).
- Recall the common infections and infestations of the skin.
- Describe acne vulgaris, rosacea and disorders of hair and nails.
- Describe the disorders of too little and too much skin pigmentation.
- Understand blistering diseases.
- Discuss the benign tumours of the skin, including the common forms of naevi.
- Describe malignant melanoma, basal cell carcinoma and squamous cell carcinoma.
- Briefly recall the other tumours of the skin.

TERMINOLOGY OF SKIN PATHOLOGY

Macroscopic appearances

Macule

This localised, flat area of altered skin colour can be hyperpigmented as in a freckle, hypopigmented as in vitiligo, or erythematous as in a capillary haemangioma.

Papule

A small, raised, solid lesion of the skin. This is generally defined as being less than 5 mm in diameter.

Nodule

This is similar to a papule but greater than 5 mm in diameter. It may be solid or oedematous and can involve any layer of the skin.

Plaque

An extended papule that forms a plateau-like elevation of skin. A plaque is usually more than 20 mm in diameter but rarely more than 5 mm in height.

Wheal

This is similar to a papule or plaque but transitory and compressible. It is caused by dermal oedema, is red or white in colour and usually signifies urticaria.

Blister

This fluid-filled space within the skin is caused by the separation of cells and the leakage of plasma into the space.

Vesicle

This small blister (less than 5 mm in diameter) contains clear fluid within or below the epidermis.

Bulla

This is similar to a vesicle but larger than 5 mm in diameter.

Pustule

A small, pus-containing blister, a pustule commonly indicates infection, but not always (e.g. those seen in psoriasis are not infected).

Scale

This thickened, horny layer of keratin forms readily detached fragments of skin. Scaling is caused by disturbances in the processes of keratinisation and usually indicates inflammation of the epidermis (Fig. 14.1A).

Lichenification

There is a thickening of the epidermis with exaggeration of the normal skin creases caused by abnormal scratching or rubbing of skin (Fig. 14.1B).

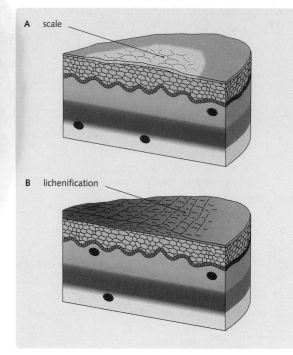

Fig. 14.1 Basic lesions of the skin showing scale and lichenification.

Excoriation

This is caused by the destruction or removal of the surface of the skin usually by scratching, but also by chemical application or other means.

Onycholysis

This is the separation of part or all of a nail from its bed. It may occur in psoriasis and in fungal infections of the skin and nail bed, and it is more common in women.

Microscopic appearances

Figure 14.2 is a diagrammatical representation of normal skin and normal epidermis.

Hyperkeratosis

Thickening of the outer horny layer of the skin (stratum corneum) occurs.

Parakeratosis

There is excessive keratin, in which nuclear remnants persist in the stratum corneum (a histological sign of increased epidermal growth).

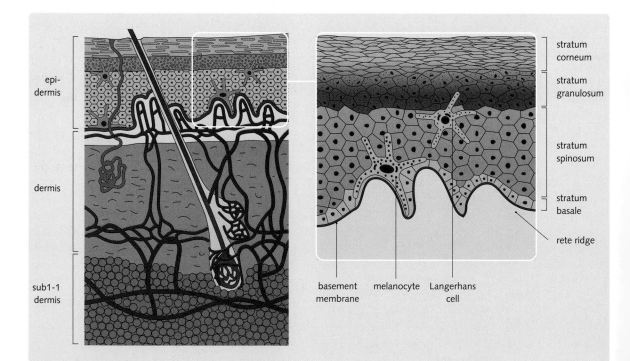

Fig. 14.2 Normal skin and epidermis.

Acanthosis

This diffuse thickening of the epidermis is caused by an increased number of prickle cells in the stratum spinosum (prickle cell layer).

Dyskeratosis

There is an abnormal premature keratinisation of cells in the prickle cell layer.

Acantholysis

The loss of cellular cohesion and separation of epidermal keratinocytes due to the rupture of intercellular bridges. Bulla formation often results.

Spongiosis

Epidermal oedema causes partial separation of keratinocytes.

Vacuolisation

This is the formation of intracellular, fluid-filled spaces (vacuoles).

Papillomatosis

In this condition, many papillomas grow on an area of skin or mucous membranes.

Lentiginous

This describes skin whose increased pigmentation is a result of increased numbers of melanocytes.

Exocytosis

Migratory inflammatory cells appear in the epidermis.

Erosion

This is the loss of all or part of the epidermis that does not extend into the dermis, but which heals without scarring.

Ulceration

A full-thickness defect (epidermis and dermis) of the skin forms.

The vocabulary of dermatology is quite distinct from that of other specialities. Learning the common dermatological terms is essential to correctly describe different skin disorders.

INFLAMMATION AND SKIN ERUPTIONS

Psoriasis

Definition

Psoriasis is a chronic, non-infectious, inflammatory disease of the skin characterised by erythematous plaques covered with thick, silvery scales.

It affects about 2% of the population in the UK and it can start at any age, but the peak onset is in the second and third decades of life.

The aetiology of psoriasis is unclear; however, about 35% of patients show a family history. It is associated with HLA haplotypes Cw6, B13 and B17.

Environmental factors are thought to trigger the disease in genetically susceptible individuals. Triggers and exacerbating factors include infection (group A *Streptococcus*), drugs, ultraviolet light, alcohol abuse and stress.

Pathogenesis:

- Epidermal cell proliferation rate is increased 20-fold or more, i.e. hyperproliferation of keratinocytes occurs.
- Epidermal turnover time is greatly reduced.
- Keratinocytes are normal, but the stem cell number is increased.

Thus, there is an increase in skin turnover and the granular layer is often absent. Epidermal cells are immature and there is accumulation of abnormal keratin, which results in scale. Characteristic histological features are:

- Long rete ridges separated by a markedly oedematous papillary dermis in which there are large numbers of dilated capillaries.
- Scale—composed of flakes of thickened surface keratin, which contain remnants of nuclei (parakeratosis).
- Neutrophil polymorphs migrate through the epidermis and they may be trapped beneath the thickened horny layer forming small aggregates (spongiform pustules).

Precipitating factors—a number of factors have been identified that can precipitate psoriasis:

- Köebner's phenomenon: trauma to skin (e.g. scratch, surgical scar or burn).
- Infection: β-haemolytic streptococcal throat infection may precipitate guttate psoriasis.

- Drugs: β-blockers, lithium and antimalarials can precipitate or worsen psoriasis.

Psoriasis most commonly affects the extensor surfaces of the knees and elbows, the trunk and the scalp (Fig. 14.3). Nail involvement is frequent. Pitting and subungual hyperkeratosis may be followed by onycholysis.

Several types of psoriasis exist, which are of variable appearance and behaviour (Fig. 14.4).

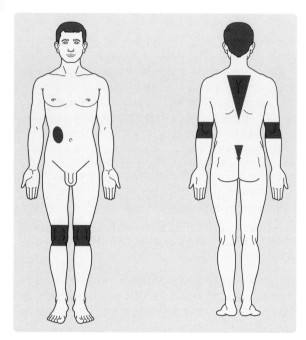

Fig. 14.3 Common sites of psoriasis.

Complications

Psoriatic arthropathy
About 7% of psoriasis patients develop arthropathy, which takes one of four forms:

1. Distal arthritis—the most common form. Affects the distal interphalangeal joints of the hands and feet, causing 'sausage-like' swelling of the digits.
2. Rheumatoid-like arthritis—polyarthropathy similar to rheumatoid disease, but usually symmetrical and negative for rheumatoid factor (seronegative arthritis). More common in women.
3. Arthritis mutilans—progressive deformity of the hands and feet caused by erosion of the small bones. Often associated with severe psoriasis.
4. Ankylosing spondylitis/sacroiliitis—in HLA-B27-positive patients.

Erythroderma
This rare complication of psoriasis (and other disorders) is characterised by a generalised reddening, flaking and thickening of all, or nearly all, of the skin surface. It is accompanied and often preceded by pyrexia, malaise and shivering. The massive loss of normal skin functioning is potentially fatal and inpatient treatment is required.

Management
Management of psoriasis includes topical therapy such as tar preparations, dithranol, topical corticosteroids and keratolytics. Systemic therapies such as photochemotherapy, retinoids and cyclosporin are used in severe cases.

Fig. 14.4 Types of psoriasis.

Fig. 14.4 Types of psoriasis	
Type	**Features**
Plaque	Most common type. Disc shaped, erythematous plaques covered with white silvery scale
Guttate	Symmetrical 'drop-like' lesions. May be associated with streptococcal infection in the young
Flexural	Smooth erythematous plaques, often glazed
Localised	Scalp, palmoplantar pustulosis, napkin (nappy area in infants), and acrodermatitis of Hallopeau (nails) types
Generalised	Rare, but potentially life threatening

Eczema and dermatitis

Definitions

Eczema and dermatitis are synonymous terms for non-infective inflammatory conditions of the skin. They are not diseases but reactive conditions occurring in response to certain stimuli, many of which are unknown. They can be acute or chronic.

Acute and chronic forms

Acute eczema/dermatitis

Acute eczema/dermatitis is characterised by:

- Erythema—caused by chronic inflammatory cell infiltrate (lymphocytes) around dilated vessels in the upper dermis.
- Spongiotic, fluid-filled vesicles—caused by epidermal oedema with separation of keratinocytes (spongiosis).
- Erythematous lesions—these are itchy (histamine release) and vesicles may weep and crust.

Chronic eczema/dermatitis

Scratching of the itchy, acute-stage lesions causes secondary changes, which result in the chronic form of the condition. It is characterised by:

- Thickening of the prickle cell layer (acanthosis).
- Thickening of the stratum corneum (hyperkeratosis).
- Elongation of the rete ridges and dermal collagenisation.
- Dilation of dermal vessels and infiltration of the dermis with inflammatory cells.

Characteristic thickening, which occurs as a result of scratching, is termed lichenification.

Atopic eczema

This chronic form of eczema is often associated with a strong family history of other atopic diseases such as asthma and hay fever. Uncontrollable itching is common. The condition follows a remitting/ relapsing course.

Although 10–15% of the population are atopic, only about 5% of these individuals will develop atopic eczema. However, the prevalence of atopic eczema is rising, for unknown reasons.

The aetiology of atopic eczema and other atopic diseases is not well understood. However, the strong family history associated with these conditions suggests at least a partial genetic cause for the disease.

The pathogenesis is as follows:

- Individuals prone to atopy have higher circulating levels of IgE antibodies than non-atopic individuals.
- On exposure to certain allergens, IgE-mediated, type I hypersensitivity reactions are triggered, causing large-scale mast-cell degranulation with the release of histamine and other inflammatory mediators.
- In the skin, this type of hypersensitivity reaction results in the histological changes of acute eczema, which on scratching becomes chronic eczema.

Atopic eczema presents at an early age, with 60% presenting before 1 year and 90% by 5 years.

The appearance of atopic eczema varies between different age groups (see below and Fig. 14.5):

- Infancy—babies develop the typical acute form of eczema on the face and hands, often with secondary infection.
- Childhood—progression from acute to chronic condition. Usually involves flexural areas such as the antecubital and popliteal fossae, neck, wrists and ankles.
- Adults—chronic condition with lichenified (and sometimes nodular) lesions. The hands are most

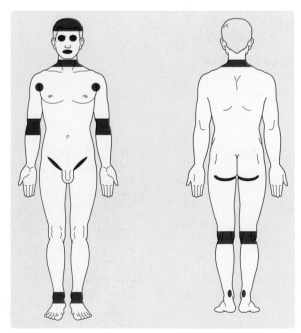

Fig. 14.5 Distribution of atopic eczema.

commonly affected but a few adults also develop the chronic, severe form of generalised atopic eczema, which is often precipitated by stressful situations.

> The prognosis from infantile eczema (starting before the age of 2) is actually pretty good—half of cases will clear by 5 years and 90% will clear by 12 years of age.

The complications are:

- Bacterial infection—typically with *Staphylococcus aureus*.
- Viral infection—increased susceptibility to the development of viral warts, molluscum contagiosum and to widespread eruption following secondary infection with herpes simplex (eczema herpeticum).
- Sleep disturbance (itchiness)—potentially causing behavioural or developmental difficulties.
- Growth retardation—may occur in children with severe eczema. The cause is unknown.
- Cataracts—rare; may occur in young adults in association with severe atopic eczema.

The treatment for atopic eczema is topical therapy (emollients, topical steroids and antibiotics), systemic therapy (antihistamines and antibiotics) and allergen avoidance (e.g. house-dust mite, rarely certain foodstuffs).

Contact dermatitis

Contact dermatitis is a form of dermatitis precipitated by exogenous agents (Fig. 14.6). It can be classified into:

- Irritant contact dermatitis—the most common form. Caused by contact of the skin with abrasives, acids, alkalis, solvents, or detergents.
- Allergic contact dermatitis—caused by a type IV (delayed-type) hypersensitivity reaction to allergens such as nickel. Previous contact with the allergen is required for sensitisation.

Lesions are localised to the site of contact, and they are most common on the hands and face.

Management is by identification and reduction in contact of the offending allergen/irritant (e.g. by protective gloves) and by topical therapy (e.g. steroids).

Other forms

Seborrhoeic dermatitis

This is a common, chronic inflammatory condition in which the skin is reddened and covered by thick,

Fig. 14.6 Distribution and causes of contact dermatitis.

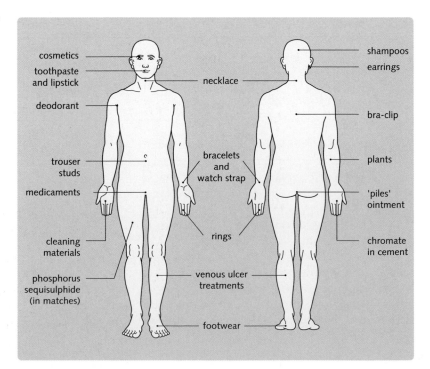

waxy or white scale. The eruption often occurs in the sebaceous gland areas of the scalp and face, although other areas may also be involved.

The aetiology is unknown but genetic factors and overgrowth of the yeast commensal *Pityrosporum ovale* have been implicated.

There are four common patterns in the clinical presentation (as shown in Fig. 14.7):

1. Scalp and facial involvement—affects the side of the nose, scalp margin, eyebrows and ears; excessive dandruff is usually present. Most common in young males. Causes 'cradle cap' in infants.
2. Petaloid—affects the presternal area.
3. *Pityrosporum folliculitis*—erythematous follicular eruption with papules or pustules, typically affecting the back.
4. Flexural—involvement of the axillae, groin and submammary areas, often secondarily colonised by *Candida albicans*.

The management is as follows:

- Medicated shampoos for scalp lesions.
- Topical antifungals for facial, truncal and flexural involvement.
- Topical hydrocortisone.

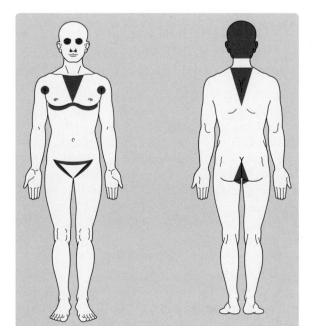

Fig. 14.7 Distribution of seborrhoeic dermatitis.

Discoid (nummular) eczema
A condition of unknown aetiology, this is characterised by 'coin-shaped', symmetrical, eczematous lesions, which typically affect the limbs of elderly men and young men who drink alcohol excessively. Secondary bacterial infection is common.

Gravitational (stasis) eczema
This typically affects the legs of middle-aged or elderly women who have venous insufficiency. It may present with haemosiderin pigmentation around the ankles or with fibrosis of the dermis and subcutaneous tissue and ulceration.

Hand dermatitis and pompholyx
This common, acute or chronic eczema may appear as a vesicular eruption known as pompholyx. 'Sago-like' vesicles appear on the sides of the fingers and on the palms.

Pompholyx is caused by the formation of eczematous vesicles that cannot rupture the thick, horny layer of the skin on the hands. The vesicles therefore persist and cause intense itching until the skin eventually peels.

Onset is usually in young adults, especially in warm weather or at times of stress, and is often recurrent.

Asteatotic eczema (eczema craquelé; winter eczema)
This dry eczema with cracking of the skin appears as a fine, 'crazy-paving' pattern of fissuring, commonly affecting the limbs and trunk of the elderly. Causes are the overwashing of patients in institutions, a dry winter climate, hypothyroidism or the use of diuretics.

Lichen striatus
A rare, self-limiting linear eczema of unknown aetiology, this typically affects the limbs of adolescents.

The terms 'dermatitis' and 'eczema' essentially describe the same reactive condition, i.e. they are histopathologically identical. Although the terms are often used interchangeably, eczema is sometimes used to describe the reaction that occurs in response to an endogenous stimulus, whereas dermatitis is used to describe the reaction that occurs in response to an exogenous stimulus.

INFECTIONS AND INFESTATIONS

Bacterial infections

Normal skin microflora

The skin is colonised by numerous microorganisms known as microflora or commensals (see Chapter 4), which may number as many as 0.5 million per cm^2. Some examples are:

- *Staphylococcus epidermidis*.
- *Staphylococcus aureus*.
- Diphtheroids.
- Streptococci.
- *Pseudomonas aeruginosa*.
- Anaerobes.
- *Candida* and *Torulopsis* species.
- *Pityrosporum* species.

Overgrowth of normal flora

Some diseases are caused by an overgrowth of normal flora:

- Erythrasma—dry, scaly, well demarcated reddish-brown eruption caused by corynebacteria. Usually asymptomatic, it can be treated with topical or oral antibiotics.
- Trichomycosis axillaris—overgrowth of corynebacteria, which form yellow concretions on axillary hair.
- Pitted keratolysis—overgrowth of micrococci, which digest keratin causing malodorous and pitted erosions with depressed discoloured areas, often on the feet. Occurs with high humidity and hyperhidrosis (increased sweating).

Staphylococcal infections

Impetigo

This highly contagious superficial skin infection is caused by either group A streptococci or *Staphylococcus aureus*. It is relatively rare in the UK, typically affecting children with poor hygiene. This means that it can spread rapidly through populations, e.g. schools.

Ecthyma

This is a full-thickness infection of epidermis by *Staphylococcus aureus*.

The clinical features of ecthyma are as follows:

- Characterised by circumscribed, ulcerated and crusted infected lesions that eventually heal with scarring.

Impetigo is characterised by the development of large, thin-walled bullae, often on the face, which leave areas of yellow crusted exudate (classically described as honey-coloured). Satellite lesions of impetigo occur due to autoinfection from the primary site.

Common differential diagnoses are herpes simplex or fungal infections.

The management of impetigo is by the removal of crusts with saline soaks and the application of topical antibiotics (usually penicillins); widespread infection can be treated with systemic antibiotics.

- Occurs most commonly on the legs, usually as a result of an insect bite or neglected minor injury.
- May also be seen in drug addicts due to the use of contaminated needles.

The management of ecthyma is by systemic and topical antibiotics.

Folliculitis

This infection of multiple hair follicles is usually caused by *Staphylococcus aureus*.

The clinical features of folliculitis are:

- Characterised by the production of tiny pustules located in the necks of hair follicles (superficial folliculitis).
- In men, it commonly affects the beard area (sycosi barbae).
- In women, it commonly affects the legs after hair removal by shaving or waxing.

A furuncle (boil) is when a deep inflammatory nodule develops within folliculitis, resulting in an expanding collection of pus that destroys the follicle and extends into the surrounding dermis.

A carbuncle is a deep abscess formed in a group of follicles with multiple drainage channels, resulting in a painful suppurating mass; it may cause systemic symptoms.

The management of folliculitis is through systemic and topical antibiotics.

Carbuncles often need surgical drainage.

Staphylococcal scalded skin syndrome

An acute toxic illness usually of infants, this is characterised by the shedding of sheets of skin, and it is caused by the potent exotoxin (exfoliatoxin) produced by a specific strain of *Staphylococcus aureus*.

The clinical presentation is as follows:

- Extensive disruption of the epidermis, with widespread confluent blistering and denuded erythematous areas resembling scalding of the skin.
- May follow impetigo, due to the spread of localised staphylococci into the bloodstream.

Management—this is a serious condition treated with potent systemic antibiotics and managed like superficial burns.

Streptococcal infections

Erysipelas

This acute, erythematous, superficial cellulitis is caused by *Streptococcus pyogenes*.

The clinical presentation is as follows:

- Usually affects the face or the lower leg and appears as a painful red swelling.
- Lesion is usually well demarcated and often oedematous and tender.
- Often preceded by fever and flu-like symptoms.
- Streptococci usually gain entry to the skin via a fissure, e.g. behind the ear or between the toes.

Severe infection requires parenteral antibiotic treatment, usually penicillin. Less severe cases can be treated with oral antibiotics.

Necrotising fasciitis

A deep-spreading infection of the fat, fascia and muscle, this is caused by *Streptococcus pyogenes*.

The condition presents as an ill-defined erythema typically affecting the leg and associated with a high fever. Infected tissues become rapidly necrotic.

It usually occurs in otherwise healthy subjects after minor trauma. It may lead to toxaemia and multisystem organ failure.

Management—is by extensive emergency surgical debridement (removal of dead tissue); systemic antibiotics are essential.

Mycobacterial infections

Tuberculosis (TB) of the skin is uncommon in the UK but is occasionally seen in the elderly and in recent immigrants from Asia.

Cutaneous manifestations of TB:

- Lupus vulgaris—the most common *Mycobacterium tuberculosis* skin infection in the UK. It usually occurs following reactivation of pre-existing disease and presents as a slowly progressive chronic skin lesion characterised by reddish-brown plaques. Typically, it affects the head or neck.
- Scrofuloderma—cutaneous involvement resulting from spread of infection from an underlying lymph node (usually cervical). Fistulae and scarring may occur.
- Warty tuberculosis—warty plaque that occurs on inoculation of the skin in an individual with immunity from a previous infection. Typically it affects the hands, knees or buttocks. Rare in Western countries, this is the most common form of cutaneous TB in developing countries.

All types are characterised by giant cell granulomatous inflammation in the dermis leading to the destruction of dermal collagen and skin appendages. Scarring is common and sometimes destruction of deeper tissues such as cartilage occurs.

Treatment is with a 6- or 9-month course of antibiotics.

Spirochaetal infections

Syphilis

Syphilis is a chronic infectious disease caused by the spirochaete *Treponema pallidum*, which is usually transmitted by sexual intercourse. It typically involves three stages: primary, secondary and tertiary.

Skin lesions may be seen in all stages, but skin manifestations tend to present during the secondary stage, in which there is an inflammatory response in the skin and mucous membranes.

The clinical presentation is as follows:

- Presents about 4–12 weeks after the onset of primary chancre (primary stage).
- Characterised by a non-itchy, pink or copper-coloured papular eruption on the trunk, limbs, palms and soles of the feet. It is often accompanied by lymphadenopathy and general malaise.
- Other signs are moist warty papules (condylomata lata) in the anogenital area, buccal erosions and diffuse patchy alopecia.
- Untreated, the eruption resolves in 1–3 months.

Management is by intramuscular penicillin. Sexual partners must be traced and they—and the patient—must be assessed for other venereal diseases.

Non-venereal treponemal infections

Rare in the UK but endemic in tropical and subtropical areas, these are transmitted by direct contact:

- Yaws—Central Africa, Central America and South-East Asia (*Treponema pertenue*).
- Pinta—Central America (*Treponema carateum*).
- Endemic syphilis (bejel) —Middle East (*Treponema pallidum*).

Lyme disease
This cutaneous and systemic infection is caused by the spirochaete *Borrelia burgdorferi* and spread by certain ticks. The majority of cases develop a slowly-extending erythematous rash at the site of the tick bite. Intermittent systemic symptoms include fever, malaise, headache, neck stiffness and muscle and joint pain.

Other bacterial infections
Anthrax
This rare infection is caused by *Bacillus anthracis* associated with farm animals, particularly cattle.

A haemorrhagic bulla forms at the site of inoculation. This may be followed by vasculitis and a necrotising, haemorrhagic inflammation of the skin.

The disease has a variable clinical course but death can occur if it is not rapidly diagnosed and treated.

Gram-negative infections
Gram-negative bacilli, such as *Pseudomonas aeruginosa*, can readily infect burns, ulcers or other moist skin lesions. They can also cause folliculitis and cellulitis (infection of subcutaneous tissues).

Figure 14.8 provides a summary of bacterial skin infections.

Viral infections
Viral warts (verrucae)
These common, benign, hyperkeratotic, papillomatous growths on the skin are caused by infection with human papillomavirus (HPV). The link between HPV infection of the skin and future skin cancer risk is currently unclear.

Keratinocytes in the stratum granulosum (granular layer) beneath the wart are often vacuolated due to the viral infection.

Common warts
Firm, dome-shaped, horny papules (1–10 mm across), and usually multiple, warts are found mainly on the hands; they can also affect the feet, face and genitalia.

Plantar warts
These occur on the soles of the feet and are often covered by callus (hyperkeratosis). Pressure causes inward growth, which results in tenderness.

Plane warts
Flat, skin-coloured papules usually found on the face. These are usually multiple. They resist treatment but eventually resolve spontaneously.

Genital warts
These affect the genitalia and the perianal region, and are linked to increased cervical cancer risk in women (see Chapter 11).

Management
Hand and foot warts frequently disappear spontaneously. Resistant varieties are treated with topical 'wart paints' (salicylic acid, lactic acid, gluteraldehyde, etc.) or with cryotherapy. Genital warts generally require cryotherapy or curettage and cautery with a local anaesthetic.

Molluscum contagiosum
This presents as discrete, multiple, pale papules with a central depression. It is caused by a DNA poxvirus.

Clinical presentation—mainly affects children or young adults. The most commonly affected areas are the face, neck and trunk, but it can affect the upper

Fig. 14.8 Summary of bacterial skin infections.

Fig. 14.8 Summary of bacterial skin infections	
Causative bacteria	**Associated skin disease**
Commensal overgrowth	Erythrasma, trichomycosis axillaris, pitted keratolysis
Staphylococci	Impetigo, ecthyma, folliculitis, scalded skin syndrome
Streptococci	Erysipelas, impetigo, necrotising fasciitis
Mycobacteria	TB (lupus vulgaris, scrofuloderma, warty tuberculosis), leprosy
Spirochaetes	Secondary syphilis, yaws/bejel/pinta, Lyme disease
Others	Anthrax, Gram-negative infections

Note: TB, tuberculosis

thighs when sexually acquired. Concomitant HIV infection results in larger skin lesions.

The virus is transmitted by contact, including sexual transmission, or on towels.

Untreated, the papules disappear in 6–9 months.

The treatment is by curettage, cryotherapy or by expressing the content of the papule (which contains a cheesy material) under local anaesthetic.

Herpes simplex

A common, acute vesicular eruption of the skin or mucous membranes, this is caused by infection with herpes simplex virus (HSV).

Pathologically:

- HSV blisters are highly contagious and they are transmitted through direct contact.
- Virus penetrates the epidermis or mucous membrane and replicates in the epithelial cells.
- Following primary infection, the virus enters a latent stage within infected cells or the dorsal root ganglion (e.g. cold sores—herpes labialis).
- Reactivation can occur at any time, even years after initial infection.
- Recurrence is thought to be precipitated by respiratory infection, sunlight, or local trauma.

Clinical presentation—there are two types of HSV:

1. HSV type 1—primary infection usually occurs in childhood and causes the common cold sore, present on or around the lips. Epithelial infection may be accompanied by fever, malaise or local lymphadenopathy. Lasts for about 2 weeks.
2. HSV type 2—this is mainly associated with genital herpes and it is sexually transmitted (see Chapter 11).

However, both type 1 and 2 viruses can cause genital herpes and cold sores, depending on the site of the initial infection.

Complications are:

- Secondary bacterial superinfection—usually staphylococcal.
- Eczema herpeticum—atopic eczema may be complicated by herpes simplex infection. Causes corneal dendritic ulceration that can threaten sight. Rarely, eczema herpeticum can be fatal.
- Disseminated herpes simplex—occasionally occurs in the newborn or in immunosuppressed patients. Active HSV is transmissible from mother to baby at birth and is an indication for elective caesarian section.

- Chronic herpes simplex—common in HIV patients.
- Herpes encephalitis—serious complication of HSV infection.
- Erythema multiforme—immune-mediated disease characterised by erythematous lesions on the hands and feet.

Management is by topical aciclovir (used for mild facial or genital herpes simplex) and oral aciclovir (prescribed for severe episodes of HSV infection).

Herpes zoster (shingles)

This acute, vesicular eruption occurs in a dermatomal distribution. It is caused by the reactivation of latent varicella zoster virus (VZV).

Following an attack of chickenpox, the virus remains dormant in the dorsal root ganglion of the spinal cord. On reactivation (the causes of which are unknown), the virus migrates down the sensory nerve to affect one or more dermatomes on the skin.

Shingles clinical presentation:
- Densely grouped vesicles and erythema in the distribution of one dermatome.
- Usually thoracic dermatomes, except in the elderly (in whom the ophthalmic division of the trigeminal nerve is more common).
- Pain, tenderness and paraesthesia may precede vesicular eruption.
- Vesicles become pustular and form crusts, which separate after 2–3 weeks to leave scarring.
- Vesicular blisters contain virus, which when shed may cause chickenpox in VZV-naïve contacts.
- Local lymphadenopathy is common.

Complications are:

- Secondary bacterial infections.
- Postherpetic neuralgia—occurs in one-third of those over 60 years old but infrequently in patients under 40 years old. Pain usually subsides within 6 months.
- Ophthalmic scarring—corneal ulcers and scarring may occur following shingles of the ophthalmic division of the trigeminal nerve.
- Motor palsy—rare; viral involvement may spread from the posterior horn of the spinal cord to the

anterior horn to infect motor nerves, resulting in palsies or paralysis of individual muscles or muscle groups.

- Disseminated herpes zoster—may occur in the immunosuppressed leading to potentially fatal varicella pneumonia or encephalitis.

Management is with oral aciclovir, which, if taken within 48 hours of onset, decreases the duration and the intensity of the disease; it may also prevent postherpetic neuralgia. Symptomatic treatment with rest, analgesia and calamine lotion is also important.

Fungal infections

Dermatophyte infections

Dermatophytes are filamentous (hyphal) fungi, which reproduce by spore formation. They commonly inhabit the keratin of the skin, hair and nails producing superficial mycoses (Fig. 14.9).

Dermatophytes are collectively termed 'ringworm' but they comprise three genera:

1. *Microsporum*, e.g. *Microsporum canis*.
2. *Trichophyton*, e.g. *Trichophyton rubrum* and *Trichophyton interdigitale*.
3. *Epidermophyton*, e.g. *Epidermophyton floccosum*.

Management is either topical or systemic depending on the extent of infection. Humid and sweaty conditions, including occlusive footwear, should be minimised.

Candida albicans

Candida albicans is a yeast-type fungus. It is a commensal of the vagina and alimentary canal and commonly produces opportunistic infections. Predisposing factors may be humidity, obesity, diabetes and oral antibiotic therapy.

Clinical presentation—in infection, hyphal forms of *Candida albicans* are seen, and the infection is termed candidosis (or candidiasis), which can present in numerous patterns as discussed below.

Genital

This is especially common in the vagina ('thrush') where white-yellowish plaques on the inflamed mucous membranes produce itching/discomfort, and sometimes a white vaginal discharge.

Oral

White plaques adhere on the tongue or inside the cheeks.

Intertrigo

A superficial inflammation of two skin surfaces that are in contact (e.g. between the thighs or under the

Fig. 14.9 Dermatophyte infections and their clinical effects

Affected area	Most common organism	Clinical presentation
Tinea corporis (trunk and limbs)	*Trichophyton verrucosum, Microsporum canis, Trichophyton rubrum*	Single or multiple ring lesions with scaling and erythema, especially at the edges Usually asymmetrical
Tinea pedis (athlete's foot)	*Trichophyton rubrum, Trichophyton interdigitale, Epidermophyton floccosum*	Redness, erosion and scaling which is often interdigital, but diffuse involvement of skin also occurs Common in young men; increased predisposition by communal washing, swimming baths, occlusive footwear, and hot weather Most common form of ringworm in the UK
Tinea capitis (scalp/hair)	*Microsporum canis, Microsporum audouinii, Trichophyton tonsurans, Trichophyton schoenleinii*	Hair loss and scaling Usually affects children
Tinea cruris (groin)	*Trichophyton rubrum, Epidermophyton floccosum, Trichophyton interdigitale*	Red, scaly, itchy rash with brown patches; more common in men and often seen in athletes ('jock itch') Starts on groin flexures and spreads to thighs
Tinea manuum (hand)	*Trichophyton rubrum*	Unilateral diffuse powdery scaling of the palm
Tinea unguium (nails)	*Trichophyton rubrum, Trichophyton interdigitale*	Thick, crumbling nails more commonly affecting toenails Incidence of onychomycosis increases with age

Fig. 14.9 Dermatophyte infections and their clinical effects.

breasts) is often aggravated by *Candida albicans* infection. Interdigital clefts are commonly affected in wet-workers.

Paronychia

The nail-fold becomes inflamed and swollen, the cuticle is lost and the nail may be ridged transversely. It is often seen in wet-workers.

Systemic

This occurs in the immunosuppressed (e.g. HIV). Red nodules appear on the skin; these have small, satellite pustules.

Mucocutaneous

This pattern of candidiasis occurs in individuals with T cell defects, most commonly occurring in Addison's disease and hypoparathyroidism. It causes chronic *Candida albicans* intertrigo and nail and mouth infections.

Management

Management is by:

- Topical therapy—for body folds and oral and genital *Candida*.
- Systemic therapy—a short course is useful for recurrent or persistent candidosis (reduces bowel carriage), also as long-term treatment for mucocutaneous candidiasis.

Infestations

Insect bites

These are a cutaneous inflammatory reaction to insect parts or to injected foreign substances. Common culprits include garden insects (gnats, etc.), insects of household pets (fleas, mites) and bedbugs (these are inactive within furniture during the day but emerge at night).

Bites are usually grouped on a limb and lesions vary from itchy wheals to quite large bullae, depending on the insect and the type of immune response elicited.

Secondary bacterial infection of excoriated insect bites is common.

It can be managed by the elimination of the cause, if within the household, and with topical hydrocortisone or calamine lotion.

Pediculosis (lice)

Lice are blood-sucking insects that, using their well-adapted legs and claws, attach to and lay eggs (nits) in the hair and clothing of humans. There are two types:

1. Pubic louse (*Pediculosis pubis*)—sexually transmitted and mostly found in young adults (colloquially known as 'crabs').

2. Body louse—associated with poor social conditions. Spread is by infested bedding or clothing. A variant, the head louse (*Pediculosis capitis*), is quite common in school children and is spread by head to head contact.

Clinical presentation—intense itching caused by bites results in excoriation and commonly in secondary bacterial infection.

Lice are found in the seams of clothes and their eggs can often be seen on hair shafts.

Scabies

Scabies is caused by the burrowing of the female mite *Sarcoptes scabiei* through the stratum corneum where she lays her eggs. After a few days the eggs hatch into larvae, which moult and mature in the epidermis. The new mites mate in the stratum corneum. The male dies and the fertilised female burrows into the skin and continues the cycle.

Clinical presentation—very itchy, raised lesions, often red and scaling, typically arise on the sides of fingers, palms, nipples and genitalia.

Linear tracks (the burrows), about 1 cm long, are often seen, and the mite can sometimes be removed by blunt needle to confirm the diagnosis.

Itching causes excoriation that frequently results in secondary bacterial infection. Untreated, the condition becomes chronic.

Management—scabies is transmitted by direct transfer and, therefore, all contacts require treatment.

Treatment—is with topical scabicides applied to the whole body.

Tropical skin infections and infestations

Leprosy (Hansen's disease)

This chronic granulomatous disease is caused by *Mycobacterium leprae*.

Leprosy is rare in the UK but is common in tropical and subtropical areas. There are about 10 million patients worldwide.

Transmission is by the inhalation of nasal droplets, after which the incubation period may be many years.

The clinicopathological features of leprosy depend on the degree of cell-mediated immunity instigated against the infection by the host. This may vary in a spectrum from strong (tuberculoid leprosy) to weak (lepromatous leprosy).

Clinical presentation—*Mycobacterium leprae* has a predilection for nerves (causing peripheral neuritis—see Chapter 5) and the skin. Figure 14.10 shows the skin involvement in the lepromatous and tuberculoid forms of leprosy.

Fig. 14.10 Skin involvement in lepromatous and tuberculoid forms of leprosy.

Fig. 14.10 Skin involvement in lepromatous and tuberculoid forms of leprosy

Lepromatous form	Tuberculoid form
Minimal immune response (occurs in patients with low cellular immunity)	Vigorous T-cell-mediated (delayed) hypersensitivity
Bacteraemia occurs to peripheral sites	Bacteraemia rare
Many skin lesions with symmetrical distribution	Few skin lesions with asymmetrical distribution
Macules, papules, plaques and nodules	Raised, red plaques with hypopigmented centre Sensation is often impaired within the plaque
Typically involves arms, legs, buttocks and face	Often affects the face
Progression causes a thickened, furrowed appearance of face (leonine facies) with eyebrow loss	Progression is slow; combined effect of extensive destruction of tissue by immune response and repeated trauma to desensitised areas results in severe disfigurement, especially to hands and feet
Untreated, this form is lethal due to the impaired immune response	Eventually heals spontaneously

Management—is by antibiotic treatment (usually multiple) for at least 2 years.

Leishmaniasis

A common disease in the tropics and subtropics caused by the protozoan *Leishmania*, this is transmitted by sand flies. Three forms of the disease exist, caused by different species of *Leishmania* (Fig. 14.11).

Management—cutaneous leishmaniasis often heals spontaneously over several months. However, other forms require pentavalent antimonials intravenously for 10–21 days.

Filariasis

This tropical disease is caused by the nematode worms *Wuchereria bancrofti* and *Brugia malayi*. The worms, which are transmitted by various mosquitoes or flies, cause inflammation and eventual blockage of the lymph vessels. The net result is gross oedema of the surrounding tissues—elephantiasis—especially of the legs or scrotum.

Larva migrans

Also known as 'creeping eruption', this is caused by the larvae of dog hookworms. Larvae burrow through

Fig. 14.11 Different types of leishmaniasis

Type of leishmaniasis	Endemic areas	Protozoan	Clinical presentation
Visceral (kala azar)	Asia, Africa and South America	*Leishmania donovani*	Affects lymphatic system, spleen and bone marrow, causing splenomegaly, hepatomegaly, anaemia and disability; patchy pigmentation may occur on face, hands and abdomen
Cutaneous	Mediterranean coast, Middle East and Asia	*Leishmania tropica*	Characterised by 'oriental sore', a red–brown nodule that appears at site of inoculation and which either ulcerates or spreads slowly to form crusty plaque
Mucocutaneous	Central and South America	*Leishmania braziliensis*	Characterised by a skin lesion similar to that of oriental sore but is followed by necrotic ulcers which cause deformity of nose, lips and palate

Fig. 14.11 Different types of leishmaniasis.

the skin (most commonly the feet), leaving intensely itchy tracks in their wake. Treatment is with topical tiabendazole, although the larvae die spontaneously after a few weeks, as they cannot complete their life cycle in humans.

Deep mycoses

These systemic diseases are caused by fungal invasion. They include:

- Blastomycosis—wart-like ulcers on the face, neck and limbs, plus lung disease.
- Histoplasmosis—lung disease plus granulomata of the skin (pathologically similar to tuberculosis).
- Mycetoma—chronic granulomata on the foot.
- Sporotrichosis—chronic granulomatous skin infection.

Onchocerciasis

This endemic disease of Africa and Central America is caused by the nematode worm *Onchocerca volvulus*, which is transmitted to humans by a gnat. The worms cause an itchy papular eruption on the skin, which progresses to form fibrous nodules with lichenification and pigmentary change. Microfilariae also invade the eye, resulting in total or partial blindness (called 'river blindness' in Africa).

- Colonisation of ducts with *Propionibacterium acnes*.
- Release of inflammatory mediators.

Figure 14.12 illustrates the pathogenesis of acne.

Clinical presentation—comedones (singular comedo) tend to be limited to the face, shoulders, upper chest and back. They are of two types:

1. Open as in blackheads—dilated pores with dark plugs of keratin and sebum.
2. Closed as in whiteheads—small, cream-coloured, dome-shaped papules formed through sebum and keratin accumulations deeper in the ducts.

The colonisation of ducts with *Propionibacterium acnes* causes the evolution of comedones into inflammatory papules, nodules or cysts, which often form scars on healing. This may persist until the early twenties and even into the fifth decade of life in a few patients, especially in women.

Management of acne is shown in Fig. 14.13.

Rosacea

This chronic inflammatory disease of the face is characterised by erythema, telangiectasia and pustules.

The aetiology of rosacea is unknown.

Telangiectatic dilatation of the upper dermal vessels is common, and it causes erythema. Fragments

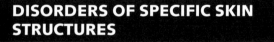

DISORDERS OF SPECIFIC SKIN STRUCTURES

Sweat and the sebaceous structures

Acne vulgaris

This inflammatory disorder of the pilosebaceous apparatus is characterised by comedones (blackheads and whiteheads), papules, pustules, nodules, cysts and scars. It is extremely common in adolescents, the peak age for clinical acne being 18 years.

Aetiopathogenesis—the cause of acne is uncertain but the androgen-sensitive sebaceous glands show a hyper-responsiveness to testosterone that results in the following sequence of events:

- Increased sebum excretion.
- Hyperkeratosis of pilosebaceous ducts.
- Blockage of pilosebaceous units with excess keratin and sebum, causing comedo formation.

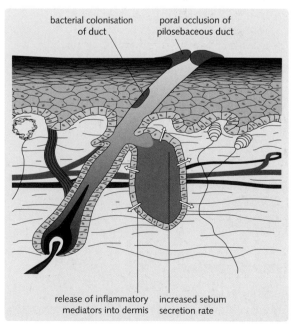

Fig. **14.12** Pathogenesis of acne.

Fig. 14.13 Management of acne vulgaris.

Fig. 14.13 Management of acne vulgaris		
Type	**Treatment**	**Comment**
Topical treatment (mild acne)	Benzoyl peroxide	Reduced numbers of *Propionibacterium acnes* but may cause irritation
	Tretinoin	Reduces number of non-inflamed lesions but may cause irritation
	Antibiotics	Used in treatment of mild or moderate acne
Systemic treatment (moderate or severe acne)	Antibiotics	e.g. tetracyclines or erythromycin for a minimum of 4 months
	Antiandrogens	Usually combined with an oestrogen and prescribed to females over a period of 6–12 months; suppresses sebum production and is also a contraceptive
	Retinoids	Isotretinoin: reduces sebum excretion, inhibits *Propionibacterium acnes* and is anti-inflammatory; 4- to 6-month course; very effective but side effects common

of the mite *Demodex folliculorum* are commonly found in follicles but its role in the pathogenesis is unclear.

Follicular pustules often develop in the markedly dilated hair follicles.

Rupture of the follicles stimulates a granulomatous reaction that leads to a florid, lumpy form of rosacea.

Rosacea typically affects the middle-aged or elderly. There is intermittent facial flushing on top of persistent erythema. Rosacea is often complicated by:
- Rhinophyma—hyperplasia of sebaceous glands and connective tissue of the nose.
- Eye involvement—blepharitis (inflammation of the eyelids) and conjunctivitis.
- The condition is exacerbated by sunlight and topical steroids.

Management is by oral tetracycline but this will not reverse telangiectasia or prevent erythema. Plastic surgery may be required for rhinophyma.

Hair disorders
Alopecia

This describes the loss of hair. It is commonly classified into three main types: diffuse non-scarring, localised non-scarring and scarring (cicatricial).

Diffuse non-scarring

There is a diffuse reduction in hair density. The patient usually notices excessive numbers of hairs on the pillow, brush or comb.

The causes of diffuse non-scarring alopecia are:

- Male pattern/androgenic alopecia—inherited, androgen-dependent hair loss. Extremely common in men but it also occurs in women, becoming more pronounced after the menopause.
- Endocrine related—hypo- and hyperthyroidism, pituitary or adrenal hypoactivity. Androgen-secreting tumours in women can produce male pattern baldness.
- Nutrition related—iron or zinc deficiency, malnutrition especially kwashiorkor (protein deficiency).
- Telogen effluvium—hair follicles, which are usually out of phase, can, under certain circumstances, become synchronised into the resting phase (telogen) and then shed in unison 3 months later. The causes of synchronisation are high fever, childbirth, surgery, drugs or stress.
- Drug induced—e.g. cytotoxics, heparin, warfarin, carbimazole, colchicine and vitamin A.

Localised non-scarring

There is patchy hair loss. The causes are:

- Alopecia areata—common condition associated with autoimmune disorders, atopy and Down syndrome. The growth phase of hair is prematurely arrested.
- Infections, e.g. with scalp ringworm (tinea capitis) or secondary syphilis.
- Trauma/traction.

It typically presents in the second or third decade of life with bald patches on the scalp, but the eyebrows and beard can also be affected. The nails may show pitting.

The course is unpredictable, varying from the progressive enlargement of bald patches to the regrowth of hair (more common).

A poor prognosis is indicated if the onset is prepubertal, associated with atopy or shows extensive involvement.

Rarely, complete scalp alopecia (totalis) or loss of all bodily hair (universalis) occurs.

Scarring (cicatricial) alopecia

This is caused by scarring of the scalp with the destruction of hair follicles.

The causes of scarring are:

- Irradiation/burns (chemical or thermal).
- Infection, e.g. shingles of the ophthalmic division of the trigeminal nerve, tinea capitis or tertiary syphilis.
- Lichen planus/lupus erythematosus—erythema, scaling and follicular changes may result in scarring.
- Pseudopelade—end stage of an idiopathic or unidentified destructive inflammatory process in the scalp.

Excess hair

Hirsutism

This is the growth of coarse, pigmented hair with an androgenic distribution in a female.

Figure 14.14 shows the aetiology of hirsutism.

Hypertrichosis

This is excessive growth of hair in a non-androgenic distribution. It is less common than hirsutism and can be:

- Localised, e.g. on melanocytic naevi or following topical steroid usage.
- Generalised—fine terminal hair appears on the face, limbs, and trunk. Mostly drug induced but it

Fig. 14.14 Aetiology of hirsutism

Idiopathic	Most common form; probably due to increased hypersensitivity of end-organ to androgens
Iatrogenic	e.g. androgens, progestogens
Virilising tumours	e.g. ovarian or adrenal tumours
Endocrine disorders	Congenital adrenal hyperplasia, Cushing's syndrome, acromegaly

Fig. 14.14 Aetiology of hirsutism.

can also be caused by anorexia nervosa (or malnutrition), porphyria, cutanea tarda or underlying malignancy.

Others

Hairshaft defects

These are rare, usually inherited, brittle hair conditions.

Dandruff

This is caused by excessive exfoliation of fine scales from an otherwise normal scalp.

Tinea capitis

Infection of the scalp with dermatophyte (see page 326); may cause scarring alopecia.

Nail disorders

Congenital disease

Congenital conditions are as follows:

- Racket nails—most common congenital nail defect characterised by broad, short, thumb nails.
- Nail–patella syndrome—nails (and patellae) are absent or rudimentary.
- Pachyonychia congenita—rare autosomal dominant condition causing thickened, discoloured nails present from birth.

Trauma

Traumatic conditions are as follows:

- Subungual haematoma—bleeding under the nail following trapping of a finger- or toenail.
- Splinter haemorrhages—almost always occur with infective endocarditis, but they may also be trauma or psoriasis induced.
- Ingrowing toenails—usually caused by ill-fitting shoes.

- Onychogryphosis—big toenails become thickened and horn-like, usually in response to trauma.
- Brittle nails—usually due to repeated exposure to detergents and water.

Nail involvement in the dermatoses

These are:

- Alopecia areata—pitting and roughness of nail surface.
- Psoriasis—pitting, nail thickening, onycholysis, brown patches, subungual hyperkeratosis, splinter haemorrhages.
- Eczema—pitting and transverse ridging. Often shiny from repeated scratching.

Infections

Infections are:

- Tinea unguium—fungal infection of the nails (Fig. 14.15).
- Chronic paronychia—*Candida albicans* infection of the nails, common in wet-workers (see page 326).
- Acute paronychia—typically, a bacterial infection of the nails usually caused by staphylococci.

Tumours of the nails

The tumours are:

- Viral warts—common around the nail-fold.
- Periungual fibroma—associated with tuberous sclerosis.
- Myxoid cysts—mucous cysts adjacent to the nail-fold that probably arise from folds of synovium.
- Malignant melanoma—subungual malignant melanoma, which produces a pigmented longitudinal streak in a nail and may cause its destruction.

Nail changes in systemic disease

Systemic disorders can often cause specific nail changes, which can help in the diagnosis of these conditions. Fig. 14.15 gives examples of nail changes and their possible causes.

DISORDERS OF PIGMENTATION

Hypopigmentation
Vitiligo

This common disorder (1% of the population) is characterised by the appearance of symmetrical white or pale macules on the skin, which are caused by focal melanocyte loss.

Aetiopathogenesis—it has been suggested that vitiligo is an autoimmune disease of melanocytes, as it is often associated with other autoimmune diseases, such as pernicious anaemia, thyroid disease and Addison's disease.

The exact aetiology is unknown but about 30% of patients have a family history.

Clinical presentation—vitiligo affects all races, but is more conspicuous in dark-skinned individuals.

Onset is usually between 10 and 30 years of age. It commonly affects the hands, wrists, knees, neck and areas around orifices (e.g. mouth), It has an unpredictable course, ranging from progression to repigmentation (rarely).

Vitiligo is managed with camouflage cosmetics and sunscreens (for both cosmetic reasons and to reduce risk of burning and skin cancer). Topical steroids occasionally induce repigmentation in darker skins. PUVA (psoralen and UV-A) is occasionally beneficial.

Albinism

This is a rare (1 in 20 000) autosomal recessive disease characterised by the lack of pigmentation in the skin, hair and eyes. Melanocyte numbers are normal but melanin production fails because of a deficiency or defect in the enzyme tyrosinase.

The skin is white or pink, the hair is white and pigmentation is lacking in the eye. It is associated with poor sight, photophobia and nystagmus. Albinos have an increased risk of skin tumours on exposure to UV light.

Prenatal diagnosis is possible.

Phenylketonuria

This autosomal recessive inborn error of metabolism is caused by a deficiency of phenylalanine hydroxylase, which normally converts phenylalanine to tyrosine.

Patients also have fair hair and skin because of impaired melanin synthesis (tyrosine is a precursor of melanin). The concentration of phenylalanine and its metabolites is increased and damages the neonatal brain. Untreated, mental retardation and choreoathetosis develop, although a low phenylalanine diet can prevent neurological damage.

The prevalence is 1 per 25 000 and it is detected by routine screening tests (heel-prick or Guthrie test performed around day 5 of life).

A summary of the causes of hypopigmentation is given in Fig. 14.16.

Fig. 14.15 Nail changes and their possible causes

Nail change	Description		Possible causes
Beau's lines	Transverse ridges		Severe illnesses that affect nail growth, e.g. pneumonia or myocardial infarction
Brittle nails	Easily broken nails		Repeated exposure to water/detergent, iron deficiency, hypothyroidism, ischaemia of digits
Colour change	Black transverse bands		Cytotoxic drugs
	Blue		Haematoma, cyanosis, antimalarials
	Blue–green		*Pseudomonas* infection
	Brown		Fungal infection, cigarette stains, chlorpromazine, gold, Addison's disease
	Brown patches		Psoriasis
	Brown longitudinal streak		Melanocytic naevus, malignant melanoma, Addison's disease
	Red–brown streaks (splinter haemorrhages)		Infective endocarditis, trauma
	White spots		Trauma to nail matrix (not calcium deficiency)
	White (leuconychia)		Hypoalbuminaemia
	Yellow		Psoriasis, tinea unguium, jaundice, tetracycline
	Yellow nail syndrome		Defective lymphatic drainage
Clubbing	Swelling of nail with loss of angle between nail-fold and nail plate	normal clubbed	Respiratory: pulmonary tuberculosis, bronchiectasis, empyema, lung cancer, fibrosing alveolitis Cardiovascular: infective endocarditis, congenital heart disease Other less common diseases, e.g. asbestosis, Crohn's disease, ulcerative colitis, cirrhosis
Koilonychia	Concave (spoon-shaped) nails		Iron deficiency anaemia Repeated exposure to detergents
Nail-fold telangiectasia	Reddened nail-folds caused by dilated capillaries		Inflammatory connective tissue disorders including systemic sclerosis and dermatomyositis
Onycholysis	Separation of part or all of nail from its bed		Psoriasis, tinea unguium, trauma, thyrotoxicosis, tetracyclines
Pitting	Small holes in nail-bed		Psoriasis, eczema, alopecia areata, lichen planus
Ridging	Transverse		Beau's lines, eczema, psoriasis, chronic paronychia
	Longitudinal		Secondary to trauma

Fig. 14.15 Nail manifestations of disease and deficiency disorders.

Fig. 14.16 Summary of causes of hypopigmentation

	Cause	Example
Generalised hypopigmentation	Genetic	Albinism and phenylketonuria
Patchy hypopigmentation	Endocrine	Hypopituitarism ($\downarrow$ACTH and $\downarrow$MSH)
	Infective	Leprosy, yaws, pityriasis versicolor
	Postinflammatory	Cyrotherapy, eczema, psoriasis, morphoea, pityriasis alba
	Chemical	Substituted phenols, hydroquinone
	Other	Vitiligo, lichen sclerosus, halo naevus

Note: ACTH, adrenocorticotrophic hormone; MSH, melanin-stimulating hormone

Fig. 14.16 Summary of causes of hypopigmentation.

Hyperpigmentation

Freckles and lentigines

Freckles (ephelides)

Freckles are small, light-brown, well-demarcated macules that darken on exposure to sunlight. They contain normal numbers of melanocytes but melanin production is increased. They are common in childhood, especially in fair-skinned children. No treatment is required.

Lentigines

Lentigines (also known as lentigos) are similar in appearance to freckles but they are more scattered and they do not darken in the sun. Their outline may be more irregular than freckles. They contain increased numbers of melanocytes and may develop in childhood, but they are more common in a sun-exposed, elderly skin. They respond to cryotherapy.

Chloasma (melasma)

This photosensitivity reaction in pregnant women (or in women taking oral contraceptives) causes the appearance of symmetrical, ill-defined brown patches on the face. These are caused by oestrogen-induced melanocyte stimulation.

Sunscreens and cosmetic camouflage can help mask the brown patches, which usually improve spontaneously.

Drug-induced pigmentation

This can be caused by stimulation of melanogenesis or by drug deposition in the skin. Drugs commonly responsible include amiodarone, bleomycin, psoralens, chlorpromazine and minocycline.

Other causes

Addison's disease

This is characterised by hypoadrenalism, with over-production of adrenocorticotrophic hormone (ACTH) by the pituitary gland. ACTH stimulates melanogenesis, resulting in hyperpigmentation of mucosae and skin creases.

Addisonian-like pigmentation is also seen in Cushing's syndrome, hyperthyroidism and acromegaly.

Peutz–Jeghers syndrome

This rare, autosomal dominant disorder is characterised by perioral lentigines and intestinal polyps.

Figure 14.17 provides a summary of the causes of hyperpigmentation.

BLISTERING DISORDERS

Blisters are fluid-filled spaces within the skin caused by the separation of two layers of tissue and the leakage of plasma into the space. The type of blister formed (Fig. 14.18) depends on the level of separation. It can be:

- Subcorneal—bullous impetigo or pustular psoriasis.
- Intraepidermal—acute eczema, herpes simplex/zoster, pemphigus, friction blisters.
- Subepidermal—pemphigoid, dermatitis herpetiformis, cold and thermal injury.

Pemphigus

This rare but potentially fatal group of autoimmune disorders is marked by successive outbreaks of blisters on the skin and in the mouth.

Fig. 14.17 Summary of causes of hyperpigmentation

Cause	Problem
Genetic	Inherited: freckles, neurofibromatosis (café-au-lait spots), Peutz–Jeghers syndrome Acquired: lentigines
Endocrine	Chloasma, Addison's disease, Cushing's syndrome, hyperthyroidism and acromegaly
Metabolic	Biliary cirrhosis (jaundice), haemochromatosis (iron deposition), porphyria
Nutritional	Carotenemia (orange discoloration), malnutrition/malabsorption, pellagra
Postinflammatory	Eczema, lichen planus, systemic sclerosis
Drugs	e.g. oestrogens, amiodarone, bleomycin, psoralens, chlorpromazine and minocycline
Other	Acanthosis nigricans, malignant melanoma, naevi, argyria (deposition of silver), chronic renal failure

Fig. 14.17 Summary of causes of hyperpigmentation.

Aetiopathogenesis—patients have circulating IgG autoantibodies that bind to intercellular junctions in the epidermis. Binding of IgG activates complement and adjacent keratinocytes are induced to release proteolytic enzymes. Cellular adhesion is lost (acantholysis), and an intraepidermal separation occurs.

This is also associated with other organ-specific autoimmune disorders,such as myasthenia gravis, and—in a minority of cases—malignancy ('paraneoplastic pemphigus').

Clinical presentation—the most common form is pemphigus vulgaris, which typically affects middle-aged people. Oral erosions precede cutaneous blistering in 50% of cases. Flaccid, superficial blisters develop over the scalp, face, back, chest and flexures.

If left untreated, the blistering is progressive and ultimately fatal (due to the loss of electrolytes and protein). Pemphigus is associated with a 15% mortality rate. It is managed with systemic steroids and other immunosuppressive agents.

Bullous pemphigoid

This is a chronic, itchy blistering disorder of the elderly.

Aetiopathogenesis—an autoimmune disorder, in which IgG antibodies are deposited at the basement membrane.

Inflammatory cells attracted by complement activation release proteolytic enzymes resulting in subepidermal bullae formation, which tend to remain intact.

Clinical presentation—large, tense blisters commonly appear on the limbs, trunk and flexures, but are occasionally localised to one site, often the lower leg. Oral lesions occur in only 10% of cases. An urticarial eruption may precede the onset of blistering.

The disease is self-limiting in about 50% of cases and is managed with systemic steroids and other immunosuppressants.

Dermatitis herpetiformis

This presents as a rare eruption of symmetrical itchy blisters on the extensor surfaces.

Aetiopathogenesis—the aetiology is unknown but associated with coeliac disease (see Chapter 8). It is characterised by granular IgA at the dermal papillae of normal-looking skin and villus atrophy of the small intestine.

It usually presents in the third or fourth decade of life, with males more often affected than females by 2 : 1. There are groups of small, intensely itchy

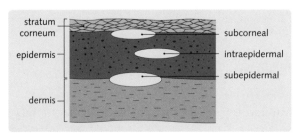

Fig. 14.18 Location of blisters within the skin.

vesicles on the knees, elbows, scalp, buttocks and shoulders.

Despite villus atrophy in most patients, symptoms of gastrointestinal (GI) disturbances are uncommon. It should be managed with a gluten-free diet with or without dapsone.

A summary of blistering disorders is given in Fig. 14.19.

Blistering diseases are rare but important because they can be severe and are potentially fatal. Pemphigus vulgaris is the most life threatening type of blistering disorder.

TUMOURS OF THE SKIN

Benign tumours of the skin

Epidermal tumours

Seborrhoeic wart

This common, benign tumour of basal keratinocytes typically occurs on the trunk, face, and arms of the elderly. The aetiology of these tumours is unknown. They are also known as basal cell papilloma:

- Warts are often greasy looking (hence seborrhoeic), but they are not associated with seborrhoea nor with sebaceous glands.
- Rare before 35 years old, then usually multiple, varying in size from a few millimetres to several centimetres.

- Progress from lightly pigmented, small papules to darkly pigmented, warty nodules.
- Often have a 'pasted on' appearance with well-defined edges.

Microscopically, all lesions show basal cell proliferation, hyperkeratosis and a variable degree of pigmentation.

Actinic keratosis

This presents as roughened, scaly brownish-to-red lesions, usually less than 1 cm across, which bleed when rubbed. They typically arise on sun-exposed areas (also known as solar keratosis), especially the face, scalp, and hands, of the middle-aged and elderly.

Histologically, they show hyperkeratosis and parakeratosis, abnormal keratinocytes with loss of maturation, and a mild to moderate degree of pleomorphism and mitotic figures.

The lesions are considered as premalignant, with 20% of them evolving into squamous cell carcinoma.

Skin tags

These common, benign, pedunculated polyps, a few millimetres in length, typically affect elderly or middle-aged individuals. They have a predilection for the neck, axillae, groin and eyelids. They consist of a fibrovascular core with an epidermal covering.

Their aetiology is unknown but they are often found in obese individuals.

Cysts

These benign, keratin-filled, firm, skin-coloured cysts are normally 1–3 cm in diameter.

Common types are epidermal cysts (derived from the epidermis) and pilar cysts (derived from the outer

Fig. 14.19 Summary of blistering disorders

Disorder	Type of bullae	Autoimmunity	Clinical features
Pemphigus vulgaris	Intraepidermal	IgG deposited on intercellular junctions	Flaccid, superficial bullae More common in middle-aged High mortality
Bullous pemphigoid	Subepidermal	IgG deposited on basement membrane	Large, tense bullae More common in elderly Self-limiting in about 50% of cases
Dermatitis herpetiformis	Subepidermal	IgA deposited on dermal papillae	Small, itchy vesicles Usually presents in 3rd or 4th decade; males > females Associated with coeliac disease

Fig. 14.19 Summary of blistering disorders.

root sheath of the hair follicle). These are often incorrectly grouped together as sebaceous cysts.

Milia

These small, white, subepidermal keratin cysts, normally 1–2 mm in diameter, often affect the eyelids and the upper cheeks. They are common in children but they can appear at any age (milia is the plural of milium).

Dermal tumours

Dermatofibroma (histiocytoma)

These firm, reddish-brown papules are common in young adults, females more than males, and usually appear on the lower legs.

Histologically, they consist of intertwining bands of collagen fibres formed by proliferating fibroblasts, with reactive hyperplasia and hyperpigmentation of overlying epidermis. Dermatofibroma can be mistaken for a melanocytic naevus or malignant melanoma.

Pyogenic granuloma

A benign, rapidly-growing, bright-red nodule arising mainly on the fingers or face, typically at a site of trauma (e.g. a thorn prick) and more commonly in young adults and children. It is neither pyogenic nor granulomatous but is a well-circumscribed dermal lesion of proliferating capillaries and inflammation that closely resembles a haemangioma.

Excision and histological examination are required to rule out malignant melanoma.

Keloid

This is an excessive proliferation of connective tissue occurring in previously injured skin (a form of scar), but extending beyond the margin of the original injury. Commonly seen in the healing of acne vulgaris. Characteristics are:

- Firm, smooth, erythematous nodules of irregular shapes, occurring mainly over the upper back, chest or ear lobes.
- More common in Black people.
- Highest incidence in second to fourth decades of life.

Treatment is by steroid injection into the keloid.

Campbell de Morgan's spot (cherry angioma)

Small, bright-red papules (1–2 mm diameter) composed of benign capillary proliferations commonly arise on the trunk in elderly or middle-aged patients.

Lipoma

A soft, subcutaneous tumour of mature adipocytes. This is often multiple and mostly found on the trunk, neck and upper extremities.

Chondrodermatitis nodularis

This small painful nodule on the upper rim of the pinna occurs usually in elderly white men. It is caused by inflammation of the underlying cartilage, and it is not a neoplasm. Excision is curative.

Figure 14.20 provides a summary of benign skin tumours.

Naevi

Definition

Naevi are benign, coloured lesions on the skin formed from a proliferation of one or more of the normal constituent cells of the skin. Although often congenital (birthmarks), they may be acquired.

Melanocytic naevi

These consist of localised benign proliferations of melanocytic cells and are the most common type of naevus (also known as 'moles'). They present in most Caucasians but they are less prevalent in those with Down syndrome; they are also less common in Black people.

The aetiology of naevi development is unknown but it seems to be an inherited trait in many families:

- About 1% of naevi are congenital.
- Majority develops during childhood or adolescence; numbers reach a peak at puberty and they have a tendency to decline during adult life.
- A few new naevi develop during the third and fourth decade of life, especially if provoked by excessive sun exposure or pregnancy.

Fig. 14.20 Summary of benign skin tumours

Tumour type	Example
Benign epidermal tumours	Viral wart Actinic keratosis Seborrhoeic wart Milia Cysts Skin tags
Benign dermal tumours	Dermatofibroma Melanocytic naevus Cherry angioma Pyogenic granuloma Keloid Lipoma Chondrodermatitis nodularis

Fig. 14.20 Summary of benign skin tumours.

Naevi can be classified according to the position of the naevus cells within the skin as follows:

- Junctional naevi—flat circular macules consisting of rounded nests of melanocytes in the lower epidermis at the dermoepidermal junction.
- Compound naevi—papules or nodules with an irregular surface, which consist of junctional nests of melanocytes combined with an intradermal mass of melanocytic cells.
- Intradermal naevi—dome-shaped papules/nodules composed entirely of melanocytic cell clusters within the upper dermis (no junctional component present).

These different types of naevi are thought to arise by progression from junctional to intradermal (Fig. 14.21).

Other variants are:

- Congenital naevi—usually over 1 cm in diameter; they may be protuberant or hairy and have a risk of malignant change, which is believed to be proportional to the size of the lesion.
- Blue naevi—steely blue intradermal naevus, usually solitary and most commonly found on the extremities.
- Halo naevi—white halo of depigmentation surrounds naevi. Represents involution of naevus following immune response against naevus cells. Mainly seen in children and adolescents.
- Becker's naevi—rare, unilateral lesion on upper back or chest. Initially hyperpigmented, it later becomes hairy. More common in adolescent males.
- Familial dysplastic naevus syndrome—familial condition characterised by large numbers of atypical and 'dysplastic' naevi. Affected individuals have a greatly increased risk of developing malignant melanoma.

The majority of naevi are entirely benign but malignant changes can occur. Junctional components of junctional or compound naevi carry the highest risk for malignancy. Invasion is preceded by nuclear pleomorphism with increased mitoses and cellular atypia. Clinically, malignant naevi appear larger than normal and have an irregular edge, surface and pigmentation. They are also more likely to be itchy and to bleed.

The management is as follows:

- Increase public awareness about significance of change in pigmented lesions.
- Excision and histological examination of suspicious naevi.

Vascular naevi

These common naevi are usually congenital or developed soon after birth. They are composed of small dermal blood vessels. There are four main types:

1. Salmon patch—most common type (present in about 50% of neonates), typically on neck or eyelids. Usually fades quickly.
2. Port wine stain naevus—irregular red/purple macule, which often affects one side of the face.
3. Capillary haemangioma (strawberry naevus)— common, red, nodular lesion, which develops during the first few weeks of life, reaches its maximum size in the first 12 months and then involutes. Most cases have regressed by 5–7 years of age.
4. Cavernous haemangioma—similar to strawberry naevus but composed of larger and deeper channels and presents as a nodular swelling. Regression is not as complete.

The treatment is by camouflage cosmetics or laser treatment for port wine stains. Strawberry naevi are

Fig. 14.21 Types of melanocytic naevi.

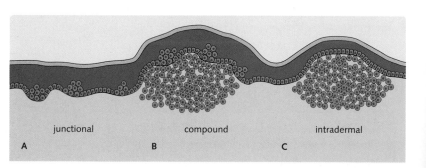

junctional

compound

intradermal

A

B

C

usually left to involute but cavernous haemangiomas may require surgery.

Epidermal naevi

These warty, pigmented and often elongated naevi are usually congenital or develop in early childhood. Most are a few centimetres long but they can be extensive.

Treatment is by excision but recurrence is common.

Connective tissue naevi

Rare, skin-coloured papules composed of coarse collagen bundles in the dermis. Common in tuberous sclerosis.

Figure 14.22 provides a summary of naevi.

Malignant melanoma (melanocarcinoma)

This malignant tumour of melanocytes usually arises in the skin. Incidence in the UK is 10 per 100 000 per year but it is rising steadily. Five-year survival is nearly 80% in males and over 90% in females, although women are more often affected than men by 2 : 1.

It occurs in all races but it is more common in Caucasian races. Incidence is proportional to geographical latitude, which suggests an effect of UV radiation. The most common site in males is on the back but in females it is the lower leg.

The aetiology is unknown but repeated exposure to UV radiation is thought to play an important role.

Major risk factors for the development of malignant melanoma (with decreasing risk) are:

- Familial dysplastic naevus syndrome—rare but lifetime risk of melanoma is over 50%.
- Multiple melanocytic naevi—50 naevi over 2 mm in diametre.
- Congenital naevus.
- Previous malignant melanoma.
- Immunosuppression.
- Fair skin—melanin pigmentation appears protective.

Classification

Four main types of malignant melanoma are recognised.

1. Superficial spreading malignant melanoma

A flat tumour with variable pigmentation and irregular edges. This is the most common type, accounting for 50% of all UK cases. There is a female preponderance and it is most common on the lower leg.

2. Lentigo malignant melanoma

A nodular lesion arising in a pre-existing lentigo maligna. This typically occurs in sun-damaged skin of the face in elderly patients. It comprises about 15% of UK cases.

Lentigo maligna is similar to a benign lentigine but it is generally larger, at over 2 cm, and it has atypical melanocytes.

3. Acral lentiginous malignant melanoma

This resembles the lentigo malignant melanoma but it affects the palms, soles and nail-beds (subungual melanoma). It comprises 10% of UK cases but it is the most common form of malignant melanoma in oriental people, suggesting it develops independently of UV radiation exposure. It is often diagnosed late and consequently has poor survival figures.

4. Nodular malignant melanoma

A pigmented nodule that may grow rapidly and ulcerate, this accounts for 25% of UK melanomas. It is more common in males, typically arising on the trunk. The preceding *in situ* phase of growth is very difficult to identify in nodular melanoma.

Fig. 14.22 Summary of naevi.

Fig. 14.22 Summary of naevi

Type of naevus	Comments
Melanocytic	Very common, usually multiple, pigmented and benign Consists of nests of melanocytic cells Classified into junctional, compound and intradermal Types are congenital, blue, halo, Becker's and dysplastic
Vascular	Common, usually congenital, composed of small dermal blood vessels Types are salmon patch, port wine stain, capillary haemangioma ('strawberry'), cavernous haemangioma
Epidermal	Warty, pigmented and often linear
Connective tissue	Rare, skin-coloured, collagenous naevi

Staging and prognosis of malignant melanoma

Local invasion of the malignant melanoma is assessed using the Breslow method (Fig. 14.23). The Breslow thickness is the measured thickness in millimetres (on a histological section) from the granular layer of the epidermis to the deepest identifiable melanoma cell.

The Breslow thickness is directly related to the risk of metastasis (Fig. 14.24). Tumours are divided into one of three prognostic groups—good, intermediate or poor—depending on their Breslow thickness.

Diagnosis—one or more of the following changes observed or reported in a naevus or pigmented lesion may suggest malignant melanoma:

- Size—usually increased.
- Shape—irregular outline.
- Colour—irregular pigmentation.
- Inflammation—at the edge of lesion.
- Crusting—oozing or bleeding lesion.
- Itchiness—a common symptom.

Malignant epidermal tumours

Basal cell carcinoma (rodent ulcer)

A malignant tumour that arises from the basal keratinocytes of the epidermis, this is the most common form of human cancer, typically seen on the face in elderly or middle-aged subjects. It is five times more common than squamous cell carcinoma (see below).

Tumours are locally very invasive, but they almost never metastasise.

Risk factors for the development of basal cell carcinoma include:

Fig. 14.24 Five-year survival rates for malignant melanomas of different Breslow thickness

Prognosis	Breslow thickness (mm)	5-year survival rate (%)
Good	< 1.0	93
Intermediate	1–3.5	67
Poor	> 3.5	31

Fig. 14.24 Five-year survival rates for malignant melanomas of different Breslow thickness.

The differential diagnosis of malignant melanoma includes:
- Benign lentigine.
- Benign melanocytic naevi.
- Dermatofibroma.
- Haemangioma.
- Pigmented basal cell carcinoma.
- Seborrhoeic wart.

Management is by surgical excision (rarely plus radiotherapy) with regular follow-up to detect recurrence, which may be:
- Local—at edge of excised site.
- Lymphatic—in regional lymph nodes or in lymphatics between tumour and nodes.
- At distant sites—due to haematogenous spread.

- Repeated UV exposure—tumours are more common in light-skinned races, with increasing incidence towards the Equator.
- X-ray irradiation.
- Chronic scarring.
- Genetic predisposition.

Tumours are typically composed of basophilic cells that invade the dermis. They appear as well-defined lobules and islands of cells.

Clinical presentation—they typically occur on sun-exposed sites, commonly around the nose, inner canthus of the eyelids and the temple.

Tumours grow slowly but relentlessly and they may destroy underlying cartilage, bone and soft tissue structures.

There are three main types of basal cell carcinoma:

1. Nodular—most common form. Skin-coloured nodule, which may show numerous telangiectatic vessels and a glistening pearly edge. Often has central ulceration with an adherent crust.

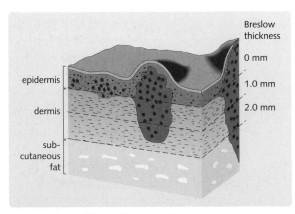

Fig. 14.23 Staging of malignant melanomas using the Breslow thickness technique.

2. Superficial (or multifocal) —flat, red plaque often with an irregular rim-like edge and light pigmentation. Often multiple and most commonly seen on the trunk.
3. Morpheic—flat, thickened, whitish-yellowish waxy plaque with indistinct edges. These may have focal areas of ulceration.

Management—complete excision is usually the best treatment but is not always possible. Radiotherapy or cryotherapy is often used for non-excisable tumours. Recurrence is about 5% at 5 years for most methods of treatment.

Squamous cell carcinoma

This malignant tumour is derived from keratinocytes of the upper layers of the epidermis. Typically seen on the face in elderly or middle-aged subjects, with a male preponderance. Tumours are locally invasive and they may also metastasise.

Its aetiology is related to:

- Chronic sunlight exposure.
- Chemical carcinogens (e.g. tar, arsenic and machine oil).
- X-ray radiation.
- Chronic ulceration and scarring.
- Smoking (lip lesions—aggressive, frequently metastasises).
- Common wart virus (HPV) in immunosuppressed individuals.
- Genetic (e.g. xeroderma pigmentosum).

Histologically, tumours consist of disorganised keratinocytes with typical malignant cytology, which destroy the dermoepidermal junction and form invading strands into the dermis. Foci of keratinisation are seen within the tumour.

The clinical presentation is:

- Dome-shaped nodules, which usually arise in sun-exposed sites such as the face, neck, forearm or hand.
- Nodules typically develop into roughened keratotic areas, ulcers or horns.
- Often difficult to distinguish from keratoacanthomas (see below).
- Less aggressive form may arise within actinic keratosis as a small papule, which progresses to ulcerate and then crust over.
- More aggressive forms may arise at the edge of chronic skin ulcers (rare).

Management—the treatment of choice is surgical excision. Radiotherapy can be used in some cases.

There are only two skin neoplasms in which metastasis is a common feature:
1. Malignant melanoma tumour of melanocytes, which metastasises early.
2. Squamous cell carcinoma tumour of upper epidermal keratinocytes, which metastasises late.

Intraepidermal carcinoma (Bowen's disease)

This carcinoma *in situ* typically occurs on the lower leg in elderly women. Its predisposition is associated with previous exposure to arsenicals. It is characterised by:

- Slowly extending, pink or lightly pigmented, scaly plaques up to several centimetres in size. Can look like psoriatic plaques.
- Full-thickness dysplasia with prominent nuclear pleomorphism and large numbers of mitoses.

Carcinomas usually remain *in situ* for many years but have the capacity to transform into squamous cell carcinomas.

Other tumours of the skin
Keratoacanthoma

This benign, self-limiting tumour typically arises on the face of elderly white males. It grows very rapidly, changing from a small, red papule to a large, domed nodule with raised edges and a central mass of keratin within a few weeks. It resembles a squamous cell carcinoma but does not invade deeply and never metastasises.

The majority spontaneously regress within a few months.

Mycosis fungoides (cutaneous T cell lymphoma)

This rare, slowly progressive (years) tumour of CD4+ (T helper) lymphocytes evolves in the skin. There are four stages:

1. Premycotic phase—erythematous eczematous lesions. May persist for 10 or more years.
2. Infiltrative phase—erythematous plaques develop, typically affecting the trunk. This stage may last for years.

3. Fungoid phase—tumour nodules or ulcers develop within the plaques suggesting systemic spread. Has a mean survival time of 2.5 years.
4. Systemic disease—involvement of lymph nodes or internal organs.

Dermatofibrosarcoma

This is a locally invasive dermal tumour of proliferating myofibroblasts with low-grade malignancy. It is similar in appearance to dermatofibromas but tends to be more invasive and is characterised by protuberant nodules on the epidermis. It does not metastasise but often recurs following excision.

Kaposi's sarcoma

This malignant disorder is characterised by bluish-brown plaques or nodules formed from a proliferation of small blood vessels and spindle cells in the dermis.

Intradermal haemorrhage with haemosiderin deposition occurs within the nodules.

It commonly occurs in association with acquired immunodeficiency syndrome (AIDS) but is also endemic with cytomegalovirus in certain African regions. The lesions may be single or multiple, often beginning on the feet and with a tendency to metastasise.

SELF-ASSESSMENT

Multiple-choice questions (MCQs)   345

Short-answer questions (SAQs)   353

Extended-matching questions (EMQs)   355

MCQ answers   359

SAQ answers   369

EMQ answers   373

Multiple-choice questions (MCQs)

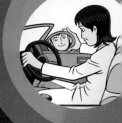

Indicate whether each answer is true or false.

Chapter 2 Inflammation, repair and cell death

1. **In acute inflammation:**
   a. The predominant cell type is the neutrophil polymorph.
   b. The inflammation is usually initiated by cell-mediated immunity.
   c. The duration may be for months.
   d. Plasma cells are frequently present.
   e. Lymphocytes are present at the start of the process.

2. **A tissue undergoing acute inflammation shows:**
   a. Vasodilatation.
   b. Decreased blood flow.
   c. Histamine release.
   d. Swelling (oedema).
   e. Nitric oxide release.

3. **Chronic inflammation:**
   a. May involve lymphocytes, plasma cells and macrophages.
   b. Is often associated with autoimmune disease.
   c. Is classically seen in hay fever.
   d. Develops rapidly.
   e. May result in the formation of granulation tissue.

4. **Wound healing:**
   a. The type of healing process depends on the extent of tissue damage.
   b. In first intention healing the margins are unapposed.
   c. In first intention healing the wound is finally covered by epidermal growth.
   d. In second intention healing the margins are apposed.
   e. Scar formation is associated with second intention healing.

5. **The systemic effects of inflammation include:**
   a. Weight loss.
   b. Leucopenia.
   c. Pyrexia.
   d. Reduced erythrocyte sedimentation rate (ESR).
   e. Enlargement of local and systemic lymph nodes.

6. **Necrosis:**
   a. Is a physiological response to injury.
   b. Maintains plasma membrane integrity.
   c. May be stimulated by oxygen free radicals.
   d. Results in an inflammatory response.
   e. Is an energy-dependent process.

7. **The following are types of necrosis:**
   a. Coagulative.
   b. Liquefactive (colliquative).
   c. Caseous.
   d. Gangrenous.
   e. Fat.

8. **Apoptosis:**
   a. Is only a pathological process.
   b. Occurs in groups of cells.
   c. Results in cell shrinkage and fragmentation.
   d. DNA is cleaved by endonucleases.
   e. Results in an inflammatory response.

Chapter 3 Cancer

9. **The following definitions are correct:**
   a. Dysplasia is a change from one type of differentiated tissue to another.
   b. Anaplasia is an almost complete lack of differentiation.
   c. Carcinoma is a malignant tumour of epithelial derivation.
   d. Metaplasia is the disordered development of cells with loss of organization.
   e. Carcinoma *in situ* is a carcinoma with stromal invasion.

10. **The following statements are correct:**
    a. Tumours arise from single cells.
    b. Lymphomas are benign lymphoid cell tumours.
    c. Cells in a tumour are always genetically identical.
    d. Transcoelomic spread occurs through the lymphatic system.
    e. Ultraviolet radiation may cause cancer.

11. **Common features of malignant tumours include:**
    a. Decreased density of nuclear chromatin.
    b. Exophytic growth.
    c. Nuclear pleomorphism.
    d. Few mitotic figures.
    e. Metastatic spread.

12. **Proto-oncogenes:**
    a. May encode proteases that are destructive to local tissue.
    b. May allow cells to grow at higher densities than normal.
    c. Cannot affect cellular orientation.
    d. Are abnormal genes not seen in normal cells.
    e. May cause cancer when hyperactive or abnormally amplified.

13. **Tumour suppressor genes:**
    a. Encode proteins that positively regulate cell growth.
    b. *p53* and *RB1* are tumour suppressor genes.
    c. Loss of function of tumour suppressor genes results in neoplastic growth.
    d. Viral proteins can deregulate tumour suppressor function.
    e. *p53* triggers apoptosis and cell cycle arrest.

14. **Angiogenesis:**
    a. Is the formation of new blood vessels.
    b. Tumours are unable to grow more than a few millimetres in diameter without angiogenesis.
    c. Is a pathological process in wound healing.
    d. VEGF is an important angiogenic factor.
    e. The angiogenic switch occurs in the vascular phase of tumour development.

Chapter 4 Infectious disease

15. **The following definitions are true:**
    a. Virulence is the degree of pathogenicity of an organism.
    b. Commensal microorganisms are those that are normally absent from the body and which cause disease.
    c. Opportunistic infections are those occurring in a fully immunocompetent host.
    d. Colonisation is the habitation of external body surfaces by harmless microorganisms.
    e. Infection is the invasion of a host by harmful microorganisms.

16. **The following are infectious organisms:**
    a. Viruses.
    b. Bacteria.
    c. Fungi.
    d. Protozoa.
    e. Prions.

17. **Viruses:**
    a. Are prokaryotes.
    b. Always possess RNA nucleic acid.
    c. If of the non-enveloped type, may release new particles by budding.
    d. Are obligate intracellular parasites.
    e. May cause cell lysis.

18. **Bacterial antibiotic resistance:**
    a. Is uncommon.
    b. Is conferred via extrachromosomal DNA.
    c. Can be directly transferred between bacteria.
    d. May occur through the alteration of the target site for an antibiotic.
    e. MRSA is virtually impossible to treat.

19. **Response to infection includes:**
    a. Suppurative polymorphonuclear inflammation.
    b. Chronic inflammation.
    c. Granulomatous mononuclear inflammation.
    d. Necrotising inflammation.
    e. Fibrinoid necrosis.

Chapter 5 Pathology of the nervous system

20. **Hydrocephalus:**
    a. Is an increase in the volume of CSF within the brain.
    b. It results in the expansion of the cerebral ventricles.
    c. Impaired absorption of CSF at the arachnoid villi is the commonest form.
    d. A ventricular shunt can be used in the management.
    e. Obstructive hydrocephalus is subdivided into non-communicating and communicating.

21. **Neural tube defects:**
    a. Spina bifida occulta is usually asymptomatic.
    b. Are the commonest congenital abnormality of the CNS.
    c. Are defined as defects of the spinal cord.
    d. Are usually associated with decreased maternal serum α-fetoprotein during pregnancy.
    e. Spina bifida cystica causes either meningomyelocele or meningocele.

22. **Extradural haemorrhage:**
    a. Occurs between the dura and outer surface of the arachnoid membrane.
    b. Is not usually associated with a skull fracture.
    c. Is due to bleeding from the cortical bridging veins.
    d. May be associated with a post-traumatic lucid period.
    e. Requires urgent surgical intervention.

23. **Creutzfeldt–Jakob disease:**
    a. Creutzfeldt–Jakob disease is a spongiform encephalitis.
    b. The disease is caused by an infectious organism called a prion.
    c. Widespread cerebral cortical atrophy is seen in affected individuals.
    d. An acute inflammatory reaction occurs.
    e. Patients present with rapidly progressive dementia.

24. **Alzheimer's disease:**
    a. Is usually familial.
    b. Is caused by senile plaques of amyloid protein.
    c. Neurofibrillary tangles occur within neurones.
    d. Affects half of all people over the age of 80 years.
    e. Is not usually associated with memory disturbance.

25. Neoplasms of the CNS:

a. Gliomas are the most common primary CNS tumour.
b. Astrocytomas rarely affect children.
c. Oligodendrogliomas are slow-growing tumours.
d. Meningiomas commonly invade deep CNS tissue.
e. Prostatic carcinoma often causes brain metastases.

Chapter 6 Pathology of the cardiovascular system

26. Ventricular septal defect:

a. Usually produces a left-to-right shunt of blood.
b. Produces respiratory depression.
c. Produces a pansystolic murmur.
d. May be of a membranous or muscular location.
e. Is the most common congenital cardiac abnormality.

27. Coarctation of the aorta:

a. Is more common in males.
b. Causes hypotension distal to the narrowing.
c. Is often associated with a bicuspid aortic valve.
d. Rarely causes serious complications.
e. Is associated with weak and delayed femoral pulsations.

28. Atherosclerosis:

a. Is characterised by the accumulation of lipid rich material in the intima of arteries.
b. Is common in the pulmonary arteries.
c. Is associated with hypercholesterolaemia and diabetes mellitus.
d. May be seen as a pathological response to endothelial injury.
e. Is characterised by neutrophil lipid uptake to form foam cells.

29. Benign hypertension is characterised by:

a. Fibrinoid necrosis of arterioles.
b. Hypertrophy of the muscular media of the arteries.
c. Fibroelastic thickening of the intima.
d. Hyaline deposition in arteriole walls.
e. Sudden and severe increase in blood pressure.

30. Myocardial infarction:

a. Results in necrosis of the myocardium following severe ischaemia.
b. Induces acute inflammatory changes.
c. The infarct tissue is replaced by new cardiac muscle.
d. Occlusion of the right coronary artery results in an inferior MI.
e. Management includes analgesics, thrombolysis and anticoagulants.

31. Mitral valve incompetence may be caused by:

a. Right ventricular dilatation.
b. Infective endocarditis.
c. Rheumatic fever.
d. Papillary muscle rupture.
e. Senile calcification.

32. Heart failure:

a. Is when the heart is unable to maintain cardiac output or can do so only by increasing filling pressure.
b. Right-sided heart failure is more common than left-sided failure.
c. Right-sided heart failure may develop as a result of left-sided failure.
d. May be a complication of myocardial infarction.
e. Is not associated with valve disease.

33. Infective endocarditis:

a. Rarely affects heart valve leaflets.
b. Rarely occurs in structurally normal valves.
c. May be caused by *Streptococcus viridens* bacteria and *Candida* species.
d. Is sometimes associated with splinter haemorrhages of the fingernails.
e. May result in multiorgan infarction.

34. The following conditions predispose to the formation of aortic aneurysms:

a. Atherosclerosis.
b. Marfan's syndrome.
c. Ehlers–Danlos syndrome.
d. Syphilis.
e. Osteopetrosis.

35. Thrombosis:

a. Thrombus is the pathological term for a clot.
b. Is predisposed by both blood stasis and turbulence.
c. Antiphospholipid antibody decreases risk of arterial and venous thrombosis.
d. The most common site of venous thrombosis is the portal vein.
e. Malignancy sometimes increases the risk of venous thrombosis.

Chapter 7 Pathology of the respiratory system

36. Carcinoma of the larynx:

a. Is usually sited in the subglottic region.
b. Has a positive association with cigarette smoking.
c. Commonly spreads by the haematogenous route.
d. Is usually of squamous cell differentiation.
e. Usually presents after the age of 40 years.

37. Chronic obstructive pulmonary disease:

a. Is characterised by chronic bronchitis, emphysema and bronchiolitis.
b. The obstructive lung disease can be completely reversed with bronchodilators.
c. Causes hypoinflated lungs.
d. Is exclusively a disease of smokers.
e. Lung fibrosis is a feature of emphysema.

38. Chronic bronchitis:

a. Defined as a productive cough on most days for three months of the year for at least two successive years.
b. Most cases are due to cigarette smoking.
c. Hypersecretion of mucus is associated with hypertrophy and hyperplasia of the bronchial mucus-secreting glands.
d. Is characterised by chronic inflammation of the bronchioles.
e. Lung function tests show a restrictive pattern.

39. Asthma:

a. Causes irreversible airway narrowing.
b. May be caused by a type I hypersensitivity reaction.
c. Bronchospasm, oedema and mucus plugging are commonly seen.
d. Is sometimes associated with α-1-antitrypsin deficiency.
e. Hypertrophy of bronchial smooth muscle may occur.

40. Cystic fibrosis:

a. Is associated with infections with *Pseudomonas*.
b. Is the most common autosomal dominant condition in Europe.
c. Is due to defective transport of chloride ions.
d. May cause malabsorption.
e. Is due to a mutation in a gene on chromosome 7.

41. Pneumonia:

a. Is most commonly viral.
b. Most cases of bacterial community-acquired pneumonia are due to Gram-negative organisms.
c. Lung fibrosis, abscess and empyema may complicate pneumonia.
d. Red hepatisation describes a pathological stage in bronchopneumonia.
e. Is more likely to occur if there is pre-existing pulmonary oedema.

42. Pulmonary tuberculosis:

a. Is most commonly due to *Mycobacterium avium intracellulare*.
b. Is caused by direct cytopathic effects of the infecting organism.
c. Has a positive association with silicosis.
d. Is a common cause of death in AIDS.
e. Is characterised histologically by granulomas.

43. Lung carcinoma:

a. Is most commonly of adenomatous differentiation.
b. Has a positive association with cigarette smoking.
c. Has a positive association with asbestos exposure.
d. Has rarely metastasised at the time of presentation.
e. Is the most common cause of death from neoplasia in the UK.

44. Idiopathic pulmonary fibrosis:

a. Is an infectious condition.
b. Causes interstitial atrophy.
c. Is a restrictive lung disease.
d. Causes peripheral lung honeycombing.
e. Causes finger clubbing.

45. Pulmonary embolism:

a. May cause pulmonary hypotension and infarction.
b. May be precipitated by mural thrombus in left ventricle.
c. Can cause pulseless electrical activity (electro-mechanical dissociation) of the heart.
d. Is always thromboembolic.
e. Is usually caused by thromboembolism from deep leg veins.

46. Malignant mesothelioma:

a. Develops rapidly after exposure to asbestos.
b. Mainly spreads via the bloodstream.
c. Is slowly progressive with a long life-expectancy.
d. Has been decreasing in incidence.
e. Is associated with recurrent pleural effusions.

Chapter 8 Pathology of the gastrointestinal tract

47. Squamous cell carcinoma of the oral cavity:

a. Occurs most commonly on the lips.
b. Is more common in women than men.
c. Has a positive association with cigarette smoking.
d. Has a positive association with moderate alcohol intake.
e. Has a 5-year survival of about 50%.

48. Oesophageal carcinoma:

a. Is most commonly adenocarcinoma.
b. May develop from Barrett's metaplasia.
c. Adenocarcinoma is the most likely pattern in heavy smokers or drinkers.
d. Has less than 10% 5-year survival.
e. Causes dysphagia.

49. Oesophageal varices:

a. Are dilated submucosal veins in the oesophagus.
b. They are commonly associated with cirrhosis of the liver.
c. Rupture causes torrential bleeding.
d. Are associated with portal vein hypotension.
e. Sclerotherapy can be used in the management.

50. Gastric ulceration:

a. Aetiology is multifactorial.
b. Gastric secretions cause damage to susceptible epithelium.
c. Patients can present with epigastric pain, nausea or heartburn.
d. There is no involvement of infectious organisms.
e. Perforation may lead to peritonitis.

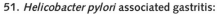

51. *Helicobacter pylori* **associated gastritis:**

a. Is an example of an acute gastritis.
b. *Helicobacter pylori* colonises the epithelium below a layer of mucus.
c. Epithelial damage is caused by the immune response against *Helicobacter pylori*.
d. Is most commonly seen at the pyloric fundus.
e. Is almost always a transient infection.

52. Gastric carcinoma:

a. Is usually of squamous cell type.
b. Is more common in females than males.
c. Occurs most commonly in the body of the stomach.
d. Is commoner in Japan than Europe.
e. Has a positive association with *Helicobacter pylori* infection.

53. Portal hypertension:

a. May be classified as prehepatic, hepatic or posthepatic.
b. Is most commonly caused by portal vein thrombosis.
c. May cause ascites and splenomegaly.
d. May cause Budd–Chiari syndrome.
e. Causes the regression of portosystemic shunts.

54. Cirrhosis:

a. A reversible condition in which the liver's normal architecture is diffusely replaced by nodules.
b. A common cause of cirrhosis is alcohol liver disease.
c. An uncommon cause of cirrhosis is autoimmune chronic hepatitis.
d. Nodules are formed from regenerated hepatocytes separated by bands of collagenous fibrosis.
e. Prothrombin time is reduced.

55. Ascites:

a. Is the accumulation of free fluid in the peritoneal cavity.
b. Cirrhosis is associated with exudative ascites.
c. Signifies liver disease.
d. The clinical sign of shifting dullness to percussion may be elicited.
e. Sodium-containing drugs are useful in the management of ascites.

56. Wilson's disease:

a. Is an autosomal dominant condition.
b. It results from a mutation in a gene for a calcium transporter protein.
c. Free copper overspills into the blood and deposits in the cornea and the brain.
d. Psychiatric disorders occur.
e. The liver is not affected.

57. Hepatitis B:

a. Is a RNA virus.
b. May be transmitted by drinking infected water.
c. Initial infection is transient and subclinical in the majority of cases.

d. Vaccination utilises the hepatitis B surface antigen (HbsAg).
e. Cirrhosis and hepatocellular carcinoma are potential complications of chronic infection.

58. Hepatocellular carcinoma (HCC):

a. Is the most common malignant tumour of the liver.
b. Has a positive association with hepatitis A.
c. Is more common in males than females.
d. Has a median survival of 3 years following diagnosis.
e. Arises from bile duct epithelium.

59. Primary biliary cirrhosis:

a. Is more common in males.
b. Is associated with autoimmune diseases.
c. Is relatively easy to treat.
d. Is strongly associated with ulcerative colitis.
e. Causes scar formation by bridging fibrosis.

60. Carcinoma of the pancreas:

a. Has a positive association with excess alcohol ingestion.
b. Is more common in women than men.
c. Is usually surgically resectable.
d. Is an adenocarcinoma.
e. Usually occurs in subjects older than 60 years of age.

61. Crohn's disease:

a. Has a positive association with erythema nodosum.
b. Has a negative association with cigarette smoking.
c. May occur anywhere from the mouth to anus.
d. Is characterised histologically by non-caseating granulomas.
e. Has a positive association with uveitis.

62. Ulcerative colitis:

a. Is characterised by transmural inflammation.
b. Has a positive association with cigarette smoking.
c. Is characterised by granulomatous inflammation.
d. Is commonly complicated by fistulae.
e. Is characterised by continuous disease distribution in the colon.

63. Coeliac disease:

a. Is caused by an abnormal immune response to gluten.
b. Is associated with intestinal villous atrophy.
c. Most commonly affects the large intestine.
d. Anti-endomyseal antibodies are a useful blood test to aid diagnosis.
e. A gluten-free diet improves symptoms but the intestinal changes are irreversible.

64. Colorectal carcinoma:

a. Is often a progression from adenoma.
b. Familial adenomatous polyposis patients almost always develop colorectal cancer if untreated.

c. Is staged by the Breslow system.
d. Usually presents earlier if affecting the left (descending) colon.
e. Most commonly develops in the caecum.

Chapter 9 Pathology of the kidney and urinary tract

65. Adult polycystic kidney disease:

a. Only one kidney is affected.
b. It is an inherited autosomal dominant disease.
c. Associations are with berry aneurysms.
d. Enlarging cysts replace and compress functioning renal parenchyma.
e. Hypertension is important for the management.

66. In glomerular disease:

a. Nephrotic syndrome in an adult is strongly suggestive of membranous nephropathy.
b. Most cases of membranous nephropathy have an identifiable cause.
c. Minimal change disease rapidly progresses to renal failure in children.
d. A focal proliferative glomerulonephritis with autoantibodies against type IV collagen is indicative of Goodpasture's syndrome.
e. Streptococcal sore throat may be a cause of proliferative glomerulonephritis.

67. Renal cell carcinoma:

a. Is more common in males.
b. Usually develops at the lower pole of the kidney.
c. Proteinuria is a common presenting feature.
d. Cigarette smoking is protective.
e. All cases are sporadic as no genetic association has been identified.

68. Bladder cancer:

a. Is largely a disease of women.
b. Is usually a squamous cell carcinoma.
c. May cause urinary obstruction.
d. Most commonly arises at the base of trigone and around the ureteric orifaces.
e. Is linked to exposure to environmental carcinogens.

Chapter 10 Pathology of the endocrine system

69. The anterior pituitary secretes:

a. Adrenocorticotrophic hormone (ACTH).
b. Antidiuretic hormone (ADH).
c. Oxytocin.
d. Thyroid-stimulating hormone (TSH).
e. Follicle-stimulating hormone (FSH).

70. Graves' disease:

a. Is equally common in males and females.
b. A minority of individuals are positive for thyroid-stimulating hormone (TSH)-receptor antibodies in their serum.
c. Causes diffuse change in the thyroid gland.
d. Only a minority of individuals show signs of exophthalmos.
e. Causes the same change in thyroid hormone levels as Hashimoto's thyroiditis.

71. Malignant thyroid tumours:

a. Include toxic adenomas.
b. May be caused by childhood radiation exposure.
c. Papillary adenocarcinomas tend to be found in elderly patients.
d. Medullary carcinoma is derived from thyroxine-secreting cells.
e. Anaplastic carcinoma is often associated with a history of multinodular goitre.

72. The following are causes of Cushing's syndrome:

a. Addison's disease.
b. Adrenocorticotrophic hormone (ACTH) administration.
c. Prednisolone administration.
d. Phaeochromocytomas.
e. Adrenal cortical adenomas.

73. Addison's disease:

a. Is characterised by a lack of glucocorticoids and mineralocorticoids.
b. Is most commonly an autoimmune phenomenon.
c. Is associated with an increased serum cortisol and decreased adrenocorticotrophic hormone (ACTH).
d. Is managed by glucocorticoid and mineralocorticoid replacement therapy.
e. May lead to an Addisonian crisis at times of sudden stress.

74. Type I diabetes mellitus:

a. Is an autoimmune-induced disorder.
b. Has a genetic predisposition.
c. Is a disease of middle-aged/elderly onset.
d. Shows destruction of insulin secreting cells of the islets of Langerhans.
e. Shows plasma insulin levels that are raised or normal.

75. Type II diabetes mellitus:

a. Is a disease most commonly of children.
b. Is thought to develop from tissue insulin resistance.
c. Is commonly treated with insulin in the first instance.
d. May be complicated by diabetic ketoacidosis.
e. Is associated with both macrovascular and microvascular complications.

Chapter 11 Pathology of the reproductive system

76. Carcinoma of the uterine cervix:

a. Is usually of adenomatous differentiation.
b. Is often preceded by cervical intraepithelial neoplasia (CIN).
c. Has a positive association with some serotypes of human papilloma virus (HPV).
d. Has a positive association with cigarette smoking.
e. Has a positive association with HIV infection.

77. Endometriosis:

a. Is defined as endometrial glands or stroma occurring outside of the uterus.
b. Commonly affects the ovaries.
c. May be caused by retrograde menstruation.
d. Worsens after the menopause.
e. Invariably causes infertility.

78. Pelvic inflammatory disease:

a. Is a combined inflammatory disorder of the fallopian tubes, ovaries and peritoneum.
b. Predisposing factors include intrauterine contraceptive devices.
c. *Neisseria gonorrhoeae* is a common aetiological agent.
d. Is characterised by chronic inflammation.
e. Pelvic inflammatory disease is an autoimmune disorder.

79. Ectopic pregnancy:

a. A fertilised ovum implants outside the uterine cavity.
b. The most common site is the fallopian tube.
c. Aetiology may be due to previous episodes of salpingitis.
d. Proliferation of the trophoblast causes erosion of the submucosa and bleeding.
e. The embryo typically survives to term.

80. Pre-eclampsia:

a. Is defined as high blood pressure during pregnancy where it was previously normal.
b. Is more common in a first pregnancy or with multiple pregnancies.
c. Is thought to be the result of placental hyperperfusion.
d. The main risks are to the mother rather than the fetus.
e. May persist for several months after delivery.

81. Breast carcinoma:

a. Most common cause of death in women aged 35–55 years of age.
b. Predisposing factors include mutation of *BRCA1* and *BRCA2* genes.
c. Screening is not carried out in the UK.

d. Tamoxifen can be used if oestrogen-receptor positive.
e. Ductal carcinoma is the most common type.

82. Prostate carcinoma:

a. Is a squamous cell carcinoma.
b. Affects the central zone of prostate.
c. Is more likely to cause urinary symptoms than benign prostatic hyperplasia.
d. Rarely extends outside of the prostatic capsule.
e. The majority have a well differentiated glandular pattern.

Chapter 12 Pathology of the musculoskeletal system

83. Osteoporosis:

a. Is an uncommon bone disorder.
b. Is a cause of pathological fractures.
c. Microscopically, bone trabeculae are thickened.
d. Diagnosis is by X-ray of the affected bones.
e. Bones appear less dense on X-ray and lumbar vertebral bodies often appear more biconcave than normal.

84. Bone fractures:

a. A fracture is a break in the continuity of the bone.
b. A simple fracture occurs without contact with the external environment.
c. A compound fracture occurs with direct contact with the external environment.
d. A pathological fracture occurs in abnormal bone.
e. Healing involves the formation of a haematoma.

85. Rheumatoid arthritis:

a. Affects 1% of the population.
b. The likelihood of onset increases with age, therefore peaking in the elderly.
c. Many, but not all, patients have circulating rheumatoid factor.
d. Causes the development of a pannus and inflammatory joint destruction.
e. Occurs with widespread extra-articular features.

Chapter 13 Pathology of the blood and immune systems

86. Systemic lupus erythematosus:

a. Is associated with autoantibodies to DNA and other nuclear components.
b. Affects females more than males.
c. Causes fibrinoid necrosis of blood vessels.
d. Malar and discoid skin rashes may be seen.
e. It is dangerous to use corticosteroids in acute SLE.

87. The human immunodeficiency virus (HIV)-1.

a. Is a DNA virus.
b. Requires reverse transcriptase from the host cell to replicate.
c. Binds to CD4 lymphocytes.
d. Is associated with *Pneumocytis carinii* infection.
e. Is associated with *Mycobacterium avium intracellulare* infection.

88. The following are primary immunodeficiencies:

a. AIDS.
b. X-linked agammaglobulinaemia of Bruton.
c. IgA deficiency.
d. Severe combined immunodeficiency.
e. Transient physiological agammaglobulinaemia.

89. Amyloidosis:

a. Amyloid is a well characterised polypeptide.
b. Amyloid takes up Congo red stain.
c. Appears to be the result of abnormal macrophage control mechanisms.
d. The most common amyloid in reactive systemic amyloidosis is the AL type.
e. May follow long-term haemodialysis.

90. Leucopenia and leucocytosis:

a. Agranulocytosis is used to describe severe neutropenia.
b. Neutropenia forms part of Kostmann's syndrome.
c. Leucocytosis is most commonly caused by an increase in lymphocytes.
d. Leucocytosis always indicates infection.
e. Basophilia is commonly seen in allergic reactions.

91. Hodgkin's disease:

a. Is characterised histologically by Reed–Sternberg cells.
b. Is more common in females than males.
c. Is staged using the Rye classification.
d. Has a better prognosis if B symptoms are present.
e. Of the mixed cellularity type has the most favourable prognosis.

92. Non-Hodgkin's lymphoma:

a. Has been linked to immunosuppression.
b. Gastric lymphoma has been linked to *Escherichia coli* gastroenteritis.
c. The majority of cases are derived from B cells.
d. Point mutations of susceptibility genes are commonly associated.
e. Extranodal presentation is more common than in Hodgkin's disease.

93. Chronic lymphocytic leukaemia:

a. Is characterised cytogenetically by the Philadelphia chromosome.
b. Is the most common leukaemia in adults.
c. Has a median survival of 9 months.
d. Is more common in males than females.
e. May affect lymph nodes.

94. Sickle-cell disease:

a. Is caused by a point mutation in the DNA coding for the α-globin chain.
b. Is more common in Europe than Africa.
c. Is associated with gallstones.
d. Is associated with hypersplenism.
e. May confer some resistance to malarial infection.

95. Haemolytic anaemia:

a. Is most commonly isoimmune.
b. May cause brain damage in neonates.
c. When autoimmune, 'warm' type results in microspherocytosis.
d. When autoimmune, 'cold' type results in red cell agglutination.
e. May be associated with lymphoma.

Chapter 14 Pathology of the skin

96. The following definitions are correct:

a. Nodule is a raised lesion less than 5 mm across.
b. Vesicle is a blister less than 5 mm across.
c. Macular describes a raised lesion of altered skin colour.
d. Pustule is a blister containing clear fluid.
e. Spongiosis means epidermal oedema.

97. Psoriasis:

a. Is an infective condition.
b. Is characterised by a reduced turnover of epithelial cells.
c. May be precipitated by lithium administration.
d. Commonly affects skin over the elbows.
e. Is associated with pitting of the nails.

98. Atopic eczema:

a. Is decreasing in incidence.
b. Is more common where there is a strong family history.
c. Is a type II hypersensitivity reaction.
d. Decreases in incidence with increasing age through childhood.
e. Increases the likelihood of skin infection.

99. Blistering disorders:

a. Pemphigoid describes subcorneal separation of skin tissue.
b. Pemphigus is associated with erosions.
c. Pemphigoid has a higher untreated mortality than pemphigus.
d. Pemphigus is associated with coeliac disease.
e. Dermatitis herpetiformis involves granular IgA deposition at the dermal papillae of normal looking skin.

100. Malignant melanoma:

a. Arises from epidermal keratinocytes.
b. Is associated with intermittent intense UV light exposure.
c. Has an increased incidence in familial dysplastic naevus syndrome.
d. With a depth of invasion of 3.5 mm has a good prognosis.
e. May arise within lentigo maligna.

Short-answer questions (SAQs)

1. What is inflammation? Compare the basic characteristics of acute and chronic inflammation.

2. List the features of apoptosis and necrosis.

3. Describe with examples the roles of proto-oncogenes and tumour suppressor genes in the aetiology of cancer.

4. Describe the characteristics of viruses and how they are classified, using common examples.

5. Describe the aetiology and pathogenesis of coeliac disease.

6. Write short notes on lung cancer.

7. Describe nephrotic syndrome and nephritic syndrome, using examples of diseases that cause them.

8. Briefly discuss the molecular and pathological features of colourectal cancer.

9. What are the differences between Hodgkin's disease and non-Hodgkin's lymphoma?

10. What is Graves' disease? Describe the aetiology and clinical features.

11. A 62-year-old woman develops a tender and swollen right calf 8 days after undergoing a lengthy surgical procedure. She suddenly presents with shortness of breath. A chest X-ray appears normal. What pathological process has occurred and why?

12. A 43-year-old woman goes to her GP complaining of painful swelling of the knuckle joints in both of her hands. On examination, the metacarpophalangeal joints are indeed swollen and warm, with erythema of the overlying skin. The lady notes that her older sister had similar problems, and that these spread to deform multiple joints. What is the most likely diagnosis in this patient, and what are the systemic consequences of this disease?

13. A 35-year-old woman presents to her GP with a lump in her breast. Examination of her left breast reveals a firm irregular mass with dimpling of the overlying skin. A lump is also palpated in the left axilla. What might the GP suspect? What are the main features of this disease and is family history important?

14. A 33-year-old woman who is pregnant complains of being woken up at night with pins-and-needles in her hands. This has gradually progressed from mild tingling sensations a few weeks earlier. What is the most likely cause of these symptoms, and where else in the body can they occur?

15. A 67-year-old retired gardener is seen in the dermatology clinic with a pigmented lesion on his back. Examination reveals a 15 mm nodule with an irregular border, crusting and surrounding erythema. The patient complains that the lesion is itchy. What is the likely cause of the lesion and how can the prognosis be determined?

16. A 42-year-old woman is referred to a gynaecologist after experiencing intermenstrual bleeding. She has a hysteroscopy at which time an endometrial biopsy is taken. The pathology report describes 'severe endometrial hyperplasia.' What does this result mean, and what is the significance for this patient?

17. A 49-year-old alcoholic presents to his GP complaining of breathlessness and tiredness over the last 6 months. The GP performs a full blood count and finds that the patient's haemoglobin is 108 g/L (normal range 130–180 g/L) and that the mean (red) cell volume is 115 fl (normal range 78–98 fl). What condition does this patient have? Assuming the history of alcoholism is responsible, what is the mechanism for the red blood cell changes?

18. A 55-year-old lorry driver experiences increasing difficulty with the physical aspects of his job. He has retrosternal chest pain when he exerts himself. This pain resolves on rest. What pathological process causes this chest pain? Comment on the risk factors.

19. A 61-year-old man with liver cirrhosis presents to the emergency department with a swollen abdomen. The doctor who examines him manages to elicit shifting dullness across the abdomen and suggests he has developed ascites. What exactly is ascites and what is the underlying mechanism by which it is likely to have developed in this patient? What are the other potential causes of ascites?

20. A 62-year-old woman with chronic obstructive pulmonary disease presents to the emergency department with increasing shortness of breath that she cannot control with her usual inhalers. She has been coughing up rusty-coloured sputum. What is likely to have happened and what are the principles of managing this patient?

Extended-matching questions (EMQs)

In each of the following questions, select the condition listed that is most likely to fit the given description.

1. Nervous system

A. Acute bacterial meningitis.
B. Viral meningitis.
C. Multiple sclerosis.
D. Subarachnoid haemorrhage.
E. Meningioma.
F. Extradural haemorrhage.
G. Guillain–Barré syndrome.
H. Alzheimer's disease.
I. Hydrocephalus.
J. HSV encephalitis.

1. The diagnosis in a patient with diffuse ventricular dilatation on CT scanning of the brain, who has had ventriculopertioneal shunt surgery.
2. A possible diagnosis in a 70-year-old woman whose husband complains that she has been getting increasingly forgetful over a period of months.
3. The diagnosis in a 23-year-old man presenting with rapidly developing focal neurological signs several hours after he sustained a head injury in a motorbike accident.
4. A condition that causes episodes of acute CNS demyelination separated in time and space.
5. The diagnosis in a patient with an infection of the leptomeninges that has caused brain abscess. Lumbar puncture revealed a cloudy CSF with increased protein and decreased glucose.

2. Cardiovascular system

A. Ventricular septal defect.
B. Angina pectoris.
C. Infective endocarditis.
D. Polyarteritis nodosa.
E. Coarctation of the aorta.
F. Myocardial infarction.
G. Dissecting aortic aneurysm.
H. Tetralogy of Fallot.
I. Giant cell arteritis.
J. Aortic stenosis.

1. A condition that causes headache, dizziness, intercostal bruits and radiofemoral pulse delay.
2. The diagnosis in a patient with sudden onset chest pain, radiating to between the scapulae, who develops asymmetry of pulses in his arms and legs. Chest X-ray reveals mediastinal widening.
3. The diagnosis in an elderly patient who has an ejection systolic murmur and a propensity for syncope. A narrow pulse pressure and slow-rising carotid pulse are also detected.

4. A condition that has the potential to cause scalp tenderness, headache and blindness. Erythrocyte sedimentation rate is significantly raised.
5. A condition that causes a left-to-right shunt with pansystolic murmur.

3. Respiratory system

A. Squamous cell carcinoma of the lung.
B. Small cell lung cancer.
C. Extrinsic (atopic) asthma.
D. Chronic obstructive pulmonary disease.
E. Pulmonary tuberculosis.
F. Cystic fibrosis.
G. Malignant mesothelioma.
H. Intrinsic (non-atopic) asthma.
I. Adenocarcinoma of lung.
J. Sarcoidosis.

1. A response to noxious agents causing reduced FEV_1, reduced FEV_1/FVC ratio and characterised by a CD8+ T-cell infiltration.
2. The likely diagnosis in a 45-year-old non-smoker, with no past history of respiratory illness, who presents with shortness of breath and wheezing. Salbutamol inhaler completely resolves the breathing difficulties.
3. The cause of abnormally thickened mucus affecting both the lung and pancreas.
4. A lung condition that may cause cough, haemoptysis, shortness of breath and chest pain, and which is exquisitely sensitive to chemotherapy and radiotherapy in its early stages.
5. The likely diagnosis in a patient with a granulomatous condition affecting the lung and other organs. Blood tests reveal hypercalcaemia and a raised serum angiotensin converting enzyme.

4. Gastrointestinal system

A. Barrett's oesophagus.
B. Wilson's disease.
C. Colourectal carcinoma.
D. Crohn's disease.
E. Coeliac disease.
F. Haemochromatosis.
G. Whipple's disease.
H. Oesophageal varices.
I. Hepatocellular carcinoma.
J. Gallstones.

1. The most likely diagnosis in a 25-year-old woman complaining of a 3-month history of diarrhoea, who has recently developed a blistering rash on her elbows.
2. The diagnosis in a 27-year-old female who presents with intermittent diarrhoea and weight loss. Endoscopy reveals multiple small bowel strictures occurring between areas of normal looking bowel.
3. A condition of metaplastic change.
4. A complication of portal hypertension.
5. The diagnosis in a 50-year-old male with leaden grey pigmentation of his groins and axillae. A liver biopsy shows increased iron deposition and some hepatic fibrosis.

5. **Renal and urinary systems**

   A. Membranous nephropathy.
   B. Alport's disease.
   C. Benign nephrosclerosis.
   D. Minimal change disease.
   E. Goodpasture's syndrome.
   F. Focal segmental glomerulosclerosis.
   G. Acute tubular necrosis.
   H. Amyloidosis.
   I. Hydronephrosis.
   J. Medullary sponge kidney.

   1. The likely diagnosis in a 5-year-old boy who develops facial swelling. Urinalysis reveals heavy proteinuria, but no blood. A kidney biopsy shows no abnormality on light microscopy.
   2. The likely diagnosis in a 25-year-old man who is being investigated for renal failure. He is complaining that he is having to change the prescription for his glasses every few weeks to see clearly and that he is struggling to hear some sounds.
   3. Describes a form of acute renal failure that is normally reversible and may be caused by an ischaemic or toxic insult.
   4. Describes a complication of urinary tract obstruction.
   5. The diagnosis in a 55-year-old man presenting with haemoptysis and haematuria. A renal biopsy shows crescentic change and IgG deposits in the basement membrane.

6. **Endocrine system**

   A. Type I diabetes mellitus.
   B. Hypoparathyroidism.
   C. Cushing's syndrome.
   D. Hypothyroidism.
   E. Addison's disease.
   F. Cranial diabetes insipidus.
   G. Hyperthyroidism.
   H. Type II diabetes mellitus.
   I. Hyperparathyroidism.
   J. Adrenal crisis.

1. The most likely diagnosis in a patient who presents with diarrhoea, vomiting, abdominal pain and profound hypotension. She has been on regular prednisolone to treat her temporal arteritis for over a year, but recently suddenly stopped taking it because she was worried about the side effects.
2. Is primarily a disorder of insulin production.
3. Is the most likely diagnosis in a patient who has recently had mumps infection, with persisting fatigue in recovery. She has now developed a painful lump in her neck, and has noticed that she has cold hands and is 'really suffering the cold weather'.
4. Is characterised by central obesity, moon face, hypertension, osteoporosis, menstrual irregularity and hirsutism.
5. Is a disorder of polyuria and polydipsia that is caused by a failure of hormone production from the posterior pituitary.

7. **Reproductive system**

   A. Pre-eclampsia.
   B. Cervical cancer.
   C. Fibroids.
   D. Choriocarcinoma.
   E. Ectopic pregnancy.
   F. Adenomyosis.
   G. Breast cancer.
   H. Benign ovarian cyst.
   I. Endometriosis.
   J. Endometrial cancer.

   1. Is a potential cause of abnormal ovarian tissue that undergoes cyclical bleeding, and commonly predisposes to infertility.
   2. Is subject to 'triple assessment' in suspicious lesions.
   3. A condition that has risk factors for development including HPV infection, combined oral contraceptive use, multiple sexual partners and smoking.
   4. Is a tumour of trophoblastic tissue.
   5. Is the most likely diagnosis in a 24-year-old female complaining of severe lower abdominal pain that came on very suddenly, and who has signs of cardiovascular collapse and shock.

8. **Musculoskeletal system**

   A. Osteogenesis imperfecta.
   B. Osteoid osteoma.
   C. Paget's disease.
   D. Dermatomyositis.
   E. Osteoarthritis.
   F. Osteoporosis.
   G. Osteosarcoma.
   H. Metastatic disease.
   I. Osteopetrosis.
   J. Duchenne muscular dystrophy.

1. The most common tumour found in bones.
2. Is the likely diagnosis in a 60-year-old man presenting with bone pain of the femur. On X-ray of the affected bone, alternating areas of increased and decreased bone density are seen. Blood tests are normal with the exception of a highly elevated alkaline phosphatase.
3. Is a degenerative disease of articular cartilage.
4. Is the term given for a group of hereditary disorders that result in abnormal type I collagen formation.
5. An X-linked inherited condition that results in failure to produce dystrophin protein.

9. **Haematological and immunological systems**

   A. Chronic lymphocytic leukaemia.
   B. Hodgkin's disease.
   C. Vitiligo.
   D. Non-Hodgkin's lymphoma.
   E. Chronic myeloid leukaemia.
   F. Myeloma.
   G. Myasthenia gravis.
   H. Thalassaemia.
   I. Acute myeloid leukaemia.
   J. Megaloblastic anaemia.

   1. Is a disorder in which the Philadelphia chromosome abnormality is detected within affected cells.
   2. Is a disease characterised by the development of Reed–Sternberg cells.
   3. Is the likely diagnosis in a 50-year-old male who presents with worsening back pain and persistent tiredness. Bone imaging show lytic bone lesions and serum electrophoresis reveals an intense gamma-globulin band.
   4. Is an autoimmune disease characterised by a raised serum titre of antiacetylcholine receptor antibodies.
   5. Is an example of a haemoglobinopathy.

10. **Dermatological system**

    A. Acantholysis.
    B. Dermatitis.
    C. Plaque.
    D. Parakeratosis.
    E. Acne vulgaris.
    F. Ulceration.
    G. Macule.
    H. Bullous pemphigoid.
    I. Blister.
    J. Pemphigus vulgaris.

    1. A localised, flat area of altered skin colour that may be hyperpigmented, hypopigmented or erythematous.
    2. A disorder that causes increased sebum excretion and blockage of pilosebaceous ducts.
    3. A disorder characterised by the development of intraepidermal bullae.
    4. Is a microscopic appearance in psoriasis.
    5. The loss of cellular cohesion and separation of epidermal keratinocytes due to the rupture of intercellular bridges.

MCQ answers

1. a. True   The neutrophil polymorph is the predominant cell type in acute inflammation.
    b. False   Acute inflammation is mediated by chemical factors.
    c. False   The duration of acute inflammation is a few hours to a few weeks.
    d. False   Plasma cells are not present. They are involved in humoral antibody-mediated immunity.
    e. False   Lymphocytes are involved in chronic inflammation.

2. a. True   Vasodilatation is a feature of acute inflammation.
    b. False   Increased blood flow (hyperaemia) is seen.
    c. True   Histamine is one of the chemical inflammatory mediators.
    d. True   Oedema occurs due to increased hydrostatic and decreased oncotic pressures.
    e. True   Nitric oxide is another inflammatory mediator that increases vascular permeability.

3. a. True   Lymphocytes, plasma cells and macrophages are chronic inflammatory cells.
    b. True   Autoimmune diseases are linked, e.g. rheumatoid arthritis.
    c. False   Hay fever classically shows acute inflammation (rhinitis).
    d. False   Chronic inflammation usually develops slowly.
    e. True   Chronic inflammation results in the formation of granulation tissue.

4. a. True   Type of healing process depends on the extent of tissue damage.
    b. False   In first intention healing the margins are closely apposed.
    c. True   In first intention the wound is finally covered by epidermal growth.
    d. False   In second intention healing the margins are unapposed due to extensive tissue damage.
    e. True   Scar formation is associated with second intention healing.

5. a. True   In severe chronic inflammation, weight loss occurs, e.g. tuberculosis.
    b. False   Inflammation is usually associated with leucocytosis.
    c. True   Pyrexia occurs and is defined as a core temperature above 38°C.
    d. False   ESR is raised by inflammatory processes.
    e. True   Lymph node involvement is a systemic sign of inflammation.

6. a. False   Necrosis is a pathological response to injury.
    b. False   Necrosis does not maintain plasma membrane integrity.
    c. True   Oxygen free radicals may stimulate necrosis.
    d. True   Necrosis is associated with a local inflammatory response.
    e. False   Necrosis is an energy-independent process.

7. a. True   Coagulative necrosis is the most common form of necrosis.
    b. True   Liquefactive (colliquative) necrosis characteristically occurs in the brain.
    c. True   Caseous necrosis is commonly seen in TB infection.
    d. True   Gangrenous necrosis occurs following invasion of putrefactive organisms.
    e. True   Fat necrosis can occur following direct trauma or enzymatic lipolysis.

8. a. False   Apoptosis can be either a pathological or physiological process.
    b. False   Single cells are usually involved.
    c. True   Cells appear fragmented and shrunk (apoptotic bodies).
    d. True   DNA fragmentation occurs in an energy-dependent process.
    e. False   There is no inflammatory response.

9. a. False   Dysplasia is the disordered development of cells resulting in an alteration in their size, shape and organization.
    b. True   Anaplasia is the almost complete lack of differentiation.
    c. True   Carcinomas are derived from epithelial cells.
    d. False   Metaplasia is an adaptive response resulting in the replacement of one differentiated cell type with another.
    e. False   Carcinoma *in situ* is an epithelial tumour with features of malignancy but it has not invaded through the basement membrane.

10. a. True   Tumours originally arise from single cells that proliferate to form a clone of cells.
    b. False   Lymphoma is a malignant lymphoreticular tumour.
    c. False   Tumours pick up additional mutations as they develop (tumour heterogeneity).
    d. False   Transcoelomic spread occurs via the pleural, pericardial and peritoneal cavities.
    e. True   Ultraviolet radiation is an important cause of many skin cancers.

11.
a. False — Malignant tumour cells show increased chromatin density.
b. False — Malignant tumours tend to show endophytic growth.
c. True — Variation in nuclear size and shape (pleomorphism) is characteristic of malignant tumours.
d. False — Malignant tumours tend to have lots of mitotic figures.
e. True — The ability of malignant tumours to invade tissue allows metastatic spread.

12.
a. True — Oncoproteins (encoded by proto-oncogenes) include proteases that help tissue invasion.
b. True — Oncoproteins may allow cells to grow at higher densities than normal.
c. False — Oncoproteins may affect the orientation of a cell.
d. False — Proto-oncogenes are expressed in normal cells.
e. True — Hyperactivity or amplification of oncoproteins contribute to cancer formation.

13.
a. False — Tumour suppressor genes encode proteins that negatively regulate cell growth.
b. True — P53 and RB1 are tumour suppressor genes located on chromosomes 17 and 13, respectively.
c. True — Loss of the protective functional role of tumour suppressor genes results in neoplastic growth.
d. True — Viral proteins such as HPV E6 can deregulate tumour suppressor function.
e. True — The so-called guardian of the genome triggers apoptosis and cell cycle arrest.

14.
a. True — Angiogenesis results in the formation of new blood vessels through budding of existing vessels.
b. True — Solid tumourigenesis requires the provision of a new blood supply.
c. False — Angiogenesis is an important physiological process in wound healing.
d. True — Vascular endothelial growth factor is an important angiogenic factor.
e. True — The angiogenic switch occurs in the transition from a prevascular to vascular phase tumour.

15.
a. True — Virulence is the degree of pathogenicity of an organism.
b. False — Commensal organisms constitute the normal flora of the healthy body.
c. False — Opportunistic infections occur in immunocompromised hosts.
d. True — Colonisation is the habitation of the body surfaces by harmless microorganisms.
e. True — Infection is the detrimental invasion of a host by harmful microorganisms.

16.
a. True — Viruses are obligate intracellular parasites, e.g. *Varicella-zoster virus* in chickenpox.
b. True — Bacteria are divided into two broad groups: Gram-negative and Gram-positive.
c. True — Fungi are eukaryotic organisms causing superficial or systemic infection.
d. True — Protozoa are unicellular eukaryotes, e.g. *Plasmodium* in malaria.
e. False — Prions are not microorganisms but infectious proteins.

17.
a. False — Viruses are neither prokaryotes nor eukaryotes.
b. False — Both RNA and DNA viruses exist.
c. False — Budding occurs in enveloped viruses, e.g. HIV.
d. True — Viruses are obligate intracellular parasites.
e. True — Host cell lysis is a method of release of new viral particles.

18.
a. False — Bacterial antibiotic resistance is very common.
b. True — Resistance is conferred through extrachromosomal DNA called plamids.
c. True — Resistance can be transferred by bacterial conjugation, transduction or transformation.
d. True — Altering the antibiotic target site is one mechanism for antibiotic resistance.
e. False — Although resistant to many common antibiotics, MRSA is still treatable (e.g. vancomycin).

19.
a. True — Suppurative polymorphonuclear inflammation is associated with pyogenic bacteria.
b. True — Chronic inflammation is associated with organisms resistant to phagocytosis or intracellular killing.
c. True — Granulomatous mononuclear inflammation occurs in response to an organism resistant to intracellular killing.
d. True — Necrotising inflammation is associated with putrefactive organisms.
e. False — Fibrinoid necrosis occurs in the arterial wall of patients with malignant hypertension.

20.
a. True — Hydrocephalus is an increase in the volume of CSF.
b. True — Cerebral ventricles become expanded and dilated.
c. False — Obstruction to the flow of CSF is the commonest form of hydrocephalus.
d. True — A ventricular shunt with one-way valve can be used in the management.
e. True — Non-communicating obstructive (within the ventricular system) and communicating (extraventricular obstruction).

21. a. True Spina bifida occulta is usually asymptomatic.

    b. True Neural tube defects are the most common congenital abnormality of the CNS.

    c. False Neural tube defects include, e.g. anencephaly, which affects the cranial hemispheres and vault.

    d. False Neural tube defects usually cause an increase in serum alpha-fetoprotein on antenatal screening.

    e. True 90% of cases of spina bifida cystica are associated with meningomyelocele, and 10% with meningocele.

22. a. False Extradural haemorrhage occurs between the skull and the dura.

    b. False Extradural haemorrhage is nearly always associated with a linear skull fracture, usually of the temporal bone.

    c. False The artery usually involved is the middle meningeal artery.

    d. True It is associated with a post-traumatic lucid interval that can last for several hours.

    e. True Prompt neurosurgery results in a good outlook.

23. a. True Creutzfeldt–Jakob disease is a spongiform encephalitis.

    b. False The disease is caused by an infectious protein called a prion (proteinaceous infectious agent).

    c. True Widespread cerebral cortical atrophy is seen in affected individuals.

    d. False No inflammatory reaction occurs.

    e. True Patients present with rapidly progressive dementia.

24. a. False Only 5% of Alzheimer's disease is familial, 95% is sporadic.

    b. True Senile plaques of amyloid protein are seen in Alzheimer's disease.

    c. True Neurofibrillary tangles occur within neurons of patients with Alzheimer's disease.

    d. False Alzheimer's disease affects 15% of those aged above 80 years old.

    e. False Memory disturbance is a common early presentation in Alzheimer's disease.

25. a. True Gliomas are the most common primary CNS tumour, accounting for 50% of cases.

    b. False Astrocytomas are more common in children than adults.

    c. True Oligodendrocytomas are slow-growing tumours.

    d. False Meningiomas commonly compress rather than invade deeper CNS tissue.

    e. False Prostatic carcinoma metastases to the brain are extremely rare.

26. a. True Ventricular septal defects cause a left to right shunt because of the higher pressure of the left side.

    b. False Ventricular septal defects cause tachypnoea.

    c. True The pansystolic murmur is caused by high pressure blood on the left side flowing to the right side.

    d. True Small defects often involve membranous areas, larger defects also involve the muscular wall.

    e. True Ventricular septal defects are the most common of all congenital heart disease (25–30%).

27. a. True Coarctation of the aorta is more common in males by 2 : 1.

    b. False Coarctation of the aorta causes hypertension distal to the stenosis.

    c. True It is associated with a bicuspid aortic valve in 50% of cases.

    d. False Serious complications in severe cases include heart failure and aortic dissection.

    e. True Coarctation of aorta causes weak femoral pulses with radiofemoral delay.

28. a. True Atherosclerosis is the accumulation of lipid rich material in the intima of arteries.

    b. False It is rare in pulmonary arteries, being seen more commonly in, for example, the aorta.

    c. True Atherosclerosis is associated with both hypercholesterolaemia and diabetes mellitus.

    d. True It may be seen as a pathological response to endothelial injury.

    e. False Macrophages take up lipid within a plaque to produce foam cells.

29. a. False Fibrinoid deposition occurs in malignant hypertension.

    b. True In benign hypertension thickening and hypertrophy of the muscular media are seen histologically.

    c. True Thickening of the elastic intima is seen histologically.

    d. True Hyaline is deposited in the arterial walls resulting in hyaline arteriosclerosis.

    e. False Benign hypertension is characterised by stable elevation of blood pressure over many years.

30. a. True Myocardial infarction results in necrosis of the myocardium following severe ischaemia.

    b. True MI induces acute inflammatory changes.

    c. False The infarct tissue is replaced by a collagenous scar.

    d. True Occlusion of the right coronary artery results in an inferior MI.

    e. True Management includes analgesics, thrombolysis, and anticoagulants.

31. a. False Left ventricular dilatation is a cause of mitral regurgitation.

b. True Infective endocarditis causes cusp damage and mitral regurgitation.

c. True Rheumatic fever is a cause of mitral stenosis.

d. True Papillary muscle dysfunction causes mitral valve regurgitation.

e. False Senile calcification causes aortic stenosis.

32. a. True Heart failure is where the heart cannot maintain adequate cardiac output, or can only do so by increasing filling pressure.

b. False Left-sided failure is more common than right-sided.

c. True The progression of left-sided heart failure is the most common cause of right-sided failure.

d. True Heart failure may be a complication of myocardial infarction due to ventricular remodelling.

e. False Heart failure commonly follows severe aortic, mitral or pulmonary valve disease.

33. a. False The valve leaflets are a very common site of infective endocarditis.

b. True Infective endocarditis rarely affects normal valves, but this is seen in, for example, intravenous drug abusers.

c. True *Streptococcus viridens* and *Candida* are recognised causes of infective endocarditis.

d. True Splinter haemorrhages of the fingernails are sometimes seen.

e. True Multiorgan infarction may be caused by infective endocarditis.

34. a. True Atherosclerosis causes thinning and fibrous replacement of the media.

b. True Marfan's syndrome is an autosomal dominant disorder of connective tissue.

c. True Ehlers–Danlos syndrome is an inherited disorder causing abnormalities in collagen.

d. True Syphilis is a rare cause of aortic aneurysm typically affecting the ascending aortic arch.

e. False Osteopetrosis is an inherited disorder affecting cartilaginous bones.

35. a. False Thrombus occurs in flowing blood, a clot occurs in non-flowing blood.

b. True Both stasis and turbulence predispose to thrombosis (one of Virchow's triad).

c. False. Antiphospholipid antibody promotes thrombosis, as seen in systemic lupus erythematosus.

d. False The most common site is the deep veins of the leg (deep vein thrombosis).

e. True Especially cancers of the breast, lung, prostate, pancreas and bowel.

36. a. False The most common affected site for carcinoma of the larynx is the glottic region (60%).

b. True Cigarette smoking is a major risk factor in the aetiology.

c. False The tumour spreads mainly through local invasion to adjacent laryngeal structures.

d. True The majority are of well-differentiated keratinizing squamous epithelium.

e. True Carcinoma of the larynx usually occurs over the age of 40 years, affecting men more than women.

37. a. True COPD is characterised by chronic bronchitis, emphysema and bronchiolitis.

b. False COPD is incompletely reversible by bronchodilators.

c. False Lungs are hyperinflated in COPD.

d. False Commonly smokers, but may occur without smoking in those occupationally exposed to dust or with α-1-antitrypsin deficiency.

e. False Emphysema causes permanent airways dilatation and tissue destruction without fibrosis.

38. a. True Chronic bronchitis is defined as a productive cough on most days for 3 months of the year for at least two successive years.

b. True Cigarette smoking is very important in the aetiology.

c. True Hypersecretion is associated with hyper-trophy and hyperplasia of the bronchial mucus-secreting cells.

d. True Is characterised by chronic inflammation.

e. False Lung function tests show an obstructive pattern.

39. a. False Asthma reverses spontaneously or with bronchodilators.

b. True Asthma may be caused by a type I hyper-sensitivity reaction.

c. True Bronchospasm, oedema and mucus plug-ging are commonly seen.

d. False α-1-antitrypsin deficiency is associated with COPD development.

e. True Bronchial smooth muscle hypertrophy may occur.

40. a. True Repeat infections occur in the stagnated secretions with organisms such as *Pseudomonas*.

b. False CF is the most common autosomal recessive condition in Europe (chromosome 7).

c. True Mutation results in a defective cystic fibrosis transmembrane regulator, impaired transport of Cl⁻ ions.

d. True   Malabsorption occurs due to reduced pancreatic secretions (mucus plugs in exocrine glands).

e. True   The most common mutation is the deletion of phenylalanine 508 on chromosome 7.

41.
a. False   Bacterial origin in 80–90% of cases.

b. False   Gram-negative bacteria are associated with hospital-acquired pneumonia, Gram-positives with community-acquired.

c. True   Lung fibrosis, abscess and empyema may complicate pneumonia.

d. False   Red hepatisation occurs in lobar pneumonia.

e. True   Pulmonary oedema does increase the risk of pneumonia.

42.
a. False   Tuberculosis is caused by the organism *Mycobacterium tuberculosis*.

b. False   Pathogenesis is due to host hypersensitivity reaction to constituents of the bacteria cell wall.

c. True   Predisposing factors include chronic lung diseases such as silicosis.

d. True   Immunocompromised patients are very susceptible to tuberculosis.

e. True   Tuberculous granulomas are called tubercles.

43.
a. False   Squamous cell carcinoma is the most common form of lung cancer.

b. True   Cigarette smoking is a major aetiological factor in the formation of lung cancer.

c. True   Occupational exposure to asbestos increases risk of lung cancer and mesotheliomas.

d. False   Metastatic spread is seen in 70% of patients at presentation.

e. True   Lung cancer is the most common cause of neoplasia in the UK.

44.
a. False   Idiopathic pulmonary fibrosis is not an infectious condition.

b. False   It causes interstitial thickening with fibrosis.

c. True   It is a restrictive airways disease.

d. True   Peripheral honeycombing describes the appearance on a cut lung surface (or CT scan).

e. True   Idiopathic pulmonary fibrosis is one of the causes of finger clubbing.

45.
a. False   Causes pulmonary hypertension and infarction.

b. False   This would cause arterial embolism.

c. True   Pulmonary embolism is a potential cause of pulseless electrical activity of the heart.

d. False   Usually thromboembolic, but can involve fat, amniotic fluid, air, foreign bodies or tumour.

e. True   This is the most common cause of pulmonary embolism.

46.
a. False   There is a long latency between asbestos exposure and mesothelioma.

b. False   Haematogenous spread is rare in mesothelioma.

c. False   Rapidly progressive with death usually occurring within 10 months of diagnosis.

d. False   The incidence has been increasing per year, and is expected to do so until at least 2010.

e. True   Mesothelioma is associated with recurrent pleural effusions.

47.
a. True   The lips are the most common site for squamous cell carcinoma of the oral cavity.

b. False   The incidence is twice as high in males as in females.

c. True   There is a direct relationship between the number of cigarettes smoked and oral cancer risk.

d. False   Moderate alcohol intake has been shown to decrease the risk of oral cancer.

e. True   Oral cancer has a 5-year survival rate of about 50%.

48.
a. False   Squamous cell carcinoma is more common.

b. True   Oesophageal adenocarcinoma may develop from Barrett's metaplasia.

c. False   Heavy smoking and drinking are associated with squamous cell carcinoma.

d. True   Five-year survival from oesophageal carcinoma is less than 10%.

e. True   Dysphagia is seen especially where the middle and upper oesophagus is affected.

49.
a. True   Oesophageal varices are dilated submucosal veins in the oesophagus.

b. True   They are commonly associated with cirrhosis of the liver.

c. True   Rupture causes torrential bleeding and haematemesis.

d. False   Are associated with portal vein hypertension.

e. True   Sclerotherapy can be used in the management by the injection of an irritant that causes thrombophlebitis.

50.
a. True   Aetiology is multifactorial (stress, *Helicobacter pylori*, NSAIDs).

b. True   The acid in gastric secretions can damage the epithelial surface of the oesophagus, stomach and duodenum.

c. True   Patients can present with epigastric pain, nausea or heartburn.

d. False   Ulcers are commonly associated with the bacterium *Helicobacter pylori*.

e. True   Complications include perforation, which may lead to peritonitis.

51. a. False   The gastritis is initially acute, but then becomes chronic.

    b. True   *Helicobacter pylori* colonises the epithelium below a layer of mucus.

    c. True   Epithelial damage is mediated by the immune response against *Helicobacter pylori*.

    d. False   Gastritis is most commonly found at the antrum.

    e. False   infection often persists for many years.

52. a. False   The vast majority of gastric tumours are adenocarcinomas.

    b. False   Males are more affected than females.

    c. False   60% of tumours are found at the pylorus.

    d. True   Interesting geographical pattern with incidence higher in East Asia than Europe.

    e. True   Patients with antibodies to *Helicobacter pylori* have a higher risk of gastric cancer.

53. a. True   The prehepatic, hepatic, posthepatic classification system is useful.

    b. False   Portal hypertension is most commonly caused by cirrhosis.

    c. True   Portal hypertension may cause ascites and splenomegaly.

    d. False   Budd–Chiari syndrome (hepatic vein thrombosis) is a cause of portal hypertension.

    e. False   Portosystemic shunts become enlarged.

54. a. False   Cirrhosis is an irreversible condition.

    b. True   A common cause of cirrhosis is alcohol liver disease (also hepatitis B and C).

    c. True   An uncommon cause of cirrhosis is autoimmune chronic hepatitis (also cystic fibrosis).

    d. True   Nodules are formed from regenerated hepatocytes separated by bands of collagenous fibrosis.

    e. False   Prothrombin time is increased due to reduced synthesis of anticoagulation factors.

55. a. True   Ascites is the accumulation of free fluid in the peritoneal cavity.

    b. False   Cirrhosis causes transudative (low protein) ascites.

    c. False   Non-hepatic causes of ascites include malignancy, nephrotic syndrome and heart failure.

    d. True   Shifting dullness on percussion of the abdomen signifies ascites.

    e. False   The treatment of ascites involves sodium restriction.

56. a. False   Wilson's disease is an autosomal recessive condition.

    b. True   It results from a mutation in a gene for a calcium transporter protein.

    c. True   Free copper overspills into the blood and deposits in the cornea and the brain.

    d. True   Psychiatric disorders occur.

    e. False   Chronic hepatitis and cirrhosis are common.

57. a. False   Hepatitis B is a DNA virus.

    b. False   Transmission routes are blood-borne, sexual contact and vertical.

    c. True   Initial infection is subclinical and transient in 65% of cases.

    d. True   Vaccination for hepatitis B utilises the surface antigen, HBsAg.

    e. True   Cirrhosis and hepatocellular carcinoma are potential complications of chronic infection.

58. a. False   The majority of malignant liver tumours are metastatic (lung, breast, colon, stomach).

    b. False   Predisposing factors include hepatitis B.

    c. True   Males are affected more than females (8 : 1 ratio).

    d. False   Prognosis is very poor with a median survival rate of less than 6 months post diagnosis.

    e. False   It is cholangiocarcinoma that arises from the bile duct epithelium, not HCC.

59. a. False   Primary biliary cirrhosis is much more common in females than males (10 : 1).

    b. True   Associations with several autoimmune diseases are seen, e.g. rheumatoid arthritis, SLE.

    c. False   Drugs are ineffective and affected individuals eventually need a liver transplant.

    d. False   Ulcerative colitis is strongly associated with primary sclerosing cholangitis.

    e. True   The scar formation in primary biliary cirrhosis is by bridging fibrosis.

60. a. True   Pancreatic cancer has a positive association with excess alcohol consumption.

    b. False   It is more common in males than females.

    c. False   Curative surgical resection is rarely possible.

    d. True   Lesions are typically moderately differentiated adenocarcinomas.

    e. True   Patients are usually over the age of 60 at presentation.

61. a. True   Systemic complications which develop in a minority of patients with Crohn's include skin disease.

    b. False   There is an increased incidence of Crohn's in cigarette smokers.

    c. True   Granulomatous inflammation can occur anywhere from the mouth to the anus.

    d. True   Non-caseating granulomas present in the bowel wall and mesenteric lymph nodes.

    e. True   There is an association between Crohn's and eye disease.

62. a. False Ulcerative colitis is characterised by superficial inflammation.

b. False Interestingly, smoking is associated with a decreased risk for UC.

c. False Inflammation is diffuse and limited to the mucosa.

d. False Features include infiltration of inflammatory cells, crypt abscesses and atrophy (Crohn's is complicated by fistulae).

e. True The disease is continuous, spreading to the whole of the large bowel.

63. a. True Coeliac disease is due to an abnormal immune response to gluten.

b. True Villous atrophy and crypt hyperplasia are seen.

c. False A disease of the small intestine.

d. True Serum screening for anti-endomyseal antibodies is a useful aid to diagnosis.

e. False There is a slow but partial or total recovery in villous structure.

64. a. True Colourectal carcinoma is thought to develop from adenomas.

b. True By the age of 45, 90% of individuals with FAP will have developed carcinoma.

c. False Staged by the modified Dukes system (A–D).

d. True Left-sided carcinomas cause early mechanical obstruction to faeces and so present earlier.

e. False The rectosigmoid is the most common area affected.

65. a. False Both kidneys are progressively replaced by cyst.

b. True It is an inherited autosomal dominant disease.

c. True Associations are with berry aneurysms of the cerebral arteries.

d. True Enlarging cysts replace and compress functioning renal parenchyma.

e. False Uncontrolled hypertension accelerates the development of renal failure.

66. a. True Membranous nephropathy is the most common cause of adult nephrotic syndrome.

b. False 80–90% of membranous nephropathy cases are idiopathic.

c. False Children with minimal change disease have a good prognosis with corticosteroids.

d. True Goodpasture's syndrome is indicated by anti-collagen IV antibodies and glomerulonephritis.

e. True Streptococcal glomerulonephritis may follow throat infection.

67. a. True Renal cell carcinoma is more common in males than females (3 : 1).

b. False Carcinoma usually occurs at the upper kidney pole.

c. False Haematuria, loin pain and a loin mass are more typical features.

d. False Smoking increases the risk of renal cell carcinoma.

e. False Renal cell carcinoma may rarely be linked to von Hippel–Lindau syndrome.

68. a. False Men are affected more often than women (3 : 1).

b. False Almost all cases are transitional cell carcinoma.

c. True Bladder cancer may obstruct urinary flow.

d. True The most commonly affected sites are the base of trigone and ureteric orifaces.

e. True Known environmental carcinogens include certain dyes, rubbers and cigarette components.

69. a. True The anterior pituitary does secrete adrenocorticotrophic hormone (ACTH).

b. False The posterior pituitary secretes antidiuretic hormone (ADH).

c. False The posterior pituitary secretes oxytocin.

d. True The anterior pituitary does secrete thyroid-stimulating hormone (TSH).

e. True The anterior pituitary does secrete follicle-stimulating hormone (FSH).

70. a. False Graves' disease is much more common in women than men (8 : 1).

b. False 95% of Graves' individuals are serum positive for TSH-receptor antibodies.

c. True Diffuse hypertrophy and hyperplasia of the acinar epithelium are seen.

d. True Only about 5% of patients show exophthalmos.

e. False Graves' disease causes thyrotoxicosis, Hashimoto's thyroiditis causes hypothyroidism.

71. a. False Toxic adenomas are benign tumours that secrete thyroid hormones.

b. True There is a link between childhood radiation exposure (e.g. Chernobyl) and thyroid cancer.

c. False Papillary carcinomas tend to develop in younger patients.

d. False Medullary carcinoma is derived from parafollicular C cells that secrete substances like calcitonin and serotonin.

e. True In about half of anaplastic carcinoma cases there is a history of multinodular goitre.

72. a. False Addison's disease results in a hypofunction of the adrenal cortex.

  b. True Iatrogenic administration of ACTH can cause Cushing's syndrome.

  c. True Iatrogenic administration of prednisolone can cause Cushing's syndrome.

  d. False Phaeochromocytoma is a tumour of the chromaffin cells that results in the secretion of catecholamines.

  e. True Adrenal cortical tumours are rare but are associated with overproduction of glucocorticoids.

73. a. True Addison's disease causes a lack of both glucocorticoids and mineralocorticoids.

  b. True It is most commonly an autoimmune disease.

  c. False Addison's disease causes increased ACTH and decreased cortisol in the serum.

  d. True It may be managed by glucocorticoid and mineralocorticoid replacement therapy.

  e. True Sudden stress placed on the chronically failing adrenal gland may cause an Addisonian crisis.

74. a. True Type 1 diabetes mellitus is an autoimmune-induced disorder, which may be triggered by a viral infection.

  b. True Genetic predisposition association with HLA-DR genotype.

  c. False Type 1 diabetes mellitus is a disease of childhood/adolescent onset.

  d. True Histologically destruction of insulin secreting cells of the islets of Langerhans is observed

  e. False Plasma insulin absent or low.

75. a. False Type II diabetes is almost exclusively a disease of adults.

  b. True Insulin resistance is an important first step in the development.

  c. False Commonly treated by diet and oral hypoglycaemic agents, although insulin may eventually be required.

  d. False Diabetic ketoacidosis is a complication of type I diabetes.

  e. True Macrovascular and microvascular complications occur in diabetes.

76. a. False The majority of cervical tumours are squamous cell carcinomas.

  b. True Cervical intra-epithelial neoplasia is a dysplastic preneoplastic proliferative state.

  c. True HPV 16, 18 and 33 have been identified in cervical carcinoma.

  d. True Cigarette smoking has a positive association with cervical cancer.

  e. True HIV infection has a positive association with cervical cancer due to its immunosuppressive action.

77. a. True Endometriosis is defined as endometrial glands or stroma occurring outside of the uterus.

  b. True The ovaries are a commonly affected site.

  c. True Retrograde menstruation is a common theory of aetiology.

  d. False Endometriosis is oestrogen dependent and therefore improves after the menopause.

  e. False It is a common cause of infertility but only 30% of those with endometriosis are infertile.

78. a. True Pelvic inflammatory disease is a disorder of the fallopian tubes, ovaries and peritoneum.

  b. True Predisposing factors include intrauterine contraceptive devices.

  c. True *Neisseria gonorrhoeae* is a common aetiological agent.

  d. False Initially inflammation is acute; untreated PID may progress to chronic inflammation.

  e. False Pelvic inflammatory disease is a disease of infection.

79. a. True Ectopic pregnancy results when a fertilised ovum implants outside the uterine cavity.

  b. True The most common site is the fallopian tube, especially the ampulla.

  c. True Aetiology may be due to previous episodes of salpingitis (inflammation of the fallopian tube).

  d. True Proliferation of the trophoblast causes erosion of the submucosa, which precipitates severe bleeding.

  e. False Tubal pregnancy invariably results in rupture of the fallopian tube and death of the fertilised ovum.

80. a. False Pre-eclampsia also requires proteinuria, otherwise it is just gestational hypertension.

  b. True First and multiple pregnancies are more commonly affected.

  c. False It is thought pre-eclampsia develops from placental ischaemia.

  d. False Pre-eclampsia is associated with fetal growth retardation and low birth weight.

  e. False It resolves within 24 hours of delivery.

81. a. True Carcinoma of the breast is the most common cause of death in women aged 35–55 years.

b. True Mutation of tumour suppressor genes *BRCA1/2* are implicated in some inherited cancers.

c. False Screening by mammography is available for all women over the age of 50.

d. True The antioestrogen tamoxifen can be used in oestrogen-receptor-positive tumours.

e. True Ductal carcinoma is the most common histological subtype.

82. a. False It is an adenocarcinoma.

b. False Prostate carcinoma affects the peripheral zone.

c. False Benign prostatic hyperplasia is more likely to cause urinary symptoms as it affects the central zone.

d. False Commonly extends outside of the prostatic capsule.

e. True The majority of prostate carcinomas have a well differentiated glandular pattern.

83. a. False Osteoporosis is very common, especially in elderly women.

b. True Osteoporosis may cause pathological fractures.

c. False Bone trabeculae are thinned and reduced in number.

d. False Diagnosis is by bone densitometry.

e. True X-ray changes include decreased bone density and 'fish' lumbar vertebrae.

84. a. True A fracture is a break in the continuity of the bone usually caused by physical trauma.

b. True A simple fracture occurs without contact with the external environment.

c. True A compound fracture occurs with direct contact with the external environment (may become infected).

d. True A pathological fracture occurs in abnormal bone.

e. True Healing involves the formation of a haematoma due to the tearing of the medullary blood vessels.

85. a. True Rheumatoid arthritis affects 1% of the UK population.

b. False Onset is normally distributed with a peak between 35–45 years old.

c. True Many, but not all, are positive for rheumatoid factor.

d. True Associated with the development of a pannus and inflammatory destruction of joints.

e. True Rheumatoid disease has widespread extra-articular manifestations.

86. a. True SLE is associated with autoantibodies against DNA and other nuclear components.

b. True SLE is 8 times more common in women than men.

c. True Fibrinoid necrosis of small arteries, arterioles and capillaries is seen.

d. True SLE may result in malar and discoid skin rashes.

e. False Corticosteroids are first-line therapy in acute SLE.

87. a. False HIV is an enveloped RNA retrovirus.

b. True Reverse transcriptase is required for viral replication.

c. True HIV binds CD4 positive cells via its gp120 cell surface glycoprotein.

d. True Opportunistic infections include *Pneumocystis carinii*.

e. True HIV infection is characterised by atypical mycobacterium infection.

88. a. False AIDS is a secondary immunodeficiency caused by HIV infection.

b. True X-linked agammaglobulinaemia of Bruton results from the inability of B cells to mature.

c. True IgA deficiency is the most common form of primary immunodeficiency.

d. True SCID is an extreme form of immunodeficiency.

e. True Transient physiological agammaglobulinaemia is due to falling levels of maternally derived IgG.

89. a. False Numerous potential proteins can fold abnormally to produce amyloid.

b. True Amyloid takes up the Congo red stain.

c. True Abnormal macrophage control systems appear to aid amyloid aggregation.

d. False The AA type is seen in reactive systemic amyloidosis.

e. True Amyloidosis may complicate long-term haemodialyis.

90. a. True Agranulocytosis describes severe neutropenia.

b. True Neutropenia is part of the autosomal recessive Kostmann's syndrome.

c. False Neutrophil increase is the most common cause of leucocytosis.

d. False Primary leucocytosis occurs in bone marrow disease, e.g. leukaemia, lymphoma.

e. False Eosinophilia is commonly seen in allergic reactions.

91. a. True   Reed–Sternberg cells are seen in Hodgkin's lymphoma.
   b. False   Males are affected more than females.
   c. False   The staging system used for Hodgkin's lymphoma is the Ann Arbor system.
   d. False   Suffix B indicates the presence of systemic symptoms and a worse prognosis.
   e. False   Mixed cellularity with numerous RS cells has a poor prognosis.

92. a. True   Non-Hodgkin's lymphoma has been linked to immunosuppression.
   b. False   *Helicobacter pylori* infection has been linked to gastric lymphoma.
   c. True   70% of non-Hodgkin's lymphomas are derived from B cells.
   d. False   Chromosomal translocations are a common feature of many lymphomas.
   e. True   Extranodal involvement is more common in non-Hodgkin's lymphoma.

93. a. False   The Philadelphia chromosome occurs in chronic myeloid leukaemia.
   b. True   Chronic lymphocytic leukaemia is the commonest leukaemia in adults.
   c. False   Survival of more than 10 years postdiagnosis is common.
   d. True   Males are affected more than females.
   e. True   Lymph nodes can be affected with normal architecture becoming effaced by infiltrating cells.

94. a. False   Sickle-cell anaemia is caused by a mutation in the gene encoding the β-globin chain.
   b. False   It is common in West and East Africa, the Mediterranean and the Middle East.
   c. True   Chronic haemolysis may result in gall stones and jaundice.
   d. False   Hyposplenism is seen (autosplenectomy).
   e. True   HbS confers protection against malaria by creating a hostile environment for the plasmodium parasite in the RBC.

95. a. False   Most commonly autoimmune.
   b. True   Causes brain damage in neonates (kernicterus).
   c. True   'Warm' type autoimmune haemolytic anaemia results in microspherocytosis.
   d. True   'Cold' type autoimmune haemolytic anaemia results in red cell agglutination.
   e. True   Autoimmune haemolytic anaemia may be associated with lymphoma.

96. a. False   A nodule is a raised lesion greater than 5 mm across.
   b. True   A vesicle is a blister less than 5 mm across.
   c. False   A macule is a localised flattened lesion of pigmented skin.
   d. False   A pustule is a small pus-containing blister, often indicating infection.
   e. True   Spongiosis means epidermal oedema.

97. a. False   Psoriasis is a chronic, non-infective inflammatory disease.
   b. False   The epidermal proliferation rate is increased 20-fold.
   c. True   Lithium may precipitate or worsen psoriasis.
   d. True   Psoriasis commonly affects the elbows, knees, trunk and scalp.
   e. True   Nail involvement is common, with pitting and thickening of the nail.

98. a. False   The incidence of atopic eczema is increasing.
   b. True   Family history is a strong risk factor for the development of atopic eczema.
   c. False   Atopic eczema is caused by a type I hypersensitivity reaction.
   d. True   Atopic eczema decreases in incidence with increasing age through childhood.
   e. True   Bacterial and viral infections complicate atopic eczema.

99. a. False   Pemphigoid is subepidermal separation of tissue.
   b. True   Pemphigus is associated with erosions.
   c. False   Pemphigus has a higher untreated mortality than pemphigoid.
   d. False   Dermatitis herpetiformis is a blistering condition associated with coeliac disease.
   e. True   Dermatitis herpetiformis involves granular IgA deposition at the dermal papillae in normal-looking skin.

100. a. False   Malignant melanoma is a tumour of melanocytes.
   b. True   Repeated exposure to UV radiation may play an aetiological role.
   c. True   Familial dysplastic naevus syndrome is a major risk factor.
   d. False   A Breslow thickness (staging of malignant melanoma) of > 3.5 mm has a poor prognosis.
   e. True   Malignant melanoma may arise in a pre-existing lentigo maligna.

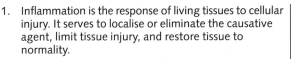

1. Inflammation is the response of living tissues to cellular injury. It serves to localise or eliminate the causative agent, limit tissue injury, and restore tissue to normality.

   Acute inflammation is the initial, rapid response of a tissue to injury. The reaction is accompanied by a prominent vascular response and the predominant cell type is the neutrophil polymorph (innate immunity). The duration of the response varies from a few hours to a few weeks.

   Chronic inflammation is the persisting, slow response of a tissue to injury. It does not involve a prominent vascular response and the predominant cell types are lymphocytes, plasma cells and macrophages (cell-mediated immunity). The duration of the response may be weeks, months or even years.

2. Apoptosis is an energy-dependent cell death process. Its features include:
   - Induction by physiological and pathological stimuli.
   - Involves the removal of single damaged or unwanted cells.
   - Endogenous endonucleases fragment DNA but lysosomes remain intact.
   - Cell membrane integrity is maintained.
   - Apoptosis does not cause an inflammatory response.
   - Cells shrink and fragment into apoptotic bodies.
   - Apoptotic bodies are phagocytosed by neighbouring cells.

   Necrosis is an energy-independent cell death process. Examples are coagulative, colliquative, caseous, gangrene, fibrinoid and fat. Its features include:
   - Induction invariably due to pathological injury.
   - Involves groups of cells.
   - Lysosomes leak lytic enzymes and ion homeostasis is dysregulated.
   - Cell membrane integrity is lost.
   - There is cell swelling and lysis.
   - Inflammatory response present.
   - Dead cells are phagocytosed by neutrophils and macrophages.

3. Cell proliferation is usually tightly regulated by two sets of opposing functioning genes: (1) proto-oncogenes are growth-promoting genes; and (2) tumour suppressor genes are negative cell-cycle regulators. Abnormal activation of proto-oncogenes and loss of function of tumour suppressor genes leads to the transformation of a normal cell into a cancer cell.

   Proto-oncogenes are genes that are expressed in normal cells. These genes encode for oncoproteins, which positively regulate cell growth and differentiation. Inappropriate expression of oncoproteins leads to abnormal cell growth and survival by, for example, gene amplification. Oncogenes include nuclear binding proteins (e.g. c-myc), tyrosine kinase proteins (e.g. src), growth factors (e.g. PDGF), receptors for growth factors (e.g. c-erbB-2/HER-2) and GTP binding proteins (e.g. ras).

   Tumour suppressor genes encode proteins that prevent or suppress the growth of tumours. Inactivation of tumour suppressor genes by, for example, gene mutation results in increased susceptibility to cancer formation. Genetically increased susceptibility to cancer formation was first proposed by Knudson. Tumour suppressor genes implicated in human cancer include the *APC* gene (colourectal tumours, chromosome 5q), *RB1* gene (retinoblastoma and others, chromosome 13q), *BRCA1* gene (breast cancer, chromosome 17q) and the *p53* gene (many tumour types, chromosome 17p).

4. Viruses carry nucleic acids but lack the synthetic material to replicate by themselves. They therefore require host cells to propagate and, as such, are termed 'obligate intracellular parasites'. They consist of a nucleic acid core protected by a protein coat (capsid), which together form the nucleocapsid. Some viruses are additionally enveloped by the outer membrane of their host cell. Viruses may be classified by morphology (icosahedral, helical, complex) but are more commonly grouped by the type of nucleic acid that they carry.

   DNA viruses include herpes simplex virus, varicella zoster virus and hepatitis B virus. These can utilise host cell polymerases to synthesise viral mRNA.

   RNA viruses include measles virus, mumps virus and influenza virus. As host cells cannot replicate RNA, these viruses encode their own replicative enzymes to form viral mRNA.

   Retroviruses are also RNA viruses but possess the enzyme reverse transcriptase, which allows the conversion of viral RNA to DNA. The newly formed viral DNA can then be inserted into the host genome, just like the replication pattern of DNA viruses. Examples of retroviruses include human immunodeficiency virus (HIV) and human T-cell lymphotropic virus (HTLV).

5. Coeliac disease is a condition of malabsorption resulting from villous atrophy of the small intestine caused by abnormal sensitivity to gluten, a protein in wheat flour.

   Autoantibodies to the protein gliadin, a component of gluten, result in inflammation of the small intestinal mucosa with loss of villous architecture.

Morphologically, the condition is characterised by a mosaic-like pattern of crypt openings with increased crypt depth and epithelial cell hyperplasia. Associations include HLA-B8 and dermatitis herpetiformis.

6. Incidence—most common cancer in the UK, affecting 30 000 individuals every year.

Age—peak incidence between 40 and 70 years of age.

Sex—males more than females, but with an increasing incidence in women.

Geography—the UK has a higher incidence than anywhere else in the world.

Risk factors—cigarette smoking.

Occupational factors—exposure to radioactive material, asbestos, nickel, chromium, iron oxides and coal-gas plants.

Environmental factors—radon (a natural radioactive gas in certain geographical areas).

Macroscopic appearance—tumours may be central (majority, all types) or peripheral (mainly adenocarcinomas).

Microscopic appearance—squamous cell carcinoma (35%), small (oat) cell (20%), adenocarcinoma (30%), large cell anaplastic carcinoma (15%).

Spread can be:

- Local—surrounding the lungs, pleura and adjacent mediastinal structures.
- Lymphatic—ipsilateral and contralateral peribronchial and hilar lymph nodes.
- Transcoelomic—across the pleural cavity.
- Haematogenous spread—brain, bone, liver and adrenal glands.

Prognosis—related to type (worse with small cell) and stage (some squamous cell and adenocarcinomas may be surgically resectable) but, overall, 5-year survival is 5%.

7. Nephrotic syndrome is defined as heavy proteinuria (more than 3.5 g per day), hypoproteinemia and peripheral oedema. Associated with these changes are an increased susceptibility to infection, hypercholesterolaemia and a greater tendency for thrombosis. Nephrotic syndrome reflects injury to podocytes and nephron architecture. The most common aetiology in adults is membranous nephropathy; minimal change disease is the predominant cause in children. These are both examples of primary disease but the syndrome can also be secondary to diseases such as diabetes mellitus, systemic lupus erythematosus (SLE) and Wegener's granulomatosis.

Nephritic syndrome describes haematuria, proteinuria (often with urinary casts) and hypertension. An affected patient usually feels unwell and may have loin pain. Haematuria always suggests an underlying inflammatory and proliferative process within the kidney. Causes of nephritic syndrome include post-streptococcal glomerulonephritis and Goodpasture's syndrome. As with nephrotic syndrome, nephritic syndrome may be secondary to vascular conditions such as SLE and Wegener's granulomatosis.

8. The genetic events resulting in colourectal carcinoma are the activation of oncogenes, loss or mutation of tumour suppressor genes and defects in DNA repair pathways leading to genomic instability. Oncogenes altered include *bcl-2*, *c-Ki-ras* and *c-myc*. Tumour suppressor genes include the *APC* and *p53* genes. Vogelstein's model of multistep genetic changes corresponds to the pathological phenotype of small and large adenoma and invasive adenocarcinoma. Familial adenomatous polyposis (FAP) is a rare autosomal dominant disorder where mutation of chromosome 5 (APC) results in colourectal cancer usually by the age of 35 years.

Approximately 50% of tumours occur in the rectum and a further 30% are found in the sigmoid colon. Microscopically, the tumours are adenocarcinomas and the extent of spread is measured by Dukes' staging.

9. Hodgkin's disease (HD) and non-Hodgkin's lymphoma (NHL) are both lymphoproliferative diseases that form solid malignant tumours of the lymph nodes. Although there are many similarities, there are also some important differences between the conditions. HD has two peaks of onset, one in early life (20–30 years old) and one in later life (50–70 years old). By contrast, NHL is a disease almost exclusively of middle and later life. The aetiology of both conditions is relatively poorly understood, but where HD has been linked to Epstein–Barr virus and the formation of Reed–Sternberg cells, NHL is associated with factors such as immunosuppression, certain viruses and radiation. Chromosomal abnormalities are also more prominent in NHL, such as those seen in Burkitt's lymphoma.

HD usually presents localised to a single peripheral lymph node region. Although systemic symptoms (B symptoms) do occur, they are less common than in NHL, in which extranodal disease is more likely. NHL has a more varied clinical presentation because of frequent involvement of multiple lymph node areas. Unlike NHL, enlarged nodes in HD are usually smooth surfaced with the capsule rarely breached.

Classification systems are also different between the diseases. HD is staged by the Ann-Arbor system and classified by the Rye system; the Kiel system is used to differentiate NHL.

10. Graves' disease is an organ-specific autoimmune disease causing thyrotoxicosis, most commonly in females. It is caused by the binding of IgG antibodies to thyroid gland receptors for TSH; these antibodies are termed TSH-receptor antibodies (TRAbs). This interaction results in the prolonged stimulation of the gland, with eventual diffuse hypertrophy and hyperplasia producing a goitre.

The symptoms of thyrotoxicosis include restlessness, anxiety, palpitations, tremor, hyperhidrosis, diarrhoea and intolerance to heat. Important signs include tachycardia, weight loss, osteoporotic bone changes and goitre formation. Additional signs seen in Graves' disease are exophthalmos, thyroid acropachy (enlarged fingernails) and pretibial myxoedema.

11. This woman has had a deep vein thrombosis. A thrombus is a solid mass of blood constituents formed within the vascular system during life. Predisposing factors for thrombosis are abnormality of the vessel wall, abnormality of blood flow and abnormality of blood constituents (Virchow's triad). This thrombus is a complication of her surgical procedure and prolonged bed rest (blood stasis). The thrombus material has dislodged and travelled to the lungs resulting in a pulmonary embolism (PE). An embolism is a mass of material in the vascular system capable of becoming lodged in a blood vessel. A PE causes the symptoms of shortness of breath. The effects of a PE depend upon the size of the dislodged fragment.

12. This patient is most likely to have rheumatoid arthritis (RA), an inflammatory joint disease that tends to start symmetrically in the metacarpophalangeal or proximal interphalangeal joints of the hands. RA has a strong genetic component, and so joint disease in her older sister is not surprising. RA causes both polyarthritis and joint deformities. However, as part of a wider systemic autoimmune disease, RA patients are also likely to develop extra-articular complications in the:

- Lungs—interstitial pulmonary fibrosis.
- Blood vessels—with the development of vasculitides.
- Eyes—secondary Sjögren's syndrome and scleritis.
- Haemopoietic system—anaemia, increased lymphoma risk and Felty's syndrome.
- Neurological system—peripheral compression neuropathies are very common.
- Heart—rarely pericardial effusions, heart block, cardiomyopathy and angina.

13. Lumps in the breast include carcinoma, fibroadenoma, fat necrosis, cysts and lipoma. Periductal mastitis and duct ectasia must also be excluded. The GP would be suspicious of a breast carcinoma due to the presence of skin dimpling and because tumour spread to the axillary lymph nodes is a common form of metastasis. Invasive carcinomas are mainly of infiltrating ductal histological type. The appearance of the tumour depends on the extent of involvement with the stroma. Tumour cells are arranged in cords. Prognosis is related to stage at presentation (using the TMN system) and the grade on histological examination.

The majority of breast cancer cases are sporadic. However, approximately 4% of breast cancers are linked to a strong family history. The genes *BRCA1*, which is located on chromosome 17, and *BRCA2*, located on chromosome 13, are associated with a family history of breast cancer. Future advances in our understanding of the molecular basis of breast cancer are likely to involve the reporting of more susceptibility genes.

14. The most likely diagnosis is carpal tunnel syndrome, a compression (entrapment) neuropathy of the median nerve as it passes through the wrist. It is a very common condition, which is more likely in pregnancy. Compressed nerves undergo segmental demyelination with reduced nerve conduction velocity, accounting for the symptoms described. Other sites affected by compression neuropathy include:

- Spinal nerve roots in the intervertebral foramina— compressed by prolapsed intervertebral discs or osteophytes.
- Ulnar nerve—compressed at the medial epicondyle of humerus.
- Common peroneal nerve—compressed at the neck of fibula.

15. This patient presents with a history of long-term sun exposure (occupational). A pigmented itchy lesion is likely to be a malignant melanoma because the major aetiological factor is UV light. (*Note*: some malignant melanomas are non-pigmented.) Malignant melanomas arise from melanocytes. Some arise from melanocytes present in a benign naevus.

Prognosis depends on the thickness of the lesion at the time of excision and is assessed using the Breslow method. Histologically, the Breslow thickness is the measured thickness in millimetres from the granular layer of the epidermis to the deepest identifiable melanoma cell. A tumour < 1 mm thick at the time of excision has a cure rate of almost 100%. However, a lesion > 3.5 mm has a poor prognosis. Consequently, as the lesion thickens, the prognosis worsens.

16. Hyperplasia of the endometrium occurs in response to ooestrogenic stimulation. The condition is thought to be preneoplastic because it is associated with an increased risk of developing endometrial adenocarcinoma. The 'severe' hyperplasia described in this case suggests prominent cellular atypia, with distorted gland structure and intraglandular polypoid formations. Cells usually show frequent mitoses. This is considered a high-risk group, with 30% of individuals progressing to adenocarcinoma, usually within about 4 years.

17. This patient has a macrocytic anaemia, shown by the abnormally low haemoglobin level (anaemia) and abnormally large mean cell volume (macrocytosis). Given the history of alcoholism, it is likely that a haematinic deficiency is responsible. Folate deficiency commonly affects alcoholics, although vitamin B_{12} levels may also rarely be reduced. Both folate and vitamin B_{12} are required for DNA synthesis; a lack of one or both of these substances therefore impairs the production of marrow precursor cells.

The result is that the bone marrow produces abnormally large red cell precursors (megaloblasts), which mature into abnormally large red cells (macrocytes). The specific name for this form of disease is megaloblastic anaemia.

Folate deficiency may also occur due to malabsorption (e.g. Crohn's disease), increased requirements (e.g. pregnancy) or drug interference (e.g. methotrexate).

---

18. This patient has ischaemic heart disease (angina pectoris) because of atherosclerotic plaques. These plaques are characterised by fibrosis, lipid deposition and chronic inflammation. Myocardial ischaemia is due to a reduction in vessel diameter because of atheroma occlusion. Atherosclerosis is a degenerative disease of large and medium-sized arteries, characterised by the focal accumulation of lipid-rich material within the intima, with associated cellular reactions. The net result is a thickening and hardening of the arterial walls, which predisposes to ischaemia, vessel rupture, aneurysms, and thrombosis.

Atherosclerotic lesions are known as atheromas. The most widely accepted theory proposes that their pathogenesis involves the following sequence of events:

A. Chronic, low-grade endothelial injury results in the entry of cholesterol-rich, low-density lipoproteins (LDLs) into the intima; migration of macrophages into the intima; platelet adhesion to the damaged endothelium.

B. Intimal macrophages phagocytose lipid, forming barely visible pale bulges or 'fatty streaks'.

C. Adhering platelets release platelet-derived growth factor (PDGF); there is a proliferation of intimal smooth muscle cells (myointimal cells).

D. Myointimal cells deposit excess collagen and elastin in the intima forming 'lipid plaques', which are raised, yellow lesions consisting of free lipid (released by macrophages) and collagen.

E. Increased collagen deposition eventually results in the formation of dense fibrous plaques—'fibrolipid plaques'—which cause pressure atrophy of the underlying media and elastic lamina, with weakening of the arterial wall.

Risk factors for atherosclerosis include increasing age, hypertension, hyperlipidaemia, diabetes, smoking, obesity, a sedentary life-style, low socioeconomic status and low birth weight.

---

19. Ascites is the accumulation of free fluid in the peritoneal cavity. The most likely cause in a patient with cirrhosis is portal hypertension. This is a continuous elevation in portal venous pressure, which causes back-pressure in the portal vascular bed. As well as causing ascites, portal hypertension may also lead to splenomegaly and the development of varicose vein channels for portosystemic shunting of blood (e.g. oesophageal varices).

Ascites may develop in conditions other than cirrhosis, including:

- Peritonitis—inflammation of the peritoneum, usually secondary to infection.
- Malignancy in the peritoneal cavity.
- Hypoproteinaemia—as seen in nephrotic syndrome.
- Heart failure—due to reduced cardiac output.

---

20. The likely diagnosis in this patient is an infective exacerbation of her chronic obstructive pulmonary disease (COPD). The principles of management involve:

- Oxygen.
- Oral corticosteroid therapy, e.g. prednisolone.
- Nebulised bronchodilators, e.g. salbutamol.
- Antibiotics—initially broad-spectrum antibiotics can be used but, ideally, a sputum sample should be sent for culturing and antibiotic sensitivity measurements.

COPD patients are at increased risk of pulmonary infection. As a general rule, infective exacerbations require hospital admission in the initial stages.

EMQ answers

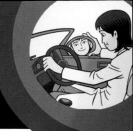

1. Nervous System

1. I. Hydrocephalus. An increase in CSF within the brain that may be congenital or acquired. Often treated with ventriculoperitoneal shunt surgery.
2. H. Alzheimer's disease. Memory disturbance is a common initial presentation of disease.
3. F. Extradural haemorrhage. Almost always the result of skull fracture, with decline in neurological function occurring after several hours of a post-traumatic lucid interval.
4. C. Multiple sclerosis. Diagnosis requires at least two episodes of CNS demyelination separated in time (i.e. recovery between episodes) and space (i.e. affecting different CNS areas).
5. A. Acute bacterial meningitis. Often presents with fever, headache, petechial rash and neck stiffness. CSF is cloudy because of increased neutrophils.

2. Cardiovascular system

1. E. Coarctation of the aorta. Causes headache, dizziness, interstitial bruits and radio-femoral pulse delay.
2. G. Dissecting aortic aneurysm. Classically causes central chest pain radiating to the back between the scapulae with pulse asymmetry. Chest X-ray changes include mediastinal widening, aortic knuckle distortion and left-sided pleural effusion.
3. J. Aortic stenosis. Syncope, angina and even sudden death are potential consequences of reduced cardiac output.
4. I. Giant cell arteritis. Affects the temporal arteries to cause scalp tenderness. Also often associated with polymyalgia rheumatica.
5. A. Ventricular septal defect. Other congenital causes of a left-to-right shunt include atrial septal defect and patent ductus arteriosus.

3. Respiratory system

1. D. Chronic obstructive pulmonary disease. Obstructive lung pattern with chronic inflammation in response to noxious stimuli (most commonly cigarette smoking) that is only partially reversible with bronchodilators.
2. H. Intrinsic (non-atopic) asthma. This is late-onset asthma that is often triggered by upper respiratory tract infection. IgE levels are normal (unlike atopic asthma).
3. F. Cystic fibrosis. A hereditary, multisystem disease that causes abnormally thick mucus. Affects several organs, but effects on the lung and pancreas are most marked.

4. B. Small cell lung cancer. Unique amongst lung cancers for its response to radiotherapy and chemotherapy, but prognosis remains very poor.
5. J. Sarcoidosis. Multisystem granulomatous disease of unknown aetiology that commonly causes lung disease. Raised serum angiotensin converting enzyme levels aid diagnosis.

4. Gastrointestinal system

1. E. Coeliac disease. A disease of malabsorption causing villous atrophy in the small intestine. The rash is that of dermatitis herpetiformis, which is strongly associated with coeliac disease.
2. D. Crohn's disease. Usually presents early in adult life causing full thickness granulomatous inflammation of any site in the GI tract. This commonly leads to strictures, but in a 'skip lesion' pattern, hence the normal areas of bowel on endoscopy.
3. A. Barrett's oesophagus. Metaplastic replacement of normal squamous epithelium with glandular columnar epithelium. Predisposes to adenocarcinoma of the oesophagus.
4. H. Oesophageal varices. Dilatation of oesophageal veins as a complication of portal hypertension.
5. F. Haemochromatosis. Caused by excessive iron deposition in the liver and elsewhere. This leads to cirrhosis if untreated. Excess melanin causes leaden grey pigmentation of skin.

5. Renal and urinary systems

1. D. Minimal change disease. Most common cause of nephrotic syndrome in children. Changes only seen on renal biopsy if examined by electron microscopy.
2. B. Alport's syndrome. A hereditary glomerulonephritis that commonly causes renal failure in the second decade of life in males affected by the X-linked form. Ocular disease and deafness to high-pitched sounds are associated features.
3. G. Acute tubular necrosis. Usually reversible renal failure caused by ischaemia or toxins.
4. I. Hydronephrosis. Dilatation of the renal pelvis and calyces in response to increased pressure from distal obstruction.
5. E. Goodpasture's syndrome. Autoimmune disease targeting type IV collagen in both the kidney and the lung.

6. Endocrine system

1. J. Adrenal crisis. A medical emergency caused by abrupt cessation of prolonged high dose corticosteroids.
2. A. Type I diabetes mellitus. Autoimmune destruction of β-cells in the pancreas result in the failure of insulin production.
3. D Hypothyroidism. Secondary to De Quervain's thyroiditis that may follow mumps infection. Causes a painfully enlarged thyroid gland with classical hypothyroid features of cold extremities and cold intolerance.
4. C. Cushing's syndrome. Caused by inappropriately elevated free glucocorticoid levels.
5. F. Cranial diabetes insipidus. Caused by failure of the posterior pituitary to produce anti-diuretic hormone.

7. Reproductive system

1. I. Endometriosis. Ectopic growth of endometrial tissue outside of the uterus.
2. G. Breast cancer. A breast lump is investigated by history/examination, imaging (mammography or ultrasound) and tissue sampling (fine-needle aspiration or core biopsy).
3. B. Cervical cancer. The same risk factors exist for development of the premalignant state, cervical intraepithelial neoplasia.
4. D. Choriocarcinoma. A malignant tumour of trophoblastic tissue, most commonly occurring from a hydatiform (molar) pregnancy.
5. E. Ectopic pregnancy. The implantation of a fertilised ovum outside the uterus. May cause severe haemorrhage from tubal rupture.

8. Musculoskeletal system

1. H. Metastatic disease. The most common tumours in bone are blood-borne metastases from other primary sites.
2. C. Paget's disease. Uncontrolled bone resorption and deposition. Most common in men over the age of 40 years.
3. E. Osteoarthritis. A very common disease of articular cartilage degeneration.

4. A. Osteogenesis imperfecta. A group of disorders characterised by the development of abnormal type I collagen. Also known as 'brittle bone disease'.
5. J. Duchenne muscular dystrophy. An inherited myopathy. The lack of dystrophin protein results in tears to muscle fibres on repeated contraction.

9. Haematological and immunological systems

1. E. Chronic myeloid leukaemia. Philadelphia chromosome is seen in 90% of cases.
2. B. Hodgkin's disease. A lymphoma characterised by painless lymphadenopathy and the presence of Reed–Sternberg cells (large binucleate cells).
3. F. Myeloma. Diagnosis here is based on skeletal lesions and characteristic serum electrophoresis.
4. G. Myasthenia gravis. Autoimmune disease of the post-synaptic acetylcholine receptor causing fatigability.
5. H. Thalassaemia. Caused by decreased α- or β-globin synthesis.

10. Dermatological system

1. G. Macule. A localised, flat area of altered skin colour that may be hyperpigmented (e.g. freckle), hypopigmented (e.g. vitiligo) or erythematous (e.g. capillary haemangioma).
2. E. Acne vulgaris. An inflammatory disorder of the pilosebaceous apparatus, characterised by comedones, pustules, papules, nodules, cysts and scars.
3. J. Pemphigus vulgaris. Causes intraepidermal bullae, which are flaccid and superficial. Erosions commonly develop.
4. D. Parakeratosis. A histological sign of increased epidermal growth, with excessive keratin and nuclear remnants persisting in the stratum corneum.
5. A. Acantholysis. Describes the loss of cellular cohesion between epidermal keratinocytes due to the rupture of intercellular bridges.

Index

A

abdominal aortic aneurysms (AAAs) 92
abetalipoproteinaemia 170
ABO incompatible blood transfusion 303
abortion, spontaneous 241–2
abscesses
   brain 51–2
   breast 244
   Brodie's 256
   intra-abdominal 178
   intrarenal 194
   liver 150
   lung 113, 114
   perivalvular 86
   skin 322
acantholysis 317
acanthosis 317
acetylcholine (ACh) 262
achalasia 132
achondroplasia 253
acne vulgaris 329, 330
acquired diseases 3
acquired immunodeficiency syndrome *see* AIDS
acromegaly 206–7
ACTH *see* adrenocorticotrophic hormone
actinic keratosis 336
acute coronary syndromes (ACS) 78
acute fatty liver of pregnancy 154
acute inflammatory demyelinating polyradiculopathy 59
acute lymphoblastic leukaemia (ALL) 289–90
acute myeloblastic leukaemia (AML) 289–90
acute nephritic syndrome 184–5, 187, 190
acute-phase proteins 12
acute respiratory distress syndrome (ARDS) 123–4
acute tubular necrosis (ATN) 193, 194
adaptive immunity 35
Addisonian crisis 223
Addison's disease 222, 277, 278, 334
adenocarcinoma
   endometrium 236–7
   fallopian tube 239
   gall bladder 158
   large bowel 177
   lung 118, 119, 122
   oesophagus 134
   pancreas 160
   renal 198–9
   stomach 138–9
   thyroid 215–16

adenohypophysis *see* pituitary, anterior
adenoma
   adrenal cortex 220
   bile duct 154
   hepatic 154
   large bowel 175, 176
   parathyroid 217
   pituitary 205–7
   renal cortex 198
   thyroid 215
   toxic thyroid 211, 215
adenoma–carcinoma sequence, large bowel 22, 23, 176
adenomatoid tumours, fallopian tube 239
adenomatous metaplasia, bladder 203
adenomatous polyps
   large bowel 176
   stomach 138
adenomyosis, endometrial 233
adenoviruses 162
ADH *see* antidiuretic hormone
adherence, bacterial 37
adhesions, small bowel 172, 178
adrenal cortex 219–23
   adenoma 220
   carcinoma 221
   hyperfunction 219–22
   hypofunction 222–3
adrenal crisis 222–3
adrenal gland
   bilateral haemorrhage 223
   disorders 73, 219–23
   hormones 219
adrenal hyperplasia, congenital 222
adrenal medulla 219, 223
adrenocortical insufficiency
   primary acute 222–3
   secondary 223
adrenocorticotrophic hormone (ACTH) 206
   deficiency 208
   ectopic secretion 120, 122, 219
   pituitary hypersecretion 207, 219
   stimulation test 206, 222
adult polycystic kidney disease (APKD) 182–3
aetiology 4
aflatoxins 24, 32, 154
agammaglobulinaemia
   transient physiological, of neonates 278, 279
   X-linked (Bruton) 279

aggressins 37
agranulocytosis 284
AIDS (HIV infection) 280–1
  gastrointestinal disorders 167
  Kaposi's sarcoma 342
  pneumonia 115
AIDS-related complex 281
airway obstruction 101
Albers–Schönberg disease 255
albinism 332
alcohol (ethanol)
  acute intoxication 57
  hepatic toxicity 151
alcohol abuse
  CNS disorders 55–6, 57
  myopathy 265
  oesophageal cancer 134
  oral cancer 131
  pancreatitis 158–9, 160
alcoholic liver disease 151
aldosterone
  deficiency 222
  excess secretion 221–2
allergic asthma 106
allergic contact dermatitis 320
allergic rhinitis 99
allopurinol 273
alopecia 330–1
  areata 331, 332
  scarring (cicatricial) 331
alpha$_1$-antitrypsin deficiency 104, 105, 147
α-fetoprotein 27, 45, 154, 250
Alport's syndrome 190–1
alveolar capillary injury 123
alveolitis, extrinsic allergic 111
Alzheimer's disease 54–5, 283
amines, vasoactive 9–10
amoebic abscess 150
amoebic dysentery 164
amyloid 282–3
amyloid precursor protein (APP) gene 54
amyloidosis 282–4
  AL 283
  hereditary 283
  localised 283–4
  myeloma 283, 294
  primary 283
  reactive systemic (AA-type) 256, 283
  renal disease 192–3
  rheumatoid arthritis 268, 283
  senile 284
  systemic 283
amyotrophic lateral sclerosis 55
anaemia 297–308
  aplastic 307
  from blood loss 298–9

causes 298
  of chronic disease 269
  classifications 297–8
  definition 297
  dyserythropoiesis 307
  haematinic deficiency 305–7
  haemolytic 299–304
  iron deficiency see iron-deficiency anaemia
  leucoerythroblastic 259
  in leukaemia 289, 291
  macrocytic 297
  megaloblastic 305–6, 309
  microcytic 297
  in myeloma 294, 295
  normocytic 297
  pernicious 135–6, 278, 305
  refractory 292
anaplastic carcinoma, thyroid 216
anaplastic neoplasm 17
androblastoma 250
androgenic alopecia 330
anencephaly 45
aneurysms 91–3
  Charcot–Bouchard 49
  dissecting 93
  false 91
  fusiform 91
  intracranial 49–50
  mycotic 86, 91
  pathogenesis 72, 92
  saccular (berry) 49–50, 91
  syphilitic (luetic) 93
  true 91
  ventricular 81
angina pectoris 78–9
  Prinzmetal's (vasospastic) 78, 79
  stable 78, 79
  unstable 78, 79
angiodysplasia, large intestinal 174
angiofibroma, nasopharyngeal 100
angiogenesis, tumour growth and 22, 23
angioma, cherry 337
angiomyolipoma, kidney 198
angiosarcoma 96
  liver 155
angular cheilitis 307
anisocytosis 297, 298
ankylosing spondylitis 270–1, 318
Ann Arbor staging system 286, 287
anorectal agenesis 162
anorectal anomalies 162
anovulatory menstrual cycle 234
anterior cerebral artery 49
anthrax 324
anti-DNA antibodies 186, 275
anti-endomyseal antibodies 169

anti-glomerular basement membrane (GBM)
    antibodies 186
anti-inflammatory drugs 9
antibiotic resistance 38
anticardiolipin antibodies 77, 275
antidiuretic hormone (ADH) 205, 206
    deficiency/unresponsiveness 208–9
    ectopic secretion 209
    inappropriate secretion 120, 122, 209–10
antimitochondrial antibodies 155
antineutrophil cytoplasmic antibodies (ANCA) 94, 95
antinuclear antibodies 275
antiphospholipid antibodies 275
antiphospholipid antibody syndrome 77
antithrombin III deficiency 77
anus, imperforate 162
aorta, coarctation 68
aortic aneurysms 91, 92–3
    abdominal (AAAs) 92
    dissecting 93
aortic atresia 68
aortic dissection 92–3
aortic isthmus 64
aortic regurgitation 83, 93
aortic stenosis 68, 83
    calcific 82–3
aortitis
    infectious 91
    syphilitic 91, 93, 94
APC gene 21
aphthous ulcers 129, 130
aplastic anaemia 307
apocrine metaplasia, breast 244
apoptosis 14, 15–16
arachidonic acid 9
Arnold–Chiari malformation 45
aromatic amines 24
arrhythmias, cardiac 80–1
arterial remodelling 72
arterial thrombosis 76
arteriolitis, necrotising 74
arteriolosclerosis 69
    hyperplastic 74
    renal 74
arteriosclerosis 69
arthritis
    enteropathic 272
    mutilans 318
    psoriatic 271, 318
    reactive 272
    Reiter's disease 271
    rheumatoid *see* rheumatoid arthritis (RA)
    sarcoid 272
    septic (infective) 268, 274
    seronegative 267, 270
    in systemic disease 271–2

systemic lupus erythematosus 277
arthropathies 265–74
    compared 271
    crystal 272–4
asbestos 111, 128, 179
asbestosis 111
Aschoff's nodules 84
ascites 142–3
Aspergillus 32, 85, 115
aspirin 126, 147, 310–11
Assmann focus 116
asteatotic eczema 321
asthma 106–9, 126
    acute severe 108
    pathogenesis 106–7, 108
astrocytes 56
astrocytoma 56–7
astroviruses 162
atelectasis 102, 126, 127
atheromas 71
atherosclerosis 69–72
    aneurysms 72, 91, 92
    arterial remodelling 72
    clinical management 70
    coronary arteries 78
    in diabetes mellitus 70, 76, 225
    hypertension and 70, 73
    pathogenesis 70–1, 72
    risk factors 70
    stages of development 71
atherosclerotic plaques 71
athlete's foot 326
atopic disease 319
atopic eczema 319–20
atrial septal defects 64, 65
atrioventricular septal defect 64, 66
Auer rods 290
autoimmune diseases 5, 275–8
    Addison's disease and 222
    hepatitis 149
    myasthenia gravis and 263
    neuromuscular junction 262–3
    organ- or cell-type specific 277–8
    parathyroid glands 219
    systemic or multisystem 275, 276
    vasculitis 94
autoimmune haemolytic anaemia 303
    cold antibody type 303, 304, 305
    warm antibody type 303, 304, 305
autonomic nervous system disorders 61–2
avascular necrosis 257–9
azathioprine 167

B
B-cell lymphomas 287, 288
Bacillus anthracis 324

Bacillus cereus 163, 164
bacteraemia 114, 256, 274
bacteria 31–2
   adherence 37
   antiphagocytic devices 37
   classification 33
   mechanisms of pathogenicity 37–8
bacterial infections
   gastrointestinal 163, 164
   infective endocarditis 85
   lower genital tract 229–30
   meningitis 51
   myocarditis 88
   neutropenic patients 284
   penis 247
   pericarditis 90
   pneumonia 112
   septic arthritis 274
   skin 320, 322–4
   urinary tract 202
bacterial overgrowth syndrome, small intestinal 170
bacteriuria 194
Baker's cyst 268
balanitis 247
balantidiasis 164
Barrett's oesophagus 132, 134
Bartholin's cyst 229
basal cell carcinoma 340–1
basal cell papilloma 336
basal ganglia disorders 55
basophilia 286
BCG vaccination 118
BCR-abl gene 290, 291
Beau's lines 333
Becker's dystrophy 264
Becker's naevi 338
bejel 324
Bence-Jones proteins 195, 294
bends, the 125
benign prostatic hyperplasia 250–1
Bernard–Soulier syndrome 310
berry aneurysms 49–50
β–blockers 126, 141
β$_2$-microglobulin 283
bile-duct adenomas 154
bile ducts, vanishing 156
bile infarcts 155, 156
bile lakes 156
biliary cirrhosis 155–6
   primary 155, 156, 157
   secondary 155–6, 157
biliary tract disorders 146–58
biliary tree disorders 155–6
bilirubin 143
   conjugated and unconjugated 144, 145

   metabolism 144
blackheads 329
bladder
   cancer 199, 203–4
   diverticula 200, 203
   metaplasia 203
   tumours 203–4
bladder neck, obstruction 201
blast cells 289, 290
blast crisis 290
blastomycosis 329
bleeding disorders 308–14
   in myeloma 295
blind loop syndrome 170
blistering disorders 334–6
blisters 315, 334, 335
blood disorders 275–314
   systemic lupus erythematosus 277
   thrombosis 77
blood flow, changes 77
blood loss, anaemia of 298–9
blood transfusion
   dilutional thrombocytopenia 310
   incompatible ABO 303
blue bloaters 106
blue naevi 338
boil 322
bone
   changes in myeloma 294
   deformity 255
   eburnation 266
   erosions, rheumatoid arthritis 268
   infections and trauma 256–9
   matrix, disorders of 253–5
   pain 254, 255, 259, 260, 295
   sclerosis 218, 259, 266
   structure, disorders of 253–6
   tumours 259–61, 262
bone marrow
   disease 309
   failure 289, 291, 307
   hyperplasia 296
   infiltration 308
   transplantation 167, 290
bone metastases 24, 259, 262
   osteolytic/osteosclerotic 259
   prostatic carcinoma 252, 259
Borrelia burgdorferi 52, 274, 324
botulism 262
Bouchard's nodes 266
Boutonnière deformity 268
bovine spongiform encephalopathy (BSE) 35, 53
bowel *see* intestine
Bowen's disease 247, 341
bradykinin 9

brain
  abscess 51–2
  contusions and lacerations 46–7
  diffuse axonal injury 47
  effects of hypertension 74
  metastatic tumours 57–8
  perinatal injury 46
  traumatic injury 46–7
  tumours 56–8
BRCA1 gene 21, 238, 245
BRCA2 gene 238, 245
breast 244–7
  abscess 244
  cysts 244
  epithelial hyperplasia 244
  fibrocystic changes 244
  inflammations/infections 244
  lumps, assessment 244
  male 247
  neoplasms 245–7
breast carcinoma 245–7, 259
  invasive 245–6
  male 247
  screening 246–7
  in situ 245
Brenner tumours, ovarian 239
Breslow thickness 340
brittle bone disease 253
brittle nails 332, 333
Brodie's abscess 256
bronchial hamartomas 122
bronchiectasis 109, 118
bronchiolitis 103, 106
bronchitis, chronic 103, 105–6
bronchoalveolar carcinoma 121
bronchodilators 104
bronchogenic carcinoma 106, 118–21
  clinical features 119, 120
  histological types 119, 122
  prognosis and staging 120, 121
  treatment 120–1
bronchopneumonia 112–13
  tuberculous 116, 117
bronze diabetes 146
brown tumours 217
bruising 308
Brunn's nests 203
Bruton's X-linked agammaglobulinaemia 279
Budd–Chiari syndrome 152–3
budding, virus particles 36
Buerger's disease 94
bulla 315
bullous pemphigoid 335, 336
Burkholderia cepacia 109
Burkitt's lymphoma 287

C
C-reactive protein (CRP) 12
C3 nephritic factor 187
CA125 27, 238
Caisson disease 125
calcium pyrophosphate deposition (pseudogout) 272, 273–4
callus 258
Campbell de Morgan's spot 337
Campylobacter jejuni 163, 164
cancer 17–27
  clinical pathology 27
  epidemiology 19, 20
  host defences 27
  molecular basis 19–22
  pericarditis 90
  thrombosis 77
  see also tumour(s)
candidosis (*Candida albicans* infections) 326–7
  genital 230, 247
  lungs 115
  mucocutaneous 327
  oral 130, 326
  skin 321, 326–7
  systemic 327
capillary haemangiomas 95, 338
Caplan's syndrome 110, 269
caput medusae 142
carbon monoxide (CO) poisoning 56
carbuncle 322
carcinogenesis 24–7
  chemical 24–5
  radiation 25–6
  viral 26–7
carcinoid heart disease 86
carcinoid tumours 121, 175
carcinoma 18–19
carcinoma *in situ* 19
  breast 245
  cutaneous 341
  penis 247
cardiac referred pain 78
cardiac tamponade 81, 89
cardiomyopathy 87–8
cardiovascular risk factors 70
cardiovascular system 63–98
carpal tunnel syndrome 59
cartilage
  articular, destruction 266, 267, 268
  forming bone tumours 260–1
caseation (caseous necrosis) 15
caspases 15
cataracts 226, 320
causalgia 61–2
cavernous haemangiomas 96, 338

CD4+ T cells 267, 280, 281
CD8+ T cells 280
cell death 13–16
    mechanisms 14
    programmed 15
cell lysis (cytolysis) 36
cell-mediated immunity
    mediating glomerular damage 188
    tumours 27
cellular transformation 31
central nervous system (CNS) 43–58
    common pathological features 43–4
    degenerative disorders 54–5
    demyelinating diseases 53–4
    infections 50–3
    malformations/developmental disease 44–6
    metabolic disorders and toxins 55–6
    neoplasms 56–8
    traumatic injuries 46–8
    see also brain; spinal cord
central pontine myelinolysis 57
centrilobular necrosis 153
cerebellar atrophy, alcohol-induced 57
cerebral arteries 49
cerebral atrophy, alcohol-induced 57
cerebral infarction 48–9, 50
cerebral oedema 43
cerebral palsy 46
cerebrovascular disease 48–50
    hypertensive 50, 74
ceruloplasmin 146, 147
cervical carcinoma 27, 232, 233
cervical intraepithelial neoplasia (CIN) 19, 27, 231–2
cervical screening 232
cervical spondylosis 267
cervicitis 231
cervix, uterine 231–2
Chagas' disease 132, 162, 163–4
chancre 230, 323
Charcot–Bouchard microaneurysms 49
Charcot–Leyden crystals 107
Charcot–Marie–Tooth disease 58
Charcot's joints 272
chemical carcinogens 24–5
chemical pathology 3
chemotaxins, neutrophil 7
chemotherapy 22
cherry angioma 337
chest pain
    ischaemic heart disease 78, 79
    lung cancer 120
chest trauma 127, 128
children
    atopic eczema 319, 320
    gait abnormalities 274
Chlamydia trachomatis 34, 229, 237

chlamydial infections 34
    genital tract 229, 233, 237, 247
    peritonitis 178
    pneumonia 114
chloasma 334
chloroquine myopathy 265
chocolate cysts 234
cholangiocarcinoma 155
cholangitis 157
cholecystitis 157, 158
choledocholithiasis 157
cholelithiasis see gallstones
cholestasis 143–5
    intrahepatic, of pregnancy 154
cholesterol
    emboli 198
    raised (hypercholesterolaemia) 70, 77
    stones 156, 157
chondroblastoma 260–1
chondrocalcinosis 273
chondrodermatitis nodularis 337
chondroma 260
chondromyxoid fibroma 261
chondrosarcoma 260
chorioadenoma destruens 243
choriocarcinoma 243
Christmas disease 312
chromaffin cells 205, 219, 223
chromosomal translocations 287, 290
chronic granulocytic leukaemia 293
chronic lymphocytic leukaemia (CLL) 291
chronic myeloid leukaemia (CML) 290–1
chronic myelomonocytic leukaemia (CMML) 292
chronic obstructive pulmonary disease (COPD)
        103–4, 107
chylocele 248
chylothorax 127
Ciacci's syndrome 59
circle of Willis 49
cirrhosis 140–1
    alcoholic 151
    biliary 155–6, 157
    classification 140, 141
    clinical features 142
    complications 141–3, 153, 154
    postnecrotic 150
clear cell carcinoma, ovarian 239
cleft palate/lip 129, 130
Clonorchis sinensis 155
Clostridium botulinum 262
Clostridium difficile-associated diarrhoea 163, 164
Clostridium perfringens 163, 164
clot, blood 76
clotting factor abnormalities 311–14
clubbing 85, 333
CNS see central nervous system

coagulation disorders 311–14
coagulative necrosis 14, 139
coal-worker's pneumoconiosis 110
coarctation of aorta 68
cobalamin deficiency *see* vitamin B_{12} deficiency
Codman's tumour 260–1
coeliac disease 169–70, 335
cold sores 325
colliquative necrosis 14
colonic diverticulosis 172–3
colonisation 29
colorectal carcinoma 176–7
    adenoma–carcinoma sequence 22, 23, 176
    inherited 176
coma, diabetic 225
comedones 329
commensals 30
common cold 99
common variable immunodeficiency 279
complement
    mediating glomerular disease 186–7
    system 8, 9
complications 4
compression neuropathies 59, 255–6, 269
concussion 46
condylomata acuminata 229, 247
condylomata lata 230, 323
congenital adrenal hyperplasia 222
congenital diseases 3
congenital heart disease (CHD) 63–9
    causes 63
    left-to-right shunts 64–6
    obstructive defects 68
    right-to-left shunts 66–8
Conn's syndrome 221
contact dermatitis 320
copper, deposition in liver 146–7
cor pulmonale 74, 104, 108, 126
coronary arteries
    occlusion, myocardial infarction 80
    spasm 78
    stenosis 78
coronary artery bypass grafting (CABG) 79
corpora amylacea 251
cortical degeneration 54–5
corticosteroids 9, 219
    adverse effects of therapy 220, 221, 222, 223
    induced myopathy 265
    induced purpura 309
    inflammatory bowel disease 166–7
corticotroph adenoma, pituitary 207, 219
corticotrophin-releasing factor (CRF)
    deficiency 207
    ectopic secretion 219
cortisol 219
    plasma 208, 221, 222

Councilman bodies 139
Courvoisier's sign 161
coxsackie virus 88
'crabs' 327
crescentic glomerulonephritis 188
cretinism 56, 212
Creutzfeldt–Jakob disease (CJD) 35, 53
    variant (vCJD) 53
Crigler–Najjar syndrome 144, 145
Crohn's disease 164–5, 272
    versus ulcerative colitis 166–7
croup 101
Cryptococcus neoformans 52
cryptorchidism 248
cryptosporidiosis 164
crystal arthropathies 272–4
Cullen's sign 159
Curschmann's spirals 107
Cushing's disease 207, 219, 221
Cushing's syndrome 219–21, 309
cutaneous T cell lymphoma 341–2
cyanocobalamin deficiency *see* vitamin B_{12} deficiency
cyanosis 66, 67
cystic fibrosis (CF) 109
cystic medial degeneration 91
cystic renal dysplasia 182
cystitis 202
    glandularis 203
    interstitial 202
cytokines 12
cytomegalovirus pneumonitis 115
cytopathic effect, direct 30
cytotoxic antibodies, mediating glomerular damage 186
cytotoxic T cells (T_C) 27, 36–7, 280

D
dandruff 331
Dandy–Walker malformation 45
De Quervain's thyroiditis 213–14
death receptors 15, 16
decompression sickness 125
deep vein thrombosis (DVT) 76, 124
definition, disease 4
dementia 54–5
    Alzheimer's disease 54–5
    multi-infarct 50
demyelinating diseases 53–4
dense deposit disease 189
dermal tumours, benign 337
dermatitis *see* eczema/dermatitis
dermatitis herpetiformis 169, 335–6
dermatofibroma 337
dermatofibrosarcoma 342
dermatological terminology 315–17
dermatomyositis 265, 276

dermatophyte infections 230, 326, 331
dermoid cysts, ovarian 240
dexamethasone suppression test 221
diabetes insipidus (DI) 208–9, 210
   cranial 208, 209
   nephrogenic 208, 209
diabetes mellitus (DM) 223–7
   atherosclerosis 70, 76, 225
   bronze 146
   chronic pancreatitis 160
   complications 225–7
   diagnosis 224, 225
   secondary 223
   type I 223–4, 277, 278
   type II 223, 224, 284
   vascular effects 76, 225
diabetic ketoacidosis (DKA) 225
diabetic maculopathy 226
diabetic nephropathy 192, 225–6
diabetic neuropathy 60, 225, 227
diabetic retinopathy 225, 226
dialysis-associated cystic kidney disease 182, 183
diarrhoea 162–4
   antibiotic-associated 163, 164
   classification 162, 163
   in graft-versus-host disease 167
   malabsorption syndromes 168, 170
   traveller's 163
DIDMOAD syndrome 209
diffuse axonal injury 47
diffuse proliferative glomerulonephritis 188
DiGeorge syndrome 30, 219, 279–80, 297
dilated (congestive) cardiomyopathy 87
disaccharidase deficiency 170
discoid eczema 321
discoid skin rash 276
disease 3
   classification 3
   features 4
disease-modifying anti-rheumatic drugs (DMARDs)
   269
disseminated intravascular coagulation (DIC) 304,
   310, 313–14
diverticulitis 173
diverticulosis, colonic 172–3
DNA damage, radiation-induced 25
DNA repair mechanisms 26
DNA viruses 32
   oncogenic 26, 27
   replication cycle 35–6
Down syndrome 162
Dressler's syndrome 81
drug-induced disorders
   alopecia 330
   haemostatic 309
   hypertension 73
   liver disease 150, 151
   lung disease 126
   malabsorption 168
   myopathies 265
   neuropathies 60
   pigmentation 334
   psoriasis 318
   renal disease 189, 194, 195
   thyrotoxicosis 211
dry eye syndrome 269
Dubin–Johnson syndrome 144, 145
Duchenne muscular dystrophy 263–4
ductal carcinoma *in situ* 245
ductal hyperplasia, breast 244
ductus arteriosus 64
   patent (persistent) 64, 65, 66
Dukes staging system 177
duodenal ulcers 136
dwarfism 253
dysautonomia, familial 59
dysentery 162, 271
dysfibrinogenemia 313
dysgerminoma 240
dyskeratosis 317
dysphagia 132, 133
dysplasia 17, 18–19
dysplastic naevus syndrome, familial 338, 339
dyspnoea 82
dystrophin 263

E
E-cadherin gene 138
ecchymosis 308
eclampsia 154, 243
ecthyma 322
ectoparasites 31, 33–4
ectopic pregnancy 239–40
eczema/dermatitis 319–21
   acute 319
   asteatotic (craquelé; winter) 321
   atopic 319–20
   chronic 319
   contact 320
   discoid (nummular) 321
   hand 321
   nail involvement 332
   seborrhoeic 320–1
   stasis (varicose) 97, 321
eczema herpeticum 320, 325
Ehlers–Danlos syndrome 309
Eisenmenger's syndrome 66
electromechanical dissociation 89
elephantiasis 98, 328
elliptocytosis, hereditary 299

Embden–Meyerhof glycolytic pathway 299, 300
embolic renal disease 198
emphysema 103, 104–5, 147
empty sella syndrome 207
empyema
    gallbladder 158
    pleural 113, 114, 127
encephalitis, viral 52, 325
encephalocele 45
enchondroma 260
enchondromatosis 260
endocarditis
    infective 84–6, 192
    Libman–Sacks 86
    non-bacterial thrombotic (marantic) 86
    rheumatic 84
endocervical polyps 231
endocrine disorders 205–28
    alopecia 330
    amyloidosis 283–4
    hypertension 73
    lung cancer 120
    myopathies 265
endometrial carcinoma 236–7
endometrial hyperplasia 235
endometrial polyps 235
endometrioid ovarian tumours 239
endometriosis 233–4
endometritis, chronic 233
endometrium 233–7
    adenomyosis 233
    contraceptives/HRT and 234–5
    functional disorders 234
endomyocardial fibrosis 87
β-endorphin 206
endoscopic retrograde cholangiopancreatography
        (ERCP) 156, 157
endothelial dysfunction 70, 71
endothelial injury 77
endotoxic shock 37
endotoxins 32, 37
Entamoeba histolytica 150, 164
enterocolitis 162–4
    bacterial 163
    infectious 162–4
    necrotising 163, 174
enterogenous cysts 179
enteropathic arthritis 272
entrapment neuropathy see nerve compression/entrap-
        ment syndromes
enzyme deficiencies, red cell 299–300
eosinophilia 284, 286
ependymal cells 56
ependymoma 57
ephelides 334

epidermal naevi 339
epidermal tumours
    benign 336–7
    malignant 340–1
epidermis 316
Epidermophyton infections 326
epidural haemorrhage 47
epinephrine (adrenaline) 205, 219
epispadias 200
epithelioid histiocytes 12
Epstein–Barr virus (EBV) 26, 27, 100, 286
c-erbB-2 (HER-2) gene 20, 238, 246
erosion 317
erysipelas 323
erythema 319
erythema multiforme 325
erythrasma 322
erythrocytes see red blood cells
erythrocytosis 308
erythroderma 318
erythroplakia (erythroplasia), oral 130
erythroplasia of Queyrat 247
erythropoietin 308
Escherichia coli
    enterohaemorrhagic (EHEC) 163, 164
    enterotoxigenic (ETEC) 163, 164
    osteomyelitis 256
    verocytotoxin-producing 197
ethanol see alcohol
Ewing's sarcoma 261
excoriation 316
exocytosis 317
exophthalmos 212
exostosis, cartilage-capped 260
exotoxins 32, 37
extradural haemorrhage 47
extrinsic allergic alveolitis 111
exudates 127
eye disease
    diabetic 226–7
    rheumatoid arthritis 269

F
Fabry's syndrome 191
factor V Leiden 77
factor VIII deficiency 311–12
factor IX deficiency 312
fallopian tube 237–9
    cysts 238
    ectopic pregnancy 240
    inflammatory disorders 237–8
    tumours 239
Fallot's tetralogy 66–7
familial adenomatous polyposis (FAP) 176
familial dysplastic naevus syndrome 338, 339

Fanconi's anaemia 307
fat necrosis 15
  breast 244
fatigability 261
fatty liver
  acute, of pregnancy 154
  alcoholic 151
  non-alcoholic 151
fatty streaks 70, 71
Felty's syndrome 269, 295
femoral hernia 172
fetal alcohol syndrome 57
fetal circulation 64
FEV_1 103
FEV_1/FVC ratio 103
fibre, dietary 173
fibrin degradation products 314
fibrinoid necrosis 15, 73, 75, 275
fibrinous inflammation 11
fibro-epithelial polyps, ureteric 203
fibroadenoma, breast 245
fibrocystic change, breast 244
fibroids, uterine 235–6
fibroma
  bone 261
  chondromyxoid 261
  periungual 332
  pleural 127
  renal 198
fibrosarcoma 261
fibrosis 10
  breast 244
  liver 140, 153
  pleural 118, 126
  pulmonary *see* pulmonary fibrosis
fibrous dysplasia 261
filariasis 98, 328
fimbriae 37
fimbrial cysts 238
finger clubbing 85, 333
fistulae 12
floppy valve syndrome 83–4
foam cells 71
focal (segmental) proliferative glomerulonephritis
    188, 191, 193
focal segmental glomerulosclerosis 190
folic acid deficiency 130, 305–6
follicle-stimulating hormone (FSH) 206, 207
  deficiency 208
follicular B cell lymphoma 287
follicular ovarian cysts 238
follicular thyroid adenocarcinoma 215–16
folliculitis 322
foramen ovale 64
forced expired volume in one second (FEV_1) 103
foreign bodies 5, 12

foreign body giant cells 12
fractures 257
  avascular necrosis after 257–9
  healing 257, 258
  pathological 254, 256, 257, 259
freckles 334
Friedreich's ataxia 55
fungal infections
  central nervous system 52
  deep mycoses 329
  infective endocarditis 85
  lower genital tract 230
  penis 247
  pneumonia 115
  skin 326–7
fungi 31, 32
  classification 33
furuncle 322

G
galactorrhoea 206
gall bladder
  carcinoma 158
  diseases 156–8
  mucocele 158
gallstones 156–8
  cholesterol 156, 157
  complications 155, 157, 158
  pigment 156
Gamna–Gandy nodules 296
ganglioneuroma 223
gangrene 15, 39
Gardnerella vaginalis 229
gas gangrene 15
gastric adenocarcinoma 138–9
gastric polyps 138
gastric ulceration 136–7
gastrinoma 137, 227, 228
gastritis 135–6
  acute 135
  autoimmune chronic 135–6, 278
  chronic 135–6
  reactive (reflux) 136
gastro-oesophageal reflux disease (GORD) 132
gastroenteritis
  bacterial 163, 272
  viral 162
gastrointestinal stromal tumours (GISTs) 139
gastrointestinal (GI) system 129–79
gastropathy, hypertrophic 137
gender differences
  atherosclerosis 70
  osteoarthritis 265
germ cell tumours
  intracranial 57
  ovary 238, 240

testis 249–50
germinomas, pineal 210
gestational trophoblastic disease 243–4
Ghon focus 116
giant cell arteritis 95
giant cell tumour 261
giant cells, multinucleate 10, 12
giardiasis 164
gigantism 206
Gilbert's syndrome 144, 145
glandular metaplasia, bladder 203
Glanzmann's disease 310
glaucoma 227
gliadin 169, 170
glial cells 56
glioblastoma 57
gliomas 56–7
glomerular disease 184–93
  aetiology 184, 185
  clinical manifestations 184–6
  diagnosis 186
  mechanisms of damage 186–8
  patterns 184
  in systemic disease 191–3
glomerulonephritis
  chronic 191
  diffuse proliferative 188
  focal (segmental) proliferative 188, 191, 193
  hereditary 190–1
  membranoproliferative (MPGN) 187, 188–9, 191
  poststreptococcal 186, 188
  proliferative 188–9
  rapidly progressive (crescentic) 188, 193
glomerulosclerosis 190
  diabetic 192, 226
  diffuse 192
  focal segmental 190
  nodular 192
glossitis 130
glucagonomas 227, 228
glucocorticoid hormones 219
  excess 219–22
  insufficiency 222
glucose
  blood, control 227
  plasma 224, 225
  red cell metabolism 299, 300
  tolerance, impaired 224, 225
glucose-6-phosphate dehydrogenase (G6PD) deficiency 300
glutathione synthetase deficiency 300
gluten 169, 170
glycolytic enzymes, deficiencies 300
glycosuria 202, 227, 230
goitre 214–15
  diffuse non-toxic (simple) 214–15

endemic 215
exophthalmic 211
multinodular 215
toxic 214
toxic multinodular 211, 214
goitrogenic agents 215
gonadoblastomas 240
gonadotrophin deficiency 208
gonadotrophin-releasing hormone (GnRH)
  agonists 236
  deficiency 207
gonorrhoea 237
Goodpasture's syndrome
  pulmonary disease 111, 126
  renal disease 185, 186, 188, 189
gout 272–3, 289
graft-versus-host disease 167
Gram-negative bacteria 31
  skin infections 324
Gram-positive bacteria 31, 33
Gram staining 31–2
granulation tissue 11, 13
granulomas 12, 13
  lethal midline 100
  pyogenic 337
  tuberculosis 115–16
granulomatous inflammation 12, 38–9
granulosa cell tumours 240
Graves' disease 211–12, 214, 277, 278
greenstick fractures 257
Grey Turner's sign 159
growth factors 12
growth hormone (GH) 206
  deficiency 208
  hypersecretion 206–7
Guillain–Barré syndrome 59
gynaecomastia 247

H
haemangiomas 95–6
  capillary 95, 338
  cavernous 96, 338
  liver 154
  sclerosing 96
haemarthrosis 312
haematemesis 134
haematinic deficiency 305–7
haematocele 248
haematological disorders see blood disorders
haematology 3
haematoma 309
haematopoietic malignancies 259, 285–95
haematosalpinx 240
haematuria
  asymptomatic 184, 187, 190
  glomerular disease 184

haemochromatosis 146
haemodialysis
    associated amyloidosis 283
    chronic 272
haemoglobin
    concentration 297
    sickle cell (HbS) 301, 302
    unstable variants 302
haemoglobinopathies 300–2
haemoglobinuria 299
    paroxysmal nocturnal 302, 309
haemolysis 299
haemolytic anaemia 299–304
    acquired red cell defects 302
    antibody-mediated 303–4, 305
    autoimmune 303, 305
    congenital 303
    hereditary red cell defects 299–302
    isoimmune antibody-mediated 303, 305
    macroangiopathic 304
    mechanical red cell damage 304
    microangiopathic 304
haemolytic disease of newborn (HDN) 303
haemolytic uraemic syndrome (HUS)
        197, 310
haemopericardium 81, 89
haemophilia 311–12
    A 311–12
    B 312
Haemophilus influenzae 101, 106, 109
haemoptysis 120
haemorrhage 298–9
haemorrhagic disease of newborn 313
haemorrhagic inflammation 12
haemorrhoids (piles) 142, 174–5
haemosiderinuria 302
haemosiderosis, idiopathic pulmonary
        111, 126
haemostatic disorders 308–14
haemothorax 127
hair disorders 330–1
hairy cell leukaemia 292
halo naevi 338
hamartomatous polyps
    large bowel 175
    stomach 138
hands
    dermatitis 321
    rheumatoid arthritis 268
Hansen's disease 59–60
hare lip 129
Hartmann's pouch 158
Hashimoto's thyroiditis 213, 214, 277, 278
hay fever 99
head and neck cancer 131
head injuries 46–8

healing
    fracture 257, 258
    tissue 11
heart
    effects of hypertension 73–4, 82
    neoplasms 88
    referred pain 78
heart disease
    carcinoid 86
    congenital see congenital heart disease
    ischaemic see ischaemic heart disease
    rheumatic 84
heart failure 81–2, 123, 127
    left-sided see left ventricular failure
    right-sided see right heart failure
heart failure cells 123
heart valve disease 82–6
    degenerative 82–4
    rheumatic 84
    see also endocarditis
heart valves
    infection 85
    prosthetic, complications 86
    regurgitation (incompetence) 82, 86
    stenosis 82
heart–lung transplants 126
heavy metals 24
Heberden's nodes 266
Heinz bodies 300
Helicobacter pylori infection
    diagnosis 136
    gastritis 135
    neoplastic complications 138, 139, 287
    peptic ulceration 137
HELLP syndrome 153–4
helminths 31, 33–4
Henoch–Schönlein purpura 192, 309
hepatic adenomas 154
hepatic disease see liver disease
hepatic encephalopathy 57, 145, 149–50
hepatic failure 123, 141, 145
    fulminant 146
hepatic steatosis see fatty liver
hepatic tumours 146
hepatic vein obstruction 151–3
hepatisation
    grey 114
    red 114
hepatitis 140
    alcoholic 151
    autoimmune 149
    fulminant 149–50
    neonatal 147
    viral 147–9
hepatitis A 147–8
hepatitis B 37, 148, 149, 154

hepatitis B virus (HBV) 26, 148, 149
hepatitis C 148–9, 154
hepatitis D 149
hepatitis E 149
hepatocellular carcinoma 148, 154
hepatocerebral degeneration, chronic 57
hepatorenal syndrome 145
hepatotoxins 151
HER-2 gene see c-erbB-2 gene
hereditary elliptocytosis 299
hereditary haemorrhagic telangiectasia 309
hereditary motor and sensory neuropathies (HMSN) 58
hereditary non-polyposis colon cancer (HNPCC)
        26, 176
hereditary sensory and autonomic neuropathies
        (HSAN) 58, 59
hereditary spherocytosis 299
hernias, abdominal 171–2
herpes simplex virus (HSV) 325
    cold sores (herpes labialis) 325
    disseminated infection 325
    encephalitis 52, 325
    genital infection (genital herpes) 229, 247, 325
    oral infection (herpetic stomatitis) 130
herpes zoster (shingles) 60, 325–6
hexose monophosphate shunt 299, 300
    enzyme deficiencies 300
hiatus hernia 133
highly active anti-retroviral therapy (HAART) 281
Hirschsprung's disease 161
hirsutism 331
histamine 10
histiocytes, epithelioid 12
histiocytoma
    cutaneous 337
    malignant fibrous 261
histopathology 3
histoplasmosis 329
HIV see human immunodeficiency virus
hoarseness 101, 102, 120, 134
Hodgkin's disease 286, 287
homocysteine 70
hormone replacement therapy (HRT) 234–5, 254
Horner's syndrome 61, 120
horseshoe kidney 181
hospital-acquired infection 38
host defences 35
HPV see human papillomavirus
HRT see hormone replacement therapy
HSV see herpes simplex virus
human chorionic gonadotrophin (hCG) 243, 250
human immunodeficiency virus (HIV) 26, 30, 280
    infection 280–1
    see also AIDS
human papillomavirus (HPV) 324
    cervical neoplasia and 231

genital tract infection 229, 247
    nasal inverted papilloma 100
    oncogenicity 26, 27
    vulval neoplasia and 230
human T cell leukaemia virus (HTLV) 26
humoral immunity, tumours 27
Hunner's ulcer 202
Hunter's syndrome 255
Huntington's disease 55
Hurler's syndrome 255
hyaline deposition 72, 73, 75
hydatidiform mole 243
hydrocele 248
hydrocephalus 43–4
hydromyelia 45–6
hydronephrosis 201
hydropic degeneration 139
hydrops fetalis 303
hydrosalpinx 237
hydrothorax 127
hydroureter 200, 201
21-hydroxylase deficiency 222
hyperaemia, acute inflammation 6
hyperaldosteronism 221–2
hyperbilirubinaemia 143
    conjugated 144, 145
    unconjugated 144, 145, 299
hypercalcaemia 120, 195, 217, 259
hypercholesterolaemia 70, 77
hypercoagulability 77
hyperemesis gravidarum 243
hyperkeratosis 316
hyperlipidaemia 71
hypernephroma 198–9
hyperosmolar non-ketotic (HONK) coma 225
hyperparathyroidism 217–18, 256
    primary 217, 218
    secondary 217–18
    tertiary 218
hyperpigmentation 334, 335
hyperpituitarism 205–7
hyperplasia 18
hyperplastic polyps
    large bowel 175
    stomach 138
hypersplenism 296, 304
hypertension 72–5
    in adrenal disorders 73, 221
    atherosclerosis and 70, 73
    benign 72–3, 74
    causes 72, 73
    cerebrovascular disease 50, 74
    classification 72–3
    complications and effects 73–4, 75
    definitions 72
    effects on heart 73–4, 82

hypertension—cont'd
  malignant (accelerated) 72, 73, 74, 196
  nephrosclerosis 74, 75, 195–6
  in pre-eclampsia 242
  primary (essential) 72, 73
  in renal disease 73, 74, 183
  renovascular 197
  secondary 72, 73
hypertensive encephalopathy 75
hyperthyroidism 210–12
  myopathy 265
  peripheral neuropathy 60
  primary 211, 215
  secondary 211, 215
hypertrichosis 331
hypertrophic cardiomyopathy 87
hypertrophic hypersecretory gastropathy 137
hypertrophic pulmonary osteoarthropathy (HPOA)
      120, 122
hypertrophy 18
hyperuricaemia 272–3
hypoalbuminaemia 123, 127
hypocalcaemia 219, 280
hypochlorhydria 136
hypoglycaemia 225, 227
hypokalaemia 221
hypoparathyroidism 218–19
hypophysectomy 207
hypophysis see pituitary
hypopigmentation 332, 334
hypopituitarism 207–8
hypoproteinaemia 123, 142
hypospadias 200
hypothalamus 205, 206
  lesions 207, 209
hypothyroidism 212–13
  congenital (cretinism) 56, 212
  myopathy 265
  nervous system effects 56, 60
  primary 215
  secondary 215
hypoxia
  cerebral 46, 48
  chronic, polycythaemia 308

I
icterus gravis neonatorum 303
idiopathic pulmonary fibrosis 109–10
IgA deficiency, isolated 279
IgA nephropathy (mesangial IgA disease) 188, 189
imatinib 291
immune complexes 186, 192
immune system disorders 275–314
immunity 35
  tumour 27
  virally infected cells 36–7

immunocompromised patients
  CNS infections 52
  lymphoma 27, 57, 287
  opportunistic infections 30
  pneumonia 114–15
  tuberculosis 115
immunodeficiency diseases 278–81, 282
  primary 278, 279–80
  secondary 278, 280–1
immunoglobulin light chains
  amyloid formation 282, 283
  monoclonal 195, 294
immunoglobulins
  monoclonal 295
  serum, of neonates 278, 279
immunopathology 3
impaired glucose tolerance 224, 225
impetigo 322
`incessant ovulation' hypothesis 239
incidence 4
inclusion body myositis 265
incomplete abortion 241
inevitable abortion 241
infantile preductal coarctation 68
infection(s)
  causing purpura 309
  diabetic predisposition 227
  general principles 29–30
  hospital-acquired 38
  in immunodeficiencies 278
  inflammatory responses 38–9
  lymphadenitis 285
  opportunistic 30, 281
infectious agents
  categories 30–5
  Koch's postulates 29–30
  mechanisms of pathogenicity 35–8
  routes of entry 35, 36
  transmission 29
infectious disease 29–39
infective endocarditis 84–6
  renal lesions 192
  sequelae 86
infertility
  female 229, 233, 234, 237
  male 248
inflammation 5–13
  acute 5–8
  chemical mediators 8–10
  chronic 5, 6, 10–11, 38
  classic signs of acute 5–6
  fibrinous 11
  granulomatous 12, 38–9
  haemorrhagic 12
  infection-associated 38–9
  necrotising 39

sequelae 6
suppurative 11–12, 38
systemic effects 13
inflammatory bowel disease 164–7, 272
infliximab 167
influenza virus 99, 114
ingrowing toenails 331
inguinal hernia 171–2, 248, 249
innate immunity 27, 35
insect bites 327
insulin
deficiency 224
resistance 224
insulinomas 227, 228
interferons 12, 37
interleukins 12
interstitial cell tumours, testis 250
interstitial cystitis 202
interstitial lung diseases 109–11
interstitial nephritis, chronic 195
intertrigo 326–7
intestinal metaplasia 136
intestine (bowel) 161–77
atresia 162
congenital abnormalities 161–2
infarction 174
infections 162–4
inflammatory disorders 164–7
neoplastic disease 175–7
obstruction 171–2, 234
pseudo-obstruction 171
stenosis 162
strangulation 171, 172, 174
vascular disorders 173–5
intracerebral haemorrhage
atraumatic 49, 50, 74, 75
traumatic 48
intracranial haemorrhage
atraumatic 49–50
perinatal 46
traumatic 47–8
intracranial herniation 43, 44
intraductal papilloma, breast 245
intraepidermal carcinoma 341
intraepithelial neoplasia 18–19
intrauterine devices (IUDs) 233, 234
intrinsic factor 136, 305
intussusception 172
invasive carcinoma 19
invasive mole 243
inverted papilloma, nasal 100
iodine
deficiency 56, 212, 213, 215
radioactive (^{131}I) 211, 216
ionising radiation 25, 26, 289
iron

accumulation, effects 146
deficiency 306–7
iron-deficiency anaemia 306–7
chronic blood loss 299
gastrointestinal features 130, 131
irritant contact dermatitis 320
ischaemia
acute tubular necrosis 193, 194
cerebral infarction 48–9
perinatal brain injury 46
renal 196–7
ischaemic bowel disease 173–4
ischaemic heart disease (IHD) 78–82
heart failure 81, 82
hypertension 74, 75
islet cell tumours, pancreatic 227, 228

J
jaundice 143–5
causes 143–4
gallstone 157
in haemolytic anaemia 299
neonatal 147
obstructive 144, 157, 160–1
JC polyomavirus 53
joint deformities, rheumatoid arthritis 267, 268
joint diseases see arthropathies
juvenile laryngeal papillomatosis 101
juvenile nephronophthisis 182, 183
juvenile rheumatoid arthritis 270

K
kala azar 328
Kallmann's syndrome 207
Kaposi's sarcoma (KS) 96, 342
Kartagener's syndrome 100, 109
Kawasaki's disease 94
keloid 337
keratoacanthoma 341
keratoconjunctivitis sicca 269
keratosis
actinic (solar) 336
oral 130
smoker's 101
kernicterus 299, 303
kidney 181–99
agenesis 181
congenital anomalies 181
diffuse cortical necrosis 198
ectopic 181
horseshoe 181
hypoplasia 181
pancake 181
structural abnormalities 181–4
see also renal disease
Kiel classification system 288

Kimmelstiel–Wilson nodules 192
kinins 9
c-KIT mutations 139
Klinefelter's syndrome 247
Knudson's two-hit hypothesis 20–1
Koch's postulates 29–30
Köebner's phenomenon 317
koilonychia 307, 333
Korsakoff's psychosis 56, 57
Krukenberg's tumour 239
kuru 35
Kussmaul's sign 89
kyphosis 254

L
lactic acidosis 225
lactose intolerance 170
Lambert–Eaton myasthenic syndrome 120, 262
Langhans' giant cells 12
large bowel
    angiodysplasia 174
    tumours 175–7
large cell anaplastic carcinoma, lung 118, 119, 122
large cell diffuse lymphoma 287
larva migrans 328–9
laryngitis
    acute 100–1
    chronic 101
larynx 100–2
    juvenile papillomatosis 101
    papillomas 101
    polyps 101
    reactive nodules 101
    squamous cell carcinoma 101–2
    verrucous carcinoma 102
laxative abuse 162
left ventricular failure 81–2, 123
left ventricular hypertrophy 73–4, 75
leiomyomas, uterine 235–6
leishmaniasis 328
lentigines 334
lentiginous 317
leprosy 59–60, 327–8
lethal midline granuloma 100
leucocytes
    classification 284
    extravasation 7
leucocytosis 284–5
    in leukaemia 289, 291
    reactive 284, 286
leucopenia 284
leucoplakia
    bladder 203
    oral 130
leukaemia 289–91
    acute 289–90

chronic 289, 290–1
    chronic granulocytic 293
    chronic myelomonocytic 292
    hairy cell 292
leukotrienes 9
LeVeen shunt 143
Lewy bodies 55
Leydig cell tumours, testis 250
Li-Fraumeni syndrome 21, 260
Libman–Sacks disease 86
lice 327
lichen planus 331
lichen sclerosus 230
lichen striatus 321
lichenification 315, 316
lifestyle, sedentary 70
lines of Zahn 76
linitis plastica 139
lipoid nephrosis 190
lipoma 337
lipotechoic acids 37
liquefactive necrosis 14
liver
    abscess 150
    circulatory disorders 151–3
    fibrosis 140, 153
    infarction 153
    inflammation 140
    necrosis 139–40
    neoplasia 154–5
    'nutmeg' 153
    regeneration 11, 140
    transplantation 145–6
liver cell carcinoma *see* hepatocellular carcinoma
liver disease 139–55
    alcoholic 151
    coagulation defects 313
    congenital errors of metabolism 146–7
    end-stage 146
    infectious and inflammatory 147–50
    patterns of injury 139–40
    in pregnancy 153–4
lobular carcinoma *in situ* 245
lobular hyperplasia, breast 244
lower genital tract infections 229–30
lung(s) 102–26
    abscess 113, 114
    cancer *see* bronchogenic carcinoma
    collapse *see* atelectasis
    fibrosis *see* pulmonary fibrosis
    function tests 103
    infections 111–18
    secondary tumours 121
    transplants 126
lung disease
    diffuse 102–11

drug-induced 126
iatrogenic 126
interstitial 109–11
neoplastic 118–22
obstructive 102–9
restrictive 103
rheumatoid 110, 111, 269
vascular 122–6
lupus anticoagulant 77
lupus erythematosus, systemic *see* systemic lupus
    erythematosus
lupus nephritis 186, 189, 191–2, 277
lupus vulgaris 323
luteal cysts, ovarian 238
luteal phase, inadequate 234
luteinizing hormone (LH) 206, 207
    deficiency 208
Lyme disease 52, 274, 324
lymph nodes, enlargement 13
lymphadenitis 284–5
lymphangiomas, cystic 179
lymphangitis 97
lymphangitis carcinomatosa 123
lymphatic disease 97–8
lymphatic obstruction, pulmonary 123
lymphocytes
    in chronic inflammation 10
    normal development 288
lymphocytosis 284, 286
lymphoedema 97–8
lymphogranuloma venereum (inguinale) 229, 247
lymphokines 12
lymphomas 285–8
    cutaneous T cell 341–2
    gastric 139
    immunocompromised patients 27, 57, 287
    lethal midline granuloma 100
    non-Hodgkin's (NHL) 286–8
    primary brain 57
    rheumatoid arthritis and 269
    small bowel 175
    testis 250
    thyroid 216

M
macrocytes 298, 305
macrophages 10–11, 12, 71
macrovascular disease, diabetic 225
macule 315
malabsorption
    causes 168
    chronic pancreatitis 160
    diarrhoea 162, 163
    megaloblastic anaemia 305, 306
    syndromes 168–70
    vitamin K deficiency 313

malakoplakia 202
malar skin rash 277
malaria 33, 301, 304
male pattern alopecia 330
malignant fibrous histiocytoma 261
Mallory bodies 151
Mallory–Weiss tears 133
malnutrition
    anaemia 305, 306
    hair disorders 330
    see also vitamin deficiencies
MALToma 139
malunion 257
mammary duct ectasia 244
mammography 246–7
marantic endocarditis 86
marble bone disease 255
mast cells 11–12, 107
mastitis, acute 244
mean cell volume (MCV) 297
measles 53
Meckel's diverticulum 161
medullary carcinoma of thyroid 216, 283–4
medullary cystic disease 182, 183
medullary sponge kidney 182, 183
medulloblastoma 57
mega-oesophagus 132
megacolon
    acquired 161–2
    congenital aganglionic 161
    psychogenic 161
    toxic 162, 165
megakaryopoiesis, ineffective 309
megaloblastic anaemia 305–6, 309
megaloblasts 305
megaloureter 200
melanocarcinoma *see* melanoma, malignant
melanocyte stimulating hormone (MSH) 206
melanocytic naevi 337–8, 339
melanoma, malignant 339–40, 341
    acral lentiginous 339
    lentigo 339
    nodular 339
    subungual 332
    superficial spreading 339
melasma 334
melatonin 210
membranoproliferative glomerulonephritis (MPGN)
    187, 188–9, 191
membranous nephropathy 189–90, 192
Ménétrier's disease 137
meningiomas 57
meningitis 50
    acute pyogenic (bacterial) 51
    aseptic (viral) 51
    chronic 52

meningitis—cont'd
  malignant 57
  tuberculous 52
meningocele 45
meningoencephalitis 50
  chronic 52
meningomyelocele 45
menopause 234
menstrual cycle
  anovulatory 234
  inadequate luteal phase 234
menstruation, retrograde 233
mesalazine 167
mesangial IgA disease 188, 189
mesenchymal tumours
  intestine 175
  lungs 122
mesenteric cysts 179
mesothelioma 128, 179
metabolic disorders
  central nervous system 55–6
  congenital errors of metabolism 146–7
  peripheral nervous system 60
metalloproteinases 23
metaplasia 17–18
metastases
  bone see bone metastases
  brain 57–8
  leukaemic 289
  liver 155
  lung 121
  ovary 239
  peritoneum 179
  pleural 127–8
  testis 250
metastasis 18, 23–4
metastatic neuropathies 61
methanol poisoning 56
metropathia haemorrhagica 235
Michaelis–Gutmann bodies 202
microbiology 3
microcyte 298
microglia 56
microorganisms
  characteristics 30
  commensal 30
  normal skin flora 322
  pathogenic 30
  routes of entry 35, 36
microspherocytes 298, 299
Microsporum infections 326
middle cerebral artery 49
milia 337
mineralocorticoids 219
  insufficiency 222–3
minimal change disease 190

minimal residual disease 22
missed abortion 241
mitral annular calcification 83
mitral regurgitation 83
mitral stenosis 83, 84
mitral valve prolapse 83–4
mole
  carneous 241
  hydatidiform 243
  invasive 243
moles (cutaneous) 337–8
molluscum contagiosum 324–5
Mönckeberg's medial calcific sclerosis 69
monoclonal gammopathy, benign 283
monocytes 7–8, 12, 71
monocytosis 284, 286
monokines 12
Morgagni, cysts of 238
morphology 4
Morvan's syndrome 59
motor neuron disease 55
mouth 129–31
  precancerous/neoplastic lesions 130–1
  in systemic disease 130
mucinous ovarian tumours 239
mucocele, gall bladder 158
mucopolysaccharidoses 255
mucormycotic infections 100
multi-organ infarction 86
multiple endocrine neoplasia (MEN) syndromes 62,
      216, 227–8
multiple sclerosis (MS) 53–4
mural thrombosis 81
muscular dystrophy
  myotonic 264
  X-linked 263–4
musculoskeletal system 253–74
myasthenia gravis 262–3, 278, 297
myc oncogene 20
mycetoma 329
mycobacterial skin infections 323
Mycobacterium leprae 327
Mycobacterium tuberculosis 52, 115
Mycoplasma 34, 114
mycoses, deep 32, 329
mycosis fungoides 341–2
mycotic aneurysms 86, 91
mycotoxins 32, 154
myelodysplastic syndromes (MDS) 291, 292
myelofibrosis 292–3
myeloma 293–5
  amyloidosis 283, 294
  multiple 195, 294
  solitary (plasmacytoma) 100, 295
myeloproliferative disorders 292–3
myocardial disease 87–8

myocardial infarction (MI) 79–81
  histological changes 14, 80
  recurrent 81
  sequelae 80–1, 90
myocardial ischaemia 78
myocardial rupture 81
myocarditis 87–8
  rheumatic 84
  versus cardiomyopathy 87
myofibroblasts 10, 11
myopathies 263–5
  endocrine 265
  idiopathic inflammatory 264–5
  inherited 263–4
  toxic 265
myotonic disorders 264
myotonic muscular dystrophy 264
myxoedema 212–13
  pretibial 212
myxoid cysts 332
myxoma 88

N
naevi 337–9
  congenital 338
  connective tissue 339
  epidermal 339
  melanocytic 337–8, 339
  vascular 338–9, 339
nail(s)
  disorders 331–2
  infections 332
  in systemic disease 332, 333
  trauma 331
  tumours 332
nail–patella syndrome 331
nasal polyps 99
nasopharyngeal angiofibroma 100
nasopharyngeal carcinoma 100
nasopharynx 99–100
  necrotising lesions 100
  neoplasms 100
natural killer (NK) cells 37
necrosis 13, 14–15
  avascular 257–9
  caseous 15
  coagulative 14, 139
  compared to apoptosis 16
  fat 15, 244
  fibrinoid 15, 74, 75, 275
  liquefactive (colliquative) 14
  liver 139–40
  pancreas 159
necrotising arteriolitis 74, 174
necrotising enterocolitis 163
necrotising fasciitis 323

necrotising inflammation 39
Neisseria gonorrhoeae 237
Neisseria meningitidis 52
neonates
  haemolytic disease 303
  hepatitis 147
  necrotising arteriolitis 174
  serum immunoglobulins 278
  transient physiological agammaglobulinaemia 278, 279
  vitamin K deficiency 313
neoplasia 17
neoplasm 17
nephritic syndrome, acute 184–5, 187, 190
nephritis
  chronic interstitial 195
  tubulointerstitial 193–5
nephroblastoma 199
nephrocalcinosis 195
nephrogenic adenoma 203
nephronophthisis, juvenile 182, 183
nephrosclerosis
  benign hypertensive 74, 75, 195–6
  malignant 196
nephrotic syndrome 185, 187, 190
  congenital 182, 191
  pulmonary oedema 123
  in systemic disease 192
nerve compression/entrapment syndromes 59, 255–6, 269
nerve injuries 58–9
nervous system 43–62
neural tube defects 44–5
neuritic plaques 54
neuroblastoma 223
  olfactory 100
neuroendocrine cells 205
neuroendocrine signalling 205
neurofibrillary tangles 54
neurofibroma 61
neurofibromatosis
  type I (von Recklinghausen's) 61, 62
  type II 61
neurohypophysis see pituitary, posterior
neuromas, traumatic 59
neuromuscular junction (NMJ) disorders 261–3
neuropathic joint disease 272
neuropathies 58–61
  hereditary 58
  infectious 59–60
  inflammatory 59
  metabolic and toxic 60–1
  metastatic 61
  traumatic 58–9
neuropil threads 54
neurosyphilis 52

neutropenia 284, 285, 289
neutrophilia 284, 286
neutrophils (neutrophil polymorphs) 7–8, 11–12
NF1 gene 21
niacin deficiency 130
nitric oxide (NO) 12
nitrosamines 24
nits 327
nodular sclerosis 287
nodule 315
non-alcoholic steatohepatitis (NASH) 151
non-Hodgkin's lymphomas (NHLs) 286–8
non-steroidal anti-inflammatory drugs (NSAIDs)
        135, 136
non-union 257
norepinephrine (noradrenaline) 219
normocytes 298
Norwalk virus 162
nose 99–100
    necrotising lesions 100
    neoplasms 100
nosocomial infection 38
nuclear radiation 26
nummular eczema 321

O
oat cell carcinoma *see* small cell carcinoma
obesity 70, 245
occupational disorders 106, 118, 266
oedema 6–7, 97
oesophagitis 132
oesophagus 131–4
    atresia 131
    cancer 134
    diverticula 133
    lacerations 133
    neoplastic disease 134
    stenosis 131
    varices 133–4, 142
    webs and rings 131
oestrogens 77, 230, 234–5, 236
olfactory neuroblastoma 100
oligodendrocytes 56
oligodendrogliomas 57
oliguria 193
Ollier's disease 260
onchocerciasis 329
oncocytoma, renal 198
oncogenes 19–21
    viral 27
onychogryphosis 332
onycholysis 316, 333
opportunistic infection 30, 281
oral cancer 131
oral contraceptive pill 154, 231, 234
oral ulceration 129, 130, 277

orchioblastoma 250
oropharynx 129–31
orthopnoea 82
Osler–Weber–Rendu syndrome 309
osteitis deformans 255–6
osteitis fibrosa 217
osteitis fibrosa cystica 217
osteoarthritis (OA) 259, 265–7
    comparative features 271
    secondary 266, 268, 273
osteoblastoma 260
osteochondroma 260
osteoclastoma 261
osteoclasts, disorders of function 255–6
osteogenesis imperfecta 253
osteolytic lesions 259, 261, 268, 294
osteoma 259–60
    giant osteoid 260
    osteoid 260
osteomalacia 218, 255, 265
osteomyelitis 256
    malignant 256
    tuberculous 256–7
osteonecrosis 257–9
osteopetrosis 255
osteophytes 266, 267
osteoporosis 253–5, 294
osteosarcoma 256, 260
osteosclerosis 218, 259, 266
ovarian cancer 238–9
ovarian cysts 238
ovarian tumours 238–9
    germ cell 238, 240
    sex-cord stromal 238, 240
    surface epithelial stromal 238, 239
ovary 237–9
oxytocin 205, 206

P
p53 gene 20, 21, 138, 238, 260
pachymeningitis 50
pachyonychia congenita 331
Paget's disease of bone 255–6, 260
Pancoast tumours 61, 118
pancreas
    carcinoma 160–1
    cystic tumours 160
    endocrine, disorders of 223–7
    exocrine, disorders of 158–61
    islet cell tumours 227, 228
    necrosis 159
    neoplasms 160–1
    pseudocysts 160
    transplantation 227
pancreatitis
    acute 158–9

chronic 159–60
gallstone 157, 158
pancytopenia 284, 285, 296
pannus 268
papillary thyroid adenocarcinoma 215, 216
papillomas, laryngeal 101
papillomatosis 317
papule 315
paracentesis, abdominal 143
paraganglia, tumours of extra-adrenal 223
parakeratosis 316
paralytic ileus 171, 178
paraneoplastic syndromes
    lung cancer 119, 120
    renal cell carcinoma 199
paraplegia 48
parasympathetic nervous system disorders 62
parathyroid gland
    adenomas 217
    carcinoma 217
    disorders 216–19
    hyperplasia 217–18
parathyroid hormone (PTH) 216
    deficiency 218–19
    hypersecretion 217–18, 256
paratubal cysts 238
Parinaud's syndrome 210
parkinsonism 55
Parkinson's disease 55
paronychia 327, 332
paroxysmal nocturnal dyspnoea 82
paroxysmal nocturnal haemoglobinuria 302, 309
patent ductus arteriosus 64, 65, 66
Paterson–Brown–Kelly syndrome 131
pathogenesis 4
pathogenicity 30
    mechanisms 35–8
pathogens 30
    classification 30–5
pathology 3
peak expiratory flow rate (PEFR) 103
peau d'orange 245
pediculosis 327
pelvic inflammatory disease (PID) 178, 229, 233,
        237–8
pelviureteric junction obstruction 200
pemphigus 334–5
pemphigus vulgaris 335, 336
pencil cell 298
penis 247–8
    carcinoma in situ 247
    infections 247
    squamous cell carcinoma 248
peptic ulceration 136–7
percutaneous coronary intervention (PCI) 79, 81
pericardial disease 88–91

pericardial effusion 88–9
pericarditis 89–91, 113
    acute 81, 89–90
    adhesive 90
    chronic 90–1
    constrictive 90
    rheumatic 84, 91
    in rheumatoid arthritis 269
perinatal brain injury 46
periodic paralysis 261
peripheral nerves
    avulsion 58–9
    lacerations 58
peripheral nervous system
    disorders 58–61
    tumours 61
peritoneum 177–9
    epithelial metaplasia 233
    infections 177–8
peritonitis 177–9
periungual fibroma 332
perivalvular abscesses 86
pernicious anaemia 135–6, 278, 305
peroneal muscular atrophy 58
persistent truncus arteriosus 67
Peutz–Jeghers syndrome 138, 334
phaeochromocytoma 62, 223
phagocytosis 7–8, 37
phenylketonuria 332
Philadelphia chromosome 20, 290, 291
phlebothrombosis 76
photosensitivity, skin 277
Phyllodes tumour 245
pica 307
Pick's disease 55
pigmentation disorders 332–4, 335
piles see haemorrhoids
pili 37
pineal gland disorders 210
pinealomas 210
pink puffers 105
pinta 324
pitted keratolysis 322
pituitary 205–10
    adenomas 205–7
    anterior 205–8
    posterior 205, 206, 208–10
Pityrosporum folliculitis 321
placental site trophoblastic tumour 244
plaque 315
plasma cells 10, 294
plasmacytoma (solitary myeloma) 100, 295
plasmids 38
platelets
    activation factors 9
    decreased production 309

platelets—cont'd
  decreased survival 309–10
  functional defects 310–11
  reduced numbers *see* thrombocytopenia
  splenic sequestration 310
pleura
  adhesions 126
  disorders 126–8
  neoplasia 127–8
pleural effusions 114
  inflammatory 126–7
  malignant 119, 126
  non-inflammatory 127
pleural fibrosis 118, 126
pleuritis
  haemorrhagic 127
  serofibrinous 126
  suppurative 127
Plummer's disease 211
Plummer–Vinson syndrome 131
pneumoconioses 110–11
Pneumocystis carinii pneumonia (PCP) 115
pneumonia 111–15
  causative organisms 112, 113
  classification 112
  immunocompromised patients 114–15
  lobar 113–14
  predisposing factors 111–12
  primary atypical 114
pneumonitis, radiation 126
pneumothorax 104, 127, 128
  spontaneous 127, 128
  tension 127
poikilocytosis 297, 298
polyarteritis nodosa 95, 193
polyarthritis, symmetrical 268
polycystic kidney disease
  adult (APKD) 182–3
  infantile (childhood) 182, 183
polycystic ovary syndrome (PCOS) 238
polycythaemia 308
  absolute 308
  relative 308
  rubra vera 292, 293, 308
polydipsia 208, 209
polymyositis 264–5, 276
polyuria 193, 208
pompholyx 321
port wine stain naevus 338
portal hypertension 141, 142, 143
portal pyophlebitis 178
portal vein obstruction 153
portosystemic shunts 141–2
posterior cerebral artery 49
posterior fossa, congenital abnormalities 44–5
postherpetic neuralgia 325

posthitis 247
poststreptococcal glomerulonephritis 186, 188
Potter's syndrome 181
Pott's disease 256–7
pre-eclampsia 153–4, 242–3
pregnancy 239–44
  ectopic 239–40
  liver disease 153–4
prevalence 4
primary biliary cirrhosis 155, 156, 157
primary sclerosing cholangitis 155, 156, 157
Prinzmetal's angina 78, 79
prions 35
progesterone 234
prognosis 4
progressive multifocal leucoencephalopathy 53
prolactin 206
prolactinomas 206
proliferative glomerulonephritis 188–9
Propionibacterium acnes 329
prostaglandins 9
prostate 250–2
prostate-specific acid phosphatase (PSAP) 252
prostate-specific antigen (PSA) 27, 252
prostatic carcinoma 251–2, 259
prostatic hyperplasia, benign 250–1
protein C deficiency 77
proteinuria
  asymptomatic 184, 187, 190
  glomerular disease 184, 185
prothrombin G20210A 77
proto-oncogenes 19, 20, 21
protozoa 31, 33, 34
protozoal infections
  central nervous system 53
  intestinal 163–4
  lower genital tract 229–30
  pneumonia 115
Psammoma bodies 239
pseudoaneurysms 91
pseudogout 272
Pseudomonas aeruginosa 109, 324
pseudopelade 331
psoriasis 317–18, 332
psoriatic arthritis 271, 318
pulmonary artery stenosis/atresia, with intact ventricular
    septum 68
pulmonary congestion 122–3
pulmonary embolism (PE) 76, 124–5
pulmonary fibrosis
  complicating pneumonia 113, 114
  complicating tuberculosis 118
  drug-induced 126
  idiopathic 109–10
  lung cancer risk 118
pulmonary haemorrhagic syndromes, diffuse 126

pulmonary haemosiderosis, idiopathic 111, 126
pulmonary hypertension 74, 75, 125–6
pulmonary infarction 125
pulmonary oedema 74, 82, 122–3
pulmonary thromboembolism 124–5
pulmonary vascular sclerosis 125–6
pulmonary venous connection, total anomalous 67–8
pulmonary venous hypertension 123
pulseless (Takayasu's) disease 94
pulseless electrical activity (PEA) 89
purpura 308
   non-thrombocytopenic 309
pus 11–12, 38
pustule 315
pyelonephritis
   acute 193–4, 226
   chronic 194–5
   obstructive 194
   reflux 194–5
pyloric stenosis 135
pyogenic granuloma 337
pyonephrosis 194
pyosalpinx 237
pyrexia 13
pyruvate kinase deficiency 300
pyuria 194

R
rabies 52
racial differences, atherosclerosis 70
racket nails 331
radiation 25–6
   ionising 25, 26, 289
   non-ionising 25
radiation pneumonitis 126
radioisotopes 26
rapidly progressive glomerulonephritis 188, 193
ras oncogene 20
Raynaud's phenomenon 61
RB1 gene 20, 21, 260
reactive arthritis 272
recurrent spontaneous abortions 241
red blood cells
   acquired defects 302
   disorders of 297–308
   enzyme deficiencies 299–300
   hereditary defects 299–302
   mechanical trauma 304
   size and shape abnormalities 297, 298
red cell antibodies 275
red cell aplasia 307
Reed–Sternberg (RS) cells 286, 287
reflux oesophagitis 132

refractory anaemia (RA) 292
   with excess blasts 292
   with excess blasts in transformation (RAEB-t) 292
   with ring sideroblasts 292
Reid index 106
Reiter's syndrome 271
renal artery stenosis 196–7
renal cell carcinoma 198–9
renal colic 201
renal cortical adenoma 198
renal cysts, simple 182, 183–4
renal disease 181–99
   cystic 182–4
   diabetic 192, 225–6
   embolic 198
   glomerular 184–93
   hyperparathyroidism 217, 218
   hypertension in 73, 74, 183
   hypertensive 74, 75, 195–6
   multiple myeloma 195, 294
   neoplastic 198–9
   systemic lupus erythematosus 186, 189, 191–2, 277
   tubular/interstitial 193–5
   vascular 195–8
   see also kidney
renal dysplasia, cystic 182
renal failure
   in amyloidosis 192–3
   chronic 185–6, 187
   in diabetes 192
   hypertensive 74, 75, 196
   uraemic neuropathy 60
renal fibroma (hamartoma) 198
renal infarction 197–8
renal medulla, cystic diseases 183
renal osteodystrophy 218
renal pelvis
   obstruction 200
   urothelial carcinoma 199
renal replacement therapy 191
renal transplantation 191
renal tubular ectasia see medullary sponge kidney
renomedullary interstitial cell tumour 198
reproductive system 229–52
respiratory failure 104, 122–3
respiratory system 99–128
restrictive cardiomyopathy 87
reticulocytes 299
retina, effects of hypertension 74, 75
retinoblastoma 21, 260
retroviruses 32
   oncogenic 26
   replication cycle 36
Reye's syndrome 147
rhesus isoimmunization 303
rheumatic disease of pericardium 84, 91

rheumatic fever 84
rheumatic heart disease 84
rheumatoid arthritis (RA) 267–70
    amyloidosis 268, 283
    extra-articular *see* rheumatoid disease
    juvenile 270
rheumatoid disease 269, 276, 277
    comparative features 271
    lungs 110, 111, 269
rheumatoid factor 267, 269, 275
rheumatoid nodules 268
rheumatoid synovitis 267, 268
rhinitis 99
rhinophyma 330
riboflavin deficiency 130
Richter's hernia 171
rickets 218, 255
Rickettsia infections 114
rickettsiae 34
right heart failure 82, 126, 152, 153
Riley-Day syndrome 59
ringworm 326
river blindness 329
RNA viruses 32
rodent ulcer 340–1
Rokitansky–Aschoff sinuses 158
rosacea 329–30
rotaviruses 162
Rotor's syndrome 144, 145
routes of entry, infectious agents 35, 36
Rye classification sytem 286, 287

S
salmon patch 338
salmonella 164, 256
Salmonella typhi 163
salpingitis 237
sarcoid arthritis 272
sarcoidosis 111
Saturday night palsy 59
scabies 327
scale 315, 316
scar formation 11, 38
schistocyte 298
Schistosoma haematobium 202
Schistosoma mansoni 164
schwannoma 61
scleroderma 94
sclerosing adenosis, breast 244
sclerosing cholangitis, primary 155, 156, 157
sclerosing haemangiomas 96
sclerosis retroperitonitis 179
scrofuloderma 323
scurvy 309
sebaceous glands, disorders of 329–30
seborrhoeic dermatitis 320–1

seborrhoeic warts 336
sedentary lifestyle 70
seminoma, testicular 249, 250
senile plaques 54
sepsis, neutropenic 284
septic arthritis 268, 274
sequelae of disease 4
seronegative arthritis 267, 270
serous ovarian tumours 239
Sertoli cell tumours 250
Sertoli–Leydig cell tumours 240
serum amyloid A (SAA) protein 282, 283
severe combined immunodeficiency (SCID) 30, 280
sex-cord and stromal tumours
    ovary 238, 240
    testis 250
sex steroids, adrenal 219
sexually transmitted infections 229–30, 237, 247
Sheehan's syndrome 207
Shigella 163, 164
shingles 60, 325–6
shunts, intracardiac 63
    left-to-right 64–6
    right-to-left 66–8
sickle-cell disease 301–2
    crises 302
    nephropathy 198
sickle cells 298, 302
silicosis 110–11
singer's nodules, larynx 101
sinusitis 99–100
Sipple's syndrome 228
Sjögren's syndrome, secondary 269
skin 315–42
    anatomy 316
    blistering disorders 334–6
    cancer 26, 340–1
    cysts 336–7
    dermatological terminology 315–17
    disorders of specific structures 329–32
    infections/infestations 322–9
    inflammation/eruptions 317–21
    normal microflora 322
    photosensitivity 277
    pigmentation disorders 332–4, 335
    in systemic lupus erythematosus 276, 277
    tags 336
    tumours 336–42
skull fractures 46
SLE *see* systemic lupus erythematosus
small bowel
    adhesions 172, 178
    bacterial overgrowth syndrome 170
    obstruction 171–2
    tumours 175
small cell carcinoma, lung 118, 119, 121, 122

small cell diffuse lymphoma 287
smoker's keratosis 101
smoking, cigarette
    atherosclerosis 70
    cervical neoplasia and 231
    chronic laryngitis 101
    lung cancer risk 118, 119, 122
    obstructive lung disease 103, 104, 105, 106
    oesophageal cancer and 134
    oral neoplastic lesions 130, 131
    renal cell carcinoma and 198–9
    thrombosis risk 77
solar keratosis 336
somatostatinomas 227, 228
somatotroph adenomas 206–7
soot 24
spherocytosis, hereditary 299
spider naevi 96
spina bifida 45
spinal cord
    injuries 48
    subacute combined degeneration 56, 305
spirochaetal skin infections 323–4
spleen 295–6
    infarction 296
    platelet sequestration 310
    red cell sequestration 304
    rupture 296
splenic vein thrombosis 153
splenic venous pressure, raised 295, 296
splenomegaly 143, 295–6
    congestive 296
splinter haemorrhages 85, 331, 333
spongiform encephalitis 53
spongiosis 317
sporotrichosis 329
squamous cell carcinoma
    bladder 203
    cervix 232
    cutaneous 341
    larynx 101–2
    lung 118, 119, 122
    mouth 131
    oesophagus 134
    penis 248
    vulva 230
squamous metaplasia
    bladder 203
    bronchial 106
src oncogene 20
staphylococcal scalded skin syndrome 322–3
Staphylococcus aureus 11, 38
    breast infections 244
    gastrointestinal infections 163, 164
    infective endocarditis 85
    musculoskeletal infections 256, 274

pulmonary infections 109, 113
    skin infections 320, 322–3
stasis (varicose) eczema 97, 321
steatorrhoea 168
steroid cell tumours 240
steroid purpura 309
stomach
    congenital abnormalities 134–5
    disorders 134–9
    inflammation 135–6
    neoplastic disease 138–9
stomatitis 129–30
storage pool disease 310
strawberry naevi 95, 338
streptococcal infections
    rheumatic fever 84
    skin 323
    throat 317
Streptococcus pneumoniae 51, 106, 113
Streptococcus pyogenes 11, 38, 323
Streptococcus viridans 85
stress fractures 257
stroke 48–50
subacute combined degeneration of spinal cord 56, 305
subacute sclerosing panencephalopathy 53
subarachnoid haemorrhage
    adult polycystic kidney disease and 183
    atraumatic 49–50
    traumatic 48
subdural empyema 52
subdural haemorrhage 47–8
subungual haematoma 331
sudden cardiac death 81
superior mesenteric artery occlusion 173–4
suppurative inflammation 11–12, 38
surfactant, pulmonary 102
swan neck deformity 268
sweat glands, disorders of 329–30
sycosis barbae 322
sympathectomies, surgical 61–2
sympathetic nervous system disorders 61–2
synovitis, rheumatoid 267, 268
syphilis 230, 247, 323
    cardiovascular complications 91, 93, 94
    CNS involvement 52
    congenital 257
    endemic 324
    skeletal 257
syringomyelia 45–6
systemic lupus erythematosus (SLE) 275–7
    clinical features 276, 277
    diagnostic criteria 276–7
    endocarditis 86
    renal disease 186, 189, 191–2, 277
    vasculitis 94
systemic sclerosis 94

T

T-cell lymphomas 288
T helper cells 280
Takayasu's disease 94
target cell 298
tear-drop cells 298
telangiectasia 96
    hereditary haemorrhagic 309
    nail-fold 333
telogen effluvium 330
temporal (giant cell) arteritis 95
Tensilon test 263
teratomas
    ovarian 240
    testicular 249–50
testes 248–50
    congenital anomalies and regression 248–9
    torsion 249
    undescended 248
testicular tumours 248, 249–50
    germ cell 249–50
    non-germ cell 249, 250
tetany 219, 280
tetralogy of Fallot 66–7
tetraplegia 48
thalassaemias 300–1
thiamine deficiency 55–6
thin glomerular basement membrane disease 191
Thorotrast 199
threatened abortion 241
thrombasthaenia 310
thromboangitis obliterans 94
thrombocythaemia, primary (essential/idiopathic) 293
thrombocytopenia 309–10
    causes 311
    dilutional 310
    in leukaemia 289
    in liver disease 313
thrombocytopenic purpura
    autoimmune 309–10
    thrombotic (TTP) 197, 310
thrombophilia 77
thrombophlebitis 76
thrombosis 76–7, 314
    arterial 76
    mural 81
    venous 76, 124
thrombotic endocarditis, non-bacterial 86
thrombotic microangiopathies 197–8
thrombotic thrombocytopenic purpura (TTP) 197, 310
thrush see candidosis
thymomas 297
thymus 296–7
    aplasia 297
    carcinoma 297
cysts 297
hyperplasia 297
hypoplasia 279–80, 297
thyroglossal cysts 210
thyroid acropachy 212
thyroid cancer 215–16, 283–4
thyroid dyshormonogenesis 212
thyroid gland 210–16
    congenital hypoplasia/absence 212
    development 210
    neoplasms 215–16
thyroid-stimulating hormone (TSH) 206, 207
    deficiency 208
    receptor autoantibodies (TRAbs) 211
thyroiditis 211, 213–14
    autoimmune 212, 213, 214
    De Quervain's 213–14
    Hashimoto's see Hashimoto's thyroiditis
    subacute giant cell/granulomatous 213–14
    subacute lymphocytic 214
thyrotoxicosis 210–12
    factitia 211
    see also hyperthyroidism
thyrotrophin-releasing hormone (TRH), deficiency 207
tinea capitis 326, 331
tinea corporis 326
tinea cruris 326
tinea manuum 326
tinea pedis 326
tinea unguium 326, 332
tissues
    healing (repair) 11
    regenerative capacity 11
TNM staging system 27, 121, 204, 246
tobacco smoke 24
toenails, ingrowing 331
tophi 273
total anomalous pulmonary venous connection 67–8
Touton giant cells 12
toxic myopathies 265
toxic neuropathies 60–1
toxins
    CNS 56
    hepatotoxic 151
    renal 195
toxoplasmosis 53
transient ischaemic attack (TIA) 48
transitional cell carcinoma 199, 203, 204
transitional cell papilloma 203
transitional cell tumours, ovary 239
transjugular intrahepatic portosystemic stent shunting (TIPSS) 134, 143
transplant patients 30
transposition of great arteries 67
transthyretin 282, 284
transudates 127

trauma
  bone 257–9
  central nervous system 46–8
  chest 127, 128
  joint 274
  nail 331
  peripheral nervous system 58–9
  sympathetic nervous system 61–2
traveller's diarrhoea 163
treatment 4
Treponema pallidum 52, 230, 247, 323
  see also syphilis
treponemal infections, non-venereal 323–4
Trichomonas vaginalis 229–30
trichomycosis axillaris 322
Trichophyton infections 326
tricuspid atresia 67
tricuspid valve incompetence 153
trophoblastic disease, gestational 243–4
tropical skin infections/infestations 327–9
tropical sprue 170
truncus arteriosus, persistent 67
Trypanosoma cruzi 132, 162, 163–4
L-tryptophan 265
TSH see thyroid-stimulating hormone
tuberculosis (TB) 115–18
  apical cavitation fibrocaseous 116–18
  arthritis 274
  genital tract 233
  meningitis 52
  miliary 116, 117, 118
  osteomyelitis 256–7
  pericarditis 90
  primary 116, 117
  pulmonary 115–18
  salpingitis 237
  secondary 116–18
  silicosis and 111
  skin 323
  warty 323
tuberous sclerosis 61, 332, 339
tubulointerstitial nephritis 193–5
tumour(s) 17
  benign 18
  grading and staging 27
  growth and spread 22–4
  immunity 27
  initiation 25
  invasion 23
  malignant 18
  metastasis 18, 23–4
  nomenclature 18, 19
  progression, multistage model 21–2, 23
  promotion 25
  see also cancer
tumour markers 27

tumour necrosis factor (TNF) 12
tumour necrosis factor (TNF)-α blockers 167, 269
tumour suppressor genes (TSGs) 19–21
tumourigenesis 21–2
tunica albuginea 248
tunica vaginalis, abnormalities 248–9

U
ulceration 13, 317
ulcerative colitis 165–7, 272
ultraviolet (UV) radiation 26
union, delayed 257
upper gastrointestinal tract disorders 129–34
upper respiratory tract disorders 99–102
uraemia, platelet defects 311
uraemic medullary cystic disease complex 182, 183
uraemic neuropathy 60
urate nephropathy 195
urea breath test 136
ureteritis 202
  cystica 202
  follicularis 202
ureteropelvic junction obstruction 200
ureters
  diverticulum 200
  double and bifid 200
  obstruction 201
  tumours 203
urethra
  congenital anomalies 200
  obstruction 201
urethritis, non-specific 271
urinary calculi 201–2
urinary retention 202
urinary tract 200–4
  congenital anomalies 200
  infections 194, 202
  inflammation 202
  neoplastic disease 203–4
  obstruction 200–1
urogenital ridge-derived cysts 179
urolithiasis 201–2
urothelial carcinoma
  bladder 203, 204
  renal pelvis 199
  ureters 203
uterus 233–7
  inflammatory disorders 233
  neoplastic disorders 235–7
  see also cervix, uterine; endometrium
  vacuolisation 317

V
vagina 229–31
  dysplasia/neoplasia 230–1
  infections 229–30

vaginal intraepithelial neoplasia (VAIN) 230–1
vaginal metaplasia, bladder 203
vagotomy 62
valvular heart disease *see* heart valve disease
varicella-zoster virus (VZV) 60, 325–6
varicocele 249
varicose leg ulcers 97
varicose veins 96–7
vascular disease
    inflammatory 93–5
    neoplastic 95–6
vascular naevi 338–9
vascular permeability, increased 6
vasculitides 93–5
vasculitis 91, 93–5
    hypersensitivity (neutrophilic) 94, 309
    idiopathic 93–4
    immune-mediated 94
    infectious 94–5
    rheumatoid disease 269
vasoactive amines 9–10
vasodilatation, acute inflammation 6
vasopressin *see* antidiuretic hormone
vegetations 84, 85, 86
veno-occlusive disease, hepatic 151
venous disease 96–7
venous thrombosis 76, 124
ventricular aneurysms 81
ventricular remodelling 81
ventricular septal defects 64–5
verrucous carcinoma, larynx 102
vesicle 315
vesicoureteric reflux 194
Vibrio cholerae 163, 164
vinyl chloride 24
VIPomas 227, 228
viral infections
    arthritis 274
    atopic eczema 320
    encephalitis 52
    gastroenteritis 162
    hepatitis 147–9
    lower genital tract 229, 230
    meningitis 51
    myocarditis 88
    penis 247
    pericarditis 90
    pneumonia 114, 115
    skin 324–6
    thyroiditis 213–14
Virchow's triad 77
virulence 30
viruses 30–1
    classification 32
    immune reaction 36–7
    inducing leukaemia 289
    inducing lymphoma 287
    mechanisms of pathogenicity 35–7
    oncogenic 26–7
    replication cycles 35–6
    triggering diabetes 224
vital capacity (VC) 103
vitamin B_1 deficiency 55–6
vitamin B_{12} deficiency 56, 130, 136, 305
vitamin C deficiency 309
vitamin D deficiency 255
vitamin deficiencies 55–6, 60, 130
vitamin K deficiency 312–13
vitiligo 278, 332
volvulus, intestinal 172, 173
von Hippel–Lindau syndrome 61, 62, 199
von Recklinghausen disease of bone 217
von Recklinghausen's disease (neurofibromatosis I)
    61, 62
von Willebrand's disease 311, 312
von Willebrand's factor 310, 311
vulva 229–30
    infections 229–30
    tumours 230
vulval intraepithelial neoplasia (VIN) 230

W
Waldenström's macroglobulinaemia 283, 295
'walled-off' infections, intra-abdominal 179
warfarin 313
warts
    genital 229, 247, 324
    plane 324
    plantar 324
    seborrhoeic 336
    viral 324, 332
warty tuberculosis 323
water deprivation test 208–9
Waterhouse–Friderichsen syndrome
    51, 223
Wegener's granulomatosis 94, 100, 126, 193
weight loss 13
Werner's syndrome 228
Wernicke–Korsakoff syndrome 56
Wernicke's encephalopathy 55, 57
wheal 315
Whipple disease 170
white blood cell disorders 284–95
whiteheads 329
Wilms' tumour 199
Wilson disease 146–7
winter eczema 321
winter vomiting disease 162
worms, parasitic 33–4
wound healing 11
    by first intention 11, 12
    by second intention 11, 12

X
X-linked agammaglobulinaemia 279
X-ray radiation 26

Y
yaws 324
yeast infections, lower genital tract 230
yellow nail syndrome 333
yolk-sac tumours 240, 250

Z
Z deformity of thumbs 268
Zenker's diverticulum 133
Ziehl–Nielsen stain 115
Zollinger–Ellison syndrome 137, 227, 228